Advanced Practice Nursing

CHANGING ROLES AND CLINICAL APPLICATIONS

SECOND EDITION

Advanced Practice Nursing

CHANGING ROLES AND CLINICAL APPLICATIONS

SECOND EDITION

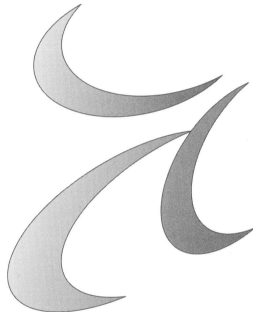

Joanne V. Hickey, *PhD, RN, CS, ACNP, FAAN*
Professor, Clinical Nursing
University of Texas-Houston, Health Science Center School
of Nursing

and

Clinical Associate Professor of Neurology
University of Texas-Houston, Health Science Center School
of Medicine
Houston, TX

Ruth M. Ouimette, *MSN, RN, ANP*
Assistant Clinical Professor
Duke University School of Nursing
Senior Fellow, Center for Aging and Human Development
Duke University Medical Center
Durham, NC

Sandra L. Venegoni, *PhD, RN*
Independent Gerontological Nurse Educator and Consultant
and Adjunct Faculty
Virginia Commonwealth University School of Nursing
Richmond, VA

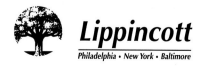

Lippincott

Philadelphia • New York • Baltimore

Acquisitions Editor: Lisa Marshall
Managing Editor: Sandra Kasko
Marketing Manager: Michelle Mulqueen
Production Editor: Lisa JC Franko
Design Coordinator: Mario Fernandez

Copyright © 2000 Lippincott Williams & Wilkins

351 West Camden Street
Baltimore, Maryland 21201-2436 USA

227 East Washington Square
Philadelphia, Pennsylvania 19106 USA

Printed in the United States of America

First Edition, 1996

Library of Congress Cataloging-in-Publication Data

Hickey, Joanne V.
    Advanced practice nursing : changing roles and clinical applications / [edited by] Joanne V. Hickey, Ruth M. Ouimette, Sandra L. Venegoni — 2nd ed.
        p.   cm.
    Includes bibliographical references and index.
    ISBN 0-781-71754-X (alk. paper)
    1. Nurse practitioners—United States.   2. Primary care (Medicine)—United States.   3. Nurse Practitioners.   4. Nurse Clinicians.   I. Hickey, Joanne V.   II. Ouimette, Ruth M.
III. Venegoni, Sandra L.   IV. Title.
    [DNLM: RT 82.8 A385 1999
    WY128 A2443   1999
    510.730692—dc21
    DNLM/DLC
    for Library of Congress   99-17479
                                                                       CIP

The publishers have made every effort to trace the copyright holders for borrowed material. If they have inadvertently overlooked any, they will be pleased to make the necessary arrangements at the first opportunity.

To purchase additional copies of this book call our customer service department at **(800) 638–3030** or fax orders to **(301) 824–7390**. International customers should call **(301) 714–2324**.

01 02
2 3 4 5 6 7 8 9 10

Preface

The pace of healthcare reformation in the United States has been unprecedented since the publication of our first edition 4 years ago. As the healthcare system continues to evolve, outdated professional practice roles and models of care are being redesigned and new ones are emerging. This is changing the way physicians, nurses, and other health professionals practice. Our goal in this second edition has been to capture the substance, as well as the excitement, of these remarkable changes in our profession.

The debate continues among nurse educators and practitioners regarding the preparation of nurses for advanced practice, with some advocating the continuation of separate nurse practitioner (NP) and clinical nurse specialist (CNS) tracks and others strongly supporting a blending of the skills and roles of the NP and the CNS. The debate aside, it is clear that the strengths of each role are required to meet the complex healthcare needs of society. The goal is an advanced practice nurse (APN) who is well prepared to provide comprehensive care and illness management in a variety of settings and at transitional points of illness and who works with physicians and other health professionals in expanded collaborative relationships. The new models of care being implemented and evaluated have one goal in common: to achieve access to quality, cost-effective care for all people, especially underserved and vulnerable populations that have either been completely excluded from healthcare or been recipients of fragmented and poor quality care. APNs must be instrumental in achieving this goal if we are to have a healthier American society in the 21st century.

Transition into advanced practice is a process of professional resocialization that requires the aspirant to attain a greater breadth and depth of knowledge not only of the existing models of practice, but also of the processes of creating new models to fully use advanced practice roles and competencies. This text is designed to facilitate this transition by providing a comprehensive resource for APN students, practitioners, and faculty. The evolution, issues, and scope of advanced practice nursing are addressed. Exemplars are provided of innovative practices by nurses who care for underserved, vulnerable, or special patient populations in a variety of settings.

Graduate nursing students and faculty will find this text appropriate for courses dealing with the roles, issues, and the future course of professional nursing and healthcare in general. For APNs engaged in actively creating the infrastructure for the new breed of professional nurses, the text can be a valuable resource for updating and validating their practice. It is for dreamers who pursue and practice excellence every day through their influence in providing care for patients and their families. We all share visions of what care can be. We hope that this text will energize and inspire nurses to envision new and exciting possibilities for the care of patients, their families, and society.

The text is organized into four sections. **Section I** provides the foundation for advanced practice nursing, beginning with a vision of practice, education, and research. A discussion of the educational preparation and socialization into advanced practice is complemented by a comprehensive chapter on the current status of licensure, approval to practice, certification, and privileging for APNs in the United States. Chapter 5, an important addition to this edition, leads us through the complexities of clinical reasoning at the advanced practice level. Four case exemplars, written by expert APNs, are used to highlight clinical reasoning competencies by engaging us in the clinical reasoning processes undertaken in the management of a particular patient.

Section II addresses changing care environments and patient diversity in healthcare delivery. Healthcare delivery systems and the changing environments of care are presented in Chapter 6, to provide a framework for discussion. Chapter 7 discusses the renaissance of primary care and new opportunities for APNs as well-prepared providers to improve the primary care needs of a nation. The influence of managed care environments on practice, as presented in Chapter 8, assists the reader in understanding the financial and insurance issues related to delivery of care. The shifting emphasis on chronic illness and long-term care along with related reimbursement issues are presented in Chapter 9. A new addition, Chapter 10, presents an overview of informatics, emphasizing its critical importance to advanced practice nursing. The section concludes with two complementary chapters that address cultural and ethnic diversity in healthcare and the growing importance and demand for complementary therapies.

Section III examines practice and economics issues that are moving APNs forward. Chapter 13 has been expanded, emphasizing the importance of accountability in practice. Chapter 14 discusses the recently enacted reimbursement for APNs and the astute political activism involved in this process. The research base for practice—both through the conduct of research and research utilization—is discussed in Chapter 15. Finally, Chapter 16 addresses the economics that influences development of a business plan for APN practice.

Section IV is a showcase of the many examples of cutting-edge practice by APNs. It is a tribute to what APNs contribute to patient care and how they are pushing the boundaries of practice to meet the needs of a diverse and complex nation. Chapter 17 includes exemplars that demonstrate models of health promotion and disease prevention provided by APNs in diverse settings and with a variety of populations. With a renewed interest in outcomes, exemplar 17D describes how outcomes are tracked in a primary care practice. Exemplars of management of high-risk and vulnerable populations are addressed in Chapter 18. Fascinating snapshots of patient care delivered to ethnically diverse populations in rural and urban areas, home healthcare, and care for person with AIDs are shared. Finally, Chapter 19 highlights the advanced practice roles and expanding boundaries of practice by a nurse–midwife, nurse anesthetist, clinical nurse specialist, and acute care nurse practitioner.

With this new edition, we continue to celebrate what APNs have accomplished and hope to stimulate a vision of what can be, as we continue to meet the healthcare needs of society in creative new ways.

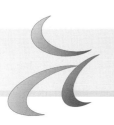

Acknowledgments

This book originally grew out of a need to provide a special textbook for graduate nursing students preparing to become advanced practice nurses (APNs). Because there was no textbook available to meet this need, a collaborative effort was initiated to write one. We are honored that the first edition quickly received acceptance and was used in many educational programs. With that success, we are pleased to present the second edition that examines the APN's role in a world of accelerated healthcare change.

There are many people to be thanked for their role in its completion. First, we thank our many contributing authors in both editions who shared their expertise and talents with this project. Each was selected for the unique piece that he or she could contribute from their individual perspective and range of experiences. Because of the in-depth presentation of their topics, the chapters can stand alone as well as contribute a critical component to the integrated whole.

We thank our editors and publication colleagues at Lippincott Williams & Wilkins for their ongoing encouragement and support throughout the project. In particular, we express our sincere appreciation to our editors, Lisa Marshall and Sandy Kasko, for their unique perspective and overall expertise; their continued assistance, sage advise, dedication, and timely electronic responses helped us meet our deadlines. It was a pleasure to collaborate with them on this journey.

We thank our families, friends, and colleagues, without whose support, understanding, and encouragement this textbook may never have reached completion. We sincerely appreciate all you did with and for us during the entire process.

And finally, we continue to thank our students—past, present, and future—whose presence reminds us of why we started this book. We dedicate this book to each of you. It is the famous line from the play *The King and I* that we understand so well in our interactions with you: "If you become a teacher, by your students you'll be taught." Thank you for continuing to teach us while we are helping you learn. May this textbook help you in your lifelong journey of learning. If it succeeds in doing that, we will have successfully completed our mission.

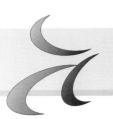

Contributors

Michael H. Ackerman, DNS, RN, CS, FCCM
Associate Professor of Clinical Nursing
Critical Care Nurse Practitioner
University of Rochester Medical Center
Rochester, NY

Anthony J. Adinolfi, MSN, ANP
Assistant Clinical Professor
Duke University Medical Center
School of Nursing
Durham, NC

Deborah Antai-Otong, MS, RN, CS
Psychiatric CNS, Director
VA North Texas Health Care System
Dallas, TX

Kristie Asimos, MSN, RN, CRNP
Team Leader—Pennsylvania Restraint Reduction
   Initiative
West Chester, PA

Janet Garvey Baradell, PhD, RN, CS
Psychiatric Clinical Nurse Specialist
Private Practice
Chapel Hill, NC

Amy Barton, PhD, RN
Associate Dean for Practice
University of Colorado Health Sciences Center
Denver, CO

Meg Bourbonniere, MSN, RN
Research Assistant
University of Pennsylvania
School of Nursing
Philadelphia, PA

Peter I. Buerhaus, PhD, RN, FAAN
Assistant Professor
Harvard School of Public Health
Department of Health Policy and Management
and
Director
Harvard Nursing Research Institute
Harvard School of Public Health
Boston, MA

Susan Burns-Tisdale, MPH, RN
Director of Community and Continuing Care Nursing
Beth Israel-Deaconess Hospitals
Boston, MA

Angeline Bushy, PhD, RN, CS
Professor, Bert Fish Endowed Chair, Community Nursing
University of Central Florida
College of Nursing
Daytona Beach, FL

Mary Chaffee, MS, RN, CNA, CCRN
Commander, Nurse Corps, United States Navy
University of Maryland at Baltimore
Gaithersburg, MD

Jean Clark, RN, MS, CS, CCRN
Critical Care Nurse Practitioner
Strong Memorial Hospital
Rochester, NY

Karen L. Dick, PhD, RN, CS
Nurse Manager, Home Care
Program Coordinator, Beth Israel-Deaconist Homecare
    Department
Beth Israel-Deaconist Hospitals
Boston, MA

Margaret A. Edmundson, MN, RN, CNM
Certified Nurse Midwife
Columbia-Presbyterian/St. Luke's Hospital
Denver, CO

Joan Engebretson, DrPH, RN, HNC
Associate Professor
University of Texas Health Science Center
School of Nursing
Houston, TX

Shotsy C. Faust, MN, RN, FNP
Associate Clinical Professor
University of California at San Francisco Medical Center
San Francisco, CA

Maria Francati, RN, MS
Critical Care Nurse Practitioner
Strong Memorial Hospital
Rochester, NY

Catherine L. Gilliss, DNSc, RN, FAAN
Dean and Professor
School of Nursing
Yale University
New Haven, CN

Jean Goeppinger, PhD, RN
Professor and Chair of Department of Psychiatric and
    Community Mental Health
School of Nursing
University of North Carolina at Chapel Hill
Chapel Hill, NC

Rosalie Hammond, PhD, RN, FNP
Assistant Professor
School of Nursing
University of North Carolina at Chapel Hill
Chapel Hill, NC

Robin M. Haskell, MSN, ACNP-CS, CCRN
Trauma Nurse Practitioner
Division of Trauma and Surgical Critical Care
University of Pennsylvania Medical Center
    Philadelphia, PA
and
Brandywine Hospital and Trauma Center
Coatesville, PA
and
Lecturer
Critical Care Nurse Practitioner Program
University of Pennsylvania School of Nursing
Philadelphia, PA

JoAnne Kirk Henry, EdD, RN,CS
Director, Offices of Health Policy
and
Associate Professor and Director of Community Nursing
    Organizations
Virginia Commonwealth University School of Nursing
Richmond, VA

M. Elizabeth Hixon, MSN, RN, A/GNP, CS
Clinical Associate
Duke University Medical Center
Durham, NC

Lori D. Johnson, MSN, RN, CCRN
Clinical Nurse Specialist, Pediatric Critical Care
Lucile Packard Children's Health Services at University
    of California
and
Assistant Clinical Professor
University of California at San Francisco
School of Nursing
San Francisco, CA

Joseph T. Kanusky, MS, RN, CRNA
Assistant Professor of Clinical Nursing
University of Texas Health Science Center
School of Nursing
Houston, TX

Maureen R. Keefe, PhD, RN, PNP, FAAN
Dean and Professor
Medical College of South Carolina
College of Nursing
Charleston, SC

Julie R. Knopp, MS, RN, C
Adult Nurse Practitioner
Beth Israel Deaconess Home Care
Boston, MA

Vicki L. Kraus, PhD, ARNP, CDE
Advanced Pracatice Nurse
Department of Nursing
The University of Iowa Hospitals and Clinics
Iowa City, IA

Jan M. Kriebs, MSN, RN, CNM
Instructor
University of Maryland School of Medicine
Department of Obstetrics, Gynecology, and
    Reproductive Sciences
Baltimore, MD

Deborah B. Kupecz, MSN, RN, NP
Nurse Practitioner
VA Medical Center
Denver, CO

Elizabeth Lawhorn, MSN, RN, COHN-S, CCM
Occupational Health Coordinator
US Medicine and Occupational Health Department
Exxon Company USA
Houston, TX

Sun Yong Lee, MD
Assistant Professor of Surgery
Division of Trauma and Surgical Critical Care
University of Pennsylvania Medical Center
Philadelphia, PA
and
Attending Trauma Surgeon
Brandywine Hospital and Trauma Center
Coatesville, PA

Carolyn K. Lewis, PhD, RN, CNAA
Executive Director
American Nurses Credentialing Center
Washington, DC

Marilyn M. Lynn, MSN, RN, NP
Adult Nurse Practitioner
VA Medical Center
Denver, CO

Ginette A. Pepper, PhD, RN, CNS, FAAN
Assistant Professor
University of Colorado Health Sciences Center
School of Nursing
Denver, CO

Mary Pat Rapp, MSN, RN, GNP-C
Instructor of Clinical Nursing
Geriatric Nurse Practitioner
University of Texas Health Science Center
School of Nursing
Houston, TX

Teresa Reed, RN, MS
Critical Care Nurse Practitioner
Strong Memorial Hospital
Rochester, NY

Bonnie Rogers, DrPH, COHN-S, FAAN
Associate Professor, Director Occupational Health
Nursing Program
School of Public Health
University of North Carolina at Chapel Hill
Chapel Hill, NC

Carol A. Romano, PhD, RN, CS, CNAA, FAAN
Chief, Clinical Informatics Services
Clinical Center, National Institutes of Health
Bethesda, MD

Leslie H. Rozier, MSN, RN, ANP
Family Nurse Practitioner/Proprietor
Prophase (Locus Tenens Contractor)
Pinedale, WY

Marjorie A. Satinsky, MBA, FACHE
Executive Director
ReXMeD PHO
Raleigh, NC

Janine J. Sherman, MSN, RN, WHNP
Women's Health Nurse Practitioner
Instructor of Clinical Nursing
University of Texas Health Science Center
School of Nursing
Houston, TX

Mary C. Smolenski, EdD, RN,CS
Director, Certification Services
American Nurses Credentialing Center
Washington, DC

Neville E. Strumpf, PhD, RN,CS, FAAN
Associate Professor and Doris Schwartz Term Chair
and
Director, Gerontological Nurse Practitioner Program
School of Nursing
University of Pennsylvania
Philadelphia, PA

Nancy L. Szaflarski, PhD, ACNP-CS, FCCM
Postdoctoral Research Fellow, Department of
    Anesthesia
University of California, San Francisco
San Francisco, CA

Nancy M. Valentine, PhD, RN, MPH, FAAN
Chief Consultant, Nursing Strategic Health Care Group
Department of Veterans Affairs
Washington, DC

Lauren Van Horn, RN, MS, CS
Critical Care Nurse Practitioner
Strong Memorial Hospital
Rochester, NY

Celeste G. Villanueva, MSN, RN, CRNA
Assistant Professor
Associate Director, Graduate Program of Nurse
    Anesthesia
Samuel Merritt College
Oakland, CA

Patricia Hinton Walker, PhD, RN, FAAN
Dean and Professor
University of Colorado Health Sciences Center
School of Nursing
Denver, CO

Anne W. Wojner, MSN, RN, CCRN
Assistant Professor of Clinical Nursing
The University of Texas Health Science Center
    School of Nursing
Houston, TX

Contents

The Foundation for Advanced Practice Nursing

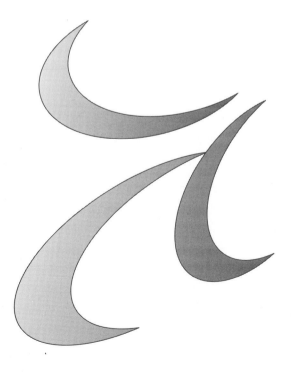

CHAPTER 1

Advanced Practice Nursing at the Dawn of the 21st Century: Practice, Education, and Research

Joanne V. Hickey

As society shifts from the postindustrial age to an information society, the dawn of the 21st century looms as a monumental landmark for reflection on the past and anticipation of an uncertain future. The future is partly amenable to shaping by visionary thinking, planning, control, or anticipatory adaptation (Pescut, 1997); however, multiple political and economic forces, as well as the complexities of life in a rapidly expanding global community, create challenges unprecedented by any faced in the past. Healthcare, the fourth largest industry in the United States, which consumes almost 14% of the gross domestic product, is being radically transformed. The response in the health disciplines and among health professionals is creating enormous change in the roles assumed by healthcare workers. This unprecedented reshaping of healthcare has enormous implications for the profession of nursing.

Subsumed under the definition of a "profession" is the notion of expertise, autonomy, commitment, and responsibility. The profession of nursing has a proud history with respect to these professional characteristics and responding effectively to changing healthcare needs. In our current climate of radical and unsettling change, advanced practice nurses (APNs) are in the forefront of the nursing profession's response by acquiring greater expertise and assuming greater autonomy and responsibility for meeting society's healthcare needs. The 21st century offers advanced practice nursing the opportunity to develop and mature as a key component in the reconfigured and redesigned, integrated, interdisciplinary healthcare delivery system. To be successful in their mission, APNs must commit to ongoing learning and to developing new skills and competencies as a means of staying competitive in the healthcare market.

Where is advanced practice nursing now, and where does it seem to be heading? This chapter examines these questions by considering the scope and standards of advanced practice nursing; the implications of the radically changing healthcare system for APNs; trends in nursing practice, education, and research; and the maturation of advanced practice nursing.

Advanced Practice Nursing

Definitions of advanced practice nursing have been proposed by many specialty professional nursing organizations. Key components in all definitions include graduate education, patient/family-focused practice, and an expanded role. The American Nurses Association published *Scope and Standards of Advanced Practice Registered Nursing* in 1996. This important document delineated advanced practice nursing and provides the basis for further discussion and refinement within the profession.

Advanced practice nurses are registered nurses who hold a master's or doctoral degree with a specialization in an area of advanced nursing; they have had "supervised practice during graduate education, and have ongoing clinical experiences" (ANA, 1996, p. 2). The curriculum includes a common core of knowledge in advanced practice nursing and an expanded core of knowledge in a specialty area of advanced nursing practice. The educational process results in an expert nurse with "an in-depth knowledge base and clinical skills" who is prepared for specialization, expansion, and advancement in practice.

> **Specialization** is a concentration in one of the four advanced practice nursing specialty areas: clinical nurse specialist, nurse practitioner, nurse midwife, or nurse anesthetist. **Expansion** refers to the commitment for ongoing learning and acquisition of new knowledge, skills, and competencies. **Advancement** involves both specialization and expansion, and results in new integration of theory, skills, and competencies to respond to the needs of patients/families and an evolving health care system. (p. 14)

Key distinguishing characteristics of APNs are listed in Table 1-1. APNs possess a "higher level of expertise in assessment, diagnosis, and treatment of complex responses of individuals, families, or communities to actual or potential health problems, prevention of illness and injury, maintenance of wellness, and provision of comfort" (ANA, 1996, p. 2). Advanced practice nursing builds on basic nursing practice, and APNs continue to perform many of the same activities employed in basic nursing practice. However, the differences in APN practice lie in the "greater depth and breadth of knowledge, a greater degree of synthesis of data, and complexity of skills and interventions" that APNs possess (ANA, 1966, p. 2).

SCOPE OF PRACTICE

Scope of practice, as it applies to advance practice nursing, delineates the boundaries of professional activities and the parameters of advanced nursing practice. Because the scope of practice is evolving and dynamic, changes will occur as APNs respond to changing so-

---

TABLE 1-1 ***Distinguishing Features of Advanced Practice Nurses***

- Manage patients with a greater depth and breadth of knowledge, skills, and competencies.
- Engage in complex clinical reasoning and decision making related to complex patient problems.
- Possess greater skills in managing organizations, systems, and environments.
- Practice with greater autonomy.
- Exercise a higher degree of independent judgement.
- Use well-developed communications skills with multidisciplinary teams and systems and across complex healthcare environments.

cietal needs and are granted expanded legal authority to practice in their roles. A common body of knowledge and scope of practice is foundational for all advanced nursing practice roles. However, distinguishing differences are also created by the particular advanced practice **specialty roles.** Currently, the recognized advanced practice nursing roles are nurse anesthetist (CRNA), nurse midwife (CNM), clinical nurse specialist (CNS), and nurse practitioner (NP). In the future, new roles may emerge and be recognized by the profession. One role currently being discussed is that of the nurse administrator or nurse manager.

Often, there is specialization beyond the four major identified APN roles, which is referred to as **subspecialization.** For example, APNs may concentrate their practice on gerontology or pediatrics (age-specific), neurology or cardiology (system-specific), heart failure or asthma (disease-specific), or wound healing or incontinence management (problem-specific).

ADVANCED PRACTICE COMPETENCIES AND ROLES

Competencies

Competencies are interpretively defined areas of skilled performance identified and described by intent, function, and meaning (Benner, 1984). A number of core competencies are common to all advanced practice nursing roles and include the following:

- Expert clinical practice
- Education, coaching, and guidance skills adaptable to individuals, families, or groups
- Consultation
- Collaboration (intradisciplinary, multidisciplinary, interdisciplinary, or across systems)
- Change agent
- Clinical and professional leadership
- Use and conduct of research
- Ethical decision making
- Evaluation of outcomes
- Quality assurance

The following additional competencies needed by all APNs should be included: commitment to "evidence-based practice" and "best practice," incorporation of evaluation into practice, outcomes management, and incorporation of informatics into all aspects of practice.

Each person expects the most effective treatment when he or she is ill. Determining what is best for a particular patient given the individual circumstances is the responsibility of healthcare providers. **Evidence-based practice (EBP)** is the explicit integrating of clinical research evidence with pathophysiologic reasoning, health provider experience, and patient preferences in the provision of care (Cook & Levy, 1998). EBP uses information technology to assemble pertinent data and determines its applicability to the given situation. **Best practice** is a combination of evidence-based practice, clinician's judgment, and patient's preference (Byers & Brunell, 1998) that has been successfully implemented and refined and that sets new standards or creates a new wave of innovation involving a cost-effective model of the work process (*AACN News,* 1998).

Advanced practice brings an enhanced level of accountability. This, in turn, means APNs must be competent to evaluate patient outcomes, practice outcomes, and the performance of themselves and others. To do this, APNs must be able to apply evaluation models appropriately and critically analyze data to make informed decisions. Outcomes research, which has emerged as a research and practice priority, is a specific type of evaluation serving as the basis for focused outcomes management programs designed to determine "best practice." Finally, competency in managing and continuously using scientific,

TABLE 1-2 *Competencies of Health Professionals for 2005*

Care for the Community's Health: Understand the determinants of health and work with others in the community to integrate a range of activities that promote, protect, and improve the health of the community. Appreciate the growing diversity of the population and understand health status and healthcare needs in the context of different cultural values.

Provide Contemporary Clinical Care: Acquire and retain up-to-date clinical skills and apply them to meet the public's healthcare needs.

Participate in the Emerging System and Accommodate Expanded Accountability: Function in the new healthcare settings and interdisciplinary team arrangement designed to meet the primary healthcare needs of the public, and emphasize high-quality, cost-effective, integrated services. Respond to increasing levels of public, governmental, and third-party participation in, and scrutiny of, the shape and direction of the healthcare system.

Ensure Cost-effective Care and Use Technology Appropriately: Establish cost and quality objectives for the healthcare process and understand any increasingly complex and often costly technology appropriately.

Practice Prevention and Promote Healthy Lifestyles: Emphasize primary and secondary preventive strategies for all people and help individuals, families, and communities maintain and promote health behaviors.

Involve Patients and Families in the Decision-making Process: Expect patients and their families to participate actively both in decisions regarding their personal healthcare and in evaluating its quality and acceptability.

Manage Information and Continue to Learn: Manage and continuously use scientific, technological, and patient information to maintain professional competence and relevance throughout practice life.

From: O'Neil, E.H. (1993). *Health professions education for the future: Schools in service to the nation.* San Francisco: Pew Health Professions Commission.

technological, and patient information is an integral part of practice and must be mastered: it is not optional; it is a must.

In addition to these competencies, the Pew Health Professions Commission Report (1993) identified competencies necessary for health professionals for 2005. These are summarized in Table 1-2. It is of interest that the competencies cited are for *all* health professionals, not just nursing. The competencies for 2005 should be reviewed in conjunction with the characteristics of the emerging healthcare system outlined by the Pew Commission (1993) and cited in Table 1-3. A key characteristic for 2005 is interdisciplinary collaboration at the local, national, and international level. To function in a truly interdisciplinary collaborative team requires significant changes in values and working relationships, thus redefining individual and team accountability and setting a new ethical framework for practice. The Pew Health Professions Commission Reports (1991, 1993, 1995) have been prominent in forecasting the future and recommending strategies for change. Other than a few minor additions (i.e., evidence-based practice, best practice) and the expansion of terms, the forecasted professional competencies and healthcare system characteristics are both on target.

The Four Major Advanced Practice Nursing Roles
Of the 2.55 million nurses in the United States, approximately 161,700 are APNs (U.S. Department of Health and Human Services, 1996). The following describes the four APN roles as they are currently viewed.

Nurse Anesthetist
The nurse anesthetist (CRNA) provides anesthesia and anesthesia-related care, including performance of the following: preanesthetic preparation and evaluation; and anesthesia induction, maintenance, and emergence, including administration of appropriate drugs and techniques and local, regional, and general anesthesia. In addition, the role of the CRNA includes establishment of invasive monitoring, postanesthesia care, acute and chronic pain

management, and associated clinical support functions such as respiratory care and emergency resuscitation (American Association of Nurse Anesthetists, 1996).

Nurse–Midwife

The nurse–midwife (CNM) is a clinical nurse expert who has the advanced knowledge, skills, competencies, and clinical reasoning for the management of care for women and newborns. The focus of practice is providing antepartum, intrapartum, and postpartum care; neonatal care; family planning; and well-women gynecological care (American College of Nurse–Midwives, 1993).

Clinical Nurse Specialist

The clinical nurse specialist (CNS) is an expert clinician who practices in a particular specialty or subspecialty area and engages in direct and indirect practice activities. The major CNS subroles include the following:

1. *Direct patient/client care,* including assessment, diagnosis, planning, and prescription of pharmacological interventions (when permitted by state laws) and nonpharmacological treatment of health problems, health promotion, and preventive care for individual patients or populations of patients within the specialty area;
2. *Education* of patients, families, nurses, and other health professionals;
3. *Consultation* to nurses, physicians, other health professionals, and other interested persons; and
4. *Research utilization* and participation in or conduct of *research.*

Nurse Practitioner

The nurse practitioner (NP) is an expert nurse clinician who conducts comprehensive health assessments, makes a diagnosis, prescribes pharmacological and nonpharmacological interventions, and evaluates outcomes in the *direct* management of individual patients with acute

TABLE 1-3 *Characteristics of the Emerging Healthcare System*

Orientation Toward Health: Greater emphasis on prevention and wellness; greater expectation for individual responsibility for healthy behaviors.

Population Perspective: New attention to risk factors affecting substantial segments of the community, including issues of access and the physical and social environment.

Intensive Use of Information: Reliance on information systems to provide complete, easily assimilated patient information, as well as ready access to relevant information on current practice.

Knowledge of Treatment Outcomes: Emphasis on the determination of the most effective treatment under different conditions and the dissemination of this information to those involved in treatment decisions.

Constrained Resources: A pervasive concern over increasing costs, coupled with expanded use of mechanisms to control or limit available expenditures.

Coordination of Services: Increased integration of providers with a concomitant emphasis on teams to improve efficiency and effectiveness across all settings.

Expectations of Accountability: Growing scrutiny by a larger variety of payers, consumers, and regulators, coupled with more formally defined performance expectations.

Growing Interdependence: Further integration of domestic issues of health, education, and public safety, combined with a growing awareness of the importance of U. S. healthcare in a global context.

From: O'Neil, E. H. (1993). *Health professions education for the future: Schools in service to the nation* (p.6). San Francisco: Pew Health Professions Commission.

and chronic illness and disease. In addition to conducting illness and disease management, the NP engages in health promotion and illness prevention activities as an integral part of practice and practices in a variety of settings, providing direct care to individuals, families, and communities by working independently or in interdisciplinary collaborative practice groups.

The subspecialty practice focus may include geriatrics, pediatrics, adults, family, primary care, acute care, or mental health.

Historical Perspective and Development of Advanced Practice Roles

The circumstances surrounding the development of each of the four advanced practice roles are quite different. The historical development of each role is discussed further in this book, and the reader is referred to those sections. The oldest advanced nursing specialty is that of the nurse anesthetist, which began in the mid-1800s. In Exemplar 19A, Kanusky discusses the historical development of the nurse anesthetist. The second advanced practice role to develop in the United States was that of the nurse–midwife, and this role is discussed by Edmundson in Exemplar 19B.

The clinical nurse specialist role was the third addition to advanced practice roles. CNSs have evolved from an original patient focus in the 1970s to an organizational and systems focus in the mid-1980s to a configuration of the role in the mid-1990s (Haddock, 1997). The CNS role is discussed in Exemplar 19C by Wojner. Finally, the last advanced practice role to emerge is that of the nurse practitioner; a brief discussion of the historical development follows.

Responding to the shortage of primary care providers who were needed to improve access to care and meet the needs for health promotion and illness management, the Surgeon General issued a report in 1963, recommending that nurses should be educated to provide primary care in collaboration with physicians. In this early stage of development, the generic term "nurse practitioner" referred to a nurse providing primary care in an ambulatory care setting such as a clinic or outpatient facility (Steel, 1997). The first graduate-level nurse practitioner program, credited to Dr. Loretta Ford and Dr. Henry Silver (1967), was established at the University of Colorado in 1965. The program prepared nurses to deliver pediatric care in rural Colorado. This program was based on a "nursing model focused on the promotion of health in daily living, growth and development for children in families as well as the prevention of disease and disability" (Ford, 1982, 1986). Other programs quickly developed and were located in a variety of settings. Programs developed that specifically focused on the adult, the family, and the older person. Some curricula were certificate programs affiliated with hospitals. However, by the mid-1980s, most nurse practitioner programs were graduate-level curricula leading to a master's degree.

Up to this time, most NPs were employed in clinics and outpatient facilities that focused on primary care. What was emerging was a demand for nurses in high-intensity acute-critical care areas who could assist with improving fragmentation of care, high resource utilization, and poorly delineated patient outcomes. In the early 1990s, acute care nurse practitioners (ACNPs) emerged to meet this need within a collaborative model of practice. The ACNP role included the following: (1) management of acutely ill individuals throughout the entire episode of acute illness; (2) diagnosis and treatment of predictable deviations in the course of illness; (3) provision of ambulatory services in the acute transitional period following discharge; and (4) monitoring responses to care (ANA & AACN, 1995). The practice of ACNPs is focused on patients' needs and is not bound to a particular care setting. Although most ACNPs practice in acute care facilities, the role is evolving into one that is centered on the intensity of patient needs—not on the environment in which care is delivered. With more high-intensity care being provided outside the traditional acute care hospital, more high-intensity care is shifting to long-term care, subacute units, ambulatory care, clinics, and the home; ACNPs will find these settings appropriate employment and practice opportunities (Walker & Sebastian, 1997).

Barriers to Practice

Although great opportunities are developing for APNs, significant barriers to practice remain. The major barriers for APNs are the scope of practice regulation and third-party reimbursement. Removal of these legal and financial barriers is essential to actualize the full potential of APNs.

Regulation of Practice

Regulation of the healthcare workforce, the Pew Commission reported, has evolved over the last century into 50 separate state systems, each with its own state practice act, creating a complex and often irrational organizational structure. The lack of uniformity in language, laws, and regulations among states limits effective professional practice and mobility; confuses the public; and presents barriers to integrated delivery systems, the use of telemedicine, and other emerging health technologies (see Chapter 4 for a complete discussion of regulation of professional practice). These inconsistencies transcend state boundaries and call for standardization across the individual states (Finocchio, Dower, McMahon, et al. 1995). Safriet (1994, p. 311) wrote the following:

> *Since health and illness are for the most part biologically and physically based, with some psychological and emotional components, it is not at all clear why licensure laws—that is, proxies for competency—should vary according to political boundaries rather than competency domains.*

The Pew Commission Report (1995) goes on to note that current statutes grant broad, near-exclusive scope of practice to a few professions and "carve-out" scopes for the remaining professions. "These (state) laws erect unreasonable barriers to high-quality and affordable care. The need for accessible healthcare calls for flexible scopes of practice that recognize the demonstrated competence of various practitioners to provide the same health services." Finally, the report states that regulatory bodies are perceived as unaccountable to the public they serve and are ineffective in protecting the public. A number of recommendations have been proposed by the Pew Commission (1995, p. ix) including:

1. Standardization of language, titles, and entry into practice to facilitate the physical and professional mobility of health professionals across state lines;
2. Requirements for practice should be based on demonstration of initial and continuing competency;
3. Allowance of different professions to share overlapping scopes of practice so that all professionals can provide services to the full extent of their current knowledge, training, experience, and skills; and
4. State regulatory boards and their functions should reflect the interdisciplinary and public accountability demands of the changing healthcare delivery system.

Changes are occurring due, in part, to astute nurses who recognize the need to participate in the political process to lobby for changes in the regulation of practice. Changes in limitations on scope of practice and in attaining prescriptive privileges are improving patients' access to affordable care and improving work opportunities for APNs.

Reimbursement

The expansion of APNs reimbursement by the Health Care and Financing Administration (HCF) as of January of 1998 has been cited as a major achievement in the struggle for reimbursement. Further discussion of reimbursement can be found in Chapters 14 and 16. In addition, many HMOs are including APNs on their panel of providers, allowing consumers to choose APNs to be their primary healthcare providers. By including APNs, HMOs are also providing reimbursement for services.

BLENDED ROLES

The CNS and NP roles share more commonalties as compared to the distinct practice focus of the CNM and CRNA roles. In the early to mid-1990s, there was much discussion about the blending the CNS role and the NP role into one advanced practice role. Precipitated, in part, by the loss of many CNS positions as cost cutting measures, the blended role appeared to be a way to prepare a multipurpose APN marketable in a changing healthcare system. Some CNS positions were converted to case manager roles. Many other CNSs flocked to NP programs to be retooled for a fickle healthcare system that seemed to favor NPs. Interestingly, many of the same institutions that cut CNS positions just a few years ago, are now attempting to rehire CNSs again as organizations experience the critical void left by the departed CNSs. There is less discussion now about blending these roles and more discussion about strengthening each role, recognizing that organizations need the unique contributions of both the CNS role and NP role.

In reviewing advanced practice roles, one notices the similarities in subroles and functions particularly for the CNS and NP. The difference lies in the primary focus of the role and the amount of time, methods, and purpose devoted to the subroles. What is unique about each role? CNSs often work through other nurses and serve as clinical experts and resources, consultants, coaches, and change agents who know how to determine and provide evidence-based practice and "best practice" for populations of patients. They are also expert in understanding systems and knowing how to navigate through systems to change practice and remove barriers to meet individual patient needs. These skills have also positioned CNSs to be excellent case managers, and many CNS positions have been converted to case manager positions. By contrast, NPs focus more on individual patients rather than populations, have more of an overlap with physicians in diagnosis and treatment of disease than CNSs, and deal more with client management in a particular setting, unlike CNSs, who are often system-focused. The roles are complementary with overlapping function, yet each role fills a unique position in delivering quality healthcare.

PUSHING THE BOUNDARIES: EMERGING PRACTICE ROLES FOR ADVANCED PRACTICE NURSES

APNs want to practice to the full extent of their current knowledge, training, experience, and skills. However, the stifling of innovation and creativity needed to nurture full actualization of advanced practice nursing is common in hospital-based practice. Aiken (1990) advocated the role of attending nurse for APNs, a role that has some similarities to the attending physician. She proposed reorganizing senior nurse clinicians into attending nurse services and integrating them into the existing medical staff organization so that each clinical service would consist of a nurse–physician group practice. Attending nurses could assume 24-hour responsibility for patients assigned to a service and make clinical decisions about nursing care for all patients on the service, regardless of location in the facility (Aiken, 1990, pp. 76–77). A few nurses have taken on the challenge of developing the attending nurse role, but it is not a common role.

A relatively new phenomenon in nursing practice concerns the appropriate role for the increased number of doctorally prepared nurses who continue to provide *direct* patient care. The major purpose of doctoral education is to prepare nurses for the conduct of research to uncover new knowledge. Increasing numbers of CNSs and NPs are joining the ranks of the doctorally prepared, and some are using their expertise in clinical practice to increase clinical research (Collins, 1992). But doctorally prepared nurses who wish to blend an academic career that includes direct patient care with the traditional roles of research and teaching find themselves without an identity, mentors, role models, career paths, and often support from their deans. Riesch (1987) proposed the academic clinician role for doctorally prepared nurses who wish to maintain a patient care practice. The academic clinician is described as an expert practitioner of a scientific discipline, prepared to teach the principles of that discipline to others, and who is a researcher working to expand the knowledge that makes up that discipline. Clinical practice is important to a researcher because it provides the experience for the generation of important research questions and access to a study population.

CHANGING ROLES IN A CHANGING HEALTHCARE ENVIRONMENT

Boundaries and scope of practice for APNs will continue to change and evolve; this is an ongoing process in any profession and is an expression of accountability to patient needs. Koerner and Burgess (1997) have summarized changing roles well:

> Nurses' roles must be adapted to a changing society that is increasingly becoming more diverse and chronically ill. Further, the isolated institutional model is giving way to an integrated continuum, and nurses' work space is expanding; wherever there are people, there is a place for nursing in preventative, primary, *tertiary,* or supportive roles. The prevailing autonomous view in all professions must give way to an interdependent one that demands a high degree of collaboration and cooperation. Finally, the notion of client as passive recipient of care from an expert professional fades when we view individuals as experts in their own health, and the healthcare system as a vehicle to support them in their efforts to maximize their life journey in the health experience. (p. 2) (italics added)

SUMMARY

The previous section has discussed advanced practice nursing and the various roles that APNs assume. The following section examines forces and trends, including healthcare financing, that create the context for advanced practice.

 Forces and Trends Affecting Healthcare

The 1990s were forecasted to be the decade of national healthcare reform legislated by the federal government. What actually occurred was reform originating at the local and regional levels. The fundamental force driving change in the United States healthcare system is cost. Healthcare is just too expensive. There is little debate about the need to control cost; the debate is how to accomplish this goal without excluding people or sacrificing quality. A brief review of the access–cost–quality framework and healthcare financing in the United States provides a perspective for discussion.

ACCESS–COST–QUALITY TRIAD

Healthcare transformation can be viewed from the perspective of an access–cost–quality triad. This relational model for the forces affecting healthcare delivery emphasizes a zero-sum interplay among the three components at a given level of system funding. The quality of the U.S. healthcare system is often touted as the best in the world although some have challenged that assertion, citing indices of health status such as high infant mortality rates and low average life expectancy in certain segments of the population. Challengers also have cited the lack of emphasis on preventive care in the United States as compared with other industrialized countries. Despite a certain amount of ambiguity and exceptions, the quality of healthcare for the bulk of the U.S. population is usually recognized as good, and there is great concern that changes in healthcare may negatively affect quality. Furthermore, the percentage of the population covered by health cost-reimbursement insurance—the de facto definition of access—is too low. An estimated 37 million Americans do not receive some level of health benefits as a condition of employment or through a government subsidy program. This includes those described as the "working poor," who cannot afford to pay out of pocket for healthcare insurance. The working poor population does receive healthcare—albeit not necessarily optimum healthcare—mostly through hospital emergency rooms and government-subsidized clinics. The cost of this care is absorbed by the system through higher insurance premiums for insured parties and through state and federal taxes for targeted health services (e.g., Indian Health Service, Frontier Nursing Service, veterans' health services). The uninsured 43.4 million Americans (16.1%) also include those who choose not to buy healthcare insurance although they could afford it. These are often young and healthy people who expect to stay healthy and are willing to pay for whatever healthcare they may need on a pay-as-you-go basis.

As a result of the rising percentage of the gross domestic product (GDP) devoted to healthcare costs, providers are compelled to do a better job of controlling costs through better management of the type and amount of care a subscriber receives. However, the concept that cost is directly linked to quality has become ingrained; a discussion of cost-effective care inevitably involves the assumption that quality is compromised by managing or controlling cost.

Two unpredictable factors may severely affect the cost of providing healthcare. The first factor is preventive health services as part of basic coverage. One argument holds that preventive health services will decrease the need for expensive future care because potentially costly medical problems will be detected at an early stage when they can be treated less expensively. Another argument predicts skyrocketing cost increases as the result of a growing volume of routine screening tests that identify conditions requiring follow-up or treatment. For example, it was recently reported that the yield of breast cancer detection through routine mammograms in women older than 70 years of age was so low that the risk of mammography outweighs the benefit of such testing. In such circumstances, re-thinking the national recommendations for screening should be considered.

The term quality, when applied to healthcare, not only refers to traditional measures of quality, such as the competence of practitioners and the accuracy of testing results, but has come to include quantity of healthcare—*how many procedures, medications, and so forth are covered by a benefits package*. Inequity in access, quality, and quantity of care has been a part of civilization since the beginning of care. Every nation, in accordance with its social conscience, must determine what amount and type of care the government (i.e., taxpayers) should and can provide and to which citizens it should be provided. Support for the traditional healthcare payment schema in the United States—as a benefit through one's employer—has eroded as a result of escalating cost, and unemployed segments of society are covered mostly by governmental programs. The problem of healthcare coverage relates not only to the provision of adequate healthcare to citizens without coverage but also to the continuing provision of meaningful healthcare to the many citizens who already have coverage.

In 1998, there was evidence of a backlash against insurers based on dissatisfaction of many enrollees who have been denied payment for services that they believe should have been provided. A "bill of rights" is being proposed for consumers that will require insurers to provide more options and services to their enrollees.

HEALTHCARE FINANCING

During the middle and latter parts of the 19th century, hospitals in the United States became the sites of healthcare delivery. However, healthcare or *sick care*—a more accurate term—was not always provided in hospitals. In the late 1800s, hospitals were dirty, unsanitary, disease-infested, deplorable institutions intended more to isolate the poor and the seriously diseased than to provide real care. Communicable diseases were the major cause of morbidity and mortality. Hospitals were places of last resort, and the ill were usually cared for in their homes by their families. Families of means employed professional nurses as private duty nurses to care for their ill family members at home.

This situation began to change with a key scientific breakthrough in healthcare in the 1860s and 1870s as a result of the work of Pasteur, Koch, and Lister (Starr, 1982, p. 135). The 1880s were a time of diffusion of knowledge based on applications of Pasteur's and Lister's work on the germ theory of disease and Koch's work in bacteriology. An understanding of sanitation and its relationship to disease emerged, and medical science developed. By 1890, the impact of Pasteur's, Koch's, and Lister's work was evident in practice. It was not until after hospital reform that sanitation and cleanliness became the hallmarks of hospitals. The influence of Florence Nightingale on nursing and the development of professional nursing in the United States promoted standards of care in hospitals. Hospitals became the desired environment for the care of the ill. Still, few hospitals existed, and the quality of care they provided varied greatly. The best hospitals were located in the larger cities and had schools of medicine and nursing. These hospitals became centers for the development of medical science, quality care, and healthcare technology.

Until relatively recently, healthcare was a scarce resource available to few. The widespread suffering that came with the Great Depression of the 1930s accentuated the need for basic healthcare for the masses. There was a public outcry for more hospitals to provide that care. The Depression came in the midst of a period of increased industrialization in which a growing number of people abandoned farming and moved to the city to work in industry. The social and family supports available during times of illness, the fiber of rural farm communities, were left behind. Independent, self-sufficient farmers were becoming employees who would now look to their employers to provide for their healthcare and other social needs. Some level of care, although not optimal, was provided through this system of corporate paternalism.

The Depression and its widespread unemployment exposed the vulnerability of these workers and led to the demand for federal government involvement in social programs. The inexorable and growing involvement of federal and state governments in the provision of basic necessities including healthcare began with the Social Security Act of 1935, enacted to assist people temporarily during times of unemployment. People now looked both to their employers and to the government to provide basic needs.

A historical review of the role of federal and state governments in healthcare provides a perspective from which to appreciate the escalation of healthcare costs over the past 40 to 50 years. With the social changes brought about by the increasing industrialization, people flocked to the cities to live and work. Communicable disease control became the focus of the federal, state, and local governments. Programs were developed for infants and children. Workers came to expect healthcare insurance from their employers. Blue Cross and healthcare insurance were born.

In response to the public demand for hospital care, the Hill-Burton legislation was enacted in late 1946. It provided federal funds for the construction of hospitals, increasing the number of hospitals exponentially. The huge Veterans' Administration hospital system was established to respond to the needs of the returning World War II veterans. After a period of national reflection about the role of government during the Eisenhower years, the Kennedy administration put forth a large-scale social and civil rights agenda with mixed success owing to lack of congressional support.

Following the assassination of President Kennedy, this mood changed, and the Great Society programs of the Johnson administration, including Medicare and Medicaid, created in 1965, were enacted with only mild resistance. Medicare increased access to healthcare for the elderly by providing basic coverage for hospitalization. In 1965, people aged 65 years and older accounted for only 10% of the population. Most coverage was for hospital-based care only; reimbursement for home-based or community-based care was excluded. Thus, Medicare promoted the use of more expensive hospital care. Medicare also created a new bureaucracy to administer the complex rules and regulations of this massive program. With Medicare, the federal government took charge of healthcare by mandating the components of coverage and setting reimbursements rates for providers. The fee schedule for the bulk of both Medicare and private services was now a matter of public record, giving government regulators the data with which to control reimbursement rates. The predominant governmental presence in healthcare was expanded through Medicaid, a state-implemented program that parallels the federally sponsored Medicare program and provides care for the poor. Medicaid includes many federally mandated state regulations that set standards for eligibility and reimbursement schedules.

Medicare/Medicaid programs did not cure all the ills of society. An increasing number of taxpayer-funded programs were enacted to provide entitlement programs for multiple purposes, such as welfare, housing, and education, as well as to provide expanded healthcare to special groups. The cost of financing these programs was sorely underestimated. Healthcare costs in particular were rising rapidly, consuming a larger percentage of the GDP each year. As concern over costs and access grew, the federal government mandated state health planning, requiring each state to develop an overall comprehensive health plan.

Among the services to be included in state health planning was the allocation of beds for people with *chronic illnesses*, a facet of medicine that was beginning to receive attention. With the advent of antibiotics and identification and control of communicable diseases, people were living longer and developing chronic illnesses. Chronic illnesses began to escalate rapidly during the 1950s. Expensive, high-tech diagnostic tools and therapeutic interventions became available at an increasing rate. A costly phenomenon was the need to replace expensive equipment every few years to take advantage of the latest improvements. Healthcare planners were considering the implications of increasingly expensive treatment options for chronic illness. The certificate of need was instituted; it was designed to address the growing problem of expensive services or resources duplicated in the same service area. A *certificate of need* required a provider to obtain approval by a government agency before purchasing expensive equipment, beginning construction, or initiating or expanding programs. This attempt to harness the escalating costs of healthcare met with spotty results because providers exerted political pressure and took advantage of loopholes to frustrate program objectives.

The next major approach to cost containment was introduced in the early 1980s: *diagnosis-related groups (DRGs)*. Under this system, each admission diagnosis and surgical procedure is assigned a designated length of stay. Based on this measure of reimbursement, the hospital receives a prospective payment for the hospitalization rather than a retrospective payment based on individualized lengths of stay judged appropriate by a provider. Because the hospital receives a flat rate for the hospitalization, it is to its advantage to be efficient in providing care within the same or in a shorter time frame than that allocated by DRGs. If the patient exceeds the length of stay, the hospital must absorb the additional cost. In essence, the DRG concept is a form of managed care adopted by the federal government for all Medicare admissions.

Since the beginning of the 1990s, the federal government has continued to have a major presence in healthcare as a provider, consumer, and regulator. As of October 1998, it has been mandated by the federal government that Medicare patients be managed by prospective payment. Control of healthcare costs continues to be a national priority.

MAJOR SOCIETAL FORCES AND TRENDS INFLUENCING HEALTHCARE

The United States healthcare system reflects a unique integration of demographic, cultural, social, technological, political, and economic trends. As these components change over time, the system responds to meet newly perceived needs and values and also to accommodate new technological and economic realities. These trends are interrelated and overlapping; they are briefly discussed in the following.

Demographics

Five demographic trends are influencing healthcare in the United States: aging population, baby boomers, decline in younger population, racial and ethnic diversity, and changes in the family unit (Pew Commission, 1991).

Aging Population

By the year 2025, the segment of the U.S. population 65 years and older will account for more than 18% of the population, a greater percentage than children (Bureau of Labor Statistics, 1998). The segments older than 75 years and older than 85 years comprise the fastest-growing segment of the population. These segments are growing not only because of the absolute increase in numbers, but also because a larger percentage of people is surviving to older ages. Survival to old age is a result of the following:

1. An improved economic condition for older Americans, together with improved access to affordable quality healthcare;
2. Strides made in the treatment of many diseases of old age, especially cancer and heart disease, which have significantly extended the life span; and
3. A new appreciation for the benefits of a healthy lifestyle, including diet, personal habits, exercise, and stress reduction.

Nevertheless, with aging eventually comes an increase in chronic illnesses such as coronary artery disease and chronic obstructive pulmonary disease and the need for use of healthcare resources.

Ethical decision making in elder care is likely to focus on the care provided for the growing number of chronically ill elderly who have a substantially decreased quality of life. It is well known that on average a person's use of healthcare resources is the highest during the last year of life and that these resources are often expended with the expectation of no gain in quality or quantity of life. The underdevelopment of less costly community-based care and support services to assist the elderly and their families in managing their needs in their homes has led to use of the high-cost alternative, hospital care. At the same time, the many elderly who are healthy, vibrant, active, and independent need help with continued health promotion and preventive measures to keep healthy. Extraordinary stress is about to be placed on the healthcare system and the country's economic resources by the "graying of America."

Baby Boomers

The nation's baby boomers, those 76 million born between the years 1946 and 1964, will drive the nation's healthcare consumption curve up steeply as they enter the age spectrum where the manifestations of chronic illness predominate. By the year 2000, the 45–54-year-old age group will number 36 million, and the onslaught of their increased healthcare needs should be well under way. The typically well-educated boomers have an appreciation for health promotion and disease prevention. Their needs will place great demands for services comparable to those of the elderly.

Decline in Birth Rate

One segment of the population is decreasing. A decline in birth rates results in a decline in the young and the accompanying needed healthcare services, at least for the short term. The long-term impact for society is that there will be fewer workers to support social services through payroll taxes at a time when there is predicted to be large numbers of elderly. What this trend means for needed changes in health economics has yet to be determined.

Racial and Ethnic Diversity

The infusion of multiple ethnic and culturally diverse groups into the United States is changing the process and structure of healthcare delivery in many communities as traditional Western healthcare values and methods are found strange and suspect by immigrants from non-American cultures. The primary migration from Western Europe in the first half of the century has been replaced by an influx of people from Asia, Africa, and Central and South America. Smaller, but growing numbers are coming from the Moslem countries of the Middle East and the countries of the former Soviet Union. A relatively small number come through the traditional and legal immigration channels. Many now come through special immigration programs. Hispanics constitute the ethnic group of most rapid growth in the United States, increasing from 8% to 11.3% by the year 2000.

Immigrant groups bring with them ethnic and cultural values that include belief-value systems about health and illness throughout the life cycle. The values and rituals of Western medicine are often held suspect by these groups and may be rejected in favor of their own ethnic and folk medicine. Culturally sensitive care is needed to meet healthcare needs of the society. Healthcare professionals must understand and respect cultural values and strive to develop and implement programs that are culturally sensitive as well as effective. This requires a blending of different, sometimes clashing, values concerning healthcare. Education of both health providers and health recipients, with the goal of easing the transition of combining native culture to U.S. culture to optimize health status, is indicated if mutual needs are to be addressed.

Immigration has been the real success story of the United States since the country's earliest days. All disciplines including healthcare disciplines are gradually becoming multicultural, thereby incorporating practitioners who will assist in the assimilation process.

Changes in the Family Unit

The traditional family unit of two married adults with children has changed over the last two decades and is no longer the dominant family structure. With a 50% divorce rate, many children are raised in a single-parent family unit. The psychological and economic impact of divorce often places children at greater risk for development of many social and psychological problems.

More than 50% of mothers are in the workforce. The choice between working outside the home and working solely in the home as a full-time homemaker/mother is difficult and is often predicated by financial need. This need may be imposed by single-parent status, a single lifestyle, or the need for two incomes for a family to make ends meet. Intermingled with financial need is the desire of some women to have careers. The reality of working mothers has a tremendous impact on family life.

Finally, Americans are very mobile; thus, both immediate and extended family members no longer live nearby. The social support and assistance in time of illness is often not available at a time when more illness management is centered in the home, with an expectation of family involvement in care.

Cultural, Social, and Political Trends

We are a multicultural society with multiculturalism evident in many nuclear and extended families. The acculturation of values and belief systems and their evolution over time and generations results in complex individuals. Last name or skin color does little to divulge these values to others. When persons seek healthcare, their cultural fiber is a driving force in the acceptance or rejection of healthcare. Culturally sensitive care is a competency for healthcare providers for the foreseeable future (see Chapters 11 and 12).

Social and political forces are fueling a demand for healthcare and a concomitant unrealistic expectation of wellness in the United States. In 1946, the World Health Organization defined health as "a state of complete physical, mental, and social well being, and not merely the absence of disease or infirmity." Most Americans believe in the right to healthcare for all. What is unresolved is to how much healthcare and to what kinds of healthcare each person is entitled. The more components included in the "basic package" for each person, the higher the cost of healthcare. High-tech, high-cost care, as has been already demonstrated in some notable studies, may be no more efficacious than less expensive traditional procedures or simple symptomatic management. Outcome studies to uncover best practice will assist health providers, payers, and consumers to make better decisions about healthcare practices.

Knowledge Explosion and Technological Trends

The knowledge explosion and extraordinary development and rate of growth of medical science and technology is unparalleled. One year's technological breakthrough often leads to the rapid development of the next year's generation of that technology often without thorough evaluation of efficacy or consideration of the appropriate uses and ethical implications of the technology. Cost of medical technology, especially new technology, is usually high, and such costs should be evaluated against the current gold standard of comparable technology to determine efficacy. However, we must not refuse to pursue new technologies aggressively because it is often the medical technological breakthroughs that set the new standards of care and provide effective treatment options to those who previously had none.

The truly revolutionary scientific breakthroughs with applications to medicine are coming predominantly from studies at the cellular and molecular level. Understanding pathophysiology at these levels, using new knowledge of gene mapping and replacement, and exploiting new sophisticated biotechnological techniques such as DNA recombination are leading to great advances in diagnosis, treatment, and disease management. One can expect work in molecular biology to be a significant healthcare factor in the next several decades.

Another significant trend in the technology of surgery uses robotics and the miniaturization of surgical instruments, together with the development of the means of visualizing microscopic structures within the body. Minimally invasive surgeries based on these developments are showing significant promise for improving outcomes while reducing recovery time and overall cost of procedures.

Sophisticated information and communications technologies are at the heart of the new systems of managing care (see Chapter 10). Medical informatics and expert systems provide rapid access to the most current information available for diagnostic and clinical reasoning and decision making. This includes access to research in progress and expert commentary as well as personal networking. Computers have allowed health providers to monitor patients, review and integrate large volumes of data, and maintain medical records electronically. Telemedicine, which is still in its early stages of development and integration and is used for distant assessment, monitoring, and treatment of patients, is increasing access to care in remote areas both nationally and internationally. These technologies are changing how health professionals practice and manage patients. It also creates new issues about confidentiality, integrity, and security of databases, which are increasingly threatened as data systems become more and more interlinked and vulnerable.

Summary

A number of societal trends, many of which are interrelated, have been discussed within the context of their impact on healthcare. The demands imposed on the U.S. healthcare system include the need not only for providing more healthcare but also for redesigning healthcare to better meet the needs of diverse peoples with changing needs.

The National Agenda for a Healthy Nation

A number of initiatives have been undertaken by governmental, private and professional organizations in an attempt to influence the future direction of healthcare for the nation. Three of the more ambitious initiatives are *Healthy People 2000,* Patient Outcomes Research Teams (PORTs), and Prevention Guidelines.

HEALTHY PEOPLE 2000 TO HEALTHY PEOPLE 2010

The quintessential document outlining a comprehensive plan for the healthcare of the nation is *Healthy People 2000* (1990), an unprecedented cooperative effort bringing together a wide spectrum of interests including government and business, voluntary and professional organizations, and private individuals. The report urges the following broad public health goals: (1) increase the span of healthy life for Americans; (2) reduce health disparities among Americans; and (3) achieve access to preventive services for all Americans. To meet these goals by the year 2000, 319 specific objectives were identified and organized around 22 priority areas. The national objectives were organized under the three broad categories of health promotion, health protection, and preventive services (p. 6). An additional priority, surveillance and data systems, addresses the need for systematic collection, analysis, interpretation, dissemination, and use of health data to understand the health status of the nation and to plan effective prevention programs (p. 79). The challenge of *Healthy People 2000* is:

> to use the combined strength of scientific knowledge, professional skill, individual commitment, community support, and political will to enable people to achieve their potential to live full, active lives. It means preventing premature death and preventing disability, preserving a physical environment that supports human life, cultivating family and community support, enhancing each individual's inherent abilities to respond and to act, and assuring that all Americans achieve and maintain a maximum level of functioning. (p. 6)

Forty-seven states, the District of Columbia, and Guam have developed their own Healthy People plans. Most states followed national objectives, but virtually all have adapted them to their specific needs.

Many reports are being generated about achievement of goals outlined in *Healthy People 2000;* there is still much work to be done. Development of *Healthy People 2010* is underway and will be published in January 2000. It will address emerging issues such as changing demographics, advances in preventive therapies, and new technologies (http://web.health. gov/healthypeople).

FROM PATIENT OUTCOMES RESEARCH TEAMS TO AN EVIDENCE-BASED PRACTICE PROGRAM

The PORT program funds multidisciplinary researchers to examine the cost-benefit relationship of clinical practices based on measurable improvements in patients' health. Funded by the Agency for Health Care Policy and Research (AHCPR), the program's ultimate goal was to disseminate the research findings to the clinical community in the form of clinical practice guidelines as a means of establishing effective standards of care. Examples of topics addressed by PORT studies are type II diabetes, management of cancer pain, and unstable angina. It was envisioned that the clinical practice guidelines would be widely disseminated to health professionals and become the standards of care for patient management. In reality, broad disseminating of a guideline does not ensure its implementation.

As a result, the clinical practice guideline program has been discontinued, and AHCPR will refocus on three activities (AHCPR, 1997a). The agency will:

1. Collect and analyze existing evidence about proven practices through the new Evidence-Based Practice Centers (EPCs). Twelve EPCs in the United States and Canada have been funded and assigned a medical topic to review the relevant scientific literature and to conduct additional analyses when needed. Their findings will be published as "evidence reports" or technology assessments.
2. Cosponsor an internet-based national guideline clearinghouse to provide broad access to information and recommendations on major guidelines as well as comparison of different guidelines on the same topic.
3. Fund new research that addresses the process of implementing guidelines into practice.

AHCPR has created the Center for Practice and Technology Assessment (CPTA) to oversee the new Evidence-based Practice Program along with the Office of the Forum for Quality and Effectiveness in Health Care (AHCPR, 1997b).

PREVENTION GUIDELINES

The *Clinician's Handbook of Preventive Services: Put Prevention into Practice* (ANA, 1994) and the second edition of *Guide to Clinical Preventive Services* (US Preventive Services Task Force, 1996) have become the gold standards for preventive services in the United States.

Preventive care is a central component within the context of primary care. The term primary care was introduced to the United States in the 1960s from Europe at a time of alarming decline of family physicians in the United States (Starfield, 1994). Starfield (1994) points out that the original definition of primary care specified four main components: the provision of first-contact care; person-focused care over time, comprehensive care, and co-ordinated care. In the 1990s, this definition of primary care was grossly inadequate. The Institute of Medicine (IOM) redefined primary care as "the provision of integrated, accessible healthcare services by clinicians who are accountable for addressing a large majority of personal healthcare needs, developing a sustained partnership with patients and practicing in the context of family and community" (Donaldson, 1996).

SUMMARY

Three key initiatives of the agenda for a healthy nation have been discussed. There is broad consensus regarding the priority of comprehensive preventive care for the nation, the need to set measurable objectives for care, and the need to disseminate clinical guidelines for the most cost effective and efficacious interventions. Building on this foundation, other broad consensus projects are sure to follow as the healthcare needs of all Americans are addressed within a cost-efficient and quality-outcome–oriented framework. Central to the refocusing of healthcare to a primary care model is the shifting of emphasis from solo clinician practice to integrated delivery systems composed of teams of clinicians working collaboratively to meet healthcare needs.

The United States Healthcare System: A Transformation in Progress

Unquestionably, the United States healthcare system is undergoing fundamental changes in structure and processes through restructuring, re-engineering, and redesigning of healthcare for the 21st century. *Restructuring* means rebuilding, reorganizing, reconfiguring, reconstructing, or changing the *structure* of an organization or system; in healthcare, restructuring refers to the organizational restructuring and is usually diagrammatically recorded on the organization chart. *Reengineering* is the fundamental rethinking and radical redesigning of *processes* to achieve dramatic improvements in critical measures of performance such as cost, quality, service, and speed (Hammer & Champy, 1993, p. 32); in healthcare, it means rethinking all of the processes involved in providing care. *Redesigning* is a term focusing on the revision in appearance, function, or content of *what people in an organization do;* in healthcare, it means redesigning who does what in providing care and services to patients. Redesigning of practice has utmost impact on nurses and nursing practice.

RESTRUCTURING OF HEALTHCARE

Major changes occurring in the restructuring of healthcare facilities have them attempting to respond to the rapidly developing capitated, managed care integrated delivery systems (IDS). An IDS combines health providers, healthcare facilities, and a health plan into one entity that assumes clinical and fiscal responsibility and accountability for providing the full spectrum of services for the enrolled population (Coddington, Moore, & Fischer, 1995; Sovie, 1995). When patients need treatment, care is provided in the least-expensive environment where the greatest value can be obtained (Sovie, 1995). Consequently, the focal point of care delivery is rapidly shifting from hospitals to community-based settings (Harrison, 1997). Hospitals, once the center of healthcare, are now a component of the continuum of care within the IDS. As a result, some hospitals have closed while others have merged or been bought by other healthcare organizations or huge health networks or systems.

Many more structures or sites of care delivery have emerged. Added to the traditional acute care hospital offering tertiary and quaternary care are an array of postacute settings such as transitional hospitals, subacute units, rehabilitation, skilled nursing care, levels of assisted living, adult day care, and home care. Long-term care facilities and nursing homes continue to provide chronic long-term care. There are many new postacute options available. Even traditional healthcare settings have been restructured to deliver care in new ways.

REENGINEERING OF HEALTHCARE

Reengineering focuses on the processes involved in providing care and services to patients/clients and their families. According to Hammer and Champy (1993), reengineering begins with asking "why do we do what we do? and why do we do it in the way we do?" (p. 32). The answer may be, "That's the way we have always done it here, or that's our policy." Development of standards of care or care maps; development of policies for visiting hours, admission, discharges, and transfers; and standards for teaching patients and families are examples of processes that can be conducted in many ways, some more efficient and with better outcomes than others.

Managed care affects the delivery of healthcare in two ways: it changes the payment structure from fee-for-service to capitation, and it switches emphasis from the care of individuals to the management of populations (Barton & Russin, 1997). Managed care is a loose term that encompasses both integrated systems such as health maintenance organizations and more decentralized arrangements such as preferred provider organizations (Yordy, 1997). Decentralization, begun in the 1980s, continues, and the business concepts of a matrix structure and product lines have been added to better delineate responsibility and accountability for managers.

The delivery of patient-centered, coordinated quality care, regardless of setting, is the goal of healthcare in a managed care environment. Managed care has created and redefined terms such as continuum of care, integrated delivery systems, partnerships, interdisciplinary care, collaborative care, population-based care, outcomes-oriented care, point-of-care, continuum-based care, and seamless healthcare, which address a fundamental rethinking of the processes for healthcare delivery (Ebeling & Groath, 1998).

Disease management, first introduced in 1991, is a comprehensive, integrated approach to care and reimbursement based on a disease's natural course (Zitter, 1997). The goal of disease management is to address the illness or condition with maximum effectiveness and efficiency regardless of treatment settings(s) or typical reimbursement patterns. This approach emphasizes management of a disease in a manner that focuses both clinical and non-clinical interventions when and where they are most likely to have the greatest positive impact. Ideally, disease management prevents exacerbation of a disease and the use of expensive resources, making prevention and proactive case management two important areas of emphasis in most disease management programs (Zitter, 1997, p. 6). Short-term and long-term patient outcomes, the cost of care throughout the course of the illness, and disease prevention and health promotion strategies are integral parts of patient management. Currently, there are some well-developed disease management programs in place for a few conditions including asthma and diabetes mellitus. With the prominence of chronic illness in healthcare today and into the future, many other chronic and disabling conditions are and will be in need of disease management programs.

REDESIGNING HEALTHCARE

Redesign is people-oriented and redefines who does what. The optimum staff mix for a given setting has been debated for many years, regardless whether the setting is institutional or community-based. From the nursing perspective, a call for an all–registered nurse (RN) staff in the 1980s was intermingled with the optimistic goal of requiring a baccalaureate nursing degree for all nursing staff. However, cost-conscious eyes scrutinizing the operating budget realized that the largest cost center is nurses' salaries. Many researchers and healthcare organizations have conducted job analyses and reexamined what types of activities are executed by the RN staff and other categories of care providers, including time spent performing each activity. Transporting some patients and answering the telephone are examples of lower level skills, which are sometimes assigned to professional staff, that could be assumed safely by non-licensed persons with supervision and at substantial cost savings. A ratio of 50:50 licensed to nonlicensed staff is not uncommon in organizations that had previously had a much higher licensed to nonlicensed ratio. Therefore, widespread changes in staff mix and redesign of roles and responsibilities have occurred and will continue to occur. In addition to the staff-mix solution came the idea for a "cross-trained" staff, i.e., nurses who have multi-skills and can move from one setting to another as needs emerge. The challenge related to cross-training is maintaining competency if skills are not used often enough to sustain a competent level.

Embedded within the redesign process is the unresolved issue of what is the appropriate differential practice for nurses prepared at the associate, baccalaureate, and graduate levels. Models of differentiated professional practice based on educational preparation have been proposed (Newman, 1990; Foss & Koener, 1997), but there has been limited success in integrating differentiated roles into nursing practice. Moreover, both nurses with master's degrees and those with doctorates have been lumped together for purposes of describing nurses with graduate education as "advanced practice nurses." Determining the role of the master's-prepared and the doctorally prepared nurses in healthcare also needs attention so that the full potential and contribution of these well-prepared nurses is realized.

Physicians are also feeling the changes of redesign imposed on their practice in a managed care, capitated environment. Many physicians recognize that the practice of medicine, as they have known it, is gone forever. Solo practice is much less common, and collaborative interdisciplinary models necessary to provide care along the continuum are increasing. In the redistribution of who does what, advanced practice nurses are assuming responsibility and accountability for care that was once the domain of the physician. Physicians, in turn, are taking on new responsibilities particularly if they are in high-tech practice environments. These transitions and renegotiations of boundaries of practice within collaborative models need to develop with care and sensitivity so that the roles are truly complementary and collaborative and not adversarial. For a win-win outcome for APNs, physicians, other health providers, and patients, everyone must work together. The key word for the 21st century is collaboration. Collaboration requires trust, respect, excellent communications skills, and a mutual commitment to a common goal (Seehafer, 1998; Lindeke & Block, 1998).

A result of healthcare redesign is more midlevel providers. Although probably not the term that APNs would choose, midlevel provider nevertheless is a broad classification, common in the literature, that includes physicians' assistants and APNs, principally NPs and some CNSs. As redesign goes forward, opportunities for APNs are challenging, numerous, and diverse. Subsequent chapters address advanced practice nursing issues in detail and provide exemplars of exciting innovative practice.

HEALTHCARE SYSTEM AT THE NEW MILLENNIUM

The Pew Commission (1995, p. I) reports that at the end of this century, the American healthcare system will have the following characteristics:

- More managed care with better integration of services and financing
- More accountable to those who purchase and use health services
- More aware of and responsive to the needs of enrolled populations
- More able to use fewer resources more effectively
- More innovative and diverse in how it provides for health
- More inclusive in how it defines health
- Less focused on treatment and more concerned with education, prevention, and care management
- More oriented to improving the health of the entire population
- More reliant on outcomes data and evidence

The 21st Century: A Vision of Advanced Practice Nursing

Predicting the future of advance practice nursing is perhaps a presumptuous exercise. On the other hand, we would be remiss not to look ahead with concern and hope at the possibilities and probabilities for the future. Unless APNs assume the risk of interpreting the present and anticipating the effects on healthcare and professional practice in the future, we will deprive ourselves of the possibility of influencing and shaping our own destiny as APNs. More importantly, we relinquish our professional responsibility and accountability for active involvement in restructuring and redesigning quality healthcare for all Americans. Trends only point a direction for a probable course given current circumstances. However, a future course is also amenable to new influences and therefore can, and most likely will, be altered. As we strive to achieve new goals and excellence in practice, change is inevitable. Pursuit of excellence toward creating something better, especially in these times of tight budgets, requires passion, courage, fortitude, imagination, creativity, commitment, visionary thinking, tireless energy, and leadership. APNs must exercise their growing power to deliberately choose and create their collective futures.

THE PROFESSION, PRACTICE, EDUCATION, AND RESEARCH

The professional triad of practice–education–research provides an organizational framework for the following discussion that explores current forces likely to affect the future development of advanced practice nursing. Predictions are made on the courses along which practice, education, and research for advanced practice nursing are likely to proceed, based mainly on a compilation of APNs' observations, experiences, and thoughts regarding key issues, trends, and projections. No particular order of priority is implied, nor is there an attempt to be all-inclusive. In addition, although certain predictions are listed in one category (e.g., practice), there will often be implications of that prediction for the other categories (e.g., education and research). The reader is invited to add, delete, and modify the list according to his or her perspective and ability to read tea leaves or interpret Bayesian theory.

The Nursing Profession

Many concerns and issues in nursing cut across all levels of professional nursing and must be addressed by the entire profession if nursing is to mature in the next millennium. The following are predictions about priorities for the profession of nursing, all of which will have a major impact on APNs.

Understand That the Future of Professional Nursing Lies in the Hands of APNs

Leadership is an earmark of APNs, and they are accountable and responsible for advanced practice nursing. More APNs will become politically active in lobbying for issues related to the healthcare needs of people, the profession of nursing, and barriers to practice for APNs. This activism will foster regulatory changes to remove barriers for APNs on the state and national levels.

Lobby for Regulatory Changes for APNs

Revamping of laws and regulations for licensure and certification is needed to protect the public and clarify nomenclature and expectations of nurses. The Pew Commission (Finocchio, Dower, McMahon, et al., 1995) recommends that states should use standardized and understandable language for health professions' regulation and should standardize entry into practice and continued practice, based on demonstrated initial and continuing competence. States should allow all professionals to provide services to the full extent of their current knowledge, training, experience, and skills. Unwieldy state laws are major barriers to advanced practice nursing in many states. Without change, APNs will not be able to practice to the full extent of their capabilities.

Consolidate the Professional Nomenclature So That There Is a Single Title for Each Level of Nursing Preparation

For the good of the profession and the consumer it is time for nursing to stop the confusion and clear up titling nomenclature. Work must be undertaken at the local, state, and national level for these changes to occur (Finocchio et al., 1995, p. vi).

Promote Interdisciplinary Collaboration to Socialize APNs

Interdisciplinary practice, education, and research will be the norm for the future. New ways must be found to work together collaboratively across disciplines and settings. New organizational partnerships are needed to foster interdisciplinary activities. Maintaining professional integrity while in the midst of interdisciplinary collaboration will take thought and skill (Lindeke & Block, 1998).

Recognize the Multiple Education Entry Points to the Professional Practice of Nursing Through Associate, Baccalaureate, and Masters Programs; Each Is Different, and Each Has a Contribution to Make to Nursing

We must address differential practice and clarify for the profession and the consumer what each level of nursing education offers. In addition, we must support appropriate utilization of each level to optimize the contribution of each level to society (Finocchio, Dower, McMahon et al., 1995, p. vi).

Accept Job Insecurity as Part of Life in a Rapidly Changing Society

The turbulence of the marketplace will affect all health professions, not only nursing. Downsizing of hospitals will eliminate nursing jobs, but there will be new opportunities in ambulatory and community-based care. Nurses will need to retool to be competitive (Hadley, 1997).

Sustain a Commitment to Lifelong Professional Learning

Commitment to ongoing learning is an earmark of any profession. Nurses must accept this commitment to stay current and to provide the best care possible to society (Hadley, 1997).

Practice

The redesign and reengineering of the healthcare delivery system are changing how APNs practice. The managed care environment, with all of the underpinnings of healthcare financing and health effectiveness, influences where and how we practice. Barriers to practice will continue to be bridged, and APNs will be able to practice to a fuller extent of their competencies. The following are predictions about practice for APNs.

Practice in a Cost Containment Environment Is Here to Stay

Economic constraints and the demand for cost-effective care are the most powerful factors influencing healthcare and advanced practice nursing. "We have no more money, now we must think." This remark, made by a British cabinet minister whose budget had been severely cut, reminds us that cost containment has become an integral and permanent part of practice for all healthcare professionals, and this forces us to think more creatively and behave differently. Economic considerations are forcing APNs to factor cost into every decision made about patients and patient care. A practitioner's attention to cost containment has become an important outcome measure in evaluating effectiveness.

Managed Care Environments Are Here to Stay and Are Expanding; Most Care Will Be Provided Through Integrated Delivery Systems

The healthcare market continues to become more saturated nationwide. Because most of healthcare will be provided through large managed care organizations, most APNs will work in managed care environments. Mega health networks formed from the buyouts of hospitals, primary care practices, extended care facilities, home care services, and multiple other components of the continuum of care profit by managing subscribers in cost-effective ways. The future will undoubtedly see a few giants emerging as the major providers of healthcare in the nation. As managed care has emerged so has the concept of "continuum-based care" where seamless care is provided—that is, care without fragmentation or duplication of services.

The Emphasis and Shift to Primary Care Will Continue

Health promotion, disease prevention, and care management have become integral parts of all healthcare. Chapter 7 discusses the important renaissance and redefinition of primary care. The shift from sickness care to wellness care is proceeding apace with the wellness concept incorporated into all care delivery settings. There will be increased emphasis on risk assessment and risk modification through healthy lifestyles education directed at keeping people in optimum health and managing chronic illness.

Most APNs will be primary care providers in collaborative practices; a few will choose independent, solo practice. Other APNs will provide care for special populations such as patients who have experienced a stroke or heart failure. Regardless of the focus of one's practice, all care will include the general health promotion and disease prevention components of primary care.

Disease Management Programs for Many Chronic Illnesses Will Become Models for Continuum-based Care

Disease management programs like those for asthma and diabetes will be developed for many other chronic illnesses. Chronic problems have become the modern healthcare epidemic, and this trend will get much stronger as the population ages and life span increases. With the merging of hospital-based care and community-based care into the all-inclusive patient-centered, continuum-based care for chronic health problems, health promotion and disease prevention will become an integral part of all care. Disease management is the perfect match for the holistic approach and patient/family–centered care characteristic of nursing. Models of care such as the trajectory of illness model proposed by Corbin and Strauss (1988) will gain prominence. **APNs will assume major leadership in the chronic illness, disease management niche of healthcare delivery.**

Meeting the Demands of Clients for Increased Patient Satisfaction

Client/patient satisfaction is at the heart of healthcare delivery. Customer satisfaction is a major determinant of success in the new competitive healthcare world. Based on consumer feedback, care and services are being restructured and redesigned to provide for customer convenience and comfort. APNs will continue to articulate the needs of patients and their families and assume a greater client advocacy role. Their input will be sought and integrated into the reengineering of healthcare to meet patient/client needs and demands more effectively.

Environments for Health and Illness Care Are Shifting From Hospital-based to Community-based Care

The Pew Commission (1995) estimates the closure of as many as half of the nation's hospitals and loss of perhaps 60% of hospital beds. Hospitals are becoming giant intensive care centers with more beds being converted to critical care beds nationally. Hospitalizations will continue to be "short stays." Once physiologically stabilized, patients will be discharged to less expensive settings of ambulatory, community-based, or home care. Rapid transitions in care will increase the risk of fragmentation of care so that increased attention will be needed to provide seamless care.

Home is where all healthcare and most of illness care will be take place as hospital-based care inevitably shifts to community-based care. Only the most sophisticated, complex, science-driven, high-technology, and experimental care will be provided in the hospital environment. Increasingly complex and technologically driven treatments will be provided in the home and community. New models of transitional, community-based, and home care will evolve to incorporate high-tech care.

The opportunities for APNs are enormous. Owing to hospital closures, 200,000 to 300,000 nurses will lose jobs; some will be APNs. The massive expansion of primary care into ambulatory care, community, and home settings will require a large increase in the number of nurses needed with the skills and competencies of generalists. The need for specialized, critical care ANPs will continue. There is a current national shortage of CNSs and NPs prepared for critical care practice. APNs employed in hospitals will assume more responsibilities requiring the use of advanced clinical reasoning skills, high-tech equipment, and complex protocols. They will require not only an increased understanding of the pathophysiology but also advanced knowledge in biological and physical sciences, instrumentation, and computer technology. The rapid and phenomenal developments in medical science and technology will require ongoing training and education to maintain competency. APNs should be at the forefront in developing new models of practice in hospital, ambulatory, community, and home care.

Population-based Care Is Emerging As a Fundamental Approach to Healthcare

Use of an epidemiological approach to a population to identify healthcare needs will become common. A population may be defined by such characteristics as age, socioeconomic status, culture/ethnicity, gender, risk factors, or illness. When the unique characteristics of a targeted population are elucidated by epidemiological methods, the healthcare needs of that population can be matched with a quality, cost-effective program of care. Such programs of care will be based on evidence-based practice and best practice. Programs for disease management of illnesses such as those established for asthma, coronary artery disease, and diabetes mellitus will develop and provide comprehensive lifelong population-centered care for major health problems. Population-centered care programs will be established for other chronic conditions, and together with health promotion and disease prevention, such programs will improve management of these illnesses. Programs for geriatric populations are emerging as important areas of care. Perhaps there is no more obvious area where increased community based health services are needed than populations in rural communities. APNs will develop and implement many of these programs. They will provide population-based care in interdisciplinary teams a focusing on a variety of populations and settings.

Outcome-oriented Care Will Undergo Profound Growth

An outcome is the consequence of an intervention or that which "comes out" of the intervention. The payer for healthcare services demands to know what the expected outcome of an intervention will be; in other words, what is being purchased? The search for outcome-oriented care will rely on evidence-based practice and best practice to provide information on expected outcomes. The need for outcome data will motivate all practitioners to develop outcomes management programs to collect, analyze, and disseminate data for the purpose of demonstrating efficacy and cost-effectiveness of care. These data will be used by the organization to determine continued funding of programs and positions. All healthcare professionals including APNs will practice in environments of new organizational and patient accountability through outcome-based practice.

Increased Development and Utilization of Practice Guidelines

Standardization of practice through guidelines, such as clinical pathways, algorithms, clinical practice guidelines, and disease-specific standards, will continue to grow. Most will be based on evidence-based practice and best practice recommendations. The Internet and other technologically driven resources will make access to this information easy. All practitioners will be held accountable to provide the best practice possible as an expected standard of care.

Interdisciplinary, Collaborative Models of Practice Will Be the Rule

Interdisciplinary, collaborative models are the cornerstone for efficient, cost-effective, high quality, seamless care. By bringing together a multidisciplinary team to work collaboratively, outcomes are optimized for the patient across continuum-based care. APNs will continue to work in interdisciplinary collaborative models in hospitals, ambulatory care, and community-based facilities, and will take on new responsibilities as the boundaries of practice are expanded.

Informatics, Computers, and Information Networks Will Erase Boundaries Created by Distances and Inaccessibility to Physical Facilities

Excellent interpersonal and verbal communications skills have always been as essential for APNs as they have for other health providers. In the 21st century, however, computer literacy will also be an absolute requirement. The application of electronic technology to practice will become pervasive as it enormously expands our access to informatics and people. For example, the very portable notebook computers will allow healthcare providers to enter standard format data from histories, physical exams, and progress notes directly into a central databank from the point of care. Computer technology also provides rapid access to the latest scientific articles and clinical texts through on-line literature searches. Computers, video cameras, remote electronic sensors, and robotic instruments provide means for healthcare providers to examine and treat patients hundreds of miles away. Communications highways and computer networks bridge urban with rural settings, generalists with specialists, national centers with international centers, and individuals with the medical libraries and special networks of the world. The bad news is that knowledge is exploding at an almost indigestible rate. The good news is that it is instantly available to the computer-literate person. As computer technology becomes more user-friendly all the time, APNs will continue to integrate computer technology and informatics into practice.

Emphasis on the Ethical Component of Care Will Continue to Increase
Technology has taken medical care so far that "a natural death," within the context of healthcare, has become a complicated and difficult event, as have decisions related to death, allocation of transplant organs, and the viability of genetically flawed fetuses. These and other equally value-ladened ethical conundrums can only become more complex as technology proceeds to scale new heights. With more medical and technological breakthroughs on the horizons, there will be a greater emphasis on integrating ethical decision making. APNs have understood the ethical component of care and have been advocates for patients' and families' wishes. In the future, APNs will need to continue to apply frameworks for ethical decision making to new technology and medical therapies and assist other health professionals in including this dimension of care within interdisciplinary practice.

Education
As is apparent from the following chapters in this book, APNs face the 21st century on a threshold of opportunity and change seldom experienced in a profession. Doors are opening, taboos are crumbling, and administrators are saying, "OK, you asked for it; let's see what you can do." To meet this challenge, APNs must be educationally prepared in a new way. New knowledge and clinical skills will indeed be required to assume the evolving advanced practice roles in primary care, tertiary care, and all areas between these anchors on the continuum of care. At a deeper level, however, curricula and the educational process of preparing APNs itself will need to be revamped to provide better methods of developing the critical thinking skills that will be so important in performing at new levels of responsibility and accountability. With this in mind, the following are predictions about formal academic programs and continuing education programs for APNs.

Major Curricular Changes Are Necessary to Prepare APNs
Most graduate programs are preparing APN students well for practice. However, there are several areas that should be strengthened to meet the challenges of practice. These areas include the biological sciences, computer literacy and informatics for evidence-based practice, clinical reasoning, health policy and financial management, outcomes management, and interdisciplinary practice.

Biological Science APNs must improve their knowledge of the biological sciences (anatomy, physiology, pathophysiology, immunology, genetics, and chemistry) to understand disease processes and therapeutic actions of pharmacological and nonpharmacological interventions. This knowledge also serves as a common ground for communicating effectively with physicians and other interdisciplinary team members regarding patient management. No one questions the need for the biological sciences. What is debated is how much science should be in the curriculum to maintain a reasonable credit structure. The strengthening in the biological sciences must not come at the expense of deemphasizing the knowledge base in the behavioral sciences. Holistic care, a hallmark of nursing, is the patient's best hope for an optimum outcome and can only be provided by the blending that results from an integration of both the biological and behavioral aspects of care.

Computer Literacy   As discussed previously, APNs require computer literacy and comfort with computer applications to clinical practice monitoring and data processing. The use of informatics is key to providing evidence-based care and best practice. The overall curriculum must be planned and implemented to ensure graduates well-developed skills and comfort with informatics and computers.

Critical Thinking   Developing skills in critical thinking and clinical reasoning is imperative for practice. These skills are best developed by using interactive teaching methods such as problem-based learning and computer-assisted interactive learning. Case presentations, seminars, and interaction with standardized patients are strategies to assist students learning in the classroom. Clinical experience with experienced preceptors, clinical logs, clinical rounds, and case analysis develop critical thinking and clinical reasoning skills in the practice setting.

Health Policy and Health Economics   Health policy and financial management form the context of healthcare delivery, and healthcare professionals who ignore these aspects will do so at their own peril. APNs will be expected to integrate this knowledge in planning and implementing programs and administering care. As healthcare policy evolves, APNs must be prepared to participate in ethical decision making that preserves patient quality of life and dignity.

Managing Chronic Illness   Management of chronic illness, vulnerable populations, and culturally sensitive care must all be included in curricula. In addition, a focus on *health* management across the life span, rather than on episodic illness or individual disease management, is needed that integrates risk modification, health promotion, and disease prevention into the curriculum.

Outcomes Measures   All APNs must understand outcomes measurement and outcomes management as a means of demonstrating effectiveness and accountability for practice. This content must be included in the curriculum with applications to practice.

Interdisciplinary Practice   Interdisciplinary care teams are becoming the norm in practice, and APNs must understand interdisciplinary teams and collaboration. In addition to didactic content, students will learn best through interdisciplinary education where students from different disciplines interact and learn together.

Evaluation   Evaluation of self, others, programs, facilities, and models is a part of practice and the pursuit of quality. APNs must be well-educated in the evaluation process and applications of evaluation.

Educational Pathways for APNs in Clinical Practice Tracts and for APNs in Management Tracts Will Become More Complementary

The nurse manager role has been de-emphasized in many schools in the past 10 years, leading to limited graduate education options for nurses. The nurse manager role must be recognized as specialty graduate nursing practice, and more programs directed at preparing nurse managers must become available to interested nurses. The nurse manager role requires advanced skills oriented toward fiscal, budgetary, personnel, and program management. More than ever before, the APN in a direct clinical practice tract needs knowledge of the business side of practice to be effective; however, the depth and scope of knowledge, as compared to the nurse manager, is different. The trilevel curriculum design of core graduate nursing, core advanced practice, and core specialty practice must have sufficient depth and breath for students to develop the advanced practice entry-level skills to be competitive. In addition, educators must design courses in which nurse manager students and direct patient care provider nursing students can learn and interact together in a way to support socialization and *intradisciplinary* practice models.

New Specialized APN Graduate Programs Will Be Offered

As new roles develop for APNs, new academic programs will be developed to prepare APNs to meet these needs. Currently, tertiary nurse practitioner and critical care nurse practitioner programs are being developed at major centers to meet shortages of house officers and attending physicians to staff ICUs and intermediate units. This trend will become stronger as more specialty residents have difficulty finding suitable openings after their residencies. Other focused APN programs will be developed as well. APN programs with foci on home health management and rural care will be the next big areas of demand for preparation.

There Will Be More Combined Education of APNs, Physician Assistants, and Medical Students

Courses open to APNs, physician assistants, and medical students will become more common. Teaching and clinical supervision will increase interdisciplinary involvement of educators and clinicians from all of these fields. This is currently occurring in some institutions successfully and is proving to be a cost-effective approach to teaching of many basic courses needed by all health providers. Additional benefits derive from the introduction of different health providers to each others' roles and from the resulting socialization that will facilitate future interdisciplinary collaborative practice.

More Doctorally Prepared Nurses Will Provide Direct Patient Care as APNs

More APNs who have been prepared as CNSs will obtain doctorates and assume the role of the academic clinician. Research programs emerging from their clinical practice will result in important findings applicable to direct patient care.

Distance Learning Will Grow to Assist APNs Become Lifelong Learners

The half-life of knowledge is already quite short and will continue to grow shorter in the future. APNs will need to be lifelong learners through continuing education programs. New cost-effective methods of teaching and learning through interactive technologies will become accessible to APNs in their homes and workplaces, utilizing personal computers, interactive teleconferences and other forms not yet contemplated. Continuing education will no longer be a "once-in-a-while" requirement, but a constant part of professional practice. Educators, as well as practitioners, need to prepare for this onslaught by completely redesigning and restructuring continuing education to meet the needs of these lifelong learners.

Research

What is best practice for a given population of patients? What factors influence patients' short-term and long-term outcomes in a variety of health problems? What are nurse-sensitive indicators of quality care? Such questions are vital to justifying the future of nursing and cannot be answered without well-designed and well-conducted research. Thus, the future of APNs is linked to the development and testing of practice patterns to demonstrate efficacy and effectiveness of nursing practice and gain new knowledge through research. The body of knowledge called *nursing science* and the growth and development of professional nursing depends on all types of research undertaken by nurses. There are also many one-time nursing studies that need to be replicated because of small sample size, design flaws, or limited generalizability. Research that is inaccessible or that is never widely applied to practice is useless. To become savvy consumers of research, nurses must be educated in the skills necessary for the critique, interpretation, and application of research findings. The following describes key trends and predications for the 21st century for nursing research.

More Researchers Will Be Applying for a Relatively Small Pool of Funds That Is Not Expected to Increase Significantly

The mission of the National Institute for Nursing Research (NINR) supports research by nurses. Unless nurses have very promising pilot studies in priority areas of research, they will not be competitive for funding of studies through the National Institutes of Health. However, more nurses will be able to conduct pilot studies through small grants from a variety of sources. It will be important for nurses to carefully explore possible funding sources through their professional organizations and private foundations. Use of computer networks to assist researchers will be another avenue for identifying potential funds.

First Research Priority: Focus on Uncovering Best Practice Through Outcome Studies Designed to Demonstrate Cost-effective Care

There is, and will continue to be, a critical need to conduct research that focuses on measurable and improved outcomes for patients that also demonstrates cost-effectiveness. Research will need to be conducted to demonstrate the efficacy of the many nursing practices that remain noninvestigated. Comparison studies will also be needed to demonstrate which of several interventions proven to be efficacious for a particular condition is the most cost-effective. Because APNs who provide direct patient care will know which important research questions need to be studied and because they will be positioned to obtain the necessary data, they will assume major roles in clinical research studies.

Second Research Priority: Gender and Ethnic Differences in Response to Various Health Problems and Cultural Sensitive Care to Better Meet the Healthcare Needs of Diverse Populations

Cultural diversity and ethnicity are responsible for differences in acceptance and response to interventions. Very little is known about these differences at a time when the United States is experiencing an unusual increase in immigrants from diverse cultural and ethnic backgrounds. As the U.S. population becomes more culturally and ethnically diverse, this area of research becomes a priority. In addition to cultural and ethnic differences, there is also a great need to understand gender differences in response to illness and interventions.

Third Research Priority: Focus on Vulnerable Populations—Those with Chronic Illnesses, Abuse Victims, the Homeless, and the Elderly—While Integrating Wellness Management Into Continuum-based Care

Chronic illness is the epidemic of the latter 20th century and will continue to be an epidemic into the 21st century, especially with the increasing number of elderly. According to Aday (1993), vulnerable populations are defined as those for whom the risk of poor physical, psychological, or social health has or is quite likely to become reality (e.g., disability, chronic illness, AIDS, or family abuse). Vulnerable populations are at-risk populations who need disease prevention, health promotion, and illness management care that is integrated to optimize health.

Emphasize Collaborative, Multidisciplinary, and Multicenter Research Studies

Well-designed collaborative, multidisciplinary, multicenter studies will have a greater chance of funding. Through the collaboration of multidisciplines, a variety of research questions can be answered for each discipline in the same well-designed study. Because so many studies have small sample sizes owing to a limited study population, multisite studies will be conducted to increase sample size while completing the study in a shorter time frame. These studies have the added advantage of increased power and reliability of the findings for generalizability. Many APNs will participate in various roles in collaborative, multidisciplinary, multicenter research. These studies will not only include facilities in the United States but will also span international projects. Barriers for protection of human subjects, translation of instruments free of cultural bias, networking, and the development and maintenance of working relationships will be challenging as nurses learn to participate in research in a global community.

More APNs Will Develop a Career Plan
for a Program of Research in a Specific Area

APNs are recognizing the need for mentors to help develop and build their careers and professional networks. They are also recognizing the value of being a mentor to help others build careers and develop the profession. As APNs learn to plan their careers, they will choose an area of interest and will plan a program of research with each study building on a previous study. This will generate new knowledge and increase the competitiveness of these research programs for funding.

Maturation of Advanced Practice Nursing: Some Final Thoughts

As we contemplate the impact of healthcare changes on advanced practice nursing, the complexities and interrelatedness of the multiple systems and contextual layers that form the fiber of healthcare delivery are both immobilizing and empowering. The restructuring, reengineering, and redesigning of healthcare is occurring around us; it cannot be stopped, and we would be foolhardy to try to stop the inevitability of change. Nurses cannot sit passively and let healthcare reform and the redesign of practice occur without a strong, active, and collective voice in shaping our own destiny. These are times of unprecedented opportunities for nursing; they are also times of risk and perils, for nothing is certain. Pursuit of excellence—especially in these times of tight budgets—requires courage, fortitude, imagination, creativity, commitment, visionary thinking, tireless energy, and leadership to create something better. APNs must exercise their growing power to deliberately choose and create their collective futures so they can participate in meeting the healthcare needs of a nation.

Nursing and nurses are broadly focused on the *healthcare needs of persons, families, communities, and populations.* By providing seamless continuum-based healthcare, people are assisted in the experience of illness and wellness across settings. Nursing has been an enduring, respected profession because nurses have stayed close to the core of our being, the human connection to the clients/patients whom we serve. It is for them and their families, as well as for the profession of nursing, that we continue to be actively involved in reshaping healthcare, our role in healthcare, and our destiny. To not be involved is to ignore the convenant that nursing has with society. Perhaps the words of Jack London capture the imperative for nurses and nursing to be actively involved:

I would rather be ashes than dust!
I would rather that my spark should burn out in a brilliant blaze than it should be stifled by dryrot.
I would rather be a superb meteor, every atom of me in magnificent glow, than a sleepy and
*   permanent planet.*
*   The proper function of man is to live, not to exist.*
I shall not waste my days in trying to prolong them.
I shall use my time.

Jack London 1876–1916

REFERENCES

Aday, L.A. (1993). *At risk in America.* San Francisco: Jossey-Bass.

AHCPR. (1997a). AHCPR to focus on strengthening the evidence based about proven clinical practices. *Research Activities 206,* 10.

AHCPR. (1997b). AHCPR merges two components and creates a new center to improve efficiency. *Research Activities 211,* 13.

Aiken, L. H. (1990). Charting the future of hospital nursing. *Image: Journal of Nursing Scholarship 22*(2), 72–78.

American Academy of Nurse Practitioners. (1993). *Scope of practice.* Austin, TX: Author.

American Association of Nurse Anesthetists (1996). *Professional practice manual for the certified registered nurse anesthetist.* Park Ridge, Illinois: Author.

American College of Nurse–Midwives. (1993). *Standards for the practice of nurse–midwifery.* Washington, DC: Author.

American Nurses Association. (1996). *Scope and standards of advanced practice registered nursing.* Washington, DC: Author.

American Nurses Association. (1994). *Clinician's handbook of preventive services: Put prevention into practice.* Washington, DC: Author.

American Nurses Association and American Association of Critical Care Nurses. (1995). *Standards of clinical practice and scope of practice for the acute care nurse practitioner.* Washington, DC: Author.

Barton, A. J., & Russin, M. M. (1997). Re-engineering intensive care: The role of informatics. *AACN Clinical Issues 8*(2), 253–261.

Benner, P. (1984). *From novice to expert* (pp. 292–293). Menlo Park, CA: Addison-Wesley.

"Best practice." (1998). *AACN News 15,* 7:5.

Bureau of Labor Statistics. (1998). US Department of Labor, Occupation Outlook Handbook, 1998–99 edition, Bulletin 2500 (p. 2, 203). Washington, DC: Superintendent of Documents, US Government Printing Office.

Byers, J. F., & Brunell, M. L. (1998). Demonstrating the value of the advanced practice nurse: An evaluation model. *AACN Clinical Issues 9*(2), 296–305.

Coddington, D. C., Moore, K. D., & Fischer, E. A. (1995). Integrating? Hang in there—The odds are in your favor. *Healthcare Forum Journal 38*(1), 14–18.

Collins, E. G. (1992). Increasing practice based-research: Doctorally prepared clinical nurse specialists may be the answer. *Clinical Nurse Specialist 6*(4), 196–200.

Cook, D. J., & Levy, M. M. (1998). Evidence-based medicine. *Critical Care Clinics 14*(3), 353–358.

Corbin, J. M., & Strauss, A. (1988). *Managing chronic illness at home.* San Francisco: Jossey-Bass.

Division of Nursing, Bureau of Health Professions, Health Resources and Services Administration, U.S. Department of Health and Human Services. Advance Notes I and II from the National Sample Survey of Registered Nurses, March, 1996.

Donaldson, M. S. (1996). *Primary care: American's health in a new era.* Washington, DC: National Academy Press.

Ebeling, T., & Groath, D. K. (1998). Nursing centers. In NONE Leadership Services: Nursing and the continuum of care. Chicago: American Hospital Publishing Co.

Finocchio, L. J., Dower, C. M., McMahon, T., Gragnola, C. M., & the Taskforce on Health Care Workforce Regulation. (1995). *Reforming healthcare workforce regulation: Policy considerations for the 21st century.* San Francisco: Pew Health Professions Commission.

Ford, L. C. (1982). Nurse practitioners: History of a new idea and predictions for the future (pp. 231–247). In L. H. Aiken & S. R. Cortner (Eds.), *Nursing in the 1980s: Crisis, Opportunities, Challenges.* Philadelphia: Lippincott.

Ford, L. C. (1986). Nurses, nurse practitioners: The evolution of primary care: Review of nurses, nurse practitioners: The evolution of primary card. Image: Journal of Nursing Scholarship, 18, 177–178.

Foss, N., & Koerner, J. (1997). The advanced practice nurse's role in differential practice: Martha's story. *AACN Clinical Issues 8*(2), 262–270.

Haddock, K. S. (1997). Clinical nurse specialists: The third generation. In S. Moorhead & D. G. Huber (Eds.), *Nursing roles: Evolving or recycled?* (pp. 139–149). Thousand Oaks, CA: Sage Publication.

Hadley, E. H. (1997). Nursing in the political and economic marketplace: Challenges for the 21st century. In C. Harrington & C. L. Estes (Eds.). *Health policy and nursing* (2nd ed., pp. 164–172). Sudbury, MA: Jones & Bartlett Publishers.

Hammer, M., & Champy, J. (1993). *Reengineering the corporation.* New York: HarperBusiness.

Harrison, J. K. (1997). Advanced practice nurses: Key to successful hospital transformation in a managed-care environment. In S. Moorhead & D. G. Huber (Eds.), *Nursing roles: Evolving or recycled?* (pp. 128–138). Thousand Oaks, CA: Sage Publication.

Healthy People 2010. (1998). http://web.health.gov/healthypeople/2010fctsht.htm.

Institute of Medicine. (1996). *Defining primary care: An Interim report.* Washington, DC: National Academy Press.

Koerner, J., & Burgess, C. S. (1997). Nursing's role and functions in a seamless continuum of care. In S. Moorhead & D. G. Huber (Eds.), *Nursing roles: Evolving or recycled?* (pp. 1–14). Thousand Oaks, CA: Sage Publication.

Lindeke, L. L., & Block, D. E. (1998). Maintaining professional integrity in the mist of interdisciplinary collaboration. *Nursing Outlook 46*(5), 213–218.

Newman, M. A. (1990). Toward an integrative model of professional practice. *Journal of Professional Nursing 6*(3), 167–173.

O'Neil, E. (1993). *Health professions education for the future: Schools in service to the nation.* San Francisco, CA: Pew Health Professions Commission, Pew Charitable Trust Foundation.

Pesut, D. J. (1997). Facilitating future thinking. *Nursing Outlook, 45*(4), 155.

Pew Health Professions Commission. (1995). *Critical challenges: Revitalizing the healthcare professions for the twenty-first century.* San Francisco: UCSF Center for the Health Professions.

Public Health Service. (1990). *Healthy People 2000* (DHHS Publication No. PHS 91-50213). Washington, DC: US Government Printing Office.

Riesch, S. K. (1987). Academic clinician: A new role for nursing's future. *Nursing and Health Care 8*(10), 583–586.

Safriet, B. (1994). Impediments to progress in health care workforce policy: License and practice laws. *Inquiry 31*, 310–317.

Seehafer, M. T. (1998). Nurse–physician collaboration. *Journal of the Academy of Nurse Practitioners 10*(9), 387–301.

Shugars, D. A., O'Neil, E. H., & Bader, J. D. (Eds.). (1991). *Healthy America: Practitioners for 2005, an agenda for action for US health professional schools.* Durham, NC: The Pew Health Professions Commission.

Sovie, M. D. (1995). Tailoring hospitals for managed care and integrated health systems. *Nursing Economics 13*, 72–83.

Starfield, B. (1994). Primary care participants or gatekeepers? *Diabetes Care 17*(Suppl. 1), 12–17.

Starr, P. (1982). *The social transformation of American medicine.* New York: Basic Books Inc.

Steel, J. E. (1997). Development of the acute care nurse practitioner role: Questions, opinions, consensus (pp. 13–28). In B. J. Daly, (Ed.), *The acute care nurse practitioner.* New York: Springer Publishing Co.

US Preventive Services Task Force. (1996). *Guide to clinical preventive services* (2nd ed). Baltimore: Williams & Wilkins.

Walker, M. K., & Sebastian, J. G. (1997). Complimentarity of advanced practice nursing roles in enhancing health outcomes of the chronically ill: Acute care nursing practitioners and nurse case managers. In S. Moorhead & D. G. Huber (Eds.), *Nursing roles: Evolving or recycled?* (pp. 170–190). Thousand Oaks, CA: Sage Publication.

Yordy, K. D. (1997). The nursing workforce in a time of change. In C. Harrington & C. L. Estes (Eds.), *Health policy and nursing* (2nd ed. pp. 141–152). Sudbury, MA: Jones & Barlett Publishers.

Zander, K. (1998). Historical development of outcomes-based care delivery. *Critical Care Nursing Clinics of North American 10*(1), 1–10.

Zitter, M. (1997). A new paradigm in health care delivery: Disease management. In W. E. Todd & D. Nash (Eds.), *Disease management: A systems approach to improving patient outcomes* (pp. 1–25). Chicago: American Hospital Publishing Inc.

CHAPTER 2

Catherine L. Gilliss

Education for Advanced Practice Nursing

As indicated in Chapter 1, significant changes in healthcare problems, their treatment, and the proposed reformation of the care and payment structure have significantly altered the demand for nurses. Although the need for staff nurses has declined, hospitals are now seeking more advanced practice nurses (APNs). Healthcare problems are more complex, and more knowledge and complex problem solving is expected of healthcare providers. Thus, as the demand for APNs grows, the profession must develop a clear understanding of what is required to prepare nurses for advanced practice. This chapter describes advanced practice nursing, identifies areas for potential growth or opportunity in advanced practice, and identifies the needed knowledge and skills for advanced practice in nursing. It also recommends one curriculum approach to preparing APNs and suggests priority areas for resource allocation for APN education.

Advanced Practice Nursing

What is advanced practice nursing? It was described by the ANA in its revised Social Policy Statement:

> Advanced practice registered nurses have acquired the knowledge base and practice experience to prepare them for specialization, expansion and advancement in practice. . . .
> As advanced practice nursing evolved in the roles of clinical nurse specialist, nurse practitioner, nurse midwife and nurse anesthetist, different components or characteristics of advanced practice nurse were adopted. . . . The nurse in advanced practice acquires specialized knowledge and skills through study and supervised practice at the master's or doctoral level in nursing. (ANA, 1995, p. 14)

As indicated above by ANA (*Nursing Facts from the ANA,* 1993), these nurses can be categorized in four principal groups:

1. Nurse Practitioners (NP). In 1993, there were approximately 25,000 to 30,000 practicing in the United States; their annual salary was approximately $35,000 to $40,000.

2. Certified Nurse Midwives (CNM). In 1993, there were approximately 5,000 midwives practicing in the Unites States; their annual salary was approximately $45,000.

3. Clinical Nurse Specialists. In 1993, there were approximately 40,000 in the United States, earning an annual salary ranging from $30,000 to $80,000.

4. Certified Registered Nurse Anesthetists. In 1993, there were approximately 25,000 practicing in the United States. Their annual salary was estimated at $78,000.

Similar figures were reported from a 1992 survey of NPs and CNMs conducted by the Washington Consulting Group (1994), which has not yet been updated.

More current figures were reported in the 1996 National Sample Survey of Registered Nurses (Moses, 1997), which indicated that 161,711 registered nurses have been prepared as APNs. Of these, 39% were prepared as nurse practitioners, 33% as clinical nurse specialists, 19% as certified registered nurse anesthetists, and 4% as certified nurse midwives.

Numerous reports indicated that these advanced practice nurses are accessible, cost-effective; they are not doctor substitutes but are capable of addressing health problems in a satisfying and qualified way (Brown & Grimes, 1992; Safriet, 1992; Office of Technology Assessment, 1986).

What are the goals of advanced practice nursing? According to Barnsteiner and colleagues (1993), the common goals of nurses in advanced pediatric nursing include:

- improved access to care;
- increased interdisciplinary and intradisciplinary collaboration within the healthcare system between providers delivering primary and specialized care for children and their families;
- an expanded knowledge base for clinical decision making, including health assessment, clinical judgement, health and social policy, scholarly inquiry, and leadership activities;
- the provision of services in new arenas; and
- increased professional autonomy and eligibility for reimbursement by various payment mechanisms.

The Pew Health Professions Commission reports have described the directions to be taken by all professions, including nursing, to meet the challenges of the year 2005 (O'Neil, 1993). Based on the Commission's projected vision of the emerging healthcare system as a system in which the orientation shifts toward health and employs a population perspective, there will be more limited resources, but these resources will address coordinated services focused on the consumer and particularly on treatment outcomes. Expectations for provider accountability will increase, as will the need for integration of domestic and global concerns for health, education, and public safety (O'Neil, 1993).

Practitioners for this emerging system must be prepared with appropriate competencies, including a focus on the community, current clinical skills, expanded accountability, the ability to use costly technology appropriately, knowledge of health promotion, and the skill to involve clients and families in decision making (O'Neil, 1993).

For nursing education, the Commission identified the following six specific strategies to address these changes:

1. Changing licensing and care delivery regulations to ensure that nurses are employed in positions for which they were trained;

2. Restructuring faculty positions in nursing schools to directly involve more faculty in patient care and nursing practice;

3. Developing interdisciplinary education, research, and service programs for the maintenance of chronically ill patient populations;

4. Redirecting resources toward the health needs of community based populations;

5. Continuing to develop graduate-level clinical training programs to prepare

nurses to deliver services that reduce costs and improve quality and access to care; and

6. Conducting comprehensive and ongoing programs of strategic planning within each nursing school.

Clearly, change is needed, and some specific directions have been offered in these documents. Beyond the world of the contemplative task force, change is occurring in the healthcare system.

McFadden and Miller (1994) surveyed 288 master's-prepared clinical nurse specialists (CNSs) regarding the implementation of their clinical practice roles and how healthcare system changes were affecting those roles. The CNSs identified that their most important responsibility, and the one requiring the greatest amount of their time, was patient care/consultation (including clinical practice; case management; patient advocacy; change agent; consultant; role modeling for staff nurses; and development of patient care standards, policies, and procedures). Four additional sets of responsibility followed: education (staff, patients, program development, and students); administration (general, committee work, budget, documentation, and quality assurance); research (consumer, identification of problems, collaboration, and nursing research committees); and professional development (continuing education, marketing, networking, and publishing). The factor reported as that most responsible for changes in the implementation of the CNS role was cost containment. Participants also acknowledged the changes in length of stay, changes in reimbursement mechanisms, and patient acuity as affecting to role implementation. However, the data collected in this survey suggest that the role of CNS, as currently implemented, is not viewed as cost-effective.

New roles are emerging, roles that combine the best of the specialty knowledge and indirect practice skills of the CNS with the primary care knowledge and direct care skills nurse practitioner (NP). Taking over house staff responsibilities (Mallison, 1993), serving as "attending nurses" (Aiken, 1990), expanding care (and collaborative) roles in critical care (Dracup & Bryan-Brown 1993), and implementing the role of tertiary care nurse practitioners (Keane & Richmond, 1993) are among the proposed changes for institutionally based nurses. Current literature calls attention to the focus on specialty practice (Lipman & Deatrick, 1997) and addresses the development of roles that draw on in-depth specialty knowledge for the care of population groups across settings. These include the critical care nurse practitioner (Watts et al., 1996), the psychiatric nurse practitioner (Dyer et al., 1997) the neonatal nurse practitioner (Kinneer & Browne, 1997), the diabetes advanced practice nurse (Melkus & Fain, 1995), and the oncological advanced practice nurse (Belcher & Shurpin, 1995).

A quiet revolution has been occurring. In 1992, 2,219 nurses reported that they were certified as both NPs and CNSs. Most of these nurses were educated in NP programs. Moreover, the nurses who held both NP and CNS certifications held the highest rate of full-time employment (Washington Consulting Group, 1994). What are the practice challenges that have led these nurses toward combining the credentials of NP and CNS?

Healthcare Reform: What Lies Ahead?

The failure of the Clinton Health Security Act shifted the impetus of current healthcare system reforms from the legislative arena to the marketplace. The last 5 years have seen significant growth in the use of the managed care organization as the principal approach to financing and delivering healthcare. Care delivery has moved from areas of high cost (high-acuity hospitals) to areas of lower cost (outpatient departments, outpatient surgery centers, transitional care center, and homes). Use of costly services has been reduced, leading to shorter length of hospital stays and greater patient acuity during hospitalization.

Patients are discharged to settings in which they require nursing support, but these supports are often not available. Rather, family members manage pain and other symptoms from the home. Thus, there is need for healthcare expertise that transcends settings, caring for patients and supporting their families wherever they may be.

The work of providing healthcare services has been shifted to the least costly safe provider. This means that nurses may be doing the work formerly assigned to physicians, and patient assistants may be doing the work formerly assigned to nurses. Additionally, a person who once had responsibility for providing direct care is sometimes assigned to develop services for groups of patients or to negotiate the appropriate payment supports from payers.

The drive to reduce costs will also spark a renewed interest in health and health education. Better funding for preventive and primary care can be anticipated. Opportunities for health education and the number of wellness and fitness centers will increase. Based on personalized assessment of individual risk (genetic, familial, and individual), dedicated centers may address the prevention of specific diseases. This approach will consider the needs of larger groups of the population and require skill in assessing, intervening, and evaluating the impact of such population-based programs.

Finally, to meet the needs of an increasingly diverse population more effectively, efforts will be made to diversify the caring professions to match the diversity of the population. Workers who are well known and influential in the community will be important allies to healthcare providers who wish to plan programs that address community need. In the interest of economy and effectiveness, outcomes of intervention will be critically evaluated; professionals able to evaluate the outcomes of care will be in demand.

By applying this forecast specifically to nursing, several predictions can be made (see also Gilliss & Mundinger, 1998). The CNS, traditionally employed in the hospital to deliver direct care and consult with the staff in the development of care plans, will accept more responsibility for direct care delivery. Consistent with the forecast of the Institute of Medicine's report on nurse staffing in hospitals (IOM, 1996), the number of APNs in hospitals can be expected to increase. Given the high-acuity and long-term needs of the hospitalized population, the APN in this setting will need to develop a more comprehensive array of direct practice skills and knowledge of the homegoing/recovery concerns of patients and families. The hospital-based advanced practice nurse will develop a continuity relationship with patients and follow the patient's need in and out of illness episodes. Additionally, the nurse can be expected to work with others on the healthcare team, which requires skills needed to develop a strong collaborative relationship.

Another developing area is providing primary care to specialty populations or providing continuity for specialty populations who suffer from functional disability or are managing difficult symptoms. This requires expertise regarding the special problem and the expanded skills to manage common problems. For instance, the diabetes expert who provided for the primary care needs of a panel of non–insulin-dependent women with diabetes sees her patients whether in the hospital or community and addresses the disease-related and healthcare maintenance needs of this group of patients.

In some institutions, we may see the advanced practice nurse substituting for physicians in well-baby nurseries, admissions areas, and emergency areas. In addition, some highly skilled nurses working in critical care and trauma units will assume even more responsibility for patient management than previously known. They will work closely with others in planning and implementing extremely sophisticated treatments.

Nurses will be well positioned to own and operate home health and extended care facilities. Because nurses do know how to keep people healthy, contracts with large managed care organizations should be available to nurses for elderly health promotion and illness treatment.

As the nation moves toward placing priority on preventive services and primary care, nursing can expect its roles in those areas to grow. More nurse practitioners, nurse–midwives, community health nurses, and health educators will be needed. The need for primary care providers to live and work in areas with a shortage of health professionals will lead to greater incentives for geographic disbursement. Faculty will be needed for education in the health professions. The need for faculty to expand primary care nurse practitioner programs is already critical. The future of community health nursing is bright, but only if nursing leaders in community health assist in the massive education program that the public health system must conduct. Few government officials or citizens realize that the proposed reforms of the healthcare system will free the public health sector for exciting news roles. The public health sector might be charged with assisting communities to identify their health needs and identify approaches to measuring outcomes of care (Pestronk et al., 1993). And, of course, we need to prepare administrators and researchers who can evaluate costs and outcomes of care. The politics of this responsibility cannot be underestimated. Nurses with an intimate knowledge of nursing practice and its intended outcomes will be critical to documenting the value of advanced nursing practice within the healthcare system.

What Knowledge and Credentials Are Required for Advanced Practice?

Currently, advanced practice in nursing requires particular credentials and skills. In addition to these, the skills that will be required in the near future should be considered. Only then will nursing be educating advanced practitioners for the future.

Advanced nursing practice is commonly described as requiring the following credentials: basic nursing education, basic licensure, graduate degree in nursing, and experience in the specialization (ANA, 1995; National Council of State Boards of Nursing, 1992).

Typically, the following are assumed to comprise the **skill base** of nurses in advanced nursing practice:

- comprehensive assessment skills;
- diagnostic ability; management of health and illness problems;
- assessment and intervention of complex systems;
- the ability to critically analyze research findings;
- leadership in healthcare;
- cooperation/collaboration skills; and
- autonomy and the ability to make critical, independent judgements.

The degree to which these abilities have been developed in traditional CNS and NP programs varies. Some even suggest that the core competencies needed to perform each of the traditional roles differs (Anderson, 1994).

A careful examination of the traditional approach to CNS and NP curricula reveals differences, which are the subject of controversy (Rasch & Frauman, 1996). Table 2-1 lists the skill areas earlier identified as necessary for advanced practice and shows how these areas have been developed in traditional curricula. Research, which usually receives equivalent coverage, has been omitted from the table.

Each curriculum has different historical strengths. The physical assessment/health assessment skills taught in CNS programs have often been limited to a particular system, whereas the NP curricula have taught comprehensive assessment skills and encouraged efficient, integrated practice of those skills. The ability to develop sound clinical reasoning skills and differentiate a diagnosis is critical to NP education because NPs have been expected to diagnose and treat previously undiagnosed conditions. CNS education has not exposed nurses to the rigors of diagnostic reasoning. The CNS relies on the nursing process and sound scientific reasoning to make clinical judgements. By the nature of their work, CNSs and NPs have different scopes of concern. Typically, the CNS works with a specialty

TABLE 2-1 *Contrasting CNS and NP Curricula for APN Preparation*

Skills	CNS Curriculum	NP Curriculum
Physical assessment	Often limited to particular system	Comprehensive
Diagnostic reasoning	Limited	Curricular thread
Management of health problems	Limited; requiring approval of others	Comprehensive
Systems focus	Usually strong; addresses consultation	Often focused on individual; limited focus on context
Leadership	Strong focus	Variable
Interdisciplinary approach	Nurse to nurse	Nurse to physician
Autonomy	Limited	Essential; contributes to role crisis

population, with a somewhat circumscribed set of conditions. Although CNSs are able to initiate management actions in the care of some patient problems, much of the management authority continues to rest with physicians. In contrast, the NP has developed as an autonomous role in which collaboration is encouraged. The scope of practice is wide, and the legal authority to implement management actions is often present. Thus, the educational program includes opportunities to develop knowledge on a wide range of problems and their treatment, as well as practice opportunities to diagnose and manage the problems presented by patients.

With respect to understanding larger systems and developing leadership abilities, traditional CNS curricula have provided more content and more practical experience. The CNS has been expected to implement a role characterized by five components: 1) direct care; 2) consultation to others; 3) education; 4) research; and 5) leadership. The NP curriculum has encouraged the development of the direct care component, usually focused on the individual. Often the focus on direct care has overwhelmed the development of leadership abilities in the NP. Fenton and Brykczynski (1993) have made similar observations.

Consistent with the expectation that the CNS would develop consultation skills as one component of the advanced practice role, the CNS learns how to supervise and collaborate with other nurses. NPs, in contrast, work with physicians as practice partners. As a result, the NP and CNS often have different views of their relationships with other nurses and with physicians.

The development of autonomy is essential to the successful implementation of the role of nurse practitioner. This shift in behavior represents a significant divergence from basic education in nursing and, for most NP students, creates a frightening role crisis. NP trainees fear that they will kill patients or that they will never know enough to practice. Once comfortable that they are able to recognize a particular condition, they panic at the prospect of selecting the treatment and a date for the patient's return visit. The practice of the CNS, like the practice of the nurse with basic preparation, is far more consultative. The autonomy exhibited in the NP role is often described by applicants to NP programs as one reason that the role is attractive.

Following graduation, CNSs and NPs now accept positions that overlap more than they once might have. Although most CNS graduates once worked in hospitals and NPs practiced in ambulatory care, there is now considerable crossover. NPs are employed in hospitals to deliver primary care to specialized groups or as physician "substitutes." CNSs are seen in group practices where their continuous care of groups with special needs complements the care offered by physicians and surgeons.

Although traditionally different in areas of emphasis, the curricula preparing CNSs and NPs include considerable common ground. A fundamental assumption underlying the discussion of educational programs in this chapter is the belief that preparation for advanced practice across areas of specialization is more similar than different. Practically, a curriculum that addresses the common competencies and permits opportunities for development of specialty-based knowledge will be efficient for faculty to teach and facilitate the socialization of nurses for advanced practice roles to further develop their common knowledge base.

Fenton and Brykczynski (1993) have described three idealogies for the future preparation of nurse practitioners and clinical nurse specialists: (1) merge the two roles into one; (2) keep the two roles separate; and (3) identify a common core for the two roles, to which specialty content can be added. Consistent with their analysis, in 1996, the American Association of Colleges of Nursing (AACN) published *The Essentials of Master's Education for Advanced Practice Nursing.*

In this document AACN proposed (1) core graduate curriculum, (2) advanced practice nursing core, and (3) specialty curriculum. The content of the graduate curriculum included research, policy (including healthcare policy, healthcare system organization, and healthcare financing), ethics, professional role development, theoretical foundations of nursing practice, human diversity and social issues, and health promotion and disease prevention. This content was proposed as foundational for all graduate students in nursing. The APN curriculum was described as essential for those providing direct patient care at an advanced level and included advanced health/physical assessment, advanced physiology and pathophysiology, and advanced pharmacology. The content of the specialization included the clinical and didactic experience defined by the specialty organizations (AACN, 1996). For instance, one example of a specialty organization's guiding document was published by the National Organization of Nurse Practitioner Faculties. *Advanced Nursing Practice: Curriculum Guidelines and Program Standards for Nurse Practitioner Education* (NONPF, 1995) provided direction of curriculum content for primary care nurse practitioner programs.

The impact of the "Essentials" document on curricular content has been significant. Many programs have reorganized their curriculum and consolidated offerings into core offerings. In addition to content, however, several authors have called for the recognition that essential *process* features must also be included in graduate preparation for advanced practice.

O'Flynn (1996) stresses the point that graduates cannot master, while they are graduate students, all the knowledge necessary to sustain a practice career; therefore, they will need to recognize that lifelong learning is essential. Lipman and Deatrick (1997) identify clinical decision making and critical thinking as essential skills to develop for advanced practice and have developed pedagogical approaches to reinforce this learning. King, Sebastian, Stanhope, and Hickman (1997) discuss problem-based learning as an approach that fosters critical thinking and reasoning skills.

An Educational Approach to Preparation of Advanced Practice Nurses

Aided by the publication of the AACN "Essentials" document and stimulated by the challenge to accommodate qualified applicants to graduate nursing programs, the curricula of nursing programs have evolved during the last 10 years. Many primary care nurse practitioner programs have opened. Specialty NP programs have begun in acute care, neonatal nursing, and psychological-mental health. The pediatric faculties at the University of Pennsylvania, Yale University, and the University of California at San Francisco have developed a curricular plan that is built on the strong clinical assessment base of the NP but prepares nurses for acute/chronic care of children or for critical care.

Case Western Reserve began a program in August 1992 to prepare NPs to offer a full range of NP services plus coordinate patient care in hospitals and clinics. The role is similar to that of a case manager. Neonatal Nurse Practitioner programs are also changing the face of specialization in nursing. In addition to meeting the needs of the hospitalized neonate, these nurses follow the family into the community setting, continuing to meet the multiple demands imposed on these families for the child's first year of life, incorporating features of the case manager. Each of these responds to the healthcare system's demand for flexible workers who provide competent care at a low cost and can work across settings.

A CURRICULUM PLAN

To plan a model curriculum or even an example requires that assumptions be made. The proposed plan assumes full-time study for 2 academic years, using a trimester structure. No academic credits have been assigned in this example. Obviously, converting the model to a semester structure would require some consolidations and reorganizations. (Full-time study is still possible for students when tuition costs are reasonable and courses are scheduled into a full 2-day block of time; however, 70% of those studying for master's degrees in nursing are studying part-time.)

Table 2-2 sets forth one example of an approach to organizing a curriculum for the preparation of advanced practice nurses. The completed program will include core content

 TABLE 2-2 *Example of an Approach to Organizing an FNP Curriculum*

	Trimester		
	Fall	*Winter*	*Spring*
Year 1	Research	Research	Pharmacology
	Health Assessment	Health Promotion/	Management I
	Clinical Lab	Disease Prevention	
		Clinical Practicum	Clinical Practicum
	Psychiatric Symptoms and Management	Family Intervention	Family Nurse Practitioner Seminar
	Family Theory	Leadership	Pediatrics Seminar
Year 2	Health Care Policy and Economics	Nutrition	
	Management II	Family Nurse Practitioner Management III	Comprehensive Exam or Thesis
	Clinical Residency	Clinical Residency	Clinical Residency
	Family Nurse Practitioner Seminar		
	Pediatrics Seminar		

required of all master's students, core advanced practice content for those preparing for roles in direct care, advanced practice, and the content of the chosen specialty. The plan appearing in Table 2-2 was developed for primary care FNPs.

The sample plan begins in the fall of the first year, with a combination of master's core courses, advanced practice core cores and specialization courses. "Research" represents content intended for inclusion in the master's core curriculum; "Health Assessment" and "Psychiatric Symptoms and Management" will be selected by all students studying for direct care advanced practice specializations; "Family Theory" represents a course taken only by the specialization or a subgrouping of specializations. In the winter of the first year, "Research" continues. The master's core curriculum also includes "Leadership." All those in the advanced practice core would begin the course "Health Promotion/Disease Prevention." In addition, a supplemental seminar would be scheduled, to be directed by faculty from the specialty. Clinical practice, under the supervision of specialty faculty, would also begin. "Family Intervention," a course particular to those caring for the family, would be included as a course for the specialty.

In the spring of the first year, the advanced practice core would include "Pharmacology" and "The Management of Common Health Problems." These courses would be supplemented by clinical practice, supervised by the specialty faculty, and specialty seminars on the management of common health problems in children and for families.

The fall of the second year begins with another master's core course, "Healthcare Policy and Economics." In addition, the advanced practice core would address "Assessment" and "Management of Complex Health Problems." In addition to the clinical residency, supervised by specialty faculty, the specialty faculty would conduct case-based seminars on the management of the complex health problems of children and families. In winter of the second year, the advanced practice core continues with "Nutrition." In addition, specialty content comes into sharper focus, with a course on the management of complex problems in family primary care and the supervised clinical residency. In the final trimester of the program, the exit assignment (comprehensive exam or thesis) can be completed in addition to more specialty-focused clinical residency hours.

In addition to explicit courses mentioned, several topic areas are threaded throughout the curriculum for all advanced practice nurses. These include clinical problem solving and decision making, collaboration in practice, communication, ethics in clinical decision making and professional behavior, sociocultural variation and cultural competency, and self-evaluation. Each should be addressed in each trimester in a deliberate fashion that builds upon the previous exposure.

How Do We Prioritize Resource Allocation in the Preparation of APNs?

A strategic approach to allocating resources for the development and redevelopment of advanced practice nurses will facilitate the development of a work force that is able to meet the needs of the population. Several areas can be identified as priority areas:

1. **Faculty development must be viewed as a top priority.** Currently, many schools are recruiting doctorate-prepared nurse practitioners or others who are clinically competent to serve as instructors for advanced practice. The demand is greater than the supply. In response, some schools are supporting the re-entry of their existing faculty in the development of clinical practice competencies, particularly for preparation as nurse practitioners. This strategy can expand faculty practice skills and enrich and enliven their teaching and research contributions. However, many faculty finish these programs and do not advance in their skill development because they do not practice.

2. **Faculty practice must be rewarded as one aspect of performance review for academic advancement.** Advanced practice education involves the advanced study of clinical care in the classroom and clinical world. Without faculty members who are masters of the clinical domain, classrooms are vulnerable to irrelevant or outdated information and students do not have models for their performance.

3. **Practicing advanced practice nurses may require post-master's education to prepare for roles in today's healthcare system.** Many nurses practicing in traditional CNS roles are returning for post-master's preparation as NPs. For many of these nurses, the underlying interest is not to become a primary care provider but to expand the scope of their practices to include health promotion and to create new opportunities for the future. Supporting the re-education of these returning nurses should be viewed as a priority for several reasons. First, they generally re-enter the work force within 1 year, rather than the 2 years required for master's study. Second, they are important consultants to the faculty in the development and implementation of educational programs. Their current clinical practice informs the curriculum and influences the relevance of what is taught. Finally, post-master's programs facilitate the creation of a community of advanced practice nurses who can advise on future curricular matters and serve as preceptors to master's students, as well as improve patient care.

4. **Nursing education must address the current curricular redundancy.** The resources of the past are no longer available to support small class offerings that are identical to each other. Where opportunities exist to combine classes and coteach or team-teach, faculty should consider creating offerings that combine students from multiple advanced practice specialties (core classes). That is not to say that small class offerings are not an important part of the curriculum; seminar work is fundamental to graduate education because it provides opportunity for the development of critical thinking and communication skills. The development of core offerings will create economies, share the workload, and aid APNs in understanding the overlap and complementary nature of their roles. Career-ladder planning should be undertaken to advance those seeking advanced practice skills. This planning should consider measures of competency in determining educational requirements.

5. **Redundancy must also be addressed on a regional level.** The need for duplicative programs within a region should be challenged. Incentives should be developed for programs to cooperate in the sharing of resources and faculty. "New" programs should be encouraged to work with existing programs in the development of complementary programs and experiences. Where possible, broadcast and interactive technologies must be employed to facilitate collaboration among programs, and to improve the availability of programs to health professional shortage areas.

6. **Access to educational preparation for advanced practice should be improved, particularly to promote diversity in the workforce and to counterbalance the aging of the advanced practice workforce.** The need to create career ladder opportunities for those entering nursing at the associate-degree levels should be obvious, but patterns that address educational mobility have not been widely adopted. Similarly, programs that permit fast-tracking to advanced practice for young people continue to be limited. Faculty members need to confront and evaluate the effect of their bias against basic prepared nurses who do not have extensive clinical experience prior to graduate study. The aging of the nursing workforce demands that new pathways for early entry be developed before the profession truly becomes extinct.

7. **Excellence in education for advanced practice nursing requires strong partnerships.** AACN has developed position papers addressing various aspects of education and practice. In their position statement on interdisciplinary education and practice, AACN states the scope of healthcare mandates that healthcare professionals work with one another and that the ability to work together is the result of shared education and practice experiences. Education for advanced practice should be planned, implemented and evaluated with our healthcare delivery partners. AACN, in their position statement on education and practice collaboration, notes that excellence in practice, education, and research is best attained when schools of nursing establish, maintain, and evaluate collaborative relationships with practice settings. Educational and service settings must work together to plan, implement, and evaluate the outcomes of our education programs for advanced practice nursing.

We sit on the edge of some of the greatest opportunities that the nursing profession has ever faced. Education has often been the tool of disenfranchised groups for self-improvement and social ascension. This is true in nursing, but our diverse educational pathways defy public understanding. As public understanding of nurse practitioners and clinical nurse specialists grows, it is important to maintain continuity in the public understanding. Thus far, the public seems to understand and accept advanced practice nursing. More important, it is important to prepare practitioners in nursing who can maintain the public trust through the competence and relevance of their practice.

REFERENCES

Aiken, L. (1990). Charting the future of hospital nursing. *Image: Journal of Nursing Scholarship, 22, 72–78.*

American Association of Colleges of Nursing (1996). *The essentials of master's education for advanced practice nursing.* Washington, DC: AACN.

American Nurses Association. (1993). *Nursing facts from the ANA.* Washington, DC: Author.

American Nurses Association. (1995). *Nursing's social policy statement.* Washington, DC: Author.

Anderson, C. (1994). Graduate education in primary care: The challenge. *Nursing Outlook 42*(3), 101–102.

Barnsteiner, J., Deatrick, J., Grey, M., et al. (1993). Future of pediatric advanced practice nursing. *Pediatric Nursing,* 196–197.

Belcher, A., & Shurpin, K. (1995). Education of the advanced practice nurse in oncology. *Oncology Nursing Forum 22*(8 Suppl.), 19–24.

Brown, S., & Grimes, D. (1992). *Meta-analysis of process of care, clinical outcomes and cost effectiveness of nurses in primary care roles: Nurse practitioners and nurse–midwives.* Kansas City, MO: American Nurses Association.

Dracup, K., & Bryan-Brown, C. (1993). Critical care and healthcare reform. *American Journal of Critical Care 2*(5), 351–353.

Dyer, J., Hammill, K., Regan-Kubinski, M., et al. (1997). The psychiatric-primary care nurse preactitioner: A futuristic model for advanced practice psychiatric-mental health nursing. *Archives of Psychiatric Nursing 11*(1), 2–12.

Fenton, M., & Brykczynski, K. (1993). Qualitative distinctions and similarities in the practice of clinical nurse specialists and nurse practitioners. *Journal of Professional Nursing 9*(6), 313–326.

Gilliss, C., & Mundinger, M. (1998). How is the role of the advanced practice nurse changing? In E. O'Neil & J. Coffman (Eds.) *Strategies for the future of nursing: Changing roles, responsibilities, and employment patterns of registered nurses* (pp. 171–191). San Francisco: Jossey-Bass.

Institute of Medicine. (1996). *Nursing staff in hospitals and nursing homes: Is it adequate?* G. S. Wunderlich. F. A. Sloan, & C. K. Davis (Eds.). Washington, DC: National Academy Press.

Keane, A., & Richmond, T. (1993). Tertiary care nurse practitioners. *Image: The Journal of Nursing Scholarship 25*(4), 281–284.

King, M., Sebastian, J., Stanhope, M., & Hickman, M. (1997). Using problem-based learning to prepare advanced practice community health nurses for the 21st century. *Family and Community Health 20*(1), 29–39.

Kinneer, M., & Browne, J. (1997). Developmental care in advanced practice neonatal nursing education. *Journal of Nursing Education 36*(2), 79–82.

Lipman, T., & Deitrich, J. (1997). Preparing advanced practice nurses for clinical decision making in specialty practice. *Nurse Educator, 22*(2), 47–50.

Mallison, M. (1993). Nurses as house staff. *American Journal of Nursing March,* 7.

McFadden, E., & Miller, M. (1994). Clinical nurse specialist practice: Facilitators and barriers. *Clinical Nurse Specialist: The Journal for Advanced Nursing Practice 8*(1), 27–33.

Moses, E. B. (1997). *The registered nurse population: Findings from the National Sample Survey of Registered Nurses, March 1996.* Rockville, Maryland: Division of Nursing, Bureau of Health Professions, Health Resources and Services Administration, US Public Health Service, Department of Health and Human Services.

National Council of State Boards of Nursing. (1992). *Position paper on the licensure of advanced practice nursing.* Chicago: Author.

National Organization of Nurse Practitioner Faculties. (1995). *Advanced nursing practice: Curriculum guidelines and program standards for nurse practitioner education.* Washington, DC: NONPF.

Office of Technology Assessment. (1986). *Nurse practitioners, physicians assistants, and certified nurse midwives: A policy analysis.* Washington, DC: GPO.

O'Flynn, A. (1996). The preparation of advanced practice nurses: Current issues. *Nursing Clinics of North America 32*(3), 429–438.

O'Neil, E. (1993). *Health professions education for the future: Schools in service to the nation.* San Francisco: Pew Health Professions Commission.

Pestronk, R., Oxman, G., Gilliss, C., et al. (1993). Managed outcomes: A strategy to improve the nation's health. *Journal of the American Academy of Nurse Practitioners 6*(3), 121–124.

Rasch, R., & Frauman, A. (1996). Advanced practice nursing: Conceptual issues. *Journal of Professional Nursing 12*(3), 141–146.

Safriet, B. (1992). Health care dollars and regulatory sense: The role of advanced practice nursing. *The Yale Journal of Regulation 9,* 417–487.

Washington Consulting Group. (1994). *Survey of certified nurse practitioners and clinical specialists: December 1992.* Washington, DC: Washington Consulting Group. (Prepared for the Division of Nursing, Bureau of Health Professions, HRSA, #240–91-0055).

Watts, R., Hanson, M., Burke, K., et al. (1996). The critical care nurse practitioner program: an advanced practice role for the critical care nurse. *Dimensions of Critical Care 15*(1), 48–56.

CHAPTER 3

Professional Development: Socialization in Advanced Practice Nursing

M. Elizabeth Hixon

Socialization refers to the learning of social roles—a process that continues throughout one's life (Kozier, Erb, & Blais, 1992; Lynn, McCain, & Boss, 1989). Socialization within advanced practice nursing can be conceptualized as three interlinked dimensions: professional socialization, organizational socialization, and role socialization. The development of the self underpins these dimensions; it is the driving force behind the synthesis of all socialization experiences in advanced practice nursing. Maximum effectiveness for advanced practice nurses (APNs) thus hinges on the development of the self.

Given the influx of master's-prepared APNs and the considerable experience with the role, rethinking how professional development can be pruned, shaped, and nourished is important. Shifting societal needs, increasingly complex patients, cost constraints, as well as actual and potential changes in healthcare delivery demand that APNs continually grow and integrate both the direct and the indirect care aspects of the role. Clinical expertise alone, although central to advanced practice nursing, is insufficient. Nursing's future healthcare delivery role in an increasingly competitive healthcare arena may well depend on the ongoing socialization of APNs.

This chapter examines the three dimensions of socialization within advanced practice nursing and the development of the personal self. It includes practical strategies for facilitating the socialization process and explores considerations that may further influence the personal and professional development of APNs.

Professional Socialization

Professional or occupational socialization is the complex process by which an individual acquires the skills, content, and sense of occupational identity characteristic of that profession. Fundamental to this process is the internalization of the profession's values, norms, and ethical standards into one's behavior and self-concept (Cohen, 1981). During professional socialization, novices must learn the technology and language of the profession, internalize the professional culture, find a personally and professionally acceptable version of the role, and integrate the professional role into all other life roles.

Each individual entering a nursing education program comes with personal values reflective of the individual's culture that frequently have influenced the choice of nursing as a profession (Kozier, Erb, & Blais, 1992; Watson, 1981). It is within this initial program that those values basic to the nursing professional are developed, clarified, and internalized. Altruism, equality, freedom, human dignity, justice, and truth are the values most often identified as essential to the practice of nursing (American Association of Colleges of Nursing, 1986; Elfrink & Lutz, 1991; Weis, Schank, Eddy, & Elfrink, 1993).

Socialization (or perhaps resocialization) at the master's level is crucial to the preservation and enrichment of these professional values for advanced nursing practice. The resocialization process denotes a continuum of steps that build on one another (Hinshaw, 1982; Malkemes, 1974) and is integral to graduate education. It is needed to help the student synthesize the changed theory base and new role expectations reflecting a redefined, internalized professional self-image. Resocialization forever alters the APN's sense of "what nursing is," but it contains elements of both the previous and the new conceptions (Leddy & Pepper, 1993).

Defining one's professional identity is a continuous and cumulative process in which interactions with reference groups play an essential part (Laing, 1993; Lum, 1988; Meleis, 1975). Reference groups provide an individual with a set of norms as well as values and a standard for the proper level of performance in a given role. They are "those groups whose perspectives constitute the frame of reference for the individual" (Lum, 1988, p. 257). Nurses within the work environment usually become the principal reference group for novices. Advanced practice nurses who are geographically isolated from other APNs oftentimes select physicians as their primary reference group. Although a reference group of APNs may become secondary or supplemental for these nurses, it remains essential to both their personal and professional development.

> By expanding into medicine, [APNs] will need, more than ever before, to increase [their] consciousness of what nursing is all about. The values of nursing must not get lost in the dominant medical culture. If they do, [APNs] justly risk the epithet of junior doctor[s]. (Bates, 1990, p. 139)

REVIEW OF THE LITERATURE

Most of the research on the socialization of nurses has focused on examining certain values and attitudes of graduating diploma, associate, and baccalaureate degree students or on measuring these same variables on a sample of nurses practicing in their first position. The resocialization of APNs is not as well described. Because of the lack of studies on the professional resocialization of clinical nurse specialists, however, research and nonresearch literature related chiefly to the nurse practitioner is included in this review.

Nursing advocates have tended to stress that the "right" personal characteristics augmented by the right educational preparation lead to an innovative and effective nurse practitioner with appropriately changed attitudes and knowledge (Davis & Olesen, 1972; Davis, Olesen, & Whittaker, 1966; Lurie, 1981; Malkemes, 1974; Oermann, 1991; Olesen & Whittaker, 1968; Simpson, 1972). Attributes such as assertiveness, independence, and decisiveness have been cited as essential for successful implementation of the nurse practitioner role (Baker, 1978; Editor, 1975; Moniz, 1978). White (1978) reported that effective nurse practitioners combine empathy, compassion, and assertion, as measured by their scores on Gough's California Psychological Inventory and Adjective Checklist. Nurse practitioners have also been found to be different from their nursing peers in that they are more self-reliant, aggressive, and competitive (Miller, 1977). In addition, "those who advocate placing nurse practitioner preparation at the graduate level emphasize that better educated nurses have different role orientations to their roles than those less well educated" (Lurie, 1981, p. 32). Better-educated nurses are less bureaucratic and more professional (Corwin, 1961; Oermann, 1991; Simpson & Simpson, 1969; Whelan, 1984), are better prepared to generalize from scientific bases in making decisions, and are better prepared to cope with uncertainty and to assume responsibility (Bucher & Stelling, 1977; Howell, 1978; Partridge, 1978; Zornow, 1977).

Beal, Maguire, and Carr (1996) surveyed 258 nationally certified neonatal nurse practitioners practicing in neonatal intensive care units across the United States to determine how they perceive their identity as APNs. Those neonatal nurse practitioners whose generic nursing education was at the master's level, who had been precepted by another neonatal nurse practitioner, who incorporated the institutional nursing philosophy into their practice, who belonged to a professional nursing organization, and who had a neonatal nurse practitioner role model were significantly more likely to have a stronger nursing identity.

A lack of confidence as well as hesitation in seeking increased responsibility and accountability have been identified as psychological barriers to the full enactment of the nurse practitioner role. Perhaps the most challenging psychological barrier facing the nurse practitioner is the insecurity that inevitably accompanies a major role change. It appears that nurse practitioners are meeting this challenge (Sullivan et al., 1978). In a national longitudinal cohort study of 497 primary care nurse practitioners and 407 of their employers, Sullivan and colleagues found that only 11.3% of the nurse practitioners and 10.3% of the employers identified "lack of confidence/willingness in taking on the responsibilities of the new role" (p. 1101) as a barrier to nurse practitioner role development. Furthermore, the reasons most frequently cited by nurse practitioners for selecting their present positions—role autonomy and a perception that the new setting offered a creative approach to healthcare delivery (Sultz, Zielenzy, Gentry, & Kinyon, 1978; 1980)—reflected a desire to maximize the potential of the new role. This finding is consistent with that of Lukacs (1982).

A study of 127 graduate students enrolled in a short-term medical nurse practitioner program between 1972 and 1976 and 31 of their physician counterparts also lends support to the assertion that nurse practitioners are overcoming psychological barriers to the role (Sullivan, 1978). Using the Edwards Personal Preference Schedule, Sullivan reported that the medical nurse practitioner students showed a noteworthy shift in identified personality needs. Whereas nurses have traditionally scored high on "order," "deference," and "endurance," the medical nurse practitioner students scored highest in the needs of "heterosexuality," "dominance," "intraception" (the need to examine one's own and others' motives), "change," and "achievement" (Sullivan, 1978, pp. 257–258). White (1975) has documented similar findings.

More recent studies of the professional socialization of APNs are noticeably absent. Longitudinal studies focusing on resocialization or perspective transformation need to extend beyond the graduate curriculum. Cutting off studies of resocialization at the point when APNs graduate from their educational programs is an arbitrary endpoint and neglects that professional socialization is a continuing, interactive, lifelong process. Resocialization is only begun in the graduate educational program, and to study it only within those boundaries is inappropriate.

The transformation process of a novice to a professional is essentially an acculturation process during which the values, norms, and symbols of the profession are internalized. Nursing education is accountable to the profession of nursing for the socialization of students into the values of the profession. "Without this initial socialization, there would be no professional at all" (Lurie, 1981, p. 46).

Organizational Socialization

When the new professional enters the workforce, another dimension of socialization occurs—organizational socialization. Organizational socialization is the process of learning what is important in an organization or a subsystem of that organization (Krcmar, 1991; Schein, 1968). The focus of this process is the interaction between a stable social system and the novice who enters the system (Krcmar, 1991). The organizational socialization new nurses and employees undergo forms the foundation for personal satisfaction and later allegiance to bureaucratic and professional standards (Ahmadi, Speedling, & Kuhn-Weissman, 1987).

On entering the work setting, novices must integrate professional beliefs acquired through education into a primarily bureaucratic setting (Hinshaw, 1982; Laing, 1993; Leddy & Pepper, 1993; Oermann, 1991). Because bureaucratic values are frequently inconsistent with professional ideals (Conway, 1983; Laing, 1993; Leddy & Pepper, 1993; Oermann, 1991), organizational socialization can result in "reality shock" (Ahmadi, Speedling, & Kuhn-Weissman, 1987; Kramer, 1974; Olsson & Gullberg, 1988). However, work setting is a powerful determinant of socialization because it is the source of one's income and social identity (Kozier, Erb, & Blais, 1992; Laing, 1993; Lum, 1988; Lurie, 1981).

Because APNs traditionally enact their role as employees in organized work settings, they are also faced with how to operationalize professional values in these settings and how to integrate into their behavior and values certain role expectations of the organizations. This issue has been labeled the professional–bureaucratic conflict (Ahmadi, Speedling, and Kuhn-Weissman, 1987; Hinshaw, 1982). The label acknowledges the existence of two dominant value systems that may require the APN to have two sets of behaviors (Hinshaw, 1982; Nyberg, 1994).

"It is not the expectation or the desire of either the profession or the work setting that professional values be changed to work–bureaucratic values" (Hinshaw, 1982, p. 31). Organizations employ APNs to use their acquired professional behaviors and standards. Concurrently, the nursing profession ensures quality by requiring that APNs have a commitment to the delivery of patient care based on its values and standards (Hinshaw, 1982; Nyberg, 1994). Thus, transition to one set of values is not a desired or an expected goal in the organizational socialization process. Resolution of value and role conflict instead must encompass an integration or adaptation of the professional and the bureaucratic value systems (Hinshaw, 1982; Nyberg, 1994).

The bureaucratic nature of work settings, however, has not always allowed nurses the opportunity or autonomy to maximize their impact on the system (Nyberg, 1994). Organizations must provide the potential for both autonomy and accountability to allow APNs to actualize their full potential. Autonomy implies independence and self-direction that will enable APNs to be accountable to both themselves and their patients without an intermediary (Conway, 1988; Hawkins & Thibodeau, 1993). Autonomy does not mean that APNs work in isolation without the benefit of consultation and collaboration from other healthcare professionals; rather, it means that they have the freedom to practice at the maximum potential permitted legally within the scope of their defined role (Conway, 1988; Hawkins & Thibodeau, 1993). Therefore,

> [advanced practice] nursing's maximum contribution . . . is dependent on . . . the organizational, legal, economic, social, and political arrangements that enable the full and proper expression of nursing values and expertise. (Styles, 1982, p. 213)

REVIEW OF THE LITERATURE

Most information on organizational socialization derives from studies of baccalaureate nursing graduates. There is, however, a dearth of literature on the organizational socialization of APNs. Some of these studies have identified organizational and structural characteristics of the practice setting that oppose maximum implementation of the advanced practice nursing role. Thus, this review primarily reflects the existing literature on variables in the practice setting that influence advanced nursing practice.

A major issue concerning the optimum performance of the clinical nurse specialist is placement in the employing agency's organizational structure. Variations of staff, line, project, and matrix placements have been described in the literature (Baird & Prouty, 1989; Blount et al., 1981; Crabtree, 1979; Fox, 1982). Although no consensus exists, authors seem to agree that the crucial point is that whatever model is used must be congruent with the goals of the organizational structure in which it is implemented, but must allow the clinical nurse specialist to move across traditional organizational lines.

Elements of the organization and structure of the healthcare system are also determinants of the employment and use of nurse practitioners. Bicknell, Walsh, and Tanner (1974) doubted whether physician assistants or nurse practitioners (terms they use interchangeably) could make a substantial contribution unless fundamental changes were made in the U.S. medical care system. Specific features of the American healthcare system, such as the fee-for-service payment structure, the emphasis on inpatient care, and the content of training programs, would militate against the effective use of nurse practitioners (Bicknell, Walsh, & Tanner, 1974). Berki (1972) also stated that "if there is any one issue relating to the introduction of [new types of health manpower] on which there is a degree of concensus, it is that both the mode of delivery and the organizational structure within which it takes place need to be altered if [new types of health manpower] are to be successfully integrated into [the practice setting]" (p. 118). The specific structural and organizational characteristics of individual delivery sites have also been recognized as critical factors in determining the ultimate success of the integration of the nurse practitioner role into a particular practice setting. Availability of examining rooms, clerical assistance, support personnel, office space, diagnostic and treatment equipment, colleague interaction, physician backup, and, of course, access to patients are required if the nurse practitioner is to practice efficiently and competently (Lewis, 1975; Sullivan et al., 1978).

"Of all the changes that must occur before the system fully incorporates the nurse practitioner, perhaps the most obvious will be the ones in the structure and organization of individual practice settings within the healthcare system" (Sullivan et al., 1978, p. 1102). In a study of barriers to the development of the nurse practitioner role in primary care, Sullivan and colleagues (1978) found that legal restrictions, limitations of space and facilities, and resistance from other providers were identified as barriers by 20% or more of the 497 nurse practitioners and 407 of their employers. Furthermore, 7 of the 15 specific barriers identified by nurse practitioners and employers were to some extent related to the physical structure or organization of the practice setting. Of these, "limitations of space and/or facilities" was the most frequently reported barrier by both the primary care nurse practitioners and their employers (Sullivan et al., 1978, p. 1100). Sullivan and colleagues (1978) asserted that nurse practitioners more frequently cited specific barriers within this group because their practice is most directly thwarted by these particular structural or organizational inadequacies.

Other impediments to APN practice that have historical precedence are the issues of prescriptive authority and third-party reimbursement. Some studies suggest that restrictive laws and regulations represent barriers to nurse practitioners' being full participants in the healthcare environment. Eliminating restrictions to allow nurse practitioners to practice at their full potential would alleviate many problems of access to primary care services (Burns

& Nochajski, 1995; Sekscenski, 1994; Straub & Pan, 1996). At the state level, scope of practice, including prescriptive authority, is the paramount issue (Osterweis & Garfinkel, 1993). Pan, Straub, and Geller (1997) analyzed the impacts of a restrictive environment on a nurse practitioner's level of authority with respect to prescribing selected categories of medications. Their analysis indicates that practice restrictiveness was the most significant independent variable related to the variation in nurse practitioner levels of prescriptive autonomy.

Lurie (1981) examined the relationship of socialization to role content, change in role attitudes and role behaviors over time, and working relationships for non–master's-prepared graduates of the University of California Adult Health Nurse Practitioner Program. She found that the socialization in training and that occurring in the work setting in enactment of the nurse practitioner role resulted in the practice of clinical assessment and management skills on which both agents of socialization were consistent. But in regard to other skills, attitudes, and expectations (e.g., patient education and counseling, expectations for collegial relations with physicians, and supportive behaviors from other nurses and healthcare professionals), the socialization received in training conflicted with socialization in the work setting (Lurie, 1981). In the areas of patient education and counseling, Lurie reported that the nurse practitioners could negotiate to practice in accord with their earlier socialization. "But practitioners were not able to change the work setting sufficiently to replicate the socialization model of their training" (p. 31). She concluded that professional socialization is therefore a two-step process in which the skills and values acquired in training must be adjusted to the demands of the work setting.

In addition, organizational socialization and role development are enhanced if role models are available and if the APN seeks out and uses these resources (Krcmar, 1991). "The period of organizational entry [a stage of organizational socialization] takes longer, involves more negatives of organizational socialization, and has a greater impact on role development for the new clinical nurse specialist than for an experienced clinical nurse specialist entering a new organization" (Krcmar, 1991, p. 38). Learning the politics of the system, having an administrator willing to share knowledge of the system, and having peer support have been noted as facilitators to role development for both novices and experienced clinical nurse specialists (Hamric & Taylor, 1989).

The organizational socialization of APNs has received little research consideration, but has significant relevance to further development of the APN role. Attention has been directed to such influential factors as the history of the practice unit, scope of the extended role, patient load, nature of physician backup, and levels of satisfaction with the nurse practitioner as the primary provider. Although other factors thought to affect APN performance, such as organizational structures and barriers, economic issues in primary care, and psychological variables, have been touched on in the literature, they continue to warrant further investigation.

Organizational socialization is the process of operationalizing or integrating the values and behaviors of both the professional and the bureaucratic work systems (Hinshaw, 1982). It is a specific dimension of socialization, distinct from but not independent of socialization in general. Today, APNs function in complex systems dealing with social, economic, ethical, professional, legal, and regulatory incentives and constraints. Each of these forces can become an obstacle to fully actualizing the APN role.

> We must now systematically begin to address those barriers in our system[s] that have hindered both the training and the autonomous practice of [APNs]. We must strive to provide appropriate regulatory flexibility to ensure that those professionals who desire to practice autonomously, whether in hospitals or birthing centers, or on an outpatient basis, can in fact do so. We must ensure that those [APNs] . . . possess viable career and reimbursement mechanisms to enhance their productivity and professionalism. (Kalisch & Kalisch, 1982, p. ix)

Role Socialization

It is through yet another dimension of socialization that one learns how to perform in a certain role, be it marital, parental, or occupational. Role socialization is described as "the training and preparation for the performance of specific tasks" (Hurley-Wilson, 1988, p. 107). It occurs through two simultaneous interactional and learning processes (Cason & Beck, 1982; Hurley-Wilson, 1988; Laing, 1993; Oermann, 1991). These processes involve multiple agents of socialization, such as one's family, peers, educators, role models, and the media.

The role socialization or role development of APNs occurs in two phases. Initial role socialization occurs during graduate nursing education and is followed by role socialization in the practice setting (Holt, 1984; Laing, 1993). Indeed, role socialization may occur more through "tacit knowledge" assimilated through work experience than through formal training (Olsson & Gullberg, 1987, 1988). V. E. Baker (1971) has identified the importance of learning the role of the APN through socialization and emphasized the need to interact with a role model in the work environment to enhance role development.

REVIEW OF THE LITERATURE

The role socialization of APNs has been the theme of little research. Information, however, has been generated related to the role and function of APNs. Thus, because of space limitation, this review comprises only the most recent literature on the role socialization of APNs and the perceptions of the role.

A number of investigators have examined what perceptions clinical nurse specialists, nurse educators, and administrators have of the role and its components. In a study examining the role expectations of students and nursing colleagues, Cason and Beck (1982) surveyed 18 practicing clinical nurse specialists, 29 graduate students, 11 faculty members, and 22 nursing service administrators for their perceptions of the role. They found that the dimensions of the role deemed important by these groups were as follows: acting from a knowledge base in a clinical specialty area, performing clinical skills competently, using a systematic approach to problem solving, promoting self-care through patient education, and collaborating with others to provide quality care. Cason and Beck also noted that there was a greater level of agreement regarding perceptions of the role between practicing clinical nurse specialists and nursing service administrators than between clinical nurse specialists and graduate faculty who were preparing students for this role.

Tarsitano, Brophy, and Snyder (1986) investigated the similarities and differences between nurse administrators and clinical nurse specialists regarding the importance of four components (clinical practice, education, administration, and research) of the clinical nurse specialist role. Using the Clifford Clinical Specialist Functions Inventory, they surveyed 54 nurse administrators and 35 clinical nurse specialists from a large metropolitan area and reported that both groups agreed on the relative importance of the components, except for research. The nurse administrators placed a higher value on the research component than did the clinical nurse specialists. Although the nurse administrators and clinical nurse specialists valued the administration role component least, both groups highly valued the consultant, education, and clinical practice components. The clinical nurse specialists, however, saw themselves as more heavily committed to direct specialized patient care than did the nurse administrators. In a study to determine the essential competency behaviors for the clinical nurse specialist role as perceived by nurse administrators, graduate nurse educators, and clinical nurse specialists, it was reported that developing an in-depth knowledge base, serving as a role model, and demonstrating clinical expertise in a selected area of clinical practice were considered the most important behaviors in the clinical nurse specialist role by all three groups (Wyers, Grove, & Pastorino, 1985).

In her landmark research, Benner (1984) identified seven domains of nursing practice that describe the clinical judgment process of expert clinicians in acute-care settings (see Table 3-1). Using Benner's approach, Fenton (1985) and Brykczynski (1985, 1989) identified the clinical competencies and skilled performance of master's-prepared clinical nurse specialists and nurse practitioners functioning in the role, respectively. Fenton and Brykczynski (1993) then compared the results of their two studies.

Fenton found that the clinical nurse specialists reported and demonstrated activities in all of Benner's (1984) areas of skilled performance, particularly in the domains of "the helping role" and "organizational and work-role competencies." A new domain, The "consulting role," was also identified as valid for the practice of clinical nurse specialist. Brykczynski (1985, 1989) identified one new domain that was interpreted as more characteristic of nurse practitioner practice. This domain, "management of patient health/illness status in ambulatory care settings," consolidates and replaces two of Benner's (1984) domains that were more typical of hospital nursing practice, namely "the diagnostic and patient-monitoring function" and "administering and monitoring therapeutic interventions and regimens." Four of the seven domains of nursing practice identified by Benner were interpreted as valid for the practice of nurse practitioners with minimal change: (1) monitoring and ensuring the quality of healthcare practices, (2) organizational and work-role competencies, (3) the helping role, and (4) the teaching–coaching function (Brykczynski, 1985, 1989; Faculty, 1993).

Brykczynski also reported that there were limited data relative to the domain "effective management of rapidly changing situations." The nurse practitioners were more health-oriented whereas clinical specialists focused more on illness. Clinical specialists were responsible for promoting the overall functions of the organization whereas the nurse practitioners focused on the patient. Lindeke, Canedy, and Kay (1997) cited similar findings.

A national survey of 94 graduate-level adult nurse practitioner students in their final semester was undertaken to determine if they were being socialized into the role of a master's-prepared nurse practitioner and to identify factors that may influence this socialization process (Hupcey, 1990). This study revealed that factors relating to the students' backgrounds (e.g., gender, age, highest nursing degree, years of nursing experience) did not significantly influence the students' expectations of nurse practitioner role behaviors. Lurie's (1981) study of non–master's-prepared nurse practitioner students also documented similar findings. The educational factor "opportunity to practice role behaviors," however, statistically increased the expectations for selected master's role behaviors, suggesting that students need the opportunity to practice role behaviors to enhance the so-

 TABLE 3-1 *Domains of Nursing Practice*

- The Helping Role
- The Teaching–Coaching Function
- The Diagnostic and Patient-monitoring Function
- Effective Management of Rapidly Changing Situations
- Administrating and Monitoring Therapeutic Interventions and Regimens
- Monitoring and Ensuring the Quality of Healthcare Practices
- Organizational and Work-role Competencies

From: *From novice to expert: Excellence and power in clinical nursing practice* (p. 46) by P. Benner, 1984, Menlo Park, CA: Addison-Wesley. Copyright 1984 by Addison-Wesley. Reprinted with permission.

cialization process (Hupcey, 1990, p. 196). Furthermore, the students placed significantly greater importance on technical-level instead of master's-level role behaviors.

In a separate study, Hupcey (1994) compared both actual and ideal role behaviors of master's-prepared and non–master's-prepared nurse practitioners and found no significant difference between the actual role behaviors of the two groups. The non–master's-prepared nurse practitioners consistently rated their ideal role behaviors higher than the master's-prepared nurse practitioners. Both groups of nurse practitioners also felt that their role placed greater emphasis on the technical-level versus the master's-level role behaviors. Hupcey (1990, 1994) thus concluded that graduate students may be inadequately socialized into the master's-prepared nurse practitioner role.

Elder and Bullough (1990) surveyed graduates from the master of science program in the School of Nursing, State University of New York at Buffalo. They asked 28 clinical nurse specialist and 46 nurse practitioner alumni of the most recent decade (1977–1987) about their current role functioning; satisfaction with their work and career choice; and opinions about various professional issues, including the merging of the two roles. The most impressive finding was the large number of overlapping activities and opinions of the graduates actually functioning in the clinical role. "Although differences in traditional areas associated with the two groups were noted, they were not nearly as large as the literature suggests" (Elder & Bollough, 1990, p. 78). The majority of the graduates also supported the merging of clinical nurse specialist and nurse practitioner preparation.

The American Nurses' Association Council of Clinical Nurse Specialists and Council of Primary Health Care Nurse Practitioners conducted a survey of all U.S. graduate nursing programs that prepare clinical nurse specialists or nurse practitioners (Forbes, Rafson, Spross, & Kozlowski, 1990). For the 195 clinical nurse specialist and the 60 nurse practitioner programs analyzed, information was obtained on the following: required courses, mean number of hours of the required courses, students' clinical practicum sites, and graduates' employment settings. Forbes and colleagues reported a marked similarity between the core curricula of clinical nurse specialist and nurse practitioner graduate programs. The only significant differences found were that nurse practitioner program curricula placed greater emphasis on pharmacology, primary care, physical assessment, health promotion, nutrition, and history taking (Forbes, Rafson, Spross, & Kozlowski, 1990). Furthermore, in both the student clinical sites and the graduate employment settings, nurse practitioners practiced chiefly in primary care settings whereas clinical nurse specialists practiced mainly in secondary or tertiary care settings (Forbes, Rafson, Spross, & Kozlowski, 1990).

Empirical studies on the role of APNs have typically examined the role behaviors in terms of medical tasks and behaviors. Although the majority of these studies have offered evidence that APNs provide safe and effective healthcare, they have not helped to define advanced practice nursing. Although additional research is needed to demonstrate the effectiveness of the APN, future studies related to the role should focus on the APN's functions (Naylor & Brooten, 1993). This research will play a significant role in distinguishing the unique services provided by APNs to different patient groups as well as the unique knowledge and skills required by APNs to meet the complex needs of vulnerable populations (Naylor & Brooten, 1993).

MODEL FOR ADVANCED PRACTICE NURSING

Implementing the APN role is a formidable challenge. Not only is the role of the nurse in advanced practice not entirely understood, but APNs are not always clear about their role (Editor, 1975). The APN role encompasses a number of direct and indirect care aspects. Identifying the competencies inherent to these care aspects can be helpful in analyzing advanced practice nursing. Although the specific practice setting influences the competencies that the APN must possess, the domains and competencies of nursing practice, as described by Benner (1984) and expanded by Fenton (1985) and Brykczynski (1985, 1989), can serve as an organizing framework for advanced practice (see Table 3-2). Advanced practice nurses can further Brykczynski's (1985; 1989) work by identifying as well as validating new domains and competencies and by refining those that have practical worth.

ROLE DEVELOPMENT OF ADVANCED PRACTICE NURSES

Advanced practice nurses prepared at the graduate level provide direct patient care in addition to indirect roles including those of educator, administrator, consultant, and researcher (Hamric, 1989; Price et al., 1992). Neither a new master's degree graduate nor a new reequipped APN can be expected to have expertise in each of these components (Holt, 1984, p. 447).

Graduate nursing education provides the academic preparation and the tools for role development in these areas (Holt, 1984, p. 447). Further development of skill in these role components, however, must also come in the practice setting following graduation (Holt, 1984, p. 447; Ryan-Merritt, Mitchell, & Pagel, 1988; Sparacino, 1990).

Several models have been developed to explain the process of socialization in professional roles. The Dreyfus model of skill acquisition is based on a study of chess players and airline pilots (Dreyfus & Dreyfus, 1980). Benner (1984) has used this model to describe the progression of skills and the competency of the staff nurse in the clinical setting. The five levels of the Dreyfus model of skill acquisition are (1) novice, (2) advanced beginner, (3) competent, (4) proficient, and (5) expert. Using this model, as applied to the nursing profession by Benner, Table 3-3 explores the transition of the APN from novice to expert practitioner, which is based on the chapter author's personal experience.

The transformation from nurse to nurse practitioner is often associated with insecurity and anxiety (Lukacs, 1982; Sullivan et al., 1978). New nurse practitioners fear incompetent performance, worry about their relationship with other healthcare providers, and struggle to avoid unconscious participation in "doctor–nurse" games (Katzman & Roberts, 1988; Lukacs, 1982; Stein, Watts, & Howell, 1990; Sullivan et al., 1978). They must also learn to delegate and to feel comfortable in not performing direct patient care. It is a precarious period of uncertain professional identity during which the novice nurse practitioner is particularly vulnerable to role challenges from other nurses, physicians, and patients (Bass, Rabbett, & Siskind, 1993; Hawkins & Thibodeau, 1993; Katzman & Roberts, 1988; Lukacs, 1982; Lurie, 1981; Sullivan et al., 1978). Confronted with the psychological barriers instilled and reinforced during past education and practice experience, the nurse practitioner must overcome nonassertive behaviors to assume the role of a decision maker and diagnostician and to become an autonomous, capable, responsible, and accountable professional (Baker, 1978; Katzman & Roberts, 1988; Lukacs, 1982; Sullivan et al., 1978).

Progression through the five stages of skill acquisition varies from APN to APN. Individual differences in the potential and the experience background of APNs, as well as the uniqueness of each practice setting, will affect their developmental patterns (Holt, 1984). Because experienced and newly reequipped APNs possess a repertoire of clinical paradigms, their transition from novice to expert practitioner may indeed be expedited. In addition, changing positions or areas of specialization returns even an experienced APN to an apprentice level (Arena & Page, 1992). Nevertheless, no one prevents APNs from reaching the expert level of development except themselves.

Role socialization, the process of learning specific skills (Hurley-Wilson, 1988), depends on the professional and the organizational dimensions of socialization as well as on the development of the personal self. The socialization or development of the APN role is characterized by continued defining, refining, and refocusing (Hamric & Taylor, 1989). It is imperative that role development be an ongoing, dynamic process for the APN to be

TABLE 3-2 ***Domains and Competencies of Nurse Practitioner Practice***

Domain	Area of Skilled Practice
Domain 1. Management of Patient Health/Illness in Ambulatory Care Settings	1. Assessing, monitoring, coordinating, and managing the health status of patients over time: a primary care provider[†] 2. Detecting acute and chronic diseases while attending to the experience of illness[†] 3. Providing anticipatory guidance for expected changes, potential changes, and situational changes[†] 4. Building and maintaining a supportive and caring attitude toward patients[†] 5. Scheduling follow-up visits to closely monitor patients in uncertain situations[†] 6. Selecting and recommending appropriate diagnostic and therapeutic interventions and regimens with attention to safety, cost, invasiveness, simplicity, acceptability, and efficacy[†]

Domain 2. Monitoring and Ensuring the Quality of Healthcare Practices	1. Providing a back-up system to ensure safe medical and nursing care
	   • Developing fail-safe strategies when concerns arise over physician consultation[†]
	 2. Assessing what can be safely omitted from or added to medical orders
	 3. Getting appropriate and timely responses from physicians
	   • Using physician consultation effectively[†]
	 4. Self-monitoring and seeking consultation as necessary[†]
	 5. Giving constructive feedback to physicians and other care providers to ensure safe care practices[†]

Domain 3. Organizational and Work-role Competencies	1. Coordinating, ordering, and meeting multiple patient needs and requests; setting priorities
	 2. Building and maintaining a therapeutic team to provide optimum therapy
	 3. Coping with staff shortages and high turnover:
	   • Contingency planning
	   • Anticipating and preventing periods of extreme work overload
	   • Using and maintaining team spirit; gaining social support from other nurses
	   • Maintaining a flexible stance toward patients, technology, and bureaucracy
	 4. Making the bureaucracy respond to patients' and families' needs[§]
	 5. Obtaining specialist care for patients while remaining the primary care provider[†]

Domain 4. Helping Role of the Nurse	1. Healing relationship: Creating a climate for and establishing a commitment to healing 2. Providing comfort measures and preserving personhood in the face of extreme breakdown 3. Presencing: Being with a patient 4. Maximizing the patient's participation and control in his or her own health/illness care[‡] 5. Interpreting kinds of pain and selecting appropriate strategies for pain management and pain control

TABLE 3-2 *Domains and Competencies of Nurse Practitioner Practice* (Continued)

Domain	Area of Skilled Practice
	6. Providing comfort and communication through touch
	7. Providing emotional and informational support to patients' families
	8. Guiding a patient through emotional and developmental change
	• Providing new options, closing off old ones
	• Channeling, teaching, mediating
	• Acting as a psychological and cultural mediator
	• Using goals therapeutically
	• Working to build and maintain a therapeutic community
Domain 5. Teaching–Coaching Function of the Nurse	1. Timing: Capturing a patient's readiness to learn • Motivating a patient to change[†]
	2. Assisting patients to integrate the implications of their illness and recovery into their lifestyle
	3. Assisting patients to alter their lifestyle to meet changing healthcare needs and capacities: Teaching for self-care[†]
	4. Eliciting an understanding of the patient's interpretation of his or her illness • Negotiating agreement about how to proceed when priorities of patient and provider conflict[†]
	5. Providing an interpretation of the patient's condition and giving a rationale for procedures
	6. Coaching function: Making culturally avoided and uncharted health and illness experiences approachable and understandable[‡]
Domain 6. Effective Management of Rapidly Changing Situations	1. Skilled performance in extreme life-threatening emergencies: Rapid grasp of a problem
	2. Contingency management: Rapid matching of demands and resources in emergency situations
	3. Identifying and managing a patient crisis until physician assistance is available

*Areas of skilled practice are adapted from Benner (1984) unless otherwise noted.
  [†]Domain and competencies identified in Brykczynski (1985).
  [‡]Competency expanded in Brykczynski (1985).
  [§]Competency identified by Fenton (1985). From: "An interpretive study describing the clinical judgement of nurse practitioners" by K. A. Brykczynski, 1989, *Scholarly Inquiry for Nursing Practice: An International Journal, 3*(2), pp. 90–91. Copyright 1989 by Springer. Reprinted with permission.

fully effective (Hamric & Taylor, 1989, p. 81). Truly, there is no shortcut in role development. By using an organizing framework for advanced practice, however, APNs can locate as well as evaluate where they are in the role development process and readily identify directions for further implementation.

Development of the Personal Self

The development of the personal self is taking time to "sharpen the saw" (Covey, 1989, p. 287). It is preserving and enhancing the greatest asset one has: one's self (Covey, 1989). The development of the personal self (or self-nurturing) underpins the three dimensions

TABLE 3-3 ***Characteristics of Performance from Novice to Expert Practitioner***

Novice	Advanced Beginner	Competent	Proficient	Expert
• Has a narrow scope of practice • Develops diagnostic reasoning and clinical decision-making skills • Needs frequent consultation and validation of clinical skills • Needs and identifies mentor • Establishes credibility • Develops confidence	• Enhances clinical competence in weak areas • Enhances diagnostic reasoning and clinical decision-making skills • Begins to develop the educator and the consultant roles • Incorporates research findings into practice • Sets priorities • Develops a reference group • Builds confidence	• Has an expanded scope of practice • Feels competent in diagnostic reasoning and clinical decision-making skills • Begins to develop administrator role • Develops organizational skills • Views situations in multifaceted ways • Senses nuances • Relies on maxims to guide practice • Feels efficient and organized • Networks	• Incorporates direct and indirect role activities into daily practice • Enhances clinical expertise • Conducts or directs research projects • Is an effective change agent • Uses holistic approach to care • Interprets nuances	• Has a global scope of practice • Cohesively integrates direct and indirect roles • Has an intuitive grasp • Has a greater sense of salience • Is a reflective practitioner • Empowers patients, families, and colleagues • Serves as a role model and mentor

of socialization within advanced practice nursing because it is the driving force that makes all the others possible.

The self is a concept of one's own person as distinguished from other objects in the external world. It is one's concept of self as a separate, whole person. The self includes individuals' appraisals of themselves as well as the appraisals others make of them. The self is never constant; it is forever changing and emerging in new ways. The emergence of self is influenced by interactions with others as well as by interactions with one's environment (Leddy & Pepper, 1993; Stuart & Sundeen, 1995).

The professional self-system emerges from the personal self (Leddy & Pepper, 1993). One's self-concept "results from previous interpersonal relationships" and affects one's future relationships (Simms & Lindberg, 1978, p. 9). "A person's view of self controls the roles he or she will be able to assume" (Simms & Lindberg, 1978, p. 9). One's self-system determines one's personal characteristics, and these personal qualities enable one to carry out professional roles (Leddy & Pepper, 1993). An individual's self-concept can, therefore, serve either as a barrier or a support for his or her professional self.

"Strength derives from a strong self-concept" (Hawkins & Thibodeau, 1993, p. 57). A strong self-concept can be linked to motivation and success in one's career (Hawkins &

Thibodeau, 1993). Horner (1975) found that women exhibit a need to avoid success. The most competent women, "when faced with a conflict between their feminine image and expressing their competencies or developing their abilities and interests, adjust their behaviors to their internalized sex-role stereotypes" (Horner, 1975, p. 219). Sex-role stereotypes convey messages that say that women are poor decision makers and are unable to assume leadership roles (Broverman et al., 1975; Edmunds, 1980; Hawkins & Thibodeau, 1993; Katzman & Roberts, 1988; Stein, Watts, & Howell, 1990). Such messages weaken women's self-concept, planting seeds of doubt about their ability to use their strength and power (Hawkins & Thibodeau, 1993; Katzman & Roberts, 1988; Stein, Watts, & Howell, 1990). Knowledge about sex-role stereotyping and the effects it has on self-concept can assist APNs to develop strategies for gaining influence in their clinical settings.

Simms and Lindberg (1978) validated that the professional self directly reflects the personal self-concept. "Responsibility for our own acts—especially toward others—will flourish in an environment which fosters growth of self and independence" (Simms & Lindberg, 1978, p. 7). "Understanding self and working to view self positively inevitable leads to more productive professional self-concepts. Negative self-concepts are barriers to the effective independent functioning vital to the successful performance of professional roles" (Leddy & Pepper, 1993, p. 67).

Self-nurturing and self-esteem are thus "necessary partners" (Bunkers, 1992, p. 155). "To feel good about themselves, [APNs] need to develop the ability to take care of themselves. At the same time, to take good care of their physical, emotional, mental, and spiritual selves, [APNs] need to feel that they are worthwhile" (p. 155). If self-nurturing is absent or deficient, self-esteem is lowered; if self-nurturing is balanced, self-esteem is raised (Bunkers, 1992, p. 155).

To a great extent, the kind of professional an individual becomes depends on the individual's self-system (Leddy & Pepper, 1993). The development of the personal self—or self-nurturing—is the single most powerful investment APNs can ever make in life: investment in themselves (Covey, 1989). "Being able to care for others, to connect with others in a meaningful way, depends fundamentally on caring for one's Self" (Chinn, 1991, p. 255). The things APNs do to "sharpen the saw" will have a positive impact on the professional, organizational, and role dimensions of socialization. The development of the personal self empowers APNs to move on an upward spiral of growth and change—of continuous improvement.

Socialization Strategies

Socialization within advanced practice nursing is a continuously evolving process that demands both time and energy. By employing proactive behaviors, APNs cannot only enhance this process but can also make it easier and less overwhelming. Thus, some practical strategies for facilitating socialization within advanced practice nursing are included in the following summary:

1. Trust your own intuitive processes.
2. Maintain your sense of humor.
3. Cultivate supportive, collegial relationships.
4. Invest your time wisely.
5. Keep abreast of local, regional, and national legislative, regulatory, and health policy issues.
6. Develop a personal mission statement and job (position) description. A considered mission statement can guide your job search. The purpose of a job description is to clarify your scope of practice and expectations of a professional position.

7. Conduct an organizational analysis. The organizational analysis enables you to understand complex systems and gives you the skills necessary to function more effectively within them (Conway, 1988; Reddecliff, Smith, & Ryan-Merritt, 1989).

8. Identify a suitable mentor. Mentorship is an intense, career-building, mutually beneficial relationship between two individuals of unequal power in an organization (Hawkins & Thibodeau, 1993; Stewart & Krueger, 1996; Yoder, 1994). Mentors serve as wellsprings of information and support. Review of the literature on the subject yields a number of tips that can be useful in choosing a mentor (Hawkins & Thibodeau, 1993; Stewart & Krueger, 1996; Yoder, 1994) (see Table 3-4). However, if a compatible individual is not readily available, networks and reference groups can also serve as mentors.

9. Continually articulate and clarify your advanced practice role to patients, families, colleagues, and the public.

10. Keep the ambiguities of your practice setting in perspective.

11. Honor your commitment to lifelong learning.

12. Develop meaning and purpose in life (Bunkers, 1992).

13. Nurture yourself without feeling guilty or selfish.

14. Take responsibility for generating satisfaction from your job and actively plan to do so without expecting the job or system to supply it.

15. Use "personal planning skills" (Davidhizar, 1994, p. 11).

16. Try to let go of the need to have all household work done a certain way.

17. Develop yearly, measurable objectives, including an implementation and an evaluation plan.

18. Conduct a periodic self-assessment of your development in the advanced practice role. You should also have a growth plan to assure continued renewal and to prevent fixation at any developmental stage.

19. Be assertive.

TABLE 3-4 *Tips for Choosing a Mentor*

A potential mentor should be:

- an individual whose company you enjoy
- an individual who is neither your direct supervisor nor a close personal friend
- an individual with whom you can communicate
- an individual who is trustworthy
- an individual who has the ability to teach and motivate you
- an individual who is respected in the area of your particular interest and in the organization
- an individual who has proven power and influence
- an individual who has confidence in his or her abilities
- an individual who is happy with his or her own career success
- an individual who is 8 to 15 years older than you
- an individual who is accessible
- an individual with whom you believe you have congruent career and life goals
- an individual who has the ability to role model
- an individual who has organizational savvy
- an individual who is ambitious

20. Recognize and deal with your own grief and loss (Bunkers, 1992).

21. Integrate continuous quality improvement (CQI) into your clinical practice.

22. Schedule weekly or biweekly meetings for direct consultation with your mentor.

Socialization within advanced practice nursing can be simultaneously frustrating and rewarding, requiring flexibility as well as determination. This summary outlines some concrete suggestions that can aid in expediting the socialization process. Furthermore, APNs can incorporate these strategies into their practice regardless of their work environment.

Considerations

Advanced practice nurses are facing countless challenges and changes as the 21st century approaches. The utmost challenge for APNs, however, will be to avoid hasty compromises in meeting future needs and to carefully plan as well as design the future role they will play (Hein & Nicholson, 1994; Price et al., 1992). The following considerations, although merely speculative, reflect the chapter author's futuristic view of advanced practice nursing.

Independent, autonomous practice will characterize nursing's role in meeting patients' increasingly complex psychological, physiologic, and social needs. Advanced practice nurses will develop sound interpersonal relationships to successfully negotiate with multidisciplinary team members for collaboration and cooperation in providing healthcare. As APNs continue to demonstrate their knowledge, competence, and skills, referrals between APNs and other healthcare professionals will increase. In addition, prescriptive authority by APNs will move beyond the currently existing pharmacologic protocols (Keane, Richmond, & Kaiser, 1994).

Nursing will continue to witness a trend toward the granting of hospital privileges to APNs who are functioning as primary healthcare providers in private practice. Privileges will enable them to not only provide clinically expert care in a holistic manner, but to also provide the link of continuity in a system that is often typified by fragmentation and impersonalization (Hayden & Rowell, 1982; Keane & Richmond, 1993). More liberal reimbursement benefits and consumer choice will lead to the spread of APNs into independent entrepreneurships: delivering healthcare to defined populations, operating managed care facilities, consulting, and creating group practice arrangements.

The movement of APNs into acute care settings will flourish. In light of future predictions for nursing (educational and hospital distribution of nurses), graduates with associate degrees will implement the plan of care developed by the APN and the multidisciplinary health team. Although APNs clearly provide quality and cost-effective care in a variety of clinical sites (Aiken, Lake, & Semaan, 1993; Brooten et al., 1986; Daly, Rudy, Thompson, & Happ, 1991; Naylor, 1990; Office of Technology Assessment, 1986; Safriet, 1992), additional research to evaluate their efficacy and acceptability in specialty areas will be essential (Keane, Richmond, & Kaiser, 1994).

The increase in chronic illnesses and an aging population will lead to greater involvement of APNs in the long-term care of older adults in various stages along the health continuum. Advanced practice nurses will care for patients in their homes, businesses, corporations, schools, churches, ambulatory health clinics, nursing homes, hospitals, hospices, health maintenance organizations, planned communities, day care centers, wellness centers, and other extended care facilities. The shifting of more APNs into these practice settings will expand patients' options for care and will also enrich the services they receive (Clochesy et al., 1994; Keane, Richmond, & Kaiser, 1994).

In addition, the importance of research to the practice and to the role of the nurse in advanced practice will be well integrated into the APN's professional value system. Advanced practice nurses will acquire the skills to conduct research through continuance of their formal education and through participation, at some level, in the research process

(Hawkins & Thibodeau, 1993). They will also prove to be knowledgeable consumers of the research generated by others and will be leaders in developing innovative ways to provide quality care in restoring, promoting, and maintaining health.

Innumerable forces at play are likely to dramatically change the shape and delivery of healthcare. "Although it is probably presumptuous to offer predictions of nursing's future, [APNs] will be better prepared to move into the next century if [they] are informed about the past, have analyzed the present, and have formed visions for the future" (Chinn, 1991, p. 251; Chinn, 1994, p. 429). Now is the time for APNs to begin to picture what their future in nursing might be like and to begin to make it happen by resolving first to improve their own personal and professional development (Chinn, 1991, p. 256; Chinn, 1994, p. 437).

Overall, socialization is a continuous and cumulative process that has significant implications for the development of APNs. It is essential that preparation for advanced practice nursing be at the master's level, facilitating a professional collegial identity (Billingsley & Harper, 1982). Graduate nursing education provides APNs with a solid foundation for advanced nursing practice. The foundation, although solid, is only a beginning. To be responsive to society's changing needs and to maintain a pivotal role in future healthcare delivery, APNs must continually strive to grow and develop. Graduate curricula can well serve both the public and the profession by instilling in APNs the belief in, as well as a desire for, constant evolution in all aspects of advanced practice nursing (Keane & Richmond, 1993).

REFERENCES

Ahmadi, K. S., Speedling, E. J., & Kuhn-Weissman, G. (1987). The newly hired hospital staff nurse's professionalism, satisfaction and alienation. *International Journal of Nursing Studies 24*(2), 107–121.

Aiken, L. H., Lake, E. T., Semaan, S., et al. (1993). Nurse practitioner managed care for persons with HIV infection. *Image: Journal of Nursing Scholarship 25*(3), 172–177.

American Association of Colleges of Nursing. (1986). *Essentials of college and university education for professional nursing.* Washington, DC: Author.

Arena, D. M., & Page, N. E. (1992). The imposter phenomenon in the clinical nurse specialist role. *Image: Journal of Nursing Scholarship 24*(2), 121–125.

Baird, S. B., & Prouty, M. P. (1989). Administratively enhancing CNS contributions. In A. B. Hamric & J. A. Spross (Eds.). *The clinical nurse specialist in theory and practice* (2nd ed., pp. 261–283). Philadelphia: W. B. Saunders.

Baker, B. A. (1978). The assertive nurse practitioner. *Nurse Practitioner 3*(2), 23, 45.

Baker, V. E. (1971). Retrospective explorations in role development (G. V. Padilla & G. J. Padilla, eds.). *Nursing Digest 6*(4), 56–63.

Bass, M., Rabbett, P. M., & Siskind, M. M. (1993). Novice CNS and role acquisition. *Clinical Nurse Specialist, 7*(3), 148–152.

Bates, B. (1990). Twelve paradoxes: A message for nurse practitioners. *Journal of the American Academy of Nurse Practitioners 2*(4), 136–139.

Beal, J. A., Maguire, D., & Carr, R. (1996). Neonatal nurse practitioners: Identity as advanced practice nurses. *Journal of Gynecologic, Obstetric and Neonatal Nursing 25*(5), 401–06.

Benner, P. (1984). *From novice to expert: Excellence and power in clinical nursing practice.* Menlo Park, CA: Addison-Wesley.

Berki, S. E. (1972). The economics of new types of health personnel. In V. W. Lippard & E. F. Purcell (Eds.). *Intermediate-level health practitioners* (pp. 104–134). New York: Josiah Macy.

Bicknell, W. J., Walsh, D. C., & Tanner, M. M. (1974). Substantial or decorative? Physicians' assistants and nurse practitioners in the United States. *Lancet 2*(7891), 1241–1244.

Billingsley, M. C., & Harper, D. C. (1982). The extinction of the nurse practitioner: Threat or reality? *Nurse Practitioner 7*(9), 22–23, 26–27, 30.

Blount, M., Burge, S., Crigler, L., et al. (1981). Extending the influence of the clinical nurse specialist. *Nursing Administration Quarterly 6*(1), 53–63.

Brooten, D., Kumar, S., Brown, L. P., et al. (1986). A randomized clinical trial of early hospital discharge and home follow-up of very low-birthweight infants. *New England Journal of Medicine 315*(15), 934–939.

Broverman, I. K., Vogel, S. R., Broverman, D. M., et al. (1975). Sex-role stereotypes: A current appraisal. In M.T.S. Mednick, S. S. Tangri, & L. W. Hoffman (Eds.). *Women and achievement* (pp. 32–47). New York: John Wiley & Sons.

Brykczynski, K. A. (1985). Exploring the clinical practice of nurse practitioners (Doctoral dissertation,

University of California, San Francisco). *Dissertation Abstracts International 46*, 3789B (University Microfilms No. DA86–00592).

Brykczynski, K. A. (1989). An interpretive study describing the clinical judgment of nurse practitioners. *Scholarly Inquiry for Nursing Practice 3*(2), 75–104.

Bucher, R., & Stelling, J. G. (1977). *Becoming professional*. Beverly Hills, CA: Sage Publications.

Bunkers, S. J. (1992). A strategy for staff development: Self-care and self-esteem as necessary partners. *Clinical Nurse Specialist 6*(3), 154–159.

Cason, C. L., & Beck, C. M. (1982). Clinical nurse specialist role development. *Nursing and Health Care 3*(1), 25–26, 35–38.

Chinn, P. L. (1991). Looking into the crystal ball: Positioning ourselves for the year 2000. *Nursing Outlook 39*(6), 251–256.

Chinn, P. L. (1994). Looking into the crystal ball: Positioning ourselves for the year 2000. In E. C. Hein & M. J. Nicholson (Eds.). *Contemporary leadership behavior: Selected readings* (4th ed., pp. 429–437). Philadelphia: J. B. Lippincott.

Clochesy, J. M., Daly, B. J., Idemoto, B. K., et al. (1994). Preparing advanced practice nurses for acute care. *American Journal of Critical Care 3*(4), 255–259.

Cohen, H. A. (1981). *The nurse's quest for a professional identity*. Menlo Park, CA: Addison-Wesley.

Conway, M. E. (1983). Socialization and roles in nursing. *Annual Review of Nursing Research 1*, 183–208.

Conway, M. E. (1988). Organizations, professional autonomy, and roles. In M. E. Hardy & M. E. Conway (Eds.). *Role theory: Perspectives for health professionals* (2nd ed., pp. 111–132). Norwalk, CT: Appleton & Lange.

Corwin, R. (1961). The professional employee: A study of conflict in nursing roles. In R. M. Pavalko (Ed.). *Sociological perspectives on occupations* (pp. 261–275). Itasca, IL: F. E. Peacock.

Covey, S. R. (1989). *The seven habits of highly effective people*. New York: Simon & Schuster.

Crabtree, M. S. (1979). Effective utilization of clinical specialists within the organizational structure of hospital nursing service. *Nursing Administration Quarterly 4*(1), 1–11.

Daly, B. J., Rudy, E. B., Thompson, K. S., & Happ, M. B. (1991). Development of a special care unit for chronically critically ill patients. *Heart and Lung 20*(1), 45–51.

Davidhizar, R. (1994). Stress can make you or break you. *Advanced Practice Nurse* (*Spring/Summer*) 10–11, 17.

Davis, F., & Olesen, V. (1972). Initiation into a women's profession: Identity problems in the status transition of coed to student nurse. In R. M. Pavalko (Ed.). *Sociological perspectives on occupations* (pp. 186–195). Itasca, IL: F. E. Peacock.

Davis, F., Olesen, V. L., & Whittaker, E. W. (1966).

Problems and issues in collegiate nursing education. In F. Davis (Ed.) *The nursing profession: Five sociological essays* (pp. 138–175). New York: Wiley.

Dreyfus, S. E., & Dreyfus, H. L. (1980). *A five-stage model of the mental activities involved in directed skill acquisition* (USAF Contract No. F49620-79-C-0063). Berkeley: University of California.

Editor. (1975). An interview with Dr. Loretta Ford. *Nurse Practitioner 1*(1), 9–12.

Edmunds, M. (1980). Non-clinical problems: Gender and the nurse practitioner role. *Nurse Practitioner 5*(6), 42–44.

Elder, R. G., & Bullough, B. (1990). Nurse practitioners and clinical nurse specialists: Are the roles merging? *Clinical Nurse Specialist 4*(2), 78–84.

Elfrink, V., & Lutz, E. (1991). American Association of Colleges of Nursing essential values: National study of faculty perceptions, practices, and plans. *Journal of Professional Nursing 7*, 239–245.

Faculty. (1993). *The status of advanced nursing practice*. Unpublished manuscript, Duke University School of Nursing, Durham, NC.

Fenton, M. V. (1985). Identifying competencies of clinical nurse specialists. *Journal of Nursing Administration 15*(12), 31–37.

Fenton, M. V., & Brykczynski, K. A. (1993). Qualitative distinctions and similarities in the practice of clinical nurse specialists and nurse practitioners. *Journal of Professional Nursing 9*(6), 313–326.

Forbes, K. E., Rafson, J., Spross, J. A., & Kozlowski, D. (1990). Clinical nurse specialist and nurse practitioner core curricula survey results. *Nurse Practitioner 15*(4), 43, 46–48.

Fox, D. H. (1982). Matrix organizational model broadens clinical nurse specialist's practice. *Hospital Progress, 63*(11), 50–53, 69.

Hamric, A. B. (1989). History and overview of the CNS role. In A. B. Hamric & J. A. Spross (Eds.). *The clinical nurse specialist in theory and practice* (2nd ed) (pp. 3–18). Philadelphia: W. B. Saunders.

Hamric, A. B., & Taylor, J. W. (1989). Role development of the CNS. In A. B. Hamric & J. A. Spross (Eds.). *The clinical nurse specialist in theory and practice* (2nd ed., pp. 41–82). Philadelphia: W. B. Saunders.

Hayden, M. L., & Rowell, P. (1982). Non-clinical problems: Hospital privileges: Rationale and process. *Nurse Practitioner 7*(1), 42–44.

Hawkins, J. W., & Thibodeau, J. A. (1993). *The advanced practitioner: Current practice issues* (3rd ed.). New York: Tiresias Press.

Hawkins, J. W., & Thibodeau, J. A. (1994). 25+ and going strong: Nurse practitioners and nursing practice. *Journal of the American Academy of Nurse Practitioners 6*(11), 525–531.

Hein, E. C., & Nicholson, M. J. (Eds.). (1994). *Contemporary leadership behavior: Selected readings* (4th ed.). Philadelphia: J. B. Lippincott.

Hinshaw, A. S. (1982). Socialization and resocialization of nurses for professional nursing practice. In E. C. Hein & M. J. Nicholson (Eds.). *Contemporary leadership behavior: Selected readings.* Boston: Little, Brown.

Holt, F. M. (1984). A theoretical model for clinical specialist practice. *Nursing and Health Care, 5*(8), 445–449.

Horner, M. S. (1975). Toward an understanding of achievement-related conflicts in women. In M. T. S. Mednick, S. S. Tangri, & L. W. Hoffman (Eds.). *Women and achievement* (pp. 206–220). New York: John Wiley & Sons.

Howell, F. J. (1978). Employers' evaluations of new graduates. *Nursing Outlook 26*(7), 448–451.

Hsiao, V., & Edmunds, M. W. (Eds.). (1982). Nonclinical problems: Master's vs. CE: The debate continues. *Nurse Practitioner 7*(10), 42–46.

Hupcey, J. E. (1990). The socialization process of master's-level nurse practitioner students. *Journal of Nursing Education 29*(5), 196–201.

Hupcey, J. E. (1994). Graduate education for nurse practitioners: Are advanced degrees needed for practice? *Journal of Professional Nursing 10*(6), 350–356.

Hurley-Wilson, B. A. (1988). Socialization for roles. In M. E. Hardy & M. E. Conway (Eds.) *Role theory: Perspectives for health professionals* (2nd ed., pp. 73–110). Norwalk, CT: Appleton & Lange.

Jacox, A. (1973). Professional socialization of nurses. *Journal of the New York State Nurses' Association 4*(4), 6–15.

Kalisch, B., & Kalisch, P. (1982). *Politics in nursing.* Philadelphia: J.B. Lippincott.

Katzman, E. M., & Roberts, J. I. (1988). Nurse–physician conflicts as barriers to the enactment of nursing roles. *Western Journal of Nursing Research 10*(5), 576–590.

Keane, A., & Richmond, T. (1993). Tertiary nurse practitioners. *Image: The Journal of Nursing Scholarship 25*(4), 281–284.

Keane, A., Richmond, T., & Kaiser, L. (1994). Critical care nurse practitioners: Evolution of the advanced practice nursing role. *American Journal of Critical Care 3*(3), 232–237.

Kozier, B., Erb, G., & Blais, K. (1992). *Concepts and issues in nursing practice* (2nd ed.). Reading: MA: Addison-Wesley.

Kramer, M. E. (1974). *Reality shock: Why nurses leave nursing.* St. Louis, MO: C. V. Mosby.

Krcmar, C. R. (1991). Organizational entry: The case of the clinical nurse specialist. *Clinical Nurse Specialist 5*(1), 38–42.

Laing, M. (1993). Gossip: Does it play a role in the socialization of nurses? *Image: The Journal of Nursing Scholarship 25*(1), 37–43.

Leddy, S., & Pepper, J. M. (1993). *Conceptual bases of professional nursing* (2nd ed.). Philadelphia: J. B. Lippincott.

Lewis, J. (1975). Structural aspects of the delivery setting and nurse practitioner performance. *Nurse Practitioner 1*(1), 16–20.

Lindeke, L. L., Canedy, B. H., & Kay, M. M. (1997). A comparison of practice domains of clinical nurse specialists and nurse practitioners. *Journal of Professional Nursing 13*(5), 281–287.

Lukacs, J. L. (1982). Factors in nurse practitioner role adjustment. *Nurse Practitioner 7*(3), 21–23.

Lum, J. L. J. (1988). Reference groups and professional socialization. In M. E. Hardy & M. E. Conway (Eds.). *Role theory: Perspectives for health professionals* (2nd ed., pp. 137–156). Norwalk, CT: Appleton & Lange.

Lurie, E. E. (1981). Nurse practitioners: Issues in professional socialization. *Journal of Health and Social Behavior 22*(1), 31–48.

Lynn, M. R., McCain, N. L., & Boss, B. J. (1989). Socialization of RN to BSN. *Image: The Journal of Nursing Scholarship 21*(4), 232–237.

Malkemes, L. C. (1974). Resocialization: A model for nurse practitioner preparation. *Nursing Outlook 22* (2), 90–94.

Meleis, A. I. (1975). Role insufficiency and role supplementation: A conceptual framework. *Nursing Research 24*(4), 264–271.

Miller, M. H. (1977). Self perception of nurse practitioners: Changes in stress, assertiveness, and sex role. *Nurse Practitioner 2*(5), 26–29.

Moniz, D. (1978). Putting assertiveness techniques into practice. *American Journal of Nursing 78*(10), 1713.

Naylor, M. D. (1990). Comprehensive discharge planning for hospitalized elderly: A pilot study. *Nursing Research 39*(3), 156–161.

Naylor, M. D., & Brooten, D. (1993). The roles and functions of clinical nurse specialists. *Image: Journal of Nursing Scholarship 25*(1), 73–78.

Nyberg, J. (1994). The nurse as professnocrat. In E. C. Hein & M. J. Nicholson (Eds.). *Contemporary leadership behavior: Selected readings* (4th ed., pp. 371–376). Philadelphia: J. B. Lippincott.

Oermann, M. H. (1991). Professional nursing practice. In M. H. Oermann (Ed.). *Professional nursing practice: A conceptual approach* (pp. 1–29). Philadelphia: J. B. Lippincott.

Office of Technology Assessment. (1986). *Nurse practitioners, physician's assistants and certified nurse–midwives: A policy analysis.* Washington, DC: Author.

Olesen, V. L., & Whittaker, E. W. (1968). *The silent dialogue.* San Francisco: Jossey-Bass.

Olsson, H. M., & Gullberg, M. T. (1987). Nursing education and professional role acquisition: Theoretical perspectives. *Nurse Education Today 7*(4), 171–176.

Olsson, H. M., & Gullberg, M. T. (1988). Nursing education and importance of professional status in the nurse role: Expectations and knowledge of the nurse role. *International Journal of Nursing Studies 25*(4), 287–293.

Pan, S., Straub, L. A., & Geller, J. M. (1997). Restrictive practice environment and nurse practitioners' prescriptive authority. *Journal of the American Academy of Nurse Practitioners 9*(1), 9–15.

Patridge, K. B. (1978). Nursing values in a changing society. *Nursing Outlook 26*(6), 356–360.

Price, M. J., Martin, A. C., Newberry, Y. G., et al. (1992). Developing national guidelines for nurse practitioner education: An overview of the product and the process. *Journal of Nursing Education 31*(1), 10–15.

Reddecliff, M., Smith, E. L., Ryan-Merritt, M. (1989). Organizational analysis: Tool for the clinical nurse specialist. *Clinical Nurse Specialist 3*(3), 133–136.

Ryan-Merritt, M. V., Mitchell, C. A., & Pagel, I. (1988). Clinical nurse specialist role definition and operationalization. *Clinical Nurse Specialist 2*(3), 132–137.

Safriet, B. J. (1992). Health care dollars and regulatory sense: The role of advanced practice nursing. *Yale Journal on Regulation 9*(2), 417–488.

Simms, L. M., & Lindberg, J. (1978). *The nurse person: Developing perspectives for contemporary nursing.* New York: Harper & Row.

Simpson, I. H. (1967). Patterns of socialization into professions: The case of student nurses. *Sociological Inquiry 37*(1), 47–54.

Simpson, I. H. (1972). Patterns of socialization into professions: The case of student nurses. In R. M. Pavalko (Ed.). *Sociological perspectives on occupations* (pp. 169–177). Itasca, IL: F. E. Peacock.

Simpson, R. L., & Simpson, I. H. (1969). Women and bureaucracy in the semi-professions. In A. Etzioni (Ed.). *The semi-professions and their organization* (pp. 196–263). New York: Free Press.

Sparacino, P. S. A. (1990). Strategies for implementing advanced practice. *Clinical Nurse Specialist 4*(3), 151–152.

Stein, L. I., Watts, D. T., & Howell, T. (1990). The doctor–nurse game revisited. *Nursing Outlook 38*(6), 264–268.

Stewart, B. M., & Krueger, L. E. (1996). An evolutionary concept analysis of mentoring in nursing. *Journal of Professional Nursing 12*(5), 311–321.

Stuart, G. W., & Sundeen, S. J. (1995). Self-concept responses and dissociative disorders. In G. W. Stuart & S. J. Sundeen (Eds.). *Principles and practice of psychiatric nursing.* St. Louis, MO: C. V. Mosby.

Styles, M. (1982). *On nursing: Toward a new endowment.* St. Louis, MO: C. V. Mosby.

Styles, M. M. (1978). Why publish? *Image: The Journal of Nursing Scholarship 10*(2) 28–32.

Sullivan, J. A. (1978). Comparison of manifest needs between nurses and physicians in primary care practice. *Nursing Research 27*(4), 255–259.

Sullivan, J. A., Dachelet, C. Z., Sultz, H. A., et al. (1978). Overcoming barriers to the employment and utilization of the nurse practitioner. *American Journal of Public Health 68*(11), 1097–1103.

Sultz, H. A., Zielenzy, M., & Kinyon, L. (1978). *Longitudinal study of nurse practitioners: Phase II* (DHEW Publication No. HRA 78–92). Washington, DC: Department of Health, Education, and Welfare.

Sultz, H. A., Zielenzy, M., & Kinyon, L. (1980). *Longitudinal study of nurse practitioners: Phase III* (DHEW Publication No. HRA 80-2). Washington, DC: Department of Health, Education, and Welfare.

Tarsitano, B. J., Brophy, E. B., & Snyder, D. J. (1986). A demystification of the clinical nurse specialist role: Perceptions of clinical nurse specialists and nurse administrators. *Journal of Nursing Education 25*(1), 4–9.

Watson, I. (1981). Socialization of the nursing student in a professional nursing education programme. *Nursing Papers 13*(2), 19–24.

Weis, D., Schank, M. J., Eddy, D., & Elfrink, V. (1993). Professional values in baccalaureate nursing education. *Journal of Professional Nursing 9*(6), 336–342.

Whelan, E. G. (1984). Role-orientation change among RNs in an upper-division level baccalaureate program. *Journal of Nursing Education 23*(4), 151–155.

White, M. S. (1975). Psychological characteristics of the nurse practitioner. *Nursing Outlook 23*(3), 160–166.

White, M. S. (1978). *Competence and commitment: The making of a nurse practitioner.* San Francisco: University of California.

Williams, C. A. (1982). Nurse practitioner research: Some neglected issues. *Nursing Outlook 23*(3), 172–177.

Wyers, M. E. A., Grove, S. K., & Pastorino, C. (1985). Clinical nurse specialist: In search of the right role. *Nursing and Health Care 6*(4), 203–207.

Yoder, L. (1994). Mentoring: A concept analysis. In E. C. Hein & M. J. Nicholson (Eds.). *Contemporary leadership behavior: Selected readings* (4th ed., pp. 187–196). Philadelphia: J. B. Lippincott.

Zornow, R. A. (1977). A curriculum model for the expanded role. *Nursing Outlook 25*(1), 43–46.

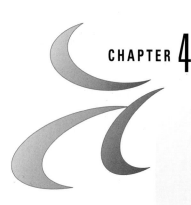

CHAPTER 4

Practice Credentials:
Licensure, Approval to Practice, Certification, and Privileging

Carolyn K. Lewis

Mary C. Smolenski

The healthcare environment in the United States has changed dramatically in the last few years. Today, more than ever before, patients in all settings—hospitals, communities, and homes—require specialized care by qualified nurses. As healthcare becomes more specialized, nursing practice similarly becomes more specific and specialized. Care by specialty nurses has become increasingly sought by the employer and the consumer; thus, more attention has focused on advanced practice nurses. Nurses in various advanced practice roles have been providing healthcare in the United States for more than 50 years. However, the practice credentials—licensure, approval to practice, certification, and privileging—have not been standardized and vary from state to state and from specialty to specialty. Historically, these mechanisms were designed to ensure quality in healthcare and as a protection for the public. Today more than ever before, the healthcare consumer is demanding that these practice credentials attest to competency of the healthcare provider to ensure public protection.

Advanced practice nurses (APNs)—comprised of clinical nurse specialists (CNSs), nurse practitioners (NPs), certified nurse midwives (CNMs), and certified registered nurse anesthetists (CRNAs)—are being incorporated into both established and innovative healthcare delivery models as they are assuming additional responsibilities in the provision of care (see Table 4-1). Because of this evolution, practice credentials and the processes involved to obtain these become even more important. While consumers and employers seek APNs with credentials to ensure public safety, the authority for voluntary credentialing ultimately rests with the nursing profession as an aspect of its social mandate to be self-governing and accountable.

Because a credential is intended to signify qualifications, responsibilities, and roles to the publics concerned, it is essential that this significance be understood in order that informed decisions and choices can be made. Increased communication and understanding between healthcare providers and society help to benefit and protect society as well as assist in ensuring accountability to the public (Committee for the Study of Credentialing in Nursing, 1979, p.50). As practicing nurses and as specialists, nurses find themselves in two environments: (1) the inner world of the clinical practice and (2) the outer world of social, political, and economic influences. Credentialing processes must respond to both of these

TABLE 4-1 *States That Recognize Clinical Nurse Specialists in Advanced Practice*

State	Statute or Regulation Citation	Requirements for Recognition	Prescriptive Authority
Alabama	Ala. code § 34-21-81 (1996)	Listed as APN—with BON given authority to outline educational requirements.	No, cannot prescribe drugs of any type.
Arizona	Ariz. Rev. Stat. Ann. § 32-1606 (1996)	Board authorized to adopt rules for the qualification and certification of clinical nurse specialists	No
Arkansas	Ark. Stat. Ann. § 17-87-102 (1995)	Master's degree in nursing and national certification	Yes
California	Cal. Wel. & Inst. Code § 14148.8 (1996)	Although California has statutorily authorized study on role of CNS as APN and has not completed such, it does allow CNS to get reimbursed under the Medi-Cal program, when providing care at alternative birth centers.	No
Colorado	Colo. Rev. Stat. § 12-38-111.5 (1996)	Requirements for registration as defined by Board of Nursing, to be based on accepted professional standards, with recognition of specialized education or experience. On or after July 1, 1995 until 2008, the requirements shall include completion of a nationally accredited education program or a passing score on a certification examination, or both, if applicable as defined in rules adopted by the board.	Yes—can prescribe as APN. If not so designated, can do so through standing order or protocol.
Connecticut	Conn. Gen. Stat. § 20-94a (1994)	Current certification by a national certifying body; 30 hours of education in pharmacology; and if certified by national certifying body after 12/31/94, hold a master's degree in nursing or in a related field recognized for certification as either a nurse practitioner, clinical nurse specialist, or nurse anesthetist by one of the certifying bodies.	Yes
Delaware	Del. Code Ann. Tit. 24 § 1902(d) (1996)	Master's degree or post-basic program certificate in a clinical specialty with national certification.	Yes
District of Columbia	D.C. Code Ann. § 2-3301.1 et seq. (1996)	Authorizes CNS as APRN. Master's degree required.	Yes
Florida	Fla. Admin. Code Ann. R. 210-11.020(7) (1997)	Completion of a formal post basic education program; current certification by a professional or national nursing specialty board recognized by the Board; and hold a master's degree in nursing clinical specialty area. Only Psychiatric Mental Health specialists can be certified as ARNPs-advanced practice.	Yes, for ARNPs.
Georgia	Ga. Code Ann. § 43-26-3 § 43-34-26.1 (1996)	Masters degree or post-basic program certificate in a clinical specialty with masters certification.	No, but can administer, order, and dispense medications.

(continued)

TABLE 4-1 *States That Recognize Clinical Nurse Specialists in Advanced Practice* *(Continued)*

State	Statute or Regulation Citation	Requirements for Recognition	Prescriptive Authority
Hawaii	HRS, Chapter 457	Law includes CNS as APRN. Master's degree or national certification	
Idaho	§ 54-1402–§ 54-1470 Idaho Code	Master's degree in nursing with current certification in a specialty.	
Illinois	PA-90-0742, Illinois Compiled Statutes, Act 65	A CNS is an APN if he or she meets the requirements for licensure, has a written collaborative agreement with a physician, and cares for patients using advanced diagnostic skills and professional judgement to initiate and coordinate care of patients. Licensure requirements are: holds a license to practice as a registered nurse in Illinois, holds national certification, successfully completed a post-basic education program in the area of the nursing specialty (after adoption of rules, a graduate degree is required).	Yes, legend drugs for advanced practice nurses.
Indiana	Ind. Code Ann. § 25-23-1-1(b)(3) (1996)	A CNS is a registered nurse qualified to practice nursing in a specialty role based upon the additional knowledge and skill gained through a formal organized program of study and clinical experience, or the equivalent as determined by the board, which does not limit but extends or expands the function of the nurse which may be initiated by the client or provider in settings that shall include hospital outpatient clinics and HMOs.	
Iowa	§ 152.6D	CNSs are ARNPs prepared at the master's level who possess evidence of current certification as clinical specialists in areas of nursing practice by a national professional nursing association approved by the board.	
Kansas	Kansas Admin. Regs. § 60-11-103 (1996)	Master's degree in a nursing clinical area that prepares the nurse to function in the expanded role; and have either graduated from a formal post-basic nursing education program approved by the board or hold a current certificate of authority to practice as a ARNP from another BON with standards equal or greater to Kansas; or prior to June 1, 1990, completed a formal education of post-basic study and clinical experience, which can be demonstrated to have sufficiently prepared the applicant for practice in the category of advanced practice for which application is made.	Yes, for ARNPs.
Kentucky	Ky. Rev. Stat. § 314.011(6, 7, 8) (Michie 1996); 201 Ky. Admin. Regs. 20:056 and 20:057 (1992) KRS 314.042 (1–4)	Completion of post-basic program of study and clinical experience and certification from a nationally established organization or agency recognized by the board to certify registered nurses for advanced practice. "ARNP" shall mean one who is registered and designated to engage in advanced registered nursing practice including but no limited to nurse anesthetist, nurse–midwife, and nurse practitioner.	Yes, as long as CNS is registered as an ARNP. Nonscheduled legend drugs (KRS 314.042).

State	Citation	Requirements/Definition	Prescriptive Authority/Reimbursement
Louisiana	La. Admin. Code 46 § 3713. See also LA. Rev. Stat. Ann. § 37.933 (1997) and La. S.B. 722 (1995)	Master's degree in a specific area of clinical nursing, certified according to national certifying body, such as the ANA, as approved by the board . . . Allow CNS to insert medical implants and "deliver" therapeutic regimen of medicine at reproduction health clinics.	Nurse Practice Act provides that RN practice may include additional acts which are recognized as proper to the practice of nursing and authorized by the Board (demonstration project).
Maine	32 Maine Rev. Stat. Ann. Tit. 2102, 2201A (1996) 24 Maine Rev. Stat. Ann. Tit. 2303 (1996)	Clinical specialist is required to have completed a formal educational program in advanced practice specialty area and hold current national certification in a program acceptable to the BON.	No, for Clinical Specialists. Yes, for ARNPs and Certified Nurse Midwives.
Maryland	Md. Regs. Code tit. 27, ch. 12	Master's degree or higher and hold current certification as a specialist in psychiatric or mental health nursing issued by the American Nurses Association or other bodies approved by the board.	Yes, for NPs. No, for nurse psychotherapists.
Massachusetts	Mass. Ann. Laws Ch. 112 § 80B; ch. 112 § 80E (1996)	Psychiatric CNSs are the only CNSs that are legally recognized.	Psychiatric mental health clinical nurse specialists have prescriptive authority, 3rd party reimbursement (indemnity only) and Medicaid reimbursement.
Michigan	BON Rules, Part 4, 338.10404	Inclusion of CNS in CNP definition.	Yes, delegated by a physician.
Minnesota	Minn. R. 6220.0100 (1991)	Master's degree, certification by professional nursing organizations approved Minnesota Board of Nursing, and completion of no less than thirty hours of formal study in the prescribing of psychotropic drugs . . . , and established has written agreement with psychiatrist based on standards estimated by MNA and Minnesota Psychiatric Association.	Yes
Missouri	Mo. Rev. Stat. § 335.016(2) (1996); Mo. Code Regs. Tit. 4 § 200-4.100 (l)(d) (1992)	Have a master's degree in the area of clinical nursing specialty practice and currently certified by the American Nurses Association as a clinical nurse specialist in the area of specialty practice. Rules allow CNS who are not certified by nationally recognized certifying body that have successfully completed, within the past 2 years, 3 graduate credit hours of post-baccalaureate pharmacology course and practice in the specialized and advanced nursing practice area a minimum of 1000 hours during the past 2 years providing direct patient care services. Must take first available certification exam after graduation. Failure to become certified requires immediate ceasing of the use of the title and practice as an advanced practice nurse.	Yes, if they are certified by ANA as CNS and have collaborative practice arrangement.
Montana	Mont. Code Ann. § 37-8-202 (1993)	Graduate degree or equivalent and certification by a certification body recognized by the BON.	Yes
Nebraska	Neb. Admin. R & Regs. 71-1, 132.05 (1992)	Clinical Nurse Specialist holds masters degree or doctoral degree in a nursing clinical specialty.	No

(continued)

TABLE 4-1 *States That Recognize Clinical Nurse Specialists in Advanced Practice* *(Continued)*

State	Statute or Regulation Citation	Requirements for Recognition	Prescriptive Authority
Nevada	Nevada Admin. Code ch. 632 § 632.037, § 632.300 (1996)	Master's or doctorate degree in nursing and educated in area of clinical specialty by completing a program designed to prepare clinical nurse specialists.	Yes, for APNs.
New Hampshire	§ RSA-326-B:10	Psych/mental only. Master's degree in nursing. CE and practice requirements. National certification.	
New Jersey	N.J. Stat. Ann. § 45:11–45 (1996)	Successful completion of an educational program, including pharmacology, approved by the board; and pass a written examination approved by the board.	Yes
New Mexico	N.M. Stat. Ann § 61-3-23.4 (new statute) (1996)	Master's degree or doctoral degree in a defined clinical nursing specialty and certification by a national nursing organization.	Yes
North Carolina	N.C. Gen. Stat. § 58-65-1 (1996)	Included CNS in definition of APN.	No
North Dakota	N.D. Admin. Code § 54-05-03.1-01 (1997)	Submit evidence of completion of an advanced nursing education program; evidence of certification by a national nursing organization in the specific area of nursing practice; and scope of practice statement.	Yes, for ARNPs.
Ohio	Ohio Rev. Code Ann. § 4723.55 (Anderson 1997) (demonstration project)	Three years of experience in RN practice and certified as a clinical nurse specialist by a national certifying organization recognized by the BON.	Yes, per formulary as approved in a manner consistent with demonstration project statute.
	Ohio Rev. Code § 4723.41–4723.44 (June 1996)	Permanent legislation authorizing advanced practice nurses includes CNS, but does not grant prescriptive authority. CNS must have master's degree upon effective date of legislation and must be certified by 2001.	
Oklahoma	Okla. Stat. Tit. § 567.3A (1996)	Included in definition of APN—must complete master's degree in nursing, have national certification by body recognized by BON, have received a certificate of recognition from BON.	Yes, supervised prescriptive authority.
Pennsylvania	40 Pa. Stat. Ann. Tit. § 3024 and § 63023 (1996)	Not specifically authorized in statute, but recognized in reimbursement statute as appropriate provider of care.	
Rhode Island	R.I. Gen. Laws § 5-34-1(l) (1996). Psychiatric and mental health nurse clinical specialist.	Psychiatric and mental health nurse clinical specialists is an expanded role utilizing independent knowledge and management of mental health and illness . . . The psychiatric and M/H clinical specialist is masters-prepared, has an active license as a RN, and is certified by a national body approved by the R.I. Board of nursing registration.	Yes, if CRNP.

State	Citation		Prescriptive Authority
South Carolina	S.C. Code Regs. 91-6 (1996)	After 1/1/95; evidence of certification by national credentialing organization acceptable to the BON and evidence of a master's degree in nursing, except for applicants who provide documentation that applicant was certified by a BON-approved national credentialing organization prior to 12/31/94 recognized by another state BON as an NP prior to 12/31/94; or graduated from advanced education program appropriate to the practice and acceptable to BON prior to 12/31/94.	Yes
South Dakota	S.D. Codified Laws Ann. § 36-9-1, 36-9-85, and 36-9-87 (1997)	Clinical nurse specialist authorization requires; (1) current licensure as RN, (2) master's in nursing and, (3) completion of examination approved by the board.	Yes
Tennessee	Tenn. Comp. R Code Tit. 22 1000-1-04(3)(b) (1996)	Rule allows for expanded role. No specific titles. Requires medical protocols if managing medical aspects of patient's care. Named in insurance law that mandates reimbursement for nurses in advanced practice.	Yes, under medical protocols if CNS has a BON Certificate of Fitness to prescribe.
Texas	Board of Nursing Regulations Sec. 221.3 See also S. Bill 673 (1995)	Completion of post-basic program of study and evidence of current certification in the area of practice by a national or state organization approved by the board. Requires completion of pharmacology program.	Yes, for APNs.
Utah	Utah Code Ann. § 58-31-6(1)(c)(iii) and § 58-31-7(5) (1996)	Master's degree from a graduate nursing education program in psychiatric nursing approved by the board; successful completion of clinical practice in psychiatric and mental health nursing, including psychotherapy after completion of master's degree required for licensure; pass examination approved by the board and meet with board, if requested to determine applicant's qualifications for licensure.	Yes
Virginia	Va. Regs. Reg. 495-01-1 § 3.10.	Master's degree in nursing for advanced practice in clinical specialty in nursing and specialty certification from a national certifying organization.	Yes, for NPs. No, for CNSs unless they are also registered as NPs.
Wisconsin	Wis. Stat. § 632.895 and § 441.01 et. Seq. (1995–1996) BON Regs Ch. 441 and Ch. N8	Must hold a master's degree in nursing for advanced practice in clinical specialty in nursing and certified as a clinical specialist by a national certifying organization.	Yes—can prescribe as an APN Prescriber (APNP).
Virgin Islands	V.I. Code Anno. Tit. 27 § 96 (1996)	Recognized as an advanced practice specialty.	Yes
Wyoming	WCWR 024-054-004 § 1 (1996)	Completion of a nationally accredited educational program for preparation as an advanced practitioner of nursing with a specific curriculum appropriate to the proposed practice, accepted by the board or certification as an advanced practitioner of nursing by a nationally recognized accrediting agency.	Yes, for APNs.

challenges. However, many challenges continue to exist that need more careful deliberation, standardization, and refinement:

1. Scope of practice;
2. Legal entanglements that exist in advanced practice legislation;
3. Titling concerns regarding name recognition;
4. Graduate programs that attest to specialty preparation;
5. Resolution of multistate licensure issues; and
6. Clearer delineation of roles through practice differentiation, thus eliminating role blurring. (Styles, 1991)

As the public seeks more information about healthcare and public safety, more emphasis is placed on the mechanisms and processes of approval to practice for the advanced practice nurse, including licensure, certification, and privileging. Practice credentials further promote accountability of the profession to the public by enforcing either national or institutional standards as determined and recognized by the profession. Inherent in this are the legal issues, the need for legislative awareness and action, and the need to ensure the continued competence of the practitioner.

Approval to Practice

The mechanism of approval to practice for the advanced practice nurse may be derived from various sources: nurse practice acts, rules and regulations promulgated by the regulatory body within each state, and institutional guidelines. The underlying purpose of these mechanisms is the protection of public health, safety, and welfare. Regulatory criteria should reflect entry-level minimum requirements for safe and competent nursing practice, and legal regulation is the joint responsibility of state legislators and boards of nursing and sometimes may include joint regulation by boards of nursing and medicine.

The history of nurse practice acts falls into three phases. The first phase, often referred to as the early nurse registration acts, was conducted in a similar manner as that of the early medical practice laws. This move was identified as a means for nursing to organize and to use the organization to promote the professionalization of nursing. The organization to promote this effort was to become the National League for Nursing (NLN), established in 1894, and was the precursor to the American Nurses' Association (ANA) in 1896. The collective goals of these organizations were to upgrade the profession educationally and to increase the power and recognition of nursing (Robinson, McKenzie, & Niemer, 1996).

The second phase started in 1938 when the first mandatory practice act was passed in New York. This practice act established two levels of nurses, registered professional and practical. This was also the first time the scope of nursing practice was defined, and the first time title protection was established (Robinson, McKenzie, & Niemer, 1996). During this time period, the American Nurses Association in 1955 defined professional practice as:

> the performance, for compensation, of any act in the observation, care and counsel of the ill, injured or infirm, or in the maintenance of health or prevention of illness in others, or in the supervision and teaching of other personnel, or the administration of medications and treatments prescribed by a licensed physician or dentist, requiring substantial specialized judgment and skill and based on knowledge and application of the principles of biological, physical and social science. The foregoing shall not be deemed to include acts of diagnosis or prescription of therapeutic or corrective measures. (ANA, 1955)

The third phase included expanding the role and scope of nursing: the development of the nurse practitioner role, nursing education, and specialization. During this phase, new legislation was implemented by several states and the definition of nursing was redefined by other states. Consequently, some states during this phase chose to use the power of boards to develop regulations to facilitate nurses' expanded role and to use agency generated protocols to guide the advanced practice role (Mezey & McGivern, 1986).

As advanced practice nurses continue to expand their scope of practice, approval to practice at the state level is determined by individual boards of nursing and may vary from state to state. Institutional approval, sometimes referred to as "privileging," is a process that is determined by the individual facility and may not necessarily parallel with those of the state boards of nursing requirements. As technology and mobility expand the geographic boundaries of nursing practice, the mechanism for approval to practice must also accommodate this expansion to ensure safe and competent practice (see Exemplar 19A for exceptions in CNRA practice).

Licensure

In the United States, each state has the jurisdiction to determine the requirements for licensure for advanced practice nurses. Licensure in the United States is the process by which an agency of state government grants permission to individuals accountable for the practice of a profession to engage in the practice of that profession and prohibits all others from legally doing so (Committee for the Study of Credentialing in Nursing, 1979). It permits the use of a particular title and defines a scope and sets the boundaries of the practice profession. Licensure further gives an individual a property right to practice his or her profession, based on fulfilling the conditions of licensure (Committee for the Study of Credentialing in Nursing, 1979). The main purpose of licensure is to protect the public by ensuring a minimum level of professional competence. Established standards and methods of evaluation are used to determine eligibility for initial licensure and for periodic renewal. Effective means are set forth for taking action against licensees for acts of professional misconduct, incompetence, and/or negligence.

As the role of nurses evolved in the 1970s, many state nurse practice acts were revised to include an advanced scope of nursing practice. Most states provided for advanced practices under their nurse practice acts under the jurisdiction of the state boards of nursing. As of 1998, all 50 boards of nursing, including the District of Columbia, have language in their nurse practice acts that addressees advanced practice. Additionally for advanced practice nurses, 19 states have sole authority in scope of practice with no requirements for physician control of supervision; 25 states have sole authority in scope of practice but the scope of practice has a requirement for physician collaboration or supervision; 5 states share the authority with the board of medicine; and 2 states allow the advanced practice function to fall under a broad nurse practice act (The Nurse Practitioner, 1998) (See Table 4-2). The above may demonstrate that advanced practice nurses are a critical link in the healthcare delivery system as the scope of practice continues to evolve. As the healthcare system moves into the 21st century, advanced practice nurses must remain at the forefront of patient delivery systems.

In 1991, the National Council of State Boards of Nursing (NCSBN) commissioned a study on the regulation of advanced nursing practice. This study revealed inconsistencies among state boards of nursing in state requirements and the approaches to the regulation of advanced practice. In 1992 NCSBN developed a statement titled "Position Paper and Model Legislation on the Licensure of Advanced Practice." This paper advocated further regulation and that regulatory authority was necessary in order to ensure minimal competency at an entry level for public safety. NCSBN asserted this was vital because of economic, legislative, and policy changes affecting healthcare (Robinson, McKenzie, & Niemer, 1996).

The nursing community reacted to this proposal with almost universal disagreement (Robinson, McKenzie, & Niemer, 1996, p.74). Edmunds (1992) asserted that although

TABLE 4-2 *Summary of Advanced Practice Nurse Legislation: Legal Authority for Scope of Practice and Prescriptive Authority*

- States with nurse practitioner (NP)* title protection and the board of nursing has sole authority in scope of practice with no statutory or regulatory requirements for physician collaboration, direction, or supervision: **AK, AR, CO, DC, HI, IN, ME, MI, MT, ND, NH, NJ, NM, OK, OR, RI, UT, WA, WV**
- States with NP* title protection and the board of nursing has sole authority in scope of practice, but scope of practice has a requirement for physician collaboration: **AL, AZ, CA, DE, IA, IL, KS, KY, MD, MO, NE, NV, NY, OH, VT, WY**
- States with NP* title protection and the board of nursing has sole authority in scope of practice, but scope of practice has a requirement for physician supervision: **CT, FL, GA, ID, LA, MA, SC, TX, WI**
- States with NP* title protection but the scope of practice is authorized by the board of nursing and the board of medicine: **MS, NC, PA, SD, VA**
- States without NP* title protection where APNs function under a broad nurse practice act: **MN, TN**
- States where NPs* can prescribe (including controlled substances) independent of any required physician involvement in prescriptive authority: **AK, AZ, DC, ME, MT, NH, NM, OR, UT,** ** **WA,** ** **WI**
- States where NPs* can prescribe (including controlled substances) with some degree of physician involvement or delegation of prescription writing: **AR, CA, CO, CT, DE, FL,*** GA, IA, ID, IL,*** IN, KS, MA, MD, MN, MS, NC, ND, NE, NJ, NY, OK, RI, SC, SD, TN,*** VA, VT, WV, WY**
- States where NPs* can prescribe (excluding controlled substances) with some degree of physician involvement or delegation of prescription writing: **AL, HI, KY, LA, MI, MO, NV, OH, PA,*** TX**
- States where NPs* have no statutory or regulatory prescribing authority: **(none)**
- States where NPs* also have the authority to dispense drug samples according to statute or rules and regulations: **AK, AZ, CO, CT, DE, GA, IA, ID, LA, ME, MD, MN, MO, MS, NC, NE, NH, NM, NV, NY, OK, OR, WI, WV, WY**

* May include other APNs (i.e., clinical nurse specialists, nurse midwives, and nurse anesthetists).
In narrowly specified situations.
** Schedule IV and/or V only.
*** Pending approval of R&R.
  k In many states, the authority by NPs to distribute/dispense samples is not legislatively specified in the statute or R&R, but it has become the community standard as accepted practice.
  (Note that Washington, DC is counted as a state in this table.)
  Adapted with permission from: Pearson, L. J. (1998). Annual Update of How Each State Stands on Legislative Issues Affecting Advanced Nursing Practice. *The Nurse Practitioner 24*(1), 18–19, Springhouse Corporation.

there is a need to promulgate consistent government standards for regulation in order to ensure public protection, this should not be done unless other sufficient mechanisms are in place such as specialty certification and continuing education and unless licensure represented more stringent regulation than that of recognition. Naturally, a logical progression to this was for NCSBN to consider the development of a second licensing examination for advance practice.

The American Nurses Association Board of Directors appointed a Blue Ribbon Committee on Credentialing in Advanced Practice. This committee was to assess and determine how to ensure consistency of standards for regulation without imposing a second license. The ANA continued to support its previous position that it is the profession's responsibility to regulate advanced nursing practice. Perceiving the essence of this critical position, the ANA strongly urged other organizations to consider the implications of this and the effects that this decision could have on the profession.

At the 1994 annual meeting of the NCSBN, the membership asked that this issue be explored further to determine the fiscal, regulatory, and political implications of developing second licensure for nurse practitioners. This task force was also charged with identifying core competencies for nurse practitioners that would serve as a basis for an examination. However, with the united efforts of many organizations and the willingness of NCSBN to come to the table to further explore these issues, the 1995 delegate assembly voted to direct NCSBN to collaborate with the NP specialty certification organizations to make "significant progress toward legally defensible, psychometrically sound NP examinations which are sufficient for regulatory purposes" (National Council of State Boards of Nursing, 1994).

After the 1995 actions of the delegate assembly, NCSBN convened a meeting to begin the process of collaborating with interested certifying bodies to develop a system that would provide evidence that the examinations were psychometrically sound, entry level, and testing at a minimal competence level. Many organizations contended that the specialty examination and competency certification was the role of the profession and the specialty certifying groups. All interested parties agreed to proceed with external accreditation by the National Commission for Certifying Agencies (NCCA), to demonstrate compliance with industry and national standards. All specialty certifying organizations for advanced practice are certified by NCCA except for the American College of Nurse Midwives Certification Council.

Because the majority of the state boards of nursing use certification examinations for regulation of advanced practice nurses, it is imperative that the testing organizations ensure periodic reviews of their processes in order to address the issue of public protection. Downing and Haladyna (1996) argue that high-stakes testing programs should be subject to routine, independent external review. This is better interpreted as those programs in which the public protection or welfare is of major concern and the consequences of the examinee failure are considerable. Examples include licensing and certification programs, college admission tests, and high school graduation tests. The authors present a five-step model for conducting an evaluation: (1) choosing an evaluator with adequate training and experience; (2) identifying the scope of the evaluation, including the data to be collected and the format of the final report; (3) collecting the data; (4) reporting to the client on issues of validity, reliability, item quality, etc.; and (5) taking corrective action to improve deficiencies.

Most states provide coverage of the advanced practice nurse under their current registered nurse license process. Three states provide either dual licenses or separate certificates for the advanced practice nurse (California, Florida, and New York).

Certification

Certification is the process by which a nongovernmental agency or association grants recognition to an individual who has met certain predetermined qualifications specified by an agency or association. Such qualifications may include (1) graduation from an accredited or approved program; (2) acceptable performance on a qualifying examination or series of examinations; and/or (3) completion of a given amount of work experience (Committee for the Study of Credentialing in Nursing, 1979). The purpose of certification is to ensure various publics that an individual has mastered a body of knowledge and acquired skills in a particular specialty.

The role of certification in the nursing profession is becoming a complex issue. Certification can be used for entry into practice, validation of competence, recognition of excellence, and/or for regulation. Certification can be mandatory or professional. The purpose of certification is often determined and set by the specialty within the profession.

Certification was introduced and accepted into the nursing profession as early as 1945 by the American Association of Nurse Anesthetists (AANA) (see Exemplar 19A). The American Nurses Association (ANA), the professional association, began to explore the relevance of certification to the profession in the 1950s but did not result in a formalized system until ANA introduced its first certification examination in 1974 in order to provide a formal recognition of achievement performance and education. In 1974 ANA administered its first advanced practice examination for pediatric nurse practitioners with the adult and family nurse practitioner examinations following shortly thereafter in 1976.

By 1979, ANA offered fifteen certification examinations, six generalist and nine advanced practice. ANA continued to administer certification examinations until in 1991, ANA's Center for Credentialing Services was separately incorporated as the American Nurses Credentialing Center (ANCC). Other organizations also certify nurses in advanced practice specialties. Some of the groups that offer certification for advanced practice nurses are as follows: Council on Certification of Nurse Anesthetist; American College of Nurse Midwives; National Certification Board of Pediatric Nurse Practitioners; National Certification Corporation for the Obstetric, Gynecologic, and Neonatal Nursing; the American Academy of Nurse Practitioners; the American Association of Critical Care Nurses Certification Corporation; and the Oncology Nursing Certification Corporation (see Table 4-3).

The ANCC certification examinations reflect practice in a particular nursing specialty that is recognized by the ANA Congress of Nursing Practice, which defines specialties by established criteria. The specialty must have a recognized scope and standards of practice in order for an examination to be developed. The advanced practice nurse is then responsible for identifying the scope of practice permitted by state and federal laws and regulations, the professional code of ethics, and professional standards.

After the definition of the specialty and scope of practice and standards are defined, test development begins. The certifying agency and the testing organization jointly plan all steps necessary to establish and administer the testing program. The program elements are as follows:

1. **Role delineation/job analysis,** as in advanced practice, defines the knowledge, skills, and abilities needed for entry-level practice;
2. **Test specifications,** which describe item and test format, test length, design of test booklets and answer sheets, and design of score reports;
3. **Item development,** which begins with the training of content experts to develop technically sound test items;
4. **Item banking,** which includes the items and the data gathered from each use that are reviewed regularly by content experts to ensure each item reflects current practice;
5. **Pretesting,** which is a method used to obtain information about the characteristics of new items before they are used to compute candidate's scores in an actual form of the test;
6. **Test assembly** of items suitable for inclusion in the certification test that have survived content review, measurement review, and pretesting;
7. **Registration,** which involves handbook and application preparation and distribution to potential examinees; and
8. **Test administration,** which involves conditions that are standardized so that all examinees take the test under the same secure conditions.

Other statistical procedures are involved in certification testing, but these are too technical to be included and are beyond the scope of this chapter; however, the above are considered to be basic universal principles of sound certification testing programs (ACT, 1988). These procedures may vary somewhat with other testing organizations.

The certification body is usually affiliated with the professional association that defines the specialty and the scope and standards for the certification examination; however with a certain degree of administrative and financial autonomy. In order to enhance their credentials, certification agencies increasingly seek accreditation/recognition of their processes to ensure adherence to rigorous national standards, such as those developed by the American

TABLE 4-3 *Certified Advanced Practice Nurses in the United States*

Specialty	Credential	# Certified	Certifying Organization	Year: 1st Exam
Clinical Specialists				
Community Health	RN,CS	437	American Nurses Credentialing Center (ANCC)	1990
Gerontology	RN,CS	878	ANCC	1989
Home Health	RN,CS	67	ANCC	1996
Medical/ Surgical	RN,CS	2268	ANCC	1976
Psychiatric–Mental Health: Adult	RN,CS	6916	ANCC	1977
Psychiatric–Mental Health: Child/ Adolescent	RN,CS	909	ANCC	1977
Oncology	AOCN	431	Oncology Nursing Certification Corp.	1995
Critical Care	CCNS		American Association of Critical-Care Nurses (AACN) Certification Corporation	1999
Other				
Anesthetist	CRNA	21,966	Council on Certification of Nurse Anesthetists	1945
Midwife	CNM	6000	American College of Nurse Midwives	1971
Nurse Practitioners				
Acute Care	RN,CS	1051	ANCC and AACN Certification Corporation	1995
Adult	RN,CS	10,224	ANCC	1976
Adult	NP-C	—[1]	American Academy of Nurse Practitioners (AANP)	1994
Family	RN,CS	17,900	ANCC	1976
Family	NP-C		AANP	1994
Gerontology	RN,CS	2938	ANCC	1979
Neonatal	RN,C	41,193[2]	National Certification Corporation for the Obstetric, Gynecologic and Neonatal Nursing Specialties (NCC)	
Pediatric	RN,CS	2890	ANCC	1974
Pediatric	CPNP	6000	National Certification Board of Pediatric Nurse Practitioners and Nurses	
School	RN,CS	240	ANCC	1979
Women's Health	RN,C	41,193	NCC	

[1]Unable to obtain number of certified nurses from AANP.
[2]NCC statistics do not differentiate between neonatal and women's health nurses.

Board of Nursing Specialties (ABNS) and the National Commission for Certifying Agencies (NCCA). The purpose of accreditation/recognition is three-fold: (1) it establishes that credentialing standards are not under the control of any other association or organization; (2) it insulates the parent organization from litigation instigated by those who are precluded from sitting for an examination, who have failed or who have lost their credential through disciplinary actions; and (3) it assists in resolving conflicts with government agencies—not the least of which is the Internal Revenue Service (Lewis, Camp, & Rothrock, 1996). A certification agency that has submitted its psychometric standards to rigorous independent scrutiny and established its independence in governance and financial matters stands on much firmer ground in this litigious society than one that self-validates.

As healthcare becomes more and more complicated and nursing more specialized, professional certification has become one mechanism to define the appropriate and safe practice privileges of differently qualified registered nurses. The initiation of healthcare reform, recognition of certification by state regulatory agencies, and third-party reimbursement for certified advanced practice nurses are major factors in the continued growth in certification programs. Certification has become a moderate form of regulation that grants recognition to individuals who have met predetermined qualifications set by a state agency. The majority of the states have developed some form of regulation of advanced practice that requires successfully passing a national certification examination. In many states, specific references to nursing certification have been incorporated into statute or into rules and regulations (see Table 4.2). However, some states such as California, Florida, and New York require state certification for advanced practice licensure.

Certification adheres to the principles of regulation promulgated by the International Council of Nursing and adopted by major nursing organizations and regulation. Thus, certification ensures national consistency of professional standards, imposes standard titles, helps the public understand scope of practice, and provides a venue for the public to raise practice grievance (American Association of Colleges of Nursing, 1996).

On the other hand, regulatory boards have been charged with protection of the public to ensure a competent work force and positive outcomes. Because most states require certification for advanced practice standing, certification must attest to entry-level competence, and recertification must attest to continued competency.

This new era approach makes the verification of the competence of the advanced practice professional an increasingly important issue—he or she must be properly licensed and certified in the area of specialty by a credible, psychometrically sound, and legally defensible examination. The characteristics of programs that provide such examinations must be:

1. Of excellent quality, meeting the high standards of the industry;
2. Document the validity of the examinations used to evaluate excellence;
3. Reflect current practice needs and educational content;
4. Incorporate flexibility in the approach to defining areas of knowledge and skills; and
5. Withstand legal review. (Styles, 1997)

Certification must continue to assure national consistency of professional standards and assist the public in understanding the advanced practice nurse's professional scope of practice. This process has become the acceptable credentialing mechanism for a specialty and in most instances is required as the regulatory mechanism for the advanced practice specialists. The professional certification process must provide recognition of a nationally uniform measure of competence that can be relied on by the public in making healthcare provider choices. As a process that facilitates communication between the healthcare providers and society, certification benefits both the public and the profession.

With certification as the regulatory mechanism for advanced practice nursing, nursing can pool resources and move forward expeditiously on the process of regulation in the interest of public safety (American Association of Colleges of Nursing, 1996).

Privileging

Another mechanism of approval to practice used to provide oversight for the scope of practice of the advanced practice nurse is privileging. Privileging is the process used by a facility or employing organization to monitor the clinical activities a provider is authorized to perform in that facility. The professional is granted privileges to practice designated clinical activities based on his or her credentials (Rustia & Bartek, 1997).

The practice of privileging has been used by the medical community for many years to verify a practitioner's preparation and competence to perform medical activities in hospitals and other medical organizations. In 1984, the Joint Commission for Accreditation of Hospitals and Organizations (JCAHO) revised its definition of medical staff and broadened scope of practice rules to include permissive language to allow hospitals to include other licensed individuals permitted by law and by the hospital to provide patient care services independently in the hospital. These privileges usually include clinical and/or admitting practices. JCAHO also established a mechanism to monitor these privileges along with charging the hospital to establish criteria for clinical privileging and a process to ensure that competent individuals are providing patient care (Quigley, Hixon, & Janzen 1991).

In most instances, a peer review board is set up by the organization to review the credentials packet of the provider, to determine criteria for granting certain privileges, and to evaluate the continued competence of the provider over time. Historically, a physician credentialing committee performed this review, and a recommendation about the awarding of the clinical privileges was then forwarded to the hospital governing board, responsible for granting the privileging. However, an alternative to this process for APNs would be to consider the development of an interdisciplinary credentialing committee. This committee would include representatives of types of providers who would be considered for clinical privileges and would make the recommendation to the governing board. All providers must have access to a process that protects them from any potential bias from economic competitors and ensures a due process mechanism (Jones-Schenk, 1998, p. 99).

Employers maintain separate files for privileging information that are distinct from the credentials files to provide confidentiality and statutory protection from discovery. For nursing, the credentials file to date has not been as in-depth as the physician's credentialing file, if it existed at all, and has not included documentation on performance measures (e.g., encounters, readmissions, and mortality rates) and financial data other than salary. The nurses credentialing file will usually consist of specific documentation as determined by the faculty (e.g., evidence of graduation from an approved nursing school) (see Table 4-4).

Providers must be able to show that they can provide quality care in a cost-effective manner; employing organizations seek outcome data on performance to validate this. Purchasers of care are demanding results of member satisfaction surveys and inquiring about how providers are selected, credentialed, and recredentialed. Care purchasers also want to know about other processes used to ensure quality and cost containment. With the growth of managed care organizations (MCOs) and the increased use of other licensed independent providers to include nurse practitioners and other advanced practice nurses, the need to verify credentials has grown. Verifying credentials has become a lucrative business that has grown out of the healthcare system with Credentials Verification Organizations (CVOs) developing to help organizations keep up with verification processes. Through the privileging and credentialing processes, the MCO delineates the scope of practice of its providers, to assure accrediting bodies that they have employed competent providers, to decrease the chances of liability for themselves and the individual, and to provide data for determining economic impact of provider practice on the healthcare system.

In 1996, the ANA identified more than 29 states in which advanced practice nurses have privileges ranging from full privileges to admitting, consulting, and performing clin-

TABLE 4-4 *Proposed Components of a Nurse Credentialing File*

Evidence of graduation from an approved nursing school

Evidence of advanced education and/or degree in the specialty

Specialized training/experience not evident in educational preparation (e.g., IUD insertion)

Experience

References

Specialty certification and history

Licensure information

DEA license number

Evidence of continuing education

Teaching appointments and references

Professional associations

Professional liability insurance data

Any liability history, judgements, settlements, disciplinary actions

Other: Physical, mental health, or chemical dependence problems that could interfere with ability

ical duties to conditional privileges based on the nursing specialty (Carson, 1996). The dynamics of today's healthcare system are forcing institutions, organizations, and individual providers of care to assess relationships and create innovative methods of assuring both quality care and safety for the consumer. One outcome of this has been the creation of formalized systematic methods of privileging, which measure and evaluate the individual advanced practice nurse's qualifications and actual performance. Nursing has been and will continue to be the discipline that will provide the types of persons and services necessary to transform the healthcare system to be responsive and accountable to the consumer.

Conclusion

Several issues affecting advanced practice nursing have been discussed: approval to practice, licensure, certification, and privileging. All of these are interrelated and assist in shaping the future of the advanced practice nurse as the enormous and rapid changes occur in healthcare delivery. Sound and credible mechanisms must be in place to ensure both the quality of care and safety for consumers in order for advance practice nurses to meet the challenges of the maturing system of healthcare. As advanced practice nurses work in their specialized areas of practice, their roles and functions will continue to evolve, and the profession will become an even more significant player in the delivery care. Glynn (1998) asserts that advanced practice nurses have played a significant role in the delivery of healthcare and continue to demonstrate increased control over the means of healthcare delivery. Should they continue to do so, there is no reason to expect anything less than their optimal utilization . . . nationwide.

REFERENCES

American Association of College of Nursing. (1996). Certification and regulation of advanced practice nurses. *Journal of Professional Nursing 12*(3), 184–186.

American College Testing. (1988). *Elements of a sound certification testing program.* Iowa City, IA: ACT.

Carson, W. Y. (1996). *Nurse privileging and advanced practice nursing.* Washington, DC: American Nurses Association.

Committee for the Study of Credentialing in Nursing. (1979). *The committee report, Vol I of the credentialing in nursing.* Kansas City, MO: American Nurses Association.

Downing, S.M., & Haladyna, T.M. (1996). A model for evaluation high-stakes testing programs: why the fox should not guard the chicken coop. *Educational Measurement: Issues and Practice 15*(1), 5–12.

Edmunds, M. W. (1992, October). Council's pursuit of national standardization for advanced practice nursing meets with resistance. *Nurse Practitioner* 81–83.

Glynn, P. M. (1998). Predicting the future of the adult nurse practitioner. *Clinical Excellence for Nurse Practitioners 2*(3), 174–182.

Jones-Schenk, J. (1998). The brave new world of advanced practice: credentialing and privileging. *Applied Nursing Research 11*(3), 99–100.

Lewis, C. K., Camp, J. , & Rothrock, J. (1996). *Nursing specialty certification in the United States of America.* Paper presented at the Trilateral Initiative for North American Nursing, Philadelphia, PA.

Mezey, M. D., & McGivern, D. O. (Eds.). (1986). *Nurses, nurse practitioners: The revolution of primary care.* Boston: Little, Brown & Co.

National Council of State Boards of Nursing, Incorporated. (1994). *National Council's book of reports.* Chicago, IL: Author.

Peterson, L.J. (Ed.). (1998). Annual update of how each state stands on legislative issues affecting advanced nursing practice [An NP Exclusive]. *The Nurse Practitioner: The American Journal of Primary Healthcare 23*(1).

Quigley, P. H., Hixon, A. H., & Janzen, S. K. (1991). Promoting autonomy and professional practice: a program of clinical privileging. *Journal of Nursing Quality Assurance 5*(3), 27–32.

Robinson, D. L., McKenzie, C., & Niemer, L. (1996). Second licensure for advanced practice: current status. *Nurse Practitioner 21*(9), 71–88.

Rustia, J. G. & Bartek, J. K. (1997). Managed care credentialing of advanced practice nurses. *The Nurse Practitioner 22*(9), 90–103.

Styles, M. M. (1991). Bridging the gap between competency and excellence. *ANNA Journal 18*(4), 353–360.

Nancy L. Szaflarski

CHAPTER 5

Clinical Reasoning

If clinical reasoning were simply a matter of pattern recognition,
a well-programmed computer might substitute for even the best clinician.
(K. Hunter, 1996)

Competent clinical reasoning is a cornerstone of advanced practice nursing because it is an essential ingredient of case-based, clinical practice. Advanced practice nurses (APNs) have been granted authority and accountability to diagnose and treat conditions, diseases, and syndromes, as well as to respond to illness of patients in primary care, home care, and acute care environments. Because the APN provides continuity of care over time, the APN's clinical reasoning of a patient's problem(s) is not restricted to an initial diagnosis or management plan; rather, the repetitive reasoning of new, unresolved, and/or chronic problems of individual patients occurs through multiple interactions encountered in outpatient clinics, hospital wards, delivery rooms, operating rooms (ORs), intensive care units (ICUs), emergency departments (EDs), and the home.

History has documented that APNs have "pressed the limit" on patient acuity because they now provide clinical reasoning necessary for medical and nursing care of unstable patients who possess minimal physiological resiliency and who are often dependent on life-support drugs and technologies (e.g., exogenous catecholamines, mechanical ventilation, and extracorporeal membrane oxygenators). This evolution has emphasized the serious nature of clinical reasoning to APN students, clinical preceptors (APNs and physicians), and graduate faculty. The serious nature has also provoked the most expert of APNs to seek counsel from other senior APNs and/or collaborating physicians to validate their reasoning of "tough" cases that present with atypical symptomatology, multiple interacting diagnoses, or tenuous physiology, and that require ever-increasing, complex treatment plans. The serious nature of learning and maintaining competence in clinical reasoning has also challenged graduate nursing programs in the United States to emphasize and integrate clinical reasoning into didactic portions of curriculums, recruit and retain high-quality clinical preceptors, and to ingrain the critical need for lifelong learning into their graduates.

This chapter provides an overview of the essential features of the cognitive processes involved in diagnostic and treatment reasoning. Although the scientific literature abounds with philosophical approaches to and probabilistic analyses of clinical reasoning, a pragmatic approach was chosen to simplify communicating the essential tenets of clinical reasoning to graduate APN students and beginning clinicians as they begin to experience the intense, case-based nature of clinical practice. As every APN has been warned to "cut to the chase" during some case presentation in their career, this chapter attempts to do the same on a topic about which volumes of medical and nursing textbooks have been written. The author's faculty experience in teaching graduate nurse practitioner students in the specialty field of adult critical care revealed that students exhibit far more difficulty in reasoning through medical problems than nursing ones. For this reason, the clinical exemplars contained in this chapter are primarily medically focused.

Finally, the integration of principles of clinical reasoning is not gained by reading chapters such as this; rather, it is only gained through repetitive clinical exposure to literally hundreds of cases to acquire the "clinical pearls" that help bring reasoning into clear focus. It is for this reason that this chapter is immediately followed by four cases that were written in a reality-based format by expert APNs, who reveal their inner clinical reasoning as their cases unfold over time.

Clinical Reasoning

Clinical reasoning is a complex thinking process that is used to acquire and evaluate data and make decisions about the diagnosis and treatment of patient problems. The terms "clinical decision making," "clinical problem solving," and "critical thinking" are often used synonymously with the term "clinical reasoning" in the health science literature. The term "clinical reasoning" will be used throughout this chapter because it emphasizes the metacognition ("thinking about thinking") of the process, which is needed to produce logical, sound clinical decisions (Table 5-1).

The outcomes of clinical reasoning are the clinical decisions of diagnosis and treatment, which should lead to problem resolution. The provision of sound and consistent clinical reasoning has serious ramifications when the consequences of inaccurate and/or inefficient clinical reasoning are considered. Cognitive error in the clinical reasoning process has been documented to result in patient anxiety, serious morbidity, excessive cost, poor clinical outcomes, and life-threatening situations (Kassirer & Kopelman, 1989a). Errors in clinical reasoning can occur at any point in the clinical reasoning process and may result in failure to begin treatment, institution of inappropriate treatment, and/or late treatment (Table 5-2).

TABLE 5-1 *Cognitive Functions Embedded in Clinical Reasoning*

▪ Collecting	▪ Formulating
▪ Organizing	▪ Analyzing
▪ Postulating	▪ Corroborating
▪ Debating	▪ Justifying
▪ Rationalizing	▪ Confirming
▪ Synthesizing	
▪ Verifying	
▪ Discriminating	

TABLE 5-2 *Effect of Errors in Clinical Reasoning*

Failure to Begin Treatment		Inappropriate Treatment		Late Treatment	
Errors	*Potential Effects*	*Errors*	*Potential Effects*	*Errors*	*Potential Effects*
▪ Failure to diagnosis	▪ Progression of disease, condition, or state ▪ Complications of disease, condition, or state	▪ Inaccurate diagnosis ▪ Inaccurate treatment	▪ Progression of disease, condition, or state ▪ Complications of disease, condition, or state ▪ Side effects of inappropriate treatment ▪ Economic cost of inappropriate treatment	▪ Inefficient diagnosis ▪ Inefficient treatment initiation	▪ Progression of disease, condition, or state ▪ Complications of disease, condition, or state ▪ Decreased treatment efficacy owing to late initiation

FACTORS CHALLENGING CLINICAL REASONING

Many patient, clinician, and healthcare factors challenge the APN's ability to perform consistent and sound clinical reasoning (Table 5-3). The factor of patient acuity is one that commonly affects clinician's ability to clinical reason. Primary care patients are seen in clinic settings where life-threatening conditions occur less commonly than in acute care settings, which is not to deemphasize that seizures, acute chest pain, anaphylactic reactions, and vasovagal syncope do occur in this setting. In primary care settings, though, clinicians are usually able to reach fairly complete diagnoses in stable patients before treatment is initiated (Goldman, 1990a). On the other hand, patients in hospital settings often possess higher acuity levels and varying degrees of physiological instability. These factors often necessitate the clinician to acquire and perform the history and physical examination, diagnostic tests, and evaluation of bedside physiological data concurrently. Clinicians practicing in critical care, perioperative care, delivery rooms, and emergency departments function under uncertain conditions due to rapidly deteriorating physiological states which often require resuscitative treatment actions before confirming laboratory data is available for diagnosis (Szaflarski, 1997). Thus, these clinicians must diagnose and treat simultaneously, attempt to achieve diagnostic closure in restricted time frames, and live with diagnostic uncertainty which is endemic to these environments (Goldman, 1990a; Goldman & Ravindranath, 1994). In these situations, treatment may also obscure signs or symptoms from developing, which would greatly assist in diagnosis (Richards, 1990).

Regardless of the practice setting, clinicians are also required to act rapidly on the basis of partial data, unconfirmed data, or even contradictory data (Goldman & Ravindranath, 1994). Comprehensive databases, which are essential to diagnostic reasoning, are often incomplete or absent. Patients may be poor historians or present with altered mental status whereby the current and past medical history is unknown or dependent on the memory of accompanying significant others or emergency medical personnel. Medical records are heavily relied on but often cannot be accessed in a timely fashion. Although laboratory point-of-care technology is frequently present in clinics and hospitals, turnaround times for other essential laboratory tests are often inadequate, resulting in frequently treating the patient before the result returns.

TABLE 5-3 *Factors Challenging the Clinical Reasoning Process of APNs*

Patient-related Factors

Poor historians (poor short-term, long-term memory)

Altered mental status (acute or chronic)

Unavailability of family or significant other(s)

Inaccurate reports of significant events from family witnesses

Unknown or unclear patient preferences in regard to:
- quality of life
- level of pain and suffering that patient is willing to endure
- advance directives

Noncompliance to treatment regimen

Increasing severity of illness

Unstable physiological status

Loss of symptoms and/or physical examination data due to treatment effects

Disease or condition with multiple systemic effects

Multiple, individual diseases, conditions, or states

Prolonged duration of disease, condition, or state (acute or chronic)

Financial constraints

Clinician–related Factors

Current and expanding scientific knowledge of:
- epidemiology of diseases, conditions, or syndromes (e.g., changing incidence, presentation patterns, or risk factors)
- diagnostic and supportive technologies (e.g., underlying science, sensitivity and specificity, risks, or efficacy)
- treatments and treatment regimens (e.g., efficacy, comparable efficacy, interaction between treatments, side effects, or complications)
- clinical practice guidelines
- clinical research findings

Managed care effects:
- increasing quantity of patients in clinical caseloads
- increasing demands for cost-effectiveness and efficiency
- increasing constraints on ordering diagnostic tests
- required justification for moderately and high expensive treatments
- increasing time limitations on clinic visits
- required justification for expensive clinic or hospital resources owing to gate-keeping control (e.g., invasive procedures, hospital and ICU admissions, or emergency surgery)

Increasing review of high-volume data streams ("data-intense" environments)

Healthcare Environment

Iatrogenicity

Uncertainty of data (incomplete databases)
- unavailable or incomplete medical records or slow retrieval of records
- slow communication of results of diagnostic or procedural tests or surgical procedures
- inaccurate or missing physiological data in medical record
- inadequate chart documentation of significant physiological events

Prolonged waiting interval for diagnostic tests or procedures

Disease complexity challenges clinical reasoning. Multiple diseases or conditions, especially in elderly adults, represent an ever-growing diagnostic challenge. The multiplicity may stem from diseases or conditions that have multisystem effects (e.g., hypertension, diabetes, and sepsis) or from multiple independent disorders. Clinicians in clinic, hospital, and home settings are thus called on to deal with simultaneous multiple problems in an individual patient or serially with clusters of problems. Signs and/or symptoms of chronic diseases may inadvertently draw the attention of the clinician away from the presenting complaint. Chronic diseases or conditions, as well as the frailty of the elderly, frequently predispose adults to developing iatrogenic problems that add to their multiplicity of problems. Iatrogenic morbidity resulting from stress, infection, ischemia, and emboli frequently complicate the clinical reasoning process because many of these interdependent processes occur simultaneously. Being assigned to care for a patient with multiple acute and/or chronic disorders in the midst of a case can be a formidable challenge for any clinician; it takes considerable skill to sift out salient data from a "2-inch thick" medical record and make sense of the available data within a short time frame.

Ethical considerations challenge clinical reasoning (Neuhaus, 1988). Issues of quality of life, pain and suffering, and advance directives may directly affect competent patients' willingness to agree to the diagnostic workup and/or treatment plan that the clinician has recommended. In these cases, the clinician is left with reconsidering other diagnostic and therapeutic options that meet the needs of patients and/or their significant others. The issue of withdrawal or withholding of therapy may arise from requests of patients or families or from the clinician who prognosticates a poor outcome. The clinician is challenged in these instances to propose a treatment plan that is aimed solely at comfort measures.

The scientific knowledge explosion greatly challenges the cognitive ability of clinicians to keep pace with new scientific evidence which postulates new mechanisms of disease or changing patterns of disease incidence, new technological advances in diagnosis and treatment, and clinical research findings of new treatments. In addition to these taxing factors, clinicians are now experiencing added stresses and constraints in clinical reasoning due to cost containment strategies instituted by managed care. Diagnostic workups are being increasingly scrutinized by insurance and hospital administrators for their cost-effectiveness and cost efficiency, which have led to mandatory algorithms in some healthcare systems. The effect of all of these factors not only challenges but places enormous added mental stress on the clinician to provide accurate and efficient clinical reasoning.

TYPES OF KNOWLEDGE

Clinical reasoning is characterized by a blend of processes that can either be systematically analyzed or escape quantitative analysis because of the intuitive nature of knowledge. Different processes are used depending on the clinical situation or the expertise of the clinician (Tanner, 1987). Systematic processes involve the use of explicit knowledge. Explicit knowledge can be systematically described, analyzed, measured, and taught. Explicit knowledge is essential to the clinical reasoning process because it provides the backbone on which reasoning takes place. Examples of explicit knowledge include epidemiology, mechanisms, clinical presentation of physical or psychological diseases, conditions or states, knowledge of physical examination, diagnostic tests and approaches, and treatment regimens.

Although some clinicians and educators believe that clinical reasoning is a fully explicit process, others believe that tacit knowledge, or intuition, is used in the complex process of clinical judgment (Goldman, 1990b; Tanner, 1987). Tacit knowledge is knowledge possessed without conscious awareness. Other researchers refer to this knowledge as intuition, describing it as understanding without a rationale (Benner & Tanner, 1987). This knowledge assists intermediate and advanced clinicians in analyzing data and making rapid, complex clinical decisions. This form of knowledge cannot be articulated in explicit terms; this becomes evident when expert clinicians attempt to reconstruct all the mental steps in making a diagnosis but are unable to provide satisfactory description of key elements of the mental process (Goldman, 1990b). Expert clinicians frequently reach a diagnosis without knowing every step used in the mental process.

The APN student unconsciously learns tacit knowledge initially through observing and working closely with clinical experts. Individual, quantitative exposure to a multitude of cases then allows the novice clinician to unknowingly use and build on this knowledge. Tacit knowledge is thus often learned through a lengthy apprenticeship or residency with a clinical expert, by listening to case presentations, defending one's clinical reasoning of cases in clinical rounds and by attending conferences where the clinical reasoning of cases is dissected (Goldman, 1990b). It is believed that some combination of these two forms of knowledge generates clinical expertise in clinical reasoning activities.

CHARACTERISTICS OF EXPERT CLINICAL REASONING

Students along with novice and intermediate-level clinicians learn how to clinically reason from expert clinicians through quantitative case analyses. Expert clinicians are masters at what they do because they possess an organized and networked knowledge, a comprehensive mental library of patients, and efficient problem-solving skills. Experts' knowledge is comprehensive and is elaborately organized so that information storage and retrieval is easy. Their clinical knowledge is linked into networks of concepts and their relationships which is then compiled into a higher-order knowledge structure that links intricate neural networks into a scheme of relationships and diagnoses (Bordage & Lemieux, 1991). Because of these neural networks, experts are able to quickly access the domain-specific information that they have stored in their long-term memory. Medical research supports that this networked organization of knowledge and its compilation is "vital" to its retention and retrieval, which are critical to successful problem solving (Mandin, Jones, Woloschuk, & Harasym, 1997). Research has demonstrated that the organization and understanding of experts' knowledge is far more important than the amount of knowledge stored in memory (Mandin, Jones, Woloschuk, & Harasym, 1997). Because the current focus of graduate education of APNs often emphasizes quantity of knowledge gained, these findings have enormous implications as to how clinical reasoning should be taught to APNs.

Expert clinicians possess comprehensive mental libraries of past cases in their specialty field of practice. Quantitative exposure to literally hundreds and thousands of patient cases over time has created mental templates of multiple clinical problems that afford experts a comprehensive memory of having seen a majority of common and uncommon clinical presentations, diagnostic conundrums, and treatment dilemmas. They possess first-hand experience in having directly seen approximately 90 to 95% of the variance that occurs in their patient population (the remaining 5 to 10% represent new variances in disease presentation or new diseases or conditions). Efficient clinical problem solving by expert clinicians is linked to the "pattern recognition" that they have developed in their mental patient libraries. Pattern recognition leads to rapid problem solving through comparison of past cases, which are instantaneously and unconsciously recalled and compared to features of the case at hand. Further aspects of pattern recognition will be discussed in the following section on diagnostic reasoning.

ℰ *Diagnostic Reasoning*

Diagnostic reasoning is a dynamic thinking process that is hypothesis-driven and targeted toward the selection of an hypothesis that best explains clinical evidence. As the initial stage in the clinical decision-making process, diagnostic reasoning results in the diagnosis of a clinical state, disorder, syndrome, or disease. Although diagnostic reasoning is one of the most critical skills of clinical decision analysis, it is the least understood among clinicians and educators and is associated with cognitive error in all steps of the diagnostic reasoning process (Kassirer & Kopelman, 1989b; Pople, 1982; Voytovich, Rippey, & Suffredini, 1985).

TYPES OF DIAGNOSTIC REASONING

Three types of diagnostic reasoning are used by clinicians throughout the diagnostic process (Kassirer, 1989). Deterministic (or categorical) reasoning relies on compiled knowledge that exists in the form of unambiguous rules. These rules outline routine clinical practices that often exist in the form of diagnostic algorithms or lists of rules. For example, the clinical finding of a diastolic blood pressure (BP) of 95 mm Hg elicits a diagnosis of mild hypertension (Type I) based on preestablished rules. Because many clinical problems occur repetitively and are often straightforward in their diagnosis, deterministic rules frequently guide diagnostic reasoning (Kassirer, 1989).

Causal, or physiologic, reasoning is based on the cause and effect relationship between clinical data (Kassirer, 1989; Epstein & Pauker, 1998). For example, if the acute deterioration of an immobile, mechanically ventilated adult with severe acute lung injury involved acute oxygen desaturation, hypotension, and a rapid rise in peak airway pressure, then these pathophysiological effects could be fully explained by the presence of a tension pneumothorax. Other diagnostic hypotheses that could be considered include pulmonary embolism and right mainstem intubation, but neither of these fully explain all of the three stated pathophysiological effects. Causal reasoning typically involves the creation of a pathophysiological hypothesis, which provides the necessary framework for further data acquisition, interpretation, and validation (Epstein & Pauker, 1998).

Lastly, probabilistic reasoning is based on associations between clinical data that trigger the potential presence of disease. Given the patient's demographics and presenting manifestations, the prevalence of all possible diseases are estimated along with the likelihood of signs and symptoms associated with a specific disease. Clinicians frequently express the likelihood of a condition by using the subjective and informal categories of quite likely, common, frequent, or rare. The use of objective estimates of probabilities of diseases or conditions may also be acquired from the medical and nursing literature (Epstein & Pauker, 1998).

DEPENDENT FACTORS

The quality of diagnostic reasoning heavily depends on the knowledge base and the ability of individuals to organize knowledge into meaningful patterns (Grant & Marsden, 1987; Lipman & Deatrick, 1997; Norman, 1988). Knowledge of conditions, states, or diseases provides clinicians with information as to their relative probability of occurrence, risk factors, pathophysiological features, mechanism of operation, and associated clinical manifestations (Connelly & Johnson, 1980). Students often lack adequate knowledge of a broad spectrum of conditions or diseases that is commonly linked to their past nursing experience in a sole specialty field; lack of knowledge is likely to result in diagnostic failure (Table 5-4). Equally ineffective is a large body of knowledge that is unorganized and memorized into long lists (Bordage & Lemieux, 1991). Other competencies that influence the effectiveness of reasoning include skill in collecting data, interpersonal skills, and the ability to involve the patient in decision making (Higgs, 1992). Nurse practitioners have been found to develop considerable diagnostic accuracy as a result of their attention to qualitative distinctions in their assessments. Such accuracy accrues through spending time with patients, listening in a focused manner, and experiencing the detection of subtle cues (Brykczynski, 1989).

Pattern recognition of conditions or diseases has been heralded as one of the most important processes that expedites economy in the diagnostic process (Bockenholt & Weber, 1993; Tanner, 1987). The acquired ability to quickly identify similarities of clusters of signs or symptoms between the presenting patient and a specific disease entity is an important probability association. Pattern recognition involves the simultaneous ability to recall the pattern of signs and symptoms for a disease and the ability to discriminate the manifestations of one disease from another (Gorry, 1970). Novice clinicians often lack depth of knowledge, confidence, prompt recall and order in reconstructing signs and symptoms of diseases, and typically have difficulty in this process (Table 5-4). Students' knowledge of disease patterns has been likened to the trunk and major branches of a tree, whereas the knowledge of master clinicians is the twigs and leaves (Riegelman, 1991).

Because of constant practice, expert clinicians retain vivid memories of previous patients as individual prototypes (Riegelman, 1991; Schmidt, Norman, & Boshuizen, 1990). These paradigm cases represent outstanding diagnostic exemplars that clinicians have solved before, which allows them to rapidly and automatically recall the diagnostic solution (Norman & Schmidt, 1992). Pattern recognition allows experts to diagnose without any type of search strategy and involves fast and unconscious recall of medical or nursing knowledge which is matched to the presenting signs or symptoms of the patient. They are able to view a new case as being similar to an archived case and retrieve diagnostic details about it. The degree of similarity between cases allows for rapid broadening or narrowing of diagnostic possibilities (Fulop, 1985).

Limitations to pattern recognition exist. The ability of clinicians to recognize patterns of diseases or conditions is often limited by the natural history of a disease because the early course of a disease may not present with any symptoms or signs (Nardone, 1990). Patients who present with incomplete or modified clinical manifestations or fail to communicate essential manifestations may lead the clinician to incorrectly identify the pattern of disease. Clinicians may try to fit clinical manifestations into one disease pattern when indeed they may result from two or more diseases. Clinicians may also not be able to fit signs and symptoms into a prototype disease pattern because their memory only recalls common manifestations, not

 TABLE 5-4 *Common Difficulties in Diagnostic Reasoning of Student and Novice APNs*

- Performance of an appropriate, time-efficient, and organized history and physical examination (H & P)
- Assimilation of H & P data
- Formulation of an appropriate and comprehensive differential diagnosis
- Limited knowledge of disease, condition, or state (e.g., probability, common initial presentations, and natural history of disease or condition)
- Slow and cumbersome pattern recognition due to underdeveloped patient library
- Backward reasoning
- Premature bias toward initial diagnostic hypotheses ("anchoring")
- Premature closure of diagnosis ("rushing the diagnosis")
- Inability to synthesize findings and commit to a diagnosis (complex database is overwhelming and leads to difficulty in assembling information and hypothesizing)
- Limited knowledge and understanding of diagnostic approach, and sensitivity and specificity of diagnostic tests

uncommon or atypical clinical manifestations (Gorry, 1970). Certain diseases may also present in a misleading fashion that lead to common diagnostic errors. Medical mirages may exist when symptoms perceived by the patient to occur in one organ system actually originate from another (Riegelman, 1991). Medical masquerades are when signs or symptoms suggest a disease that is not the true disease (Riegelman, 1991). Common examples of these entities include syphilis, subacute bacterial endocarditis, miliary tuberculosis, aortic aneurysm, ectopic pregnancy, and pulmonary emboli.

HEURISTICS

Heuristics, "rules of thumb," are mental strategies that are used as shortcuts to reduce the complex task of assessing diagnostic probabilities to a simple, judgmental process (Goldman, 1990b; O'Neill, 1995). Heuristics are frequently used to assess subjective probabilities. Clinicians rely heavily on heuristics especially when a large degree of uncertainty exists (Goldman, 1990b). Although effective and popular, heuristics often improve the efficiency of diagnostic reasoning but may also lead to biases and errors that can result in poor decision making (Gifford, Mittman, & Vickrey, 1996).

The heuristic "When you hear hoofbeats, don't think zebras" is the most frequently heard and chief epitome of medicine's practical wisdom (Hunter, 1996). It implies that diagnostic hypotheses involving common diseases should receive more credence when they fully explain clinical manifestations. With the clinical finding of systemic hypertension, the clinician should thus initially assign more weight to the diagnostic possibility of essential hypertension than renovascular stenosis because the likelihood of essential hypertension is 95% (Kaplan, 1990). Common diseases occur commonly; thus, clinicians need to remain appropriately focused unless discord among the data become evident.

The use of heuristics should serve to provoke thinking, not restrict it (Hunter, 1996). If one hears hoofbeats while residing in Kansas, one should appropriately think horses. This clinical aphorism serves to remind us of the ordinary real world of common diseases, conditions, and states that exist in most outpatient clinic and hospital settings. On the other hand, if one hears hoofbeats and lives in Africa, one should begin to think zebras. If one practices in an academic tertiary care medical center that operates as a referral center, zebras are apt to be more commonplace. Rare diseases and conditions (e.g., transposition of the great vessels, Creutzfeldt-Jakob disease, and rare leukemias) may be commonplace in referral settings. Regardless of this, however, it should be stressed that atypical presentations of common diseases still occur more frequently than classical presentations of rare diseases (Riegelman, 1991).

THE HYPOTHESIS-DRIVEN STRATEGY

Many models exist to explain the cognitive thinking involved in the diagnostic process. The hypothetical-deductive reasoning strategy is commonly used by clinicians, and initial evidence has shown that nurse practitioners use it in practice (Barrows, & Feltovich, 1987; White, Nativio, Kobert, & Engberg, 1992). Hypotheses are used to progressively rule out conditions or diseases on the basis of the history, physical examination, and/or diagnostic tests; modification and refinement of hypotheses occurs until a working diagnostic hypothesis is defined. Early generation of hypotheses within the diagnostic process serves to efficiently direct the search (Joseph & Patel, 1990). A hypothesis-driven model will be used to review the process of diagnostic reasoning (Figure 5-1) (Nordone, 1990; Szaflarski, 1997).

Problem Identification

The first step in the diagnostic reasoning process is identifying the existence of symptoms or physical signs of importance. No greater substitute for acquiring data exists than the verbal expression of symptoms by the patient (Nardone, 1990). Research has documented that only 18 seconds of free or open-ended expression by the patient elapsed before clinicians took control of the interview (Burack & Carpenter, 1983). The dangers of inhibiting the patient's free expression during the interview are that all symptoms and signs do not get expressed and clinicians become biased by focusing on a single symptom or sign. The importance of clinical information obtained from the history and physical also is underestimated by clinicians who often weight diagnostic test data more owing to its quantitative nature (Panzer, Black, & Griner, 1991). Success or failure in the diagnostic process depends on the relationship that develops between the clinician and patient (Nardone, 1990). A caring and trustful environment with the exhibition of clinical competence often enhances the interchange.

Problem identification depends on the ability of the patient to effectively communicate their symptoms and their report of present illness. The psychological state of the patient along with their short-term memory will affect the quality and reliability of their reporting. Denial of symptoms and/or incomplete presentations can occur secondary to fear or stigmas surrounding diseases and their prognosis.

Patients may present with multiple symptoms. The clinician then becomes responsible for prioritizing the diagnostic workup of the patient's symptoms based on the seriousness and the probability of the diagnostic possibility. During history-taking and the physical examination, clinicians often use shortcuts in gathering data. Novices tend to use nonselective "search and seek" strategies that produce volumes of quantitative data; questions are often nonfocused and nonspecific as to any initial hunches. Research has documented that nurse practitioners (NPs) made diagnostic errors stemming from inconsistent use of clini-

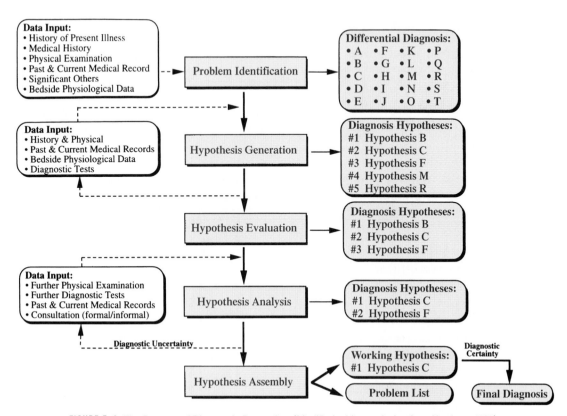

FIGURE 5-1 The Process of Diagnostic Reasoning. (Modified with permission from Nardone, 1990).

cal cues and collection of cues that were unrelated to the diagnostic problem (Rosenthal et al., 1992). Novices often fail to perform additional specific maneuvers on physical examination that would enhance and delimit diagnostic thinking. Experts, on the other hand, are astute clinicians who know the associated physical findings of symptoms. For example, although the novice clinician who evaluates a 68-year-old male with chest pain is mainly suspicious of angina pectoris, the expert, after auscultating a crescendo-decrescendo, systolic murmur in the second right intercostal space that radiates to the carotid arteries, places the entity of aortic stenosis at the top of the list of differential diagnoses.

Differential Diagnosis

Differential diagnosis is a process that involves logical analysis of all possible causes of the patient's complaint. The initial list of differentials must be all-inclusive because elimination of selected disorders involves prejudgment (Tumulty, 1973). Research has demonstrated that if the correct diagnosis is not in the initial list of differential diagnoses, then the correct diagnosis was less likely to be reached at the end of the case (Gruppen et al., 1993). Deciding on which conditions should be included in the list of differentials frequently depends on what conditions come easily to mind (Riegelman, 1991). Errors in differential diagnosis most frequently result from errors of omission resulting from haphazard guessing games used to create the list (Ledley & Lusted, 1959). Thus, clinicians need to have an organized, systematic method of bringing to mind other diagnostic possibilities. Purposeful thinking of disease categories and/or organ systems will assist in providing structure for the clinician to review (Table 5-5).

Formulation of the differential diagnosis should include consideration of several factors. Thought should be given to the most life-threatening disease that would explain the patient's complaint (Riegelman, 1991). Because common diseases occur commonly, serious consideration should be given to frequently occurring diseases because of their high probability of occurrence. The age and sex of the patient should be factored into the thinking about common diseases because diagnostic possibilities of agitation in a 75-year-old male will clearly be different in a 20-year-old female. The clinician must possess current knowledge of the probability of a disease because the probability of a given disease may change over time (e.g., acquired immune deficiency syndrome and nosocomial infections).

Consideration of rare diseases in the list of differentials should occur in the following cir-

TABLE 5-5 *Disease Categories and Organ Systems Used to Formulate a Differential Diagnosis*

Disease Categories	Organ Systems
▪ Congenital	▪ Neurological
▪ Environmental (toxic)	▪ Muscular
▪ Endocrinologic (metabolic)	▪ Pulmonary
▪ Genetic	▪ Cardiac
▪ Infectious	▪ Vascular
▪ Inflammatory (immunologic)	▪ Gastrointestinal
▪ Mechanical (e.g., pulmonary embolism)	▪ Genitourinary
▪ Neoplastic	▪ Skin
▪ Psychologic–Psychiatric	▪ Psychological
▪ Traumatic	
▪ Unknown	

cumstances (Riegelman, 1991). A rare disease should be considered when it could be altered by early therapy or when the presentation of symptoms is not usual. If unexplained symptoms are present, rare diseases may help to explain their presence. If the initial workup for common diseases proves negative, the likelihood of an uncommon disease becomes greater.

Common errors exist in formulating the differential diagnosis. Failure to accrue thorough information from the patient interview and physical examination often leaves essential details and findings undiscovered whereby salient diseases and conditions may be omitted from the differential ("errors of omission"). Evidence gained from the history and physical examination may be misinterpreted. Lack of familiarity with the full spectrum of disease mechanisms and the likelihood of disease probabilities may contribute to inadvertent omission of conditions from the list as well as improper weighting of diagnoses, a common error of students and novice clinicians. Clinicians may assign the presence of new signs and symptoms to a preexisting chronic disease, thus failing to perceive a new potential disease or a complication resulting from the chronic disease process. Impetuosity may result in the clinician concluding that all clinical manifestations are superficially explained by a disease without considering all disease mechanisms (Tumulty, 1973). The clinician may also become biased to a single diagnosis early on despite evidence that weakens its presence (known as "anchoring"). Out of frustration, clinicians may inadvertently force nonsupporting data to fit a diagnostic category.

Information gained from the history and physical examination generates most of the diagnostic hypotheses. Results of diagnostic tests contribute very little to the generation of hypotheses but prove useful in future steps to rule in or rule out hypotheses. When the clinician constructs the differential diagnosis, a rigorous and thorough search must occur to delineate all possible causes that could explain clinical findings. The best predictor of diagnostic accuracy is the inclusion of the correct diagnosis among the initial list of differential diagnoses being consideration.

Hypothesis Generation

The major function of generating a hypothesis is to guide subsequent information gathering and interpretation by providing a context within which information can be methodically gathered and evaluated (Kassirer & Kopelman, 1991). Early generation of hypotheses is preferred because it provides efficiency to the diagnostic process. Hypotheses allow the clinician to focus on a clinical entity and tailor questions or perform physical examination techniques to prove or disprove its existence. Hypotheses are used to predict cues in the data that can further refine the problem and yield an accurate solution. Data collection, data processing, and hypothesis formulation are highly dependent processes (Samiy & Akman, 1987). Consistency of a hypothesis is constantly evaluated to determine whether the collected data upholds the hypothesis. Candidate hypotheses that are not consistent with the available data are rejected. Hypotheses linked with clusters of data, rather than just a single data bit, are retained (Kassirer & Kopelman, 1989a).

Expert clinicians generate initial hypotheses rapidly and often select a single, working hypothesis based only on the patient's age, sex, and presenting symptom. Research has documented that the earlier a good hypothesis is made, the more predictive it is of the quality of the diagnosis (Joseph & Patel, 1990). Studies of expert clinicians report that an average of five to seven diagnostic hypotheses are initially generated; this small number is attributed to the limitations of human memory (Kassirer & Kopelman, 1991). Research in primary care settings has revealed that nurse practitioners use diagnostic hypotheses in driving subsequent data acquisition (White, Nativio, Kobert, & Engberg, 1992).

Two patterns of diagnostic reasoning are used in generating diagnostic hypotheses (Figure 5-2). Forward reasoning uses a data item or data set to generate a hypothesis (Arocha, Patel, & Patel, 1993). Forward reasoning is characteristic of expert clinicians when they encounter an unusual or difficult clinical problem. Forward reasoning is dependent on a solid knowledge of symptomatology and is highly efficient in leading from

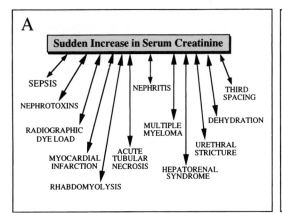
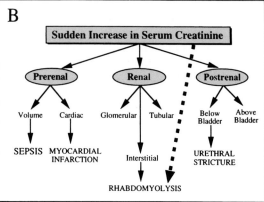

FIGURE 5-2 Patterns of Diagnostic Reasoning. A. Backward reasoning. A search-and-scan form of inquiry that is time-intensive and typical of novice clinicians. Two-headed arrows indicate that each diagnostic hypothesis is sequentially tested. B. Forward reasoning. A scheme-driven form of inquiry in which experts employ pattern recognition (dashed line) to efficiently identify conditions. See text for further explanation. (Modified and with permission from: Mandin, Jones, Woloschuk, & Harasym, 1997).

data to diagnosis (Patel, Groen, and Norman, 1991). For example, forward reasoning allows the clinician to assimilate the data of "nonradiating stomach pains that occur before meals, which is relieved by eating" and generate a hypothesis of duodenal ulcer.

Backward reasoning involves first generating a hypothesis and then examining the available data to see if the data conform to it (Figure 5-2). Backward reasoning is a characteristic of novice clinicians (Arocha, Patel, & Patel, 1993). Lack of knowledge prohibits the clinician from constructing a hypothesis from the data alone and involves generating a single diagnostic hypothesis and then acquiring data to see if it upholds the hypothesis. Backward reasoning is thus inefficient and depends primarily on memory. If hypotheses are slow to come to mind for novice clinicians, conducting the review of systems at an earlier time in the interview may trigger the development of hypotheses (Sox, 1988).

Hypothesis Evaluation

Hypothesis evaluation involves clarifying, refining, and reformulating diagnostic hypotheses through the methodical collection of further data. Each hypothesis is evaluated as to its coherency in explaining all of the clinical manifestations. Physiologic linkages, predisposing factors, and complications are evaluated as to their appropriateness to each hypothesis. Hypotheses are tested by further interviewing and conducting specific physical examination maneuvers. Hypotheses that cannot be tested by these methods are tested through conducting diagnostic tests. Hypotheses are mentally assigned a probability that is adjusted upward or downward, depending on new information gained from the history, physical examination, and diagnostic tests (Kaplan, 1990). Thus, evaluation of hypotheses is dynamic, continuous, and iterative. New information can confirm an existent hypothesis, reject an existent hypothesis, or help create a new hypothesis (Sox, 1988). New information reduces the state of diagnostic uncertainty. The greatest reduction in the degree of diagnostic uncertainty usually occurs following the initial contact with the patient.

Common Errors in Hypothesis Evaluation

Common cognitive errors exist when evaluating diagnostic hypotheses. Clinicians often fail to search for confirming evidence of a disease process. This often occurs when clinicians become biased in favor of a certain diagnosis and do not collect essential data for other hypotheses or misinterpret results (Harvey, Bordley, & Barondess, 1979). Clinicians may become oversensitized to irrelevant clinical manifestations and place enormous weight on inappropriate diagnostic hypotheses (Bockenholt & Weber, 1993). APN students tend to commit to a diagnosis too early in the reasoning process, which is known as premature diagnostic closure (Lipman and Deatrick, 1997).

Hypothesis Analysis

The process of analyzing hypotheses involves the modification of hypotheses, the elimination of diagnostic hypotheses, the discrimination between competing hypotheses, and the confirmation of a leading hypothesis (Nardone, 1990). Here, the clinician searches for further signs or symptoms that are highly specific to the leading hypotheses to help confirm it. A rigorous search for coherency among physiologic linkages, predisposing factors, and complications of the disease, as well as consistency between clinical findings, is conducted (Kassirer, 1989). A search for etiologic clues is performed that will help determine the cause of the disease. Case-building is prominent; it involves consolidating clinical data to solidify hypotheses and distinguishing features between two likely hypotheses. This stage results in the production of one or two working hypotheses.

Principles exist for discriminating between two competitive diagnostic hypotheses. When two competitive hypotheses exist, favoring the one that is most common in the general population will prove fruitful. If the evidence for a high fever in a 4-year-old male who presents with depressed level of consciousness points to the two diagnoses of community-acquired pneumonia and brain abscess, the diagnosis of pneumonia should clearly receive higher diagnostic weight, in the absence of focal neurological findings. A second principle involves the diagnosis of exclusion. This implies that if evidence argues strongly against one competing hypothesis, the chance of the other hypothesis being correct is greatly increased.

The question of how much clinical data is enough to substantiate a diagnostic hypothesis frequently arises. Clinicians often develop "thresholds" to assist them in deciding when a conclusion for a diagnosis has been reached (Black, Panzer, Mayewski, & Griner, 1991). When the probability of disease rises above the set threshold, the diagnosis has been confirmed, and no further hypothesis evaluation is necessary. If the probability of disease is below the threshold level, the diagnostic hypothesis can be eliminated. When diagnostic thresholds are set too high, extensive diagnostic workups become indefensible, delaying treatment and increasing cost (Voytovich & Rippey, 1982). Premature diagnostic closure is a risk when thresholds are set too low, resulting in misdiagnosis and potential inappropriate treatment and disease progression.

Hypothesis Assembly

Assembly of the leading hypothesis or hypotheses involves the refinement of a product of impressions and attenuation of diagnostic uncertainty (Bolinger & Ahlers, 1975). If uncertainty still exists, consultation is appropriate to achieve diagnostic closure. The working diagnosis should be concordant with all clinical data, including atypical features and discordant facts, the course of illness, and the clinician's knowledge of the disease process (Samiy & Akman, 1987).

Problem listing is a feature of the hypothesis assembly stage (Nardone, 1990). The clinician uses the signs and symptoms to develop a list of clinical problems. This list must account for all clinical findings. The identification of the clinical problems along with working hypotheses identifies a course of action. Courses of action include ordering additional diagnostic tests, observing the patient to see if additional evidence arises from the natural course of the disease, obtaining a consult, referring the patient, or initiating treatment (Sox, 1988).

DIAGNOSTIC REASONING OF SIGNIFICANT EVENTS

APNs are directly faced with difficult clinical problems whose diagnosis may be aided through the temporal analysis of a clinically significant, physiological event that has occurred. Frequently, these problems present to the APN in the form of an acute episode (e.g., hypotension, seizure, cardiopulmonary arrest, or oxygen desaturation) that requires immediate diagnosis and treatment. In these instances, the sequence of temporal events must be accurately defined, temporally ordered, and analyzed. Event analysis clearly depends on the memory and astuteness of the attendants who witnessed the significant event. Witnesses may vary depending on the setting in which the event occurred (e.g., family members in a home setting, staff nurses in a hospital setting, or paramedics at a trauma scene).

The clinician needs to first assess the witnesses for their level of astuteness, reporting ability, and recall of the significant event. Table 5-6 details a case of a postoperative adult with significant cardiac disease who sustains cardiopulmonary arrest 18 hours following surgery in a monitored stepdown unit. In this example, two witnesses claim that they observed the demise of this patient. The licensed practical nurse (LPN) states that she first observed ventricular tachycardia (VT) that subsequently led to hypotension and, ultimately, the arrest state. The registered nurse (RN), however, critically notes that hypotension was present before the onset of VT. The important difference between these two witnesses' observations is the time at which their observations of the event began (the LPN missed observing the initial hypotension). What is critical to appreciate in this example is how different the differential diagnosis was when each witness's account was considered (Table 5-6). Electrolyte imbalances, acidosis, digitalis toxicity, and myocardial ischemia/infarction are likely diagnoses to account for primary VT in a postoperative patient receiving digoxin. On the other hand, the critical observation of initial hypotension by the RN leads one to rank hypovolemia, myo-

TABLE 5-6 *Analysis of a Significant Physiological Event.* This event involved a 58-year-old male who underwent successful repair of a suprarenal abdominal aortic aneurysm. Past medical history revealed coronary artery disease with two previous myocardial infarctions (preoperative ejection fraction 39%). Intraoperative course was unremarkable except for prolonged aortic cross-clamp time of 70 minutes. The significant event occurred 18 hours postoperatively while the patient was receiving digoxin and while the patient was monitored in a stepdown unit bed. See text for interpretation.

	Time and Observed Events			
	10:10 a.m.	*10:16 a.m.*	*10:17 a.m.*	*Differential Diagnosis*
LPN Witness	▪ None	▪ VT ▪ Hypotension	▪ VT ▪ Cardiopulmonary arrest	#1 Electrolyte depletion (K^+, Mg^{++}, Ca^{++}) #2 Digitalis toxicity #3 Myocardial ischemia +/or infarction #4 Metabolic +/or respiratory acidosis
RN Witness	▪ Hypotension	▪ Hypotension ▪ VT	▪ VT ▪ Cardiopulmonary arrest	#1 Hypovolemia #2 Myocardial ischemia +/or infarction #3 Pulmonary embolism #4 Tension pneumothorax

cardial ischemia/infarction, and pulmonary embolism high on the differential of hypotension in a postoperative patient. Emergency and subsequent treatment for the top diagnostic entities in each differential list is very different in this patient's case. Autopsy results of this patient revealed a massive pulmonary embolism that straddled both right and left main pulmonary arteries despite the prophylactic use of perioperative and postoperative pneumatic thigh and calf compression. This complex case demonstrates two points: first, the need to assess discrepancies among the accounts of witnesses, and second, that the report from an inaccurate or unreliable witness can confound the diagnostic and treatment reasoning instead of clarifying it.

SELECTION AND INTERPRETATION OF DIAGNOSTIC TESTS

An essential part of the diagnostic reasoning process requires thorough knowledge of how to select and interpret diagnostic tests. Proper selection and interpretation of diagnostic tests is an iterative process with the goal of decreasing uncertainty about diagnostic hypotheses that cannot be resolved through interview and physical examination. Diagnostic tests establish or exclude the presence of disease and narrow the list of differential diagnosis. Diagnostic tests are part of a good diagnostic strategy only if the results reduce the error of misdiagnosis (Gorry, 1970). Overreliance on and abuse of diagnostic tests is often related to fear of malpractice (Riegelman, 1991).

The intelligent selection of diagnostic tests depends on several factors. The clinician needs a working knowledge of the characteristics of diagnostic tests to facilitate selection. Selection of diagnostic tests should be based on the clinician's estimate of pretest likelihood of a disease(s) that is the most unlikely or probable diagnosis (Black, Panzer, Mayewski, & Griner, 1991). The accuracy of diagnostic tests along with the costs of tests will be the major influences in the decision-making process. Given the current cost-contained era of healthcare, the monetary cost of the test must be examined along with psychologic distress, time costs, and risk of morbidity or mortality associated with the test. The cost of diagnostic tests must be weighed in view of the current degree of diagnostic uncertainty (Gorry, 1970). The availability of tests and their processing time are also considerations.

Several strategies for selecting diagnostic tests exist to optimize the reduction of diagnostic uncertainty. The use of "rule out" testing is frequently employed when clinicians face a complex diagnostic problem with a broad differential diagnosis. This strategy is best for eliminating diseases that are highly probable on the list of differentials. Using "parallel tests" employs a variety of diagnostic tests that are ordered simultaneously. Parallel testing is used with suspected emergencies in which a diagnosis must be made quickly so that life-saving treatment can be initiated (Bluestein & Archer, 1991). This shotgun approach is used frequently in acute and critical care when time is of the essence. "Serial testing" is when the clinician proceeds from simple to more complex tests; the test result of the first test will then determine which subsequent test should be used (Bluestein & Archer, 1991). Serial testing is often used when patients are studied over time, as in primary care settings. Finally, "repeating tests" are when multiple repetitions of the same test occur over time. Examples include repetitive blood cultures or stool occult blood tests. With these tests, either a positive or negative result can be used to confirm or rule out a disease respectively.

Diagnostic tests possess varying degrees of accuracy and are discussed elsewhere in detail (Bluestein & Archer, 1991; Panzer, Black, & Griner, 1991). Characteristics of accuracy of diagnostic tests will assist the clinician in deciding which diagnostic tests are more likely to produce a higher diagnostic yield and which are liable to errors (Table 5-7) (Harvey, Bordley, & Barondess, 1979). A sensitive test rarely yields a false-negative result and is therefore often the first ordered in a diagnostic workup to detect all individuals with disease (to rule out disease) (Fletcher, Fletcher, & Wagner, 1988). Two or more tests are often used to evaluate a diagnostic possibility because few diagnostic tests exist that are both highly sensitive and specific (Black, Panzer, Mayewski, & Griner, 1991).

TABLE 5-7 *Characteristics of Accuracy of Diagnostic Tests*

Sensitivity:	The likelihood that a diseased patient has a positive test ("positive in disease"). A diagnostic test with high sensitivity has few false negative results and thus will confirm the presence of disease. A sensitive test is often used to exclude a diagnosis or rule out a disease.
Specificity:	The likelihood that a healthy patient has a negative test ("negative in health"). A diagnostic test with high specificity has few false-positive results and thus will confirm the absence of disease. A specific test is often used to confirm a diagnosis or to rule in a disease.
Positive Predictive Value:	The likelihood of having a disease or condition, given a diagnostic test result.
Negative Predictive Value:	The likelihood of not having a disease or condition, given a diagnostic test result.
Likelihood Ratios:	An expression of the probability that a given diagnostic test would occur in a patient with, as opposed to without, the disease or condition. A likelihood ratio of greater than 1.0 denotes that disease probability is increased; a likelihood ratio of less than 1.0 denotes that disease probability is decreased.

Adapted from: Bluestein & Archer, 1991; Nicoll & Detmer, 1997.

Problems exist in interpreting diagnostic test results. If multiple diagnostic tests are ordered, the chance of obtaining a falsely abnormal result is increased. It has been estimated that if 20 independent tests are conducted on a healthy person, a 64% probability exists of having at least one abnormal test result (Nicoll & Detmer, 1997). This is related to the reference or normal range of diagnostic tests. Because reference ranges are determined for 95% of the population, the other 5% of healthy patients will have a test result that falls outside the normal range (Nicoll & Detmer, 1991). Although the test result may be abnormal, it does not imply the presence of disease.

Diagnostic tests cannot be interpreted correctly without determining the suspected probability of the disease before obtaining the test result (Panzer, Black, & Griner, 1991). If the suspected probability of a disease is high, a positive test result helps to confirm the diagnosis, but a negative test result is not convincing in ruling out the disease. If the suspected probability is low, a normal test value helps confirm the absence of disease, while a positive result is not convincing in ruling in the disease.

Unexpectedly, abnormal laboratory results should be repeated if they would result in prompt treatment (Black, Panzer, Mayewski, & Griner, 1991). For example, a high serum potassium level or a high partial prothrombin time would often be repeated first before significant and immediate changes in therapy were implemented. Spurious factors affecting test results include bedside collection errors, equipment errors, and laboratory human error.

Normal test values reflect normal states but may heavily contribute in establishing a diagnosis based on the trend of values. For example, consider the respective levels of an arterial carbon dioxide tension ($PaCO_2$) of 31 and 45 mm Hg occurring in a spontaneously breathing patient with worsening, severe pneumonia on admission and one hour later. Although a $PaCO_2$ level of 44 mm Hg is considered normal, the temporal trend might suggest beginning ventilatory failure that would warrant further close monitoring. Normal values offer no security, especially in unstable patients. Clinicians often also fail to fully use normal values to their greatest potential as negative test results (Riegelman, 1991). Negative test results should assist in ruling out diseases as well as raising the probability of other possible diseases.

The proper selection and interpretation of diagnostic tests will contribute to accurate and efficient diagnostic thinking as well as cost efficiency and effectiveness. The steady growth of diagnostic technology in acute and critical care settings challenges clinicians to keep up-to-date with knowledge of new diagnostic tests as well as their place in the diagnostic evaluation of clinical problems.

Treatment Reasoning

Treatment is the ultimate goal of the patient-clinician encounter, not the diagnosis (Barrows, 1991). Clinicians often consider treatment approaches early in the patient encounter when they are evaluating the patient. Initial thoughts are often placed on considering the alternative general approaches to treatment; examples include medicine versus surgery, medicine as opposed to physical therapy, classes of drugs, and conventional versus complimentary therapies. Subsequently, the clinician reasons through therapeutic possibilities and formulates explicit treatment recommendations that complement the patient's requests and preferences. The quality of reasoning surrounding the prescription of therapy is heavily dependent on the breath and depth of the clinician's knowledge of treatments and their mechanisms of actions, indications, contraindications, efficacy, side effects, and complications. Maintaining a state-of-the-art knowledge base of therapeutic alternatives remains a challenge for every clinician because of the current and future exponential growth of approved pharmaceutical agents and new treatment technologies in the new millennium.

Treatment reasoning begins with first establishing the goal(s) of treatment (Table 5-8; Figure 5-3). If the goals or objectives of treatment are never defined, the clinician will never know if his or her reasoning or the treatment was effective (Barrows, 1991). A common exemplar, which highlights the critical need to set treatment goals before starting treatment, occurs with treatments that are ordered to be "given as needed" (i.e., PRN). Intravenous sedation is a prime example because treatment goals may range widely from decreasing anxiety without affecting airway reflexes, "conscious sedation" for procedures, antegrade amnesia, or decreased motor movement to prevent loss of artificial airway in

TABLE 5-8 *Goals of Therapy*

- Preventitive
  — risk factor modification
    - symptomatic disease, condition, or state
    - asymptomatic disease, condition, or state
  — counselling
  — education
- Curative
- Supportive
  — maintenance of current physiological and/or psychological state
  — improvement in natural course of disease/condition
  — symptom management
    - alleviation of symptoms
    - provision of comfort
    - education
    - psychological support

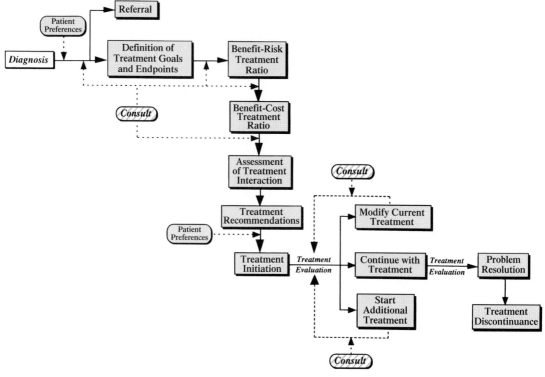

FIGURE 5-3 The Process of Treatment Reasoning.

intubated patients. If a specific goal(s) is not established, then intravenous sedation may inadvertently result in morbidity and negative patient outcomes (e.g., drug side effects, prolonged ICU or hospital stays, tracheal aspiration, or patient dissatisfaction).

The determination of treatment goals needs to be based on an assessment of health-related values, perceptions of quality of life, and preferences of the patient, family, or parents early in the initial patient contact. Such assessment will not only save the clinician time in formulating treatment recommendations, but it will also establish the role that patients, families, and parents are willing to take regarding treatment decision making. Active engagement of patients, families, and parents in discussing and deciding on therapeutic options should be strongly encouraged (Forrow, Wartman, & Brock, 1988). The appraisal of the current quality of life along with advance directives are decisions that patients and families make that can have great impact on the clinician's reasoning in developing a treatment plan. Table 5-9 details factors that clinicians should consider when tailoring a treatment for a specific patient.

The term "treatment" usually evokes thoughts of medical and nursing interventions that prevent, cure, and/or support the condition for which the patient is seeking help. Common treatment options include drug therapy, patient education, counselling, physical therapy, exercise prescriptions, procedures, surgery, and complementary therapies. Other treatment options may not be as apparent because their therapeutic effect may be not as direct. Admission of a patient to a stepdown or intensive care unit can itself be therapeutic because the inherent nursing care rendered in those environments provides a standardized level of monitoring and therapy. The same effect occurs with admission to a hospital or with an order for home nursing care visits.

TABLE 5-9 *Factors to Consider When Prescribing a Treatment for an Individual Patient*

Preferences of patient, family, or parents

Factors underpinning patient treatment compliance

- short-term and long-term memory
- understanding of disease/condition and treatment regimen
- psychomotor ability (e.g., insulin administration)
- psychological stability
- current psychological and social support systems
- insurance coverage
- financial status

Complexity of existent treatment plan (e.g., home drug regimen, home ventilation, and outpatient hemodialysis)

Current status of:

- quality of life rating (e.g., functional capacity, cognitive function, work performance, and
- overall "well-being")
- dietary intake
- substance abuse (e.g., cigarette smoking or drug abuse)
- physiological stability and status
  —age
  —body weight
  —current diagnostic test reports
  —current organ function

Treatment can imply a single treatment prescribed to a patient or be used with the noun "regimen" to connote the full management plan for a particular disease, condition, or state. A common example of a treatment regimen concerns asthma treatment. In this disease, the treatment regimen often consists of an inhaled bronchodilator to relax airway obstruction from constricted bronchioles, an inhaled corticosteroid to reduce airway inflammation and edema, and an inhaled anticholinergic agent to block bronchiole constriction that results from increased vagal activity. Treatment regimens commonly involve multiple treatments that are aimed at a variety of pathophysiological mechanisms underpinning a single disease characteristic; in the previous example, the trifold management plan for asthma is aimed at attacking the three known mechanisms that underpin increased airway resistance. Treatment regimens may also consist of multiple treatments that affect different disease mechanisms. An example is the treatment of an acute myocardial infarction where a thrombolytic agent, heparin, acetylsalicylic acid (ASA), beta-adrenergic blocking agent, nitroglycerin, and an angiotensin-converting enzyme inhibitor (ACEI) may be concurrently administered (assuming no absolute contraindications). Whatever the multipronged attack against the disease or condition is, treatment regimens make reasoning more complex owing to the number of treatments involved.

Many questions need to be answered before starting a treatment (Table 5-10). In many patient encounters, the selection of treatment is automatic and straightforward because the clinician's extensive experience may have confirmed the efficacy and safety of a given treatment (Burgus & Hamm, 1995). Clinicians have developed treatments of choice for

TABLE 5-10 *Treatment Considerations and Decisions*

- Is the treatment necessary or not?
- What are the benefits and risks of a treatment?
- What is the most appropriate treatment(s) for an individual patient, given all appropriate alternatives?
- How will the new treatment affect existing treatments or treatment regimens?
- How should a treatment be administered (e.g., dose, frequency, and route)?
- What sequence of treatments is appropriate?
- How should the treatment be evaluated (e.g., symptom and/or diagnostic monitoring)?
- How often should the treatment be evaluated?
- How should a treatment be modified to enhance its efficacy (i.e., modification of what parameter: dose, frequency, and route)?
- When should treatment be discontinued?

common conditions or diseases that they see on a daily basis (e.g., treatment of a sexually transmitted disease in a clinic setting). However, atypical characteristics of patients (e.g., morbid obesity, organ dysfunction, or comorbid illness), will challenge the clinician in selecting the most appropriate therapy and mandate more rigorous methods of treatment reasoning.

RISK–BENEFIT RATIOS

When patients and families are presented with treatment options, they expect clinicians to provide the scientific information relevant to the proposed treatment (e.g., probability of benefit and risks) and to summarize their clinical experience with the proposed treatment in their patients (Forrow, Wartman, & Brock, 1988). The risk–benefit calculation involves a probability analysis in which the advantages of using specific treatment options are weighed against their disadvantages (Degner & Beaton, 1987). The risk–benefit ratio is an essential step in the treatment reasoning process (Figure 5-3). The calculation of risk and benefits of treatment involves considering all appropriate treatment options for the individual patient; specifying the probability of the efficacy of each treatment tailored to the individual patient; specifying the risks, complications, burdens, and costs of each treatment; and then making a calculation from these data to determine the optimal treatment recommendation for the intended patient. Formal methods for performing decision analysis and probability analyses exist in the medical literature (Epstein & Pauker, 1998; Schwartz & Griffin, 1986). The "thinking through" and weighing the alternatives of a therapeutic option is often typified by "invisible" reasoning because many clinicians unconsciously and simultaneously entertain both diagnostic and treatment options during the initial patient workup (Barrows, 1991).

Some risk–benefit calculations are easier to assess. If the risks of a treatment are very low and the benefits are either questionable or not very high, the treatment may be chosen with the rationale that "it can't hurt and might help." Determination of therapeutic risk–benefit ratios becomes increasingly complicated when the number of major health problems multiplies and the number of available treatment options increases (Degner & Beaton, 1987). For example, the antibiotic treatment of a hospitalized adult who develops acute renal failure from ongoing gram-negative sepsis is exceedingly complex. Other risk–benefit calculations that are difficult and risky occur when the risk and benefits appear to be of equal weight ("50–50" situation) and when the risks of treatment are high but the patient will clearly benefit from the treatment (Degner & Beaton, 1987). The benefits of some treatments may clearly increase life expectancy but at the cost of creating extraordinary burden to the patient and family. Many of these interventions are related to technological advances (e.g., chronic ventilatory support, intravenous infusion pumps, and continuous monitoring) that are instituted in the home and are frequently related to chronic and terminal illness.

The issue of timing is an important feature in calculating treatment risk–benefit ratios. Most treatments work best with greatest efficacy when administered early in the course of disease. If the patient presents late or the clinician makes the diagnosis late in the disease course, the efficacy of a treatment option may be greatly decreased, without necessarily decreasing the treatment's risks.

The risk–benefit ratio of the entire therapeutic plan for a specific patient needs to be determined before new treatment is implemented or before the existent treatment plan is modified. This step is critical because many patients require multiple new treatments or have a new treatment added to an existent complex treatment regimen. The clinician must reason through each individual treatment and determine the probability that each treatment will positively or negatively affect each other. This is known as "treatment interaction." Potential negative or adverse interaction among treatments must be addressed before treatment initiation and the clinician must ensure that attempts to eliminate or minimize negative or adverse interactions have been taken. The determination of the risks and benefits of a complex therapeutic plan requires state-of-the-art knowledge of known interactions among therapies.

Drug interactions represent a source of serious concern for the clinician due to the ever-growing number of new pharmaceutical agents on the market, the polypharmacy of specialty populations, and the serious morbidity associated with drug interactions. A drug interaction refers to an event in which the usual therapeutic effect of a drug is modified by other factors, such as diet, environment, or other drugs; mechanisms of drug interactions are multiple have been described in the literature (Malseed, Goldstein, & Balkon, 1995). A drug interaction between two drugs may result in synergism (e.g., additive effect or potentiation) or antagonism (e.g., competitive, chemical, or physiologic effects). As the growing occurrence and complexity of polypharmacy rises among geriatric, chronic organ failure, and transplanted patients, clinicians are increasing the frequency of consultation with clinical pharmacists before implementing new or changed drug regimens.

Errors in calculating risk–benefit ratios of potential treatment in the past have primarily stemmed from judgment bias in risk perception (Dawson & Arkes, 1987; Hamm & Zubialde, 1995; Schwartz & Griffin, 1986). The perception of a certain risk of a treatment is often influenced by the clinician's objective clinical experience with risk. Because of errors associated with treatment reasoning, a new approach arose in the 1980s to assist in the determination of risk–benefit ratios based on scientific evidence. This approach has been termed "evidence based medicine."

EVIDENCE-BASED MEDICINE

Therapeutic recommendations are becoming increasingly based on the results of peer-reviewed scientific studies. Large prospective controlled clinical trials, which demonstrate that a certain treatment lowers morbidity and mortality in a specific population, give clinicians the necessary support to recommend a treatment (Forrow, Wartman, & Brock, 1988). In the hierarchy of evidence, randomized controlled clinical trials have been recognized as providing the best evidence. Meta-analysis is also gaining increasing popularity and acceptance as a method for summarizing the results of a number of clinical trials focused on an intervention. However, the problems facing clinicians are keeping up with research results of clinical trials and integrating their implications into their daily clinical practice. One method created to enhance treatment reasoning and decision making as a result of the knowledge explosion is evidence-based medicine.

Evidence-based medicine (EBM) is "the conscientious, explicit, and judicious use of current best evidence in making decisions about the care of individual patients" (Sackett et al., 1996). EBM attempts to shift the basis of decision making away from clinical experience, intuition, and pathophysiological rationale toward a critical examination of scientific findings (Wijetunge & Baldock, 1998). Through a process of systematically finding and appraising research findings, EBM stresses the need to look for evidence to judge the effectiveness of medical treatments and to be cautious in acting purely from unsystematic clinical experience, intuition, and untested pathophysiologic reasoning in clinical decision making (Chessare, 1998; Rosenberg & Donald, 1995). EBM helps clinicians by enhancing skills involving acquisition of scientific literature through clinical informatics and critical appraisal. EBM also highlights determinants of clinical decisions including caregiver knowledge, pathophysiology, research evidence, patient and societal values, and care costs (Cook, 1998). The EBM movement has promoted the format of "integrated reviews," which compile results of clinical trials into relevant evaluative summaries for clinicians. EBM has gained momentum in the past 5 years as a result of enthusiasm from clinicians and from pressures to contain healthcare costs.

The methods underpinning EBM are currently not taught in conventional graduate nursing curriculums. Whether APNs will embrace the EBM movement remains to be determined. The integration of this method in medicine is, however, becoming increasingly clear as it is becoming a standard part of medical school curriculums (Chessare, 1998). APNs can learn EBM methods through continuing educational coursework that typically emphasizes strategies on how to search the literature and critically appraise the evidence for its validity and usefulness; these courses are usually taught in small groups. EBM requires the real-time availability of scientific information in order to search medical and nursing databases and search for evidence-based integrated reviews via the Internet in order to gain the best evidence available (Chessare, 1998). EBM represents one significant method for potentially improving the reasoning underpinning treatment decision making.

BENEFIT–COST RATIOS

In the era of managed care, the economic costs of individual treatments as well as the full therapeutic plan must be balanced in relation to their potential benefits. The APN has a responsibility to provide cost-effective care not only within the healthcare institution or health plan, but also to the patient directly. Patients and their families face a multitude of sources in which they directly are responsible for healthcare costs (Table 5-11). In formulating the treatment plan, the APN must retain a current knowledge of many of the sources of patient costs within individual health plans in order to provide cost-effective care to the patient. For example, an awareness of which outpatient prescription drugs are categorized as "formulary" and "nonformulary" by a certain health plan may directly affect treatment compliance due to differences in copayments for the patient, as well as knowing which brand name drugs have equally effective generic equivalents. Other copayment structures in regard to office visits and outpatient laboratory test copayments may directly affect the clinician's treatment reasoning in recommending a therapeutic plan and in altering the frequency of evaluation of a particular treatment. A current knowledge of community resources that offer free or reduced charges for surgical services, substance abuse programs, and used medical equipment is essential when treating indigent or homeless patients who may otherwise be unable to afford prescribed treatments. Establishing a close relationship with a social worker in the clinic or hospital environment will assist the APN in recommending a cost-effective treatment plan.

For APNs practicing within hospital environments, expensive and/or extensive diag-

TABLE 5-11 *Potential Sources of Treatment Costs to Patients*

A. Outpatient services
- Office visit copayments
- Outpatient diagnostic test copayments
- Outpatient prescription drug copayments
- Outpatient physical medicine
- Ambulance services
- Emergency room services
- Pregnancy-related services
- Ambulatory surgical services
- Home care
- Home medical equipment
- Nutritional supplements
- Prosthetic appliances
- Rehabilitation care
- Psychiatric care
- Speech therapy
- Family planning services
- Substance abuse and alcoholic treatment programs

B. Inpatient services
- Room rates
- Professional fees
- Operative and delivery procedures
- Pharmacy charges
- Diagnostic test services
- Physical therapy/occupational therapy

C. Other services
- Hospice care
- Skilled nursing care

nostic workups and treatment plans may be challenged by case managers employed by individual health plans or healthcare institutions. Specific algorithms for diagnosis and treatment may be enforced by health plans or institutions as cost-curbing measures surrounding "expensive" diagnoses or treatments. Although some APNs may possess admission privileges, decisions to admit patients to "high-cost" care environments (e.g., OR, ICU, and ER) may be challenged by gate-keeping personnel whereby the APN is forced to rethink alternative strategies. In these situations, the cost–benefit ratios of alternative strategies may be best developed and optimized through consultation with members of the medical or nursing team with whom the APN works intensely.

TREATMENT AS DIAGNOSIS

Treatment reasoning can be aided by interventions that are therapeutic as well as diagnostic. If treatment provides relief of the presenting problem, then the list of differential diagnoses may become narrowed or a specific diagnosis may be confirmed. For example, a diagnostic conundrum that commonly arises is in differentiating the causes of chest pain. If the administration of sublingual nitroglycerin relieves chest pain, then the problem is likely owing to esophageal spasm or myocardial ischemia. If further therapy of antacid administration at a different time relieves chest pain, then fairly strong evidence points toward esophageal pain. The effect of therapy in aiding diagnosis may also save considerable time, pain, suffering, and cost in the diagnostic workup.

Clinicians frequently overlook the ability of simple treatments to aid in diagnosis. An example is the application of 100% oxygen via a nonrebreather face mask to a hospitalized adult who develops acute shortness of breath who concurrently exhibits acute arterial oxygen desaturation (80% by pulse oximeter) in the face of increased spontaneous minute ventilation. If the application of oxygen results in briskly raising arterial oxygen saturation levels back to normal, then the differential diagnosis of the arterial hypoxemia can be quickly limited to causes surrounding ventilation/perfusion mismatch. On the other hand, if oxygen administration does not raise arterial oxygen saturation values, then a diagnosis of intrapulmonary shunt is strongly supported, which can greatly hasten the treatments of airway intubation, mechanical ventilation, and application of positive end-expiratory pressure (PEEP). Another common example of how treatment can help diagnosis is when intravenous (IV) fluids are administered for hypotension when the source of hypotension is unknown and reliable clinical parameters of intravascular volume status are not available. If the administration of IV fluids resolves hypotension, then a diagnosis of hypovolemia can be inferred.

CONDITIONS OF UNCERTAINTY AND URGENCY

Diagnostic uncertainty can occur because of insufficient or nonsupporting data that do not corroborate each other. Treatment decisions often must be made before a diagnosis has been confirmed. If the risk of treatment is low or if the efficacy of therapy is high, then administration of treatment should occur. If the risk of treatment is unusually high, then the treatment should be given only if the probability of the suspected disease or condition is high (Kassirer & Kopelman, 1991). In these cases, the decision to continue with further diagnostic workup may precede treatment.

The need to administer treatment before the diagnosis is established frequently occurs in practice settings where patients present with or develop acute conditions. If a 4-month-old, lethargic baby presents to an emergency clinic with a temperature of 41°C, the decision to treat the fever is very likely to even preceed the full history and physical examination for three reasons. First, a child with a high fever is at risk of developing seizures; second, the treatment of fever in a child carries low risk and high efficacy; and third, the presence of fever-related lethargy may obscure focal or general findings on the neurologic examination and delay diagnosis.

Clinicians face other dilemmas in urgent situations when administering treatment before establishing a diagnosis. Administration of treatment may greatly obscure signs or symptoms that may assist in making the diagnosis. Common examples of treatments that result in loss of symptoms and other physical examination data include intravenous sedation, neuromuscular blockade, and airway intubation. The tenuous balance that exists among the probability of complications, degree of physiological instability, and the degree of diagnostic uncertainty guides clinicians in making the decision whether to treat or not to treat.

EVALUATION OF TREATMENT

Treatment goals or objectives serve an important purpose in the evaluation of the efficacy of treatment. Treatment objectives help clinicians to decide whether the treatment has resulted in improved or worsened status within a specified time frame and whether treatment end points have been achieved. The serial use of clinical indicators is needed to estimate the degree of improvement or deterioration in the patient's condition after a chosen treatment has begun. Objective clinical indicators commonly include diagnostic tests (e.g., blood counts, serum drug levels, chest X-rays, and blood gases), physical examination criteria, or other physiological criteria (e.g., body weight, blood pressure, and pulse oximeter readings). Subjective criteria include ratings from the patient in regard to specific symptoms or overall ratings related to general health (e.g., functional ability and quality of life). Evaluation of parameters will guide decisions on whether the current treatment is adequate, whether the treatment plan needs to modified or changed altogether, or whether treatment needs to be discontinued (Figure 5-3).

A Few Words About Learning Clinical Reasoning

No method of learning clinical reasoning will ever replace the one-on-one interchange and experience that occurs between a patient and an APN. Learning clinical reasoning is a "time-in-grade" phenomenon that can be accelerated through direct exposure to quantitative cases, actively observing the clinical reasoning of experts, and other methods detailed in the literature (Fonteyn, 1995; Lange et al., 1997; Prion & Graby, 1995; Tryssenar, 1995; Van Leit, 1994). The use of practice guidelines and diagnostic and treatment algorithms, developed by governmental and medical and nursing organizations, are often beneficial to students and beginning APNs in learning clinical reasoning because diagnostic and treatment pathways are dissected and outlined in their format. Although these aids may assist in providing novice clinicians with beginning templates of standard care, their scientific validity is often unproved. Their use has been criticized by many because of their "cookbook" approach, which can lead clinicians to think that the approaches are a means to an end (Epstein & Pauker, 1998). These aids were intended to "guide" the management of clinical problems and never to substitute for independent reasoning.

Another primary method of learning clinical reasoning is the study of clinical cases. Many case studies, however, are written in a full-disclosure format in which the entire case (diagnosis and treatment) is revealed and then followed by expert commentary. Although full-disclosure formats are beneficial to many intermediate and expert clinicians, this format has not proven fruitful to students or beginning clinicians because step-by-step reasoning is not explicitly revealed. A case format that has proven beneficial to students and beginning clinicians is the "progressive disclosure format" (Ryan-Wenger & Lee, 1997). The progressive disclosure format discusses a specific case in a format that mimics the reality of an actual case evolving across time. Clinical data of a case are revealed in sequential stages with expert commentary being given at each stage which details reasoning at each point in time. A well-known exemplar of this format is the running feature in the *New England Journal of Medicine* titled, "Clinical Problem-Solving." The reader is encouraged to examine and experience this format in the four case exemplars that immediately follow this chapter. The "bold" text in these case exemplars delineates the data as it unfolds across time. The "regular" text represents the clinician's reasoning underpinning the most recent aliquot of data.

Conclusion

Clinical reasoning is a difficult, complex process that advanced practice nurses are performing daily in their practices. It is a process that APNs must learn and master for them to be successful in their roles. Mastering clinical reasoning comes with time, multiple case exposure, and actively listening to clinical experts who unknowingly share their "clinical pearls" of wisdom through casual case discussion. Sound clinical reasoning can only be maintained through constant practice and the infusion of new scientific knowledge; safe clinical reasoning comes with knowing when to seek consultation or refer the patient to a physician.

Because diagnostic and treatment reasoning heavily depends on scientific knowledge, new time-efficient learning strategies are necessary to keep pace with the scientific knowledge explosion that has already begun and will continue into the new millennium. Integrated reviews in the form of either hard copy publications or audio tapes as well as meta-analyses are becoming increasingly available in a number of clinical specialty fields and hold enormous potential for becoming a key method of knowledge acquisition. APNs are also accessing the Internet for a variety of knowledge resources including acquisition to online clinical practice guidelines published by governmental or organizational agencies, as well as to free issues of electronic nursing and medical journals. State-of-the-art information on new pharmaceuticals, drug interactions, and enrollment criteria into multicenter clinical drug trials can also be accessed online within minutes. EBM web pages, electronic journal clubs, and online discussion groups are also potentially powerful, new learning tools for APNs to explore to rapidly gain knowledge surrounding advances in diagnosis and treatment. Graduate faculty members also play a critical role in molding current and future APN curriculums that will instill the value of lifelong learning into their graduates and the knowledge and information management skills needed to independently and effortlessly pursue new scientific knowledge.

The effects of clinical reasoning ultimately become evident in the subjective and objective outcomes of patients. The monitoring of patient outcomes of APNs occurs through self-review, peer review, and institutional review. Regardless of which review process is conducted, APNs need to critically examine and evaluate their past diagnoses and treatments that were associated with suboptimal patient outcomes in order to improve their reasoning skills. Through peer evaluation and self-evaluation, APNs will be able to improve the soundness and safety of their clinical reasoning, which will grant them the ability to further improve patient outcomes and gain even greater acceptance in their clinical roles.

REFERENCES

Arocha, J. F., Patel, V. L., & Patel, Y. C. (1993). Hypothesis generation and the coordination of theory and evidence in novice diagnostic reasoning. *Medical Decision Making* 13, 198–211.

Barrows, H. S. (1991). Therapeutic decision making. In H. S. Barrows (Ed.), *Developing clinical problem-solving skills* (pp. 162–176). New York: W.W. Norton & Company.

Barrow, H. S., & Feltovich, P. J. (1987). The clinical reasoning process. *Medical Education* 21, 86–91.

Benner, P., & Tanner C. (1987). How expert nurses use intuition. *American Journal of Nursing* 87(1), 23–28.

Black, E. R., Panzer, R. J., Mayewski, R. J., & Griner, P. F. (1991). Characteristics of diagnostic tests and principles for their use in quantitative decision making. *Diagnostic strategies for common medical problems* (pp. 1–16). American College of Physicians.

Bluestein, D. A., & Archer, L. R. (1991). The sensitivity, specificity and predictive value of diagnostic information: A guide for clinicians. *Nurse Practitioner* 16(7), 39–45.

Bockenholt, U., & Weber, E. U. (1993). Toward a theory of hypothesis generation in diagnostic decision making. *Investigative Radiology* 28, 76–80.

Bolinger, R. E., & Ahlers P. (1975). The science of "pattern recognition." *Journal of the American Medical Association* 233, 1289–1290.

Bordage, G., & Lemieux, M. (1991). Semantic structures and diagnostic thinking of experts and novices. *Academic Medicine* 66, S70–S72.

Brykczynski, K. A. (1989). An interpretive study describing the clinical judgment of nurse practitioners. *Scholarly Inquiry for Nursing Practice: An International Journal* 3(2), 75–104.

Burack, R. C., & Carpenter, R. R. (1983). The predictive value of the presenting complaint. *Journal of Family Practice* 16(4), 749–754.

Burgus, G. R., & Hamm, R. M. (1995). Clinical practice: How physicians make medical decisions and why medical decision making can help. *Medical Decision Making* 22, 167–180.

Chessare, J. B. (1998). Teaching clinical decision making to pediatric residents in an era of managed care. *Pediatrics* 101, 762–767.

Connelly, D. P., & Johnson, P. E. (1980). The medical problem solving process. *Human Pathology* 11(5), 412–419.

Cook, D. (1998). Evidence-based critical care medicine:

A potential tool for change. *New Horizons,* 6(1), 20–25.

Dawson, N. V., & Arkes, H. R. (1987). Systematic errors in medical decision making. *Journal of General Internal Medicine* 2, 183–187.

Degner, L. F., & Beaton, J. I. (1987). Decision making. In L. F. Degner & J. I. Beaton (Eds.), *Life-death decisions in health care* (pp.49–65). Cambridge: Hemisphere Publishing Corporation.

Epstein, S. K., & Pauker, S. G. (1998). Principles of clinical decision making. In M.J. Tobin (Ed.), *Principles and practice of intensive care monitoring* (pp. 149–160). New York: McGraw-Hill, Inc.

Feinstein, A. R. (1973). An analysis of diagnostic reasoning: II. The strategy of intermediate decisions. *Yale Journal of Biological Medicine* 46, 264–83.

Fletcher, R. H., Fletcher, S. W., & Wagner, E. H. (1988). *Clinical epidemiology: The essentials* (pp. 66–68). Baltimore: Williams & Wilkins.

Fonteyn, M. (1995). Use of think aloud method to study nurses' reasoning and decision making in clinical practice settings. *Journal of Neuroscience Nursing* 27, 124–128.

Forrow, C., Wartman, S. A., & Brock, D. W. (1988). Science, ethics, and the making of clinical decisions. *Journal of the American Medical Association* 259(21), 3161–3167.

Fulop, M. (1985). Teaching differential diagnosis to beginning clinical students. *American Journal of Medicine* 79, 745–749.

Gifford, D. R., Mittman, B. S., & Vickrey, B. G. (1996). Diagnostic reasoning in neurology. *Neurologic Clinics,* 14(1), 223–238.

Goldman, G. M. (1990a). Judgmental error in intensive care practice. *Journal of Intensive Care Medicine* 5, 93–103.

Goldman, G. M. (1990b). The tacit dimension of clinical judgment. *Yale Journal of Biology* 63, 47–61.

Goldman, G. M., & Ravindranath, T. M. (1994). The contextual nature of critical care judgment. *Journal of Intensive Care Medicine* 9, 58–63.

Gorry, G. A. (1970). Modelling the diagnostic process. *Journal of Medical Education* 45, 293–302.

Grant, J., & Marsden, P. (1987). The structure of memorised knowledge in students and clinicians: An explanation for diagnostic expertise. *Medical Education* 21, 92–98.

Gruppen, L. D., Palchik, N. S., Wolf, F. M., Laing, T. J, Oh, M. S., & Davis, W. K. (1993). Medical student use of history and physical information in diagnostic reasoning. *Arthritis Care and Research* 6(2), 64–70.

Hamm, R. M., & Zubialde, J. (1995). Physicians' expert cognition and the problem of cognitive biases. *Medical Decision Making* 22, 181–212.

Harvey, A. M., Bordley, J., & Barondess, J. A. (1979). Introduction. In A. M. Harvey, J. Bordley, J. A. Barondess (Eds.), *Differential diagnosis: The interpretation of clinical evidence* (pp. 1–16). Philadelphia: W. B. Saunders.

Higgs, J. (1992). Developing clinical reasoning competencies. *Physiotherapy* 78(8), 575–581.

Hunter, K. (1996). "Don't think zebras": Uncertainty, interpretation,and the place of paradox in clinical education. *Theoretical Medicine* 17, 225–241.

Joseph, G. M., & Patel, V. L. (1990). Domain knowledge and hypothesis generation in diagnostic reasoning. *Medical Decision Making* 10, 31–46.

Kaplan, C. (1990). Use of the laboratory. In H. K. Walker, W. D. Hall, & J. W. Hurst (Eds.), *Clinical methods: The history, physical, and laboratory examinations* (pp. 40–48). Boston: Butterworth.

Kassirer, J. P. (1989). Diagnostic reasoning. *Annals of Internal Medicine* 110, 893–900.

Kassirer, J. P., & Kopelman, R. I. (1989a). Generation of diagnostic hypotheses. *Hospital Practice* 24(4), 27–34.

Kassirer, J. P., & Kopelman, R. I. (1989b). Cognitive errors in diagnosis: Instantiation, classification, and consequences. *The American Journal of Medicine* 86, 433–441.

Kassirer, J. P., & Kopelman, R. I. (1991). *Learning clinical reasoning.* Baltimore: Williams & Wilkins.

Lange, L. L., Haak, S. W., Lincoln, M. J., Thompson, C. B., Turner, C. W., Weir, C., Foerster, V., Nilasena, D., & Reeves, R. Use of Iliad to improve diagnostic performance of nurse practitioner students. *Journal of Nursing Education* 36, 36–44.

Ledley, R. S., & Lusted L. B. (1959). Reasoning foundations of medical diagnosis. *Science* 130(3366), 7–12.

Lipman, T. H., & Deatrick, J. A. (1997). Preparing advanced practice nurses for clinical decision making in specialty practice. *Nurse Educator* 22(2), 47–50.

Malseed, R. T., Goldstein, F. J., & Balkon, M. (1995). Drug interactions. In R. T. Malseed, F. J. Goldstein, & N. Balkon (Eds.), *Pharmacology: Drug therapy and nursing considerations* (pp. 35–39). Philadelphia: J.B. Lippincott Company.

Mandin, H., Jones, A., Woloschuk, W., & Harasym, P. Helping students learn to think like experts when solving clinical problems. *Academic Medicine* 72, 173–179.

Nardone, D. A. (1990). Collecting and analyzing data: Doing and thinking. In H. K. Walker, W. D. Hall , & J. W. Hurst JW (Eds.), *Clinical methods: The history, physical, and laboratory examinations* (pp. 22–28). Boston: Butterworth.

Neuhaus, B. E. (1988). Ethical considerations in clinical reasoning: The impact of technology and cost containment. *The American Journal of Occupational Therapy* 42(5), 288–294.

Nicoll, D., & Detmer, W. M. (1997). Basic principles of diagnostic test use and interpretation. In D. Nicoll, S. J. McPhee, T. M. Chou, & W. M. Detmer (Eds.), *Pocket guide to diagnostic tests* (pp. 1–16). Stamford, CT: Appleton & Lange.

Norman, G. R. (1988). Problem-solving skills, solving problems, and problem-based learning. *Medical Education* 22, 279–286.

Norman, G. R., & Schmidt, H. G. (1992). The psychological basis of problem-based learning: A review of the evidence. *Academic Medicine* 76(9), 557–565.

O'Neill, E. S. (1995). Heuristics reasoning in diagnostic judgment. *Journal of Professional Nursing* 11(4), 239–245.

Panzer, R. J., Black, E. R., & Griner, P. F. (1991). Interpretation of diagnostic tests and strategies for their use in quantitative decision making. *Diagnostic strategies for common medical problems* (pp. 17–28). American College of Physicians.

Patel, V. L., Groen, G. J. & Norman, G. R. (1991). Effects of conventional and problem-based medical curricula on poroblem solving. *Academic Medicine* 66, 380–389.

Pople, H. E. (1982). Heuristic methods for imposing structure on ill-structured problems: The structuring of medical diagnostics. In P. Szolovits (Ed.), *Artificial intelligence in medicine.* Boulder, CO: Westview Press.

Prion, S., & Grady, R. P. (1997). The case study as an instructional method to teach clinical reasoning. In J. Higgs & M. Jones, *Clinical Reasoning in the Health Professions* (pp.193–202). Boston: Butterworth-Heineman Medical.

Richards, E. P. (1990). Living with uncertainty: Information theory and critical care decision making. *Journal of Intensive Care Medicine* 5, 91–92.

Riegelman, R. K. (1991). Alternatives: Developing a differential diagnosis. In R. K. Riegelman (Ed.), *Minimizing medical mistakes: The art of medical decision making* (pp. 37–45). Boston: Little, Brown, & Company.

Rosenberg, W., & Donald, A. (1995). Evidence based medicine: An approach to clinical problem-solving. *British Medical Journal* 310, 1122–1126.

Rosenthal, G. E., Mettler, G., Pare, S., Riegger, M., Ward, M., & Landerfeld, C. S. (1992). Diagnostic judgments of nurse practitioners providing primary gynecologic care: A quantiative analysis. *Journal of General Internal Medicine* 7, 304–311.

Ryan-Wenger, N. A., & Lee, J. E. (1997). The clinical reasoning case study: A powerful teaching tool. *The Nurse Practitioner* 22, 66–70.

Sackett, D. L., Rosenberg, W. M., Gray, J. A., Haynes, R. B., & Richardson, W. S. (1996). Evidence-based medicine: What it is and what it isn't. *British Medical Journal* 312, 71–72.

Samiy, A. H., & Akman, W. V. (1987). Principles of clinical diagnosis. In A. H. Samiy, R. G. Douglas, & J. A. Barondess (Eds.), *Textbook of diagnostic medicine.* Philadelphia: Lea & Febiger.

Schmidt, H. G., Norman, G. R., & Boshuizen, H. P. (1990). A cognitive perspective on medical expertise: Theory and implications. *Academic Medicine* 65, 611–621.

Schwartz, S., & Griffin, T. (1986). Choosing actions. In S. Schwartz & T. Griffin (Eds.), *Medical thinking: The psychology of medical judgment and decision making* (pp.97–153). New York: Springer-Verlag.

Sox, H. (1988). Differential diagnosis. In H. Sox (Ed.), *Medical decision making* (pp. 9–26). Boston: Butterworth-Heineman Medical.

Szaflarski, N. L. (1997). Diagnostic reasoning in acute and critical care. *AACN Clinical Issues in Advanced Practice in Acute and Critical Care* 8(3), 291–302.

Tanner, C. A. (1987). Teaching clinical judgment. In J. J. Fitzpatrick R. L.Taunton (Eds.), *Annual review of nursing research.* New York: Springer Publishing Company.

Tryssenar, J. (1995). Interactive journals: An educational strategy to promote reflection. *The American Journal of Occupational Therapy* 49, 695–702.

Tumulty, P. A. (1973). A systematic approach to differential diagnosis. *The effective clinician* (pp. 189–199). Philadelphia: W. B. Saunders Company.

VanLeit, B. (1994). Using the case metod to develop clinical reasoning skills in problem-based learning. *The American Journal of Occupational Therapy* 49, 349–353.

Voytovich, A. E., & Rippey, R. M. (1982). Knowledge, realism, and diagnostic reasoning in a physical diagnosis course. *Journal of Medical Education* 57, 461–467.

Voytovich, A. E., Rippey, R. M., & Suffredini, A. (1985). Prematuare conclusions in diagnostic reasoning. *Journal of Medical Education* 60, 302–307.

White, J. E., Nativio, D. G., Kobert, S. N., & Engberg, S. J. (1992). Content and process in clinical decision making by nurse practitioners. *IMAGE: Journal of Nursing Scholarship* 24(2), 153–158.

Wijetunge, A., & Baldock, G. J. (1998). Evidence-based intensive care medicine. *Anaesthesia* 53, 419–421.

Internet Resources of Evidence-based Medicine

1. Centre for Evidence-based Medicine: The Centre was established in Oxford, England as the first of several centers around the country whose aim broadly is to promote evidence-based healthcare and provide support and resources.

http://cebm.jr2.ox.ac.uk/

2. McMaster University EBM Site: McMaster University in Canada sponsors this large website that contains a large inventory of evidence-based resources, an online database, user guides, and bibliographies.

http://hiru.hirunet.mcmaster.ca/ebm/

3. The Cochrane Library: The Cochrane Library is an electronic publication designed to supply high quality evidence to inform people providing and receiving care, and those responsible for research, teaching, funding and administration at all levels.

http://www.cochrane.de/cc/cochrane/cdsr.htm

4. Journal of Evidence-based Medicine: Published bimonthly, Evidence-based Medicine surveys a wide range of international medical journals (at least 70) to identify the key research papers that are scientifically valid and relevant to practice.

http://www.bmjpg.com/data/ebm.htm

5. Resources for Practicing EBM: A comprehensive and concise bibliography of EBM resources on the web.

http://intensivecare.com/EBM.html

6. Evidence-based Nursing: Evidence-based Nursing is a new high quality international journal. This journal provides access to the best research related to nursing with the most important new evidence within nursing.

http://www.bm.jpg.com/data/ebn.htm

7. Core Library for Evidence-based Practice: This Virtual Library has been put together by assembling links to full text documents on how to learn about Evidence-based Practice.

http://www.shef.ac.uk/~scharr/ir/core.html

8. Centre for Evidence-based Nursing: The University of York has established a Centre for Evidence-based Nursing as part of the national network of Centres for Evidence-Based Clinical Practice.

http://omni.ac.uk/submit-url/archive/0169.html

9. The Alberta Clinical Practice Guidelines Program: The Alberta Clinical Practice Guidelines Program is supporting appropriate, effective and quality medical care in Alberta through promotion, development and implementation of evidence-based clinical practice guidelines.

http://www.amda.ab.ca/general/clinical-practice-guidelines/index.html

10. Netting the Evidence: A ScHARR Introduction to Evidence Based Practice on the Internet: A comprehensive website containing links to other EBM sites, journals, clinical practice guidelines, systematic reviews, and appraisal guides.

http://www.shef.ac.uk/uni/academic/R-Z/scharr/ir/netting.html

11. Agency for Healthcare Policy and Research EBM: The AHCPR sponsors 12 related EBM practice centers.

http://www.ahcpr.gov/browse/evidmed.htm

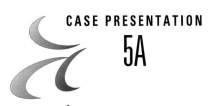

CASE PRESENTATION
5A

Adult Trauma Case: Adding Insult to Injury

Robin M. Haskell

Sun Yong Lee

An 80-year-old male was transported via helicopter to a surburban Level II trauma center after a high-speed motor vehicle collision in which he was an unrestrained passenger. No loss of consciousness was reported, and the patient had full recollection of events. Paramedics noted one hypotensive episode (80/60 mm Hg) en route, which improved with intravenous (IV) fluids. His past medical and surgical history included coronary artery disease, hypertension (usual blood pressure 150/80 mm Hg), non–insulin-dependent diabetes (diet-controlled), five-vessel coronary artery bypass grafting 4 months prior to admission, and tissue aortic valve replacement for aortic stenosis 5 years ago. Home medications included metoprolol and enteric coated aspirin.

On arrival to the emergency department (ED) at 1630 hours, the patient was alert and oriented, with complaints of low anterior left-sided chest pain. His primary survey revealed a patent airway, equal breath sounds, and +2 pulses throughout. Glasgow Coma Scale (GCS) score was 15. Secondary survey was notable for blood pressure (BP) 90/60 mm Hg, heart rate (HR) 88 beats per minute (BPM), respiratory rate 22 per minute, and temperature 36.9° C. Abnormal physical examination findings included left lower anterolateral chest wall tenderness. The abdomen was soft, flat, and nontender. After the secondary survey was completed, a central venous catheter was inserted in the right internal jugular vein. An indwelling bladder catheter was also inserted.

Diagnostic tests in the trauma resuscitation area included cervical spine and pelvic films, which were normal, and an anteroposterior (AP) chest radiograph, which revealed multiple left lateral rib fractures with underlying pulmonary contusion and a small hemothorax (Figure 5A-1). Serum magnesium was 1.0 mg/dL; other chemistry values were within normal limits (Table 5A-1). Hematologic data included hemoglobin (Hgb) 11.4 G/dL, hematocrit (Hct) 33.2%, prothrombin time (PT) 14 seconds, and partial thromboplastin time (PTT) 38 seconds. Subsequent computed tomography (CT) of the abdomen and pelvis revealed a splenic laceration, left renal laceration, and hemoperitoneum (Figure 5A-2).

Immediately following the CT scan, at 1730 hours, the patient underwent left thoracostomy, exploratory laparotomy, evacuation of large hemoperitoneum, and splenectomy (a large splenic hilar laceration was found) under general endotracheal anesthesia. Because the left perinephric hematoma was stable (nonpulsatile, nonex-

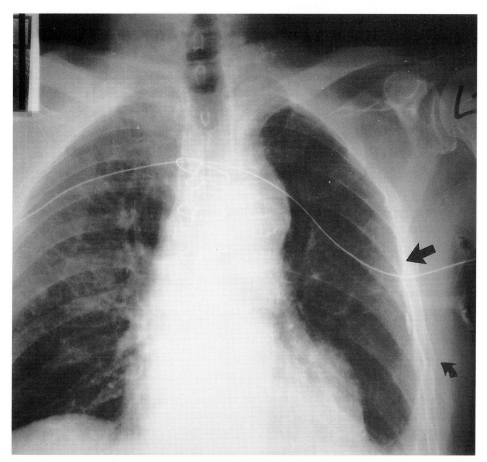

FIGURE 5A-1 Anteroposterior (AP) chest radiograph on admission to the emergency department, showing left lateral rib fractures, numbers 6 (small arrow) through 8, and a small hemothorax. There is haziness along the middle and lower lateral margins of his left lung field (large arrow) consistent with pulmonary contusion. Also note the presence of sternal wires from recent cardiac surgery.

panding), nonoperative management was elected. The intraoperative course was uneventful, except for an increased lactate level (3.3 mmol/L) and abnormal coagulation studies (PT 21 seconds, PTT 60 seconds). Four units of fresh frozen plasma (FFP) were ordered and were thawing. Six grams of magnesium sulfate ($MgSO_4$) were administered intravenously. A total of 4 units (1200 mL) of packed red blood cells (PRBCs) and 4 liters of lactated ringers were administered during the case. The estimated blood loss was 1400 mL. Invasive devices in place at the end of the case included a radial arterial line, nasogastric tube, left chest tube, and indwelling bladder catheter.

The patient, still chemically paralyzed and sedated, was transported to the intensive care unit (ICU) at 1945 hours. Initial vital signs were BP 146/71 mm Hg, HR 104 BPM, and temperature 36.4°C. The patient remained intubated and ventilated on assist control mode with a rate of 10, fraction of inspired oxygen (FiO_2) 0.50, and positive end-expiratory pressure (PEEP) 5 cm. Breath sounds were clear. Extremities were cool and dusky with 5-second (delayed) capillary refill. Postoperative 12-lead electrocardiogram (ECG) showed normal sinus rhythm with a right bundle branch block and

TABLE 5A-1 *Serum chemistries, complete blood counts, coagulation studies, lactate levels, and arterial blood gas (ABG) analyses on admission to the emergency department (ED), intraoperatively (OR), and during the first 24 hours of the patient's hospital course in the intensive care unit (ICU). For all ABGs, the fraction of inspired oxygen (FiO$_2$) was 0.50, and positive end-expiratory pressure (PEEP) 5 cm.*

Time	Na$^+$ (meq/L)	K$^+$ (meq/L)	Cl (meq/L)	CO$_2$ (meq/L)	BUN (mg/dL)	Cr (mg/dL)	Glu (mg/dL)	Mg (mg/dL)	Hgb (g/dL)	Hct (%)	Plt ($\times$ 1000)	PT (sec)	PTT (sec)	Lactate (mmol/L)	pH	PaCO$_2$ (mm Hg)	PaO$_2$ (mm Hg)	HCO$_3$ (mmol/L)	BE (mmol/L)
1630 (ED)	138	4.5	105	28	15	1.5	144	1.0	11.4	33.2	181	14	38						
1750 (OR)	137	4.4	110	21	14	1.2	153		9.1	26	109	21	60	3.3	7.40	36	315	22	−1.8
2030 (ICU)	139	4.3	110	22					11.6	33.5	101			2.9	7.40	37	299	22	−1.8
2300 (ICU)	138	4.4	113	19	16	1.2	159	1.8	11.5	32.9	53	19	49	2.6	7.39	39	184	24	−1.9
0500 (ICU)	140	4.0	111	18	12	1.2	132	2.2	12.7	37	86	14	43	4.5	7.40	34	77	23	−3.3
1400 (ICU)	138	4.3	111	19	15	1.2	149		10.8	31.1	153	14	43	2.5	7.41	39	83	24	−0.9

Na$^+$, sodium; K$^+$, potassium; Cl, chloride; CO$_2$, carbon dioxide; BUN, blood urea nitrogen; Cr, creatinine; Glu, glucose; Mg, total magnesium; Hgb, hemoglobin; Hct, hematocrit; Plt, platelet; PT, prothrombin time; PTT, partial thromboplastin time; PaCO$_2$, partial pressure of carbon dioxide; PaO$_2$, partial pressure of oxygen; HCO$_3$, bicarbonate; BE, base excess.

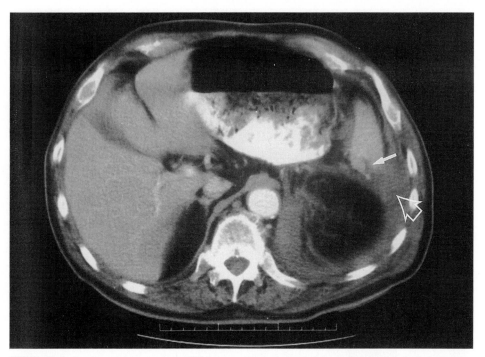

FIGURE 5A-2 A computed tomography (CT) image of the upper abdomen, showing a splenic laceration (small arrow) and significant hemoperitoneum (open arrow), which extends downward along the lateral abdomen and posterior to an air-filled bowel loop. Note the stomach distended with air and radiopaque contrast material.

first degree AV block, which were both present on an ECG performed 1 month prior to admission. See Table 5A-1 for results of sequential laboratory studies.

As the acute care nurse practitioner admitting this critically ill patient to the ICU, I would approach each clinical problem, both actual and potential, in a systematic fashion to ensure efficient, comprehensive diagnosis and treatment. My immediate concerns are assessment of airway patency, oxygenation, and ventilation. A chest radiograph would be needed to evaluate endotracheal tube (ETT), central line, and chest tube placement (Figure 5A-3). I would also send blood specimens for complete blood count (CBC), electrolytes, and arterial blood gases (ABGs).

Although there was no loss of consciousness and the admission neurologic examination was normal, my primary concern in regard to his neurologic status is that he may be harboring a potentially severe intracranial injury that has simply not had time to manifest itself because of the presence of extensive age-related cerebral atrophy. Narcotic analgesics and sedatives would be withheld until the patient arouses and a neurologic examination is performed. Persistent coma or a focal neurologic deficit would warrant an urgent head CT scan to rule out traumatic intracerebral hemorrhage.

The implications of the prehospital hypotensive episode are significant for this normally hypertensive patient with severe atherosclerotic coronary vascular disease. Any episode of hypotension could result in decreased myocardial oxygen delivery, which would increase vulnerability to myocardial ischemia and dysrhythmias. Preexisting beta-blockade therapy in this patient would undermine attempts by the autonomic nervous system to compensate for hypovolemia via β-1 receptor-mediated increases in heart rate and contractility. Thus, the severity of shock may be underestimated by the absence of compensatory tachycardia. Hem-

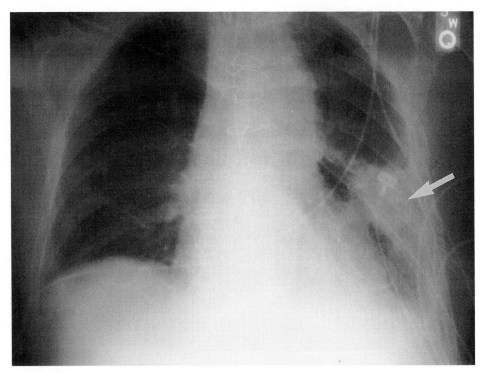

FIGURE 5A-3 Chest radiograph performed postoperatively on admission to the intensive care unit, showing a blossoming left pulmonary contusion (arrow). Note the presence of an endotracheal tube, right internal jugular catheter, and left thoracostomy tube. The left lateral rib fractures are not identifiable on this film because the patient is somewhat rotated and the lateral chest wall is obscured by cardiac monitoring leads.

orrhage may cause rapid intravascular volume shifts, hypotension, and anemia, increasing his risk of myocardial ischemia. It will be important to maintain a relatively normal hematocrit to augment O_2 carrying capacity and myocardial O_2 delivery. I will need to watch closely for hypovolemia and cardiac dysfunction in the immediate postoperative period.

The intraoperative monitoring devices are not adequate to address all of these concerns. Given the patient's cardiac history, hypotension, coagulopathy, injury severity, advanced age, and pulmonary contusion, a pulmonary artery (PA) catheter should be inserted immediately. Frequent monitoring of his cardiac index (CI), systemic vascular resistance (SVR), central venous pressure (CVP), and pulmonary capillary wedge pressure (PCWP) will enable informed clinical decision making regarding the diagnosis and management of intravascular volume status and cardiac function. ST segment monitoring might also be indicated but is unavailable in this ICU. Serial ECGs will be important for both detection of ischemic changes and increases in PR interval relative to the preexisting AV block.

The finding of pulmonary contusion is a potentially lethal injury because its natural course is associated with worsening hypoxemia for the first 24 to 72 hours. Radiographic findings are typically delayed; therefore, his pulmonary contusion is considered severe because the parenchymal hemorrhage was already visible on the admission chest radiograph. Judicious use of PEEP and incremental increases in FiO_2 will inevitably be required to maintain adequate oxygen saturation. Rib fractures cause severe pain leading to splinting and restriction of ventilation, which will have later implications for his postoperative pain control and weaning from mechanical ventilation. Continuous pulse oximetry adequately monitors arterial oxygenation status, but serial ABGs would be needed to assess ventilation and acid–base status.

Splenic hemostasis in this patient has been surgically assured with a splenectomy; however, the left kidney is still at risk for hemorrhage from potential disruption of the protective perinephric hematoma. Because the most important tenet of early nonoperative management of a solid organ injury is monitoring for ongoing intraabdominal hemorrhage, I would examine him frequently for the presence of peritoneal signs as well as perform serial Hgb and Hct checks. Renal function should not be affected by the renal injury per se, but his advanced age, history of diabetes and cardiac disease, and injury severity mandates close monitoring of urine output and at least once daily measurement of blood urea nitrogen and creatinine.

The development of his intraoperative coagulopathy is most likely related to hemodilution from IV crystalloid and red blood cell administration. Additionally, his home aspirin therapy has probably caused some degree of platelet dysfunction for which the only treatment is discontinuation of the drug. Hypothermia, a common comorbidity in trauma patients, can cause or aggravate coagulopathy. Although hypothermia has not occurred in this patient, I would monitor his temperature closely and prevent heat loss by initiating active and passive rewarming measures, such as using warmed blankets and fluids.

The most common cause of nonsurgical bleeding in trauma patients is dilutional thrombocytopenia. His intraoperative platelet count remained above 100,000, but I would expect further decline as fluid resuscitation continues, and would monitor platelet count frequently. Even in the absence of hemorrhage, it is important to keep the PT and PTT within normal limits and the platelet count greater than 50,000 in the patient with solid visceral injury (kidney, liver, or spleen) who is managed nonoperatively. Because FFP requires 30 to 45 minutes to thaw, it is crucial to anticipate the need for FFP transfusion.

At 2015 hours, a PA catheter was inserted without complications. The following initial hemodynamic parameters were noted: CVP 10 mm Hg, PCWP 12 mm Hg, cardiac index (CI) 1.8 L/min/m², SVR 2100 dynes/sec/cm⁵, BP 137/73 mm Hg, and HR 118 BPM. A chest radiograph performed after line insertion showed the ETT, chest tube, and PA catheter to be in good position. The pulmonary contusion remained unchanged. The patient was awake, following commands and moving all four extremities. The abdomen was soft and flat with incisional tenderness. A morphine infusion was started at 2 mg/hour.

The hemodynamic profile shows that this patient is unable to maintain adequate systemic blood flow. His blood pressure is "normal" as a result of a catecholamine-induced peripheral vasocontriction caused by decreased cardiac output, as manifested by his increased SVR. The negative chronotropic effect of the beta-blocker is wearing off, as evidenced by his tachycardia. Although a tachycardiac response is appropriate with this hemodynamic profile, it will place him at added risk of myocardial ischemia because of decreased myocardial diastolic filling time.

Although the CVP and PCWP are within normal limits, his elevated SVR tells us that he still has inadequate preload and is underresuscitated. He will need IV fluids that will stay in the intravascular space. Isotonic solutions (normal saline or lactated ringers) are the most readily available, safest, and economical fluids for treatment of acute volume deficit. Because only about 25% of administered isotonic crystalloid volume remains in the intravascular space, successful resuscitation with crystalloid requires giving four times the estimated intravascular deficit. Because this patient has already received almost four times the volume of operative blood loss and is manifesting laboratory signs of hemodilution and clotting factor depletion, I would plan to use colloids in the form of blood component therapy directed at correcting red blood cell, platelet, or clotting factor deficiencies. Assuming that his capillary permeability has not increased, colloids offer additional theoretical advantage over crystalloids in that a majority of the administered volume remains in the intravascular space for a longer period of time. His cardiac history and injury complex mandate frequent monitoring of hemodynamic parameters as fluid resuscitation proceeds. The monitoring devices in place should be utilized dynamically to gauge the patient's hemodynamic response to fluid boluses.

I would plan to administer a 1000 mL bolus of saline over 30 minutes while we are waiting for the FFP to thaw. A rapid bolus will effect more pronounced changes in preload. According to the Frank-Starling phenomenon, the preload (or diastolic volume) is the principle force that governs the strength of myocardial ventricular contraction. Thus, increasing preload may help to reduce compensatory peripheral vasoconstriction while increasing systolic performance, which would in turn decrease his afterload and improve cardiac output and oxygen delivery. I would also plan to give him 4 units of FFP because a PT greater than 20 seconds usually requires at least 4 units for correction.

By 2130 hours, the patient had received 1000 mL additional normal saline and 4 units (940 mL total) of FFP. Repeat hemodynamic parameters were CVP 12 mm Hg, PCWP 13 mm Hg, CI 2.1 L/min/m², SCR 1980 dynes/sec/cm⁵, BP 130/80 mm Hg, and HR 108 BPM. Oxygen saturation (SpO$_2$) was 98%. Abdominal examination was unchanged. Urine output was 100 mL over the last hour. Hemoglobin was 11.3 G/dL.

Following the fluid boluses, his heart rate, SVR, and cardiac index have improved, indicating that his heart responded positively to increases in preload although there were only minor increases in cardiac filling pressures. Unfortunately, all responses were less than expected after nearly 2 liters of fluid. Ongoing hemorrhage or the development of third-space losses could account for this, but I would also be concerned about altered cardiac systolic or diastolic function. He may need further augmentation of preload to improve ventricular contractility. However, no obvious source of hemorrhage exists and the cardiac parameters and urine output are trending in the right direction, reflecting adequate organ perfusion. Thus, I would elect to continue to closely monitor the patient's hemodynamic parameters and urine output.

At 2300 hours, 4 hours postoperatively, the patient became hypotensive (70/41 mm Hg). Hemodynamic parameters were CVP 9 mm Hg, PCWP 12 mm Hg, CI 1.7 L/min/m², and SVR 2120 dynes/sec/cm⁵. Temperature was 37.2° C. The patient was lethargic but arousable and able to follow commands. He denied chest pain. Breath sounds were clear and equal. SpO$_2$ was 97% on the same ventilator settings. The abdomen was soft and nondistended. Urine output was 40 to 70 cc per hour. Repeat ECG showed sinus rhythm at 96 BPM; right bundle branch block; and acute aVF 1 to 2 mm ST segment elevation in leads II, III, and aVF (Figure 5A-4). Repeat chest radiograph showed minimal enlargement of the left pulmonary contusion. Hemoglobin was 11.5 G/dL. Platelet count had decreased to 53,000. PT and PTT remain elevated after FFP transfusion (see Table 5A-1). The morphine infusion was discontinued with the onset of hypotension.

Hypotension after blunt trauma implicates an extensive list of differential diagnoses. I would be most concerned about ongoing hemorrhage; however, the patient's physical examination and chest radiograph are inconsistent with external bleeding or major cavitary bleeding into the chest or abdomen. The Hgb is also stable. His thrombocytopenia and persistent coagulopathy are probably dilutional as would be expected with the large volume of IV fluids given. These abnormalities are not inconsequential in this critically ill patient even if there are no signs of bleeding. Because platelets are usually ordered in 6-unit aliquots ("a 6-pack"), I would start with this amount and anticipate the need to give more. I would order 6 additional units of FFP because the patient had a less-than-expected re-

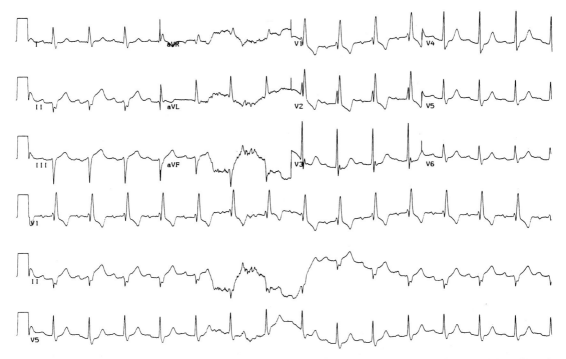

FIGURE 5A-4 12-lead electrocardiogram performed subsequent to the patient's hypotensive episode at 2300 hours. There is a first-degree heart block, right bundle branch block, and 1 to 2 mm ST elevation in leads II, III, and aVF. The underlying rhythm is sinus with a heart rate of 96 BPM.

sponse to 4 units given previously. Lethargy in association with hypotension is an important sign, indicating that compensatory mechanisms are failing to maintain adequate systemtic blood flow. I would need to use an isotonic crystalloid bolus for immediate treatment as the blood products would not be readily available for transfusion.

There were no major dysrhythmias or vasodilating medications given to explain the sudden drop in cardiac output. Importantly, his ECG tracings are consistent with acute inferior wall myocardial injury. I would obtain an echocardiogram (ECHO) to evaluate for wall motion abnormalities, pericardial fluid, or valvular incompetence. I would also obtain cardiac enzymes profiles, recognizing that elevated creatine kinase (CK) or creatine kinase-MB isoenzyme (CK-MB) values in blunt trama patients are nonspecific, arising from cardiac or skeletal muscle injury or both. The CK-MB relative index would be more helpful, but it is not 100% sensitive. Troponin-I has been shown to be a more sensitive marker than CK-MB relative index for early detection of myocardial injury, even in patients with "minor" myocardial damage, in which CK-MB mass may be normal. Therefore, I would include troponin-I levels as part of the cardiac enzyme profile.

The patient's acute myocardial injury pattern is very worrisome both in terms of potential pump failure and the intimation of oxygen debt in other organs as well. I would suspect that his myocardial O_2 consumption is increased because of the high systemic vascular resistance. While attempting to optimize preload with fluid boluses, I would start a dobutamine infusion in an effort to increase myocardial contractility and decrease afterload, to improve cardiac output. Vasopressors are usually withheld until intravascular volume has been repleted; however, this patient has had a discouraging response to substantial fluid resuscitation and is at risk for multiple organ failure if his tissue perfusion deficit is not rapidly corrected.

At 2300 hours, a transthoracic echocardiogram was ordered but will be unavailable for several hours. A cardiac enzyme panel was sent to the laboratory. One liter of normal saline was given over 15 minutes. A dobutamine infusion was initiated at 5 mcg/kg/min. Additional blood products (2 units PRBCs, 6 units FFP, and 6 units of platelets) were given over 2 hours.

At 0100 hours, BP was 150/70 mm Hg, CVP 12 mm Hg, PCWP 14 mm Hg, CI 3.5 L/min/m², SVR 975 dynes/sec/cm⁵, and HR 104 BPM. The patient was alert and somewhat restless but denied pain (including chest pain) and settled down with verbal reassurance. His neurologic examination was nonfocal. Ventilator settings were unchanged, and the SpO_2 was 96%. Breath sounds were coarse and diminished at the left base. Urine output was 80 to 120 mL per hour.

The patient responded well to volume resuscitation and inotropic support, confirming the earlier diagnoses of hypovolemia and decreased myocardial contractility. At this point, I would continue frequent reassessment of the patient's vital signs, urine output, and hemodynamic profiles to ensure the continued adequacy of intravascular volume resuscitation. I would begin to consider resuscitation end points to avoid significant fluid overload in this patient with myocardial injury and pulmonary contusion. Just as volume deficits can adversely affect systolic performance according to the Frank-Starling phenomenon, fluid overload can overdistend cardiac muscle with the same end result. I would order right-sided chest lead (V_{3R}, V_{4R}) tracings with his next ECG. Because the inotropic and chronotropic effects of dobutamine can vary widely in critically ill patients, the infusion should be titrated according to hemodynamic profiles rather than preselected dose rates, especially because the elderly are relatively resistant to the drug.

Restlessness can be an early indicator of hypoxemia, but I would be reassured by his stable SpO_2 and lack of significant change in the chest radiograph performed 2 hours prior. Restlessness and anxiety can also be normal behavioral reactions to invasive monitors, lack of control, pain, and overstimulation. I would be concerned about the effects of his increased motor activity on myocardial and systemic oxygen consumption. At this point in the resuscitation, small intermittent bolus doses of a benzodiazepine agent should be administered hourly on an as-needed basis. A short-acting agent such as midazolam would enable periodic neurologic reassessment.

At 0500, the patient's cardiac index declined again to 1.4 L/min/m². Concurrent hemodynamic parameters included CVP 13 mm Hg, PCWP 14 mm Hg, SVR 1370 dynes/sec/cm⁵, BP 114/70 mm Hg, and HR 116 BPM. Cardiac enzyme results from 2300 hours included CK 737 U/L, CK-MB 17.8 ng/mL, with a relative index of 2.4%. Cardiac troponin-I was 0.55 ng/dL at 0500 (Table 5A-2). The patient was sedated but was easily arousable to voice and able to follow commands. He continued to deny chest pain. Neck veins were somewhat distended. Lung auscultation and ventilator settings were unchanged. SpO_2 was 93%. ABGs were remarkable for a partial pressure of arterial oxygen (PaO_2) of 77 mm Hg on FiO_2 0.50. The abdomen was soft and flat. Echocardiogram showed moderate right heart dilitation with moderate right ventricular systolic dysfunction, ejection fraction of 30%, and mild tricuspid regurgitation. The prosthetic aortic valve had normal mobility and no insufficiency or regurgitation was seen. ECG showed 3–4 mm ST segment elevations in leads II, III, aVF, V_{3R}, and V_{4R}. CXR showed the left pulmonary contusion, which was unchanged. Hgb, Hct, and coagulation studies were now normal. Platelet count had increased to 86,000. Lactate level (4.5 mmol/L) and base deficit (−3.3 mmol/L) had worsened. Urine output was 30–60 mL per hour.

The patient's adequate cardiac filling pressures and normal Hgb/Hct suggest that aggressive resuscitation has repleted the intravascular volume deficit. However, the relative

TABLE 5A-2 *Results of Serum Cardiac Injury Markers.* Normal range for Troponin-I is 0.0 to 0.4 ng/dL.

Date	Time	CK (U/L)	CK-MB (ng/mL)	Relative Index (%)	Troponin-I (ng/dL)
Date of Injury	2300	737	17.8	2.4	
Postoperative Day 1	0500	824	15.8	1.9	0.55
	1100	1184	8.5	0.7	
	1700	1122	5.9	0.4	11.8
	2300	998	4.0	0.4	
Postoperative Day 2	0500	802	2.1	0.3	4.1
	2100	455	1.0	0.2	
Postoperative Day 3	0500	350	0.3	0.1	2.6

CK, creatine kinase; CK-MB, creatine kinase; MB, isoenzyme.

hypotension, inability to clear lactate, worsened base deficit, and decreased urine output indicate persistent tissue hypoperfusion. CK-MB relative indices were normal, but cardiac troponin-I was elevated, which strongly suggests a diagnosis of myocardial injury. The ECHO results, ECG tracing, and cardiac isoenzyme profiles support a diagnosis of acute inferior wall myocardial infarction (MI) with probable resultant right heart failure. The right-sided chest lead tracings confirm the presence of an acute right ventricular myocardial injury pattern, which probably reflects an evolving right-ventricular myocardial infarction (RV MI).

Many of the current management strategies for acute myocardial infarction would be contraindicated in this patient owing to recent trauma and surgery. Thrombolytic therapy and antithrombotic agents (aspirin, heparin) are contraindicated. Relief of chest pain is also a mainstay of MI treatment, but the patient denies pain at this time. Nitroglycerin is not recommended in right ventricular infarction because of the risk of hypotension. Although beta-blockers have been shown to reduce infarct size and the incidence of dysrhythmias if given within a few hours of the onset of MI, several contraindications exist in this case, including AV block, hypotension, and systolic heart failure. Magnesium sulfate administration can dilate coronary arteries, inhibit platelet aggregation, and suppress dysrhythmias; the patient's serum magnesium level is currently within normal limits, but this should be monitored closely.

In acute RV MI, the compliance of the right ventricle is increased. Because the right ventricle acts as a passive conduit, a higher preload is required for adequate ventricular filling so that adequate stroke volume can be maintained. The treatment goal in acute RV MI is to maintain high preload, but care must be taken since overzealous fluid administration will overdistend cardiac muscle and decrease systolic performance. Volume should be infused until the PCWP or CVP increases by approximately 5 mm Hg, followed by reassessment of cardiac parameters. I would prefer to use blood component therapy, but because hematologic deficiencies have been corrected, normal saline boluses would be sufficient. If signs of right heart failure (hepatomegaly, neck vein distention, pulmonary edema, or ECG changes) persist or worsen with optimal filling pressures (as incident to adequate CI), I would increase the dobutamine dosage because this is a good inotropic agent for the acute management of low output states secondary to right heart failure. SVR and BP must be monitored closely with dobutamine administration because profound peripheral vasodilation would decrease preload, which would have a diametrical effect on cardiac output in the setting of right ventricular failure. If the patient becomes hypotensive, a dopamine infusion at intermediate or high doses (5 to 10 mcg/kg/min) will activate alpha receptors and augment preload through vasoconstriction. A phosphodiesterase inhibitor (amrinone) may be added if increases in dobutamine do not increase cardiac index.

The patient received 2 liters of normal saline over 1 hour. PCWP increased to 19 mm Hg, but cardiac index remained low (1.6 L/min/m^2). Dobutamine was then increased to 8.25 mcg/kg/min with immediate improvement in cardiac index (2.4 L/min/m^2). Other hemodynamic parameters on this dobutamine infusion included BP 146/80 mm Hg, HR 92 BPM, and SVR 942 dynes/sec/cm^5. The patient was lightly sedated but arousable without neurologic deficit. Breath sounds were unchanged, and the SaO$_2$ was 95%. Normal saline with 40 meq KCL/L and 16 meq MgSO$_4$/L was ordered to infuse at 120 mL/hr.

The patient is now stable, but inattention to subtle physiologic changes might result in extension of the myocardial infarct and further loss of functional cardiac muscle mass. Hemodynamic parameters should be assessed every 2 to 4 hours until the patient no longer requires titration of inotropic support and fluid boluses. I would obtain troponin-I levels in about 12 hours to ascertain a peak value, and then daily for the next 3 days to assure that the values are decreasing as expected.

At 1400, the dobutamine infusion remained at 8.25 mcg/kg/min. Hemodynamic parameters included CI 2.9 L/min/m^2, PCWP 18 mm Hg, CVP 16 mm Hg, SVR 1049 dynes/sec/cm^5, BP 130/60 mm Hg, and HR 84 BPM. The patient was awake, alert, and cooperative. FiO$_2$ was increased to 0.60 and PEEP increased to 7.5 cm H$_2$O owing to progressive hypoxemia (see Table 5A-1). Chest radiograph reveals mild progression of the left pulmonary contusion. The abdomen was soft and nondistended with mild incisional tenderness and no bowel sounds. Urine output was 100 mL/hr. Repeat ECG was unchanged. Lactate level and base deficit were decreasing (2.5 mmol/L and −0.9 mmol/L respectively). CBC, platelet count, and coagulation profiles were normal.

The patient's cardiac index continued to improve with inotropic support. The pulmonary contusion is worsening but less severely than anticipated. I expect the need for further increases in FiO$_2$ or PEEP over the next 24 to 48 hours. There are no signs of ongoing abdominal hemorrhage, and his tissue perfusion deficit has resolved. I would decrease the frequency of phlebotomy to twice daily.

This patient's mechanism of injury (high-velocity motor vehicle collision with lack of safety restraints) suggests a high potential for yet undetected associated injuries. Now that he has recovered from anesthesia and can reliably communicate and cooperate during physical examination, I would perform a complete tertiary survey, with particular scrutiny of the musculoskeletal system. Findings of pain, swelling, or deformity of the spine, pelvis, or extremities should be evaluated radiographically.

No new abnormalities were found on tertiary survey. On postoperative day 2, the patient remained on dobutamine at 8.25 mcg/kg/min. Hemodynamic parameters, vital signs, and oxygenation had been stable although an earlier attempt to wean the dobutamine resulted in hypotension and decreased cardiac index. The patient complained of left anterior chest wall pain on inspiration despite a morphine infusion at 2 mg/hr. His neurologic examination was normal. Breath sounds were equal with fine crackles in both bases. Ventilator settings include intermittent mandatory ventilation mode with rate of 12, FiO$_2$ 0.60, and PEEP of 7.5. Spontaneous tidal volumes range from 200 to 500 mL. The abdomen was soft and mildly distended, with

hypoactive bowel sounds and incisional tenderness. The midline abdominal incision had no inflammation or drainage. Urine output was 60 to 80 mL/hr. Extremities were warm with +2 edema noted at the ankles. Chest radiograph showed mild pulmonary edema; the pulmonary contusion was unchanged. Hematologic studies were stable. The troponin-I peaked at 11.8 ng/dL 24 hours after injury and had decreased to 4.1 ng/dL.

The PA catheter should remain in place until the dobutamine can be discontinued. I would continue to monitor his hemodynamic parameters every 6 hours as the patients fluid requirements and cardiac performance will be unpredictable as fluid shifts occur.

The patient's rib fractures are causing pain and splinting, resulting in impaired ventilation while increasing the risk of atelectasis and pneumonia. Systemic opiates are usually effective but may cause significant respiratory depression and gastrointestinal problems such as nausea, vomiting, and paralytic ileus. Now that the the patient is no longer coagulopathic and hypovolemic, I would consult the pain service for insertion of a thoracic epidural catheter. Continuous epidural analgesia will provide local pain relief, minimize systemic narcotic side effects, prevent pulmonary complications, and facilitate weaning from mechanical ventilation.

After massive fluid resuscitation, gentle diuresis helps to both decrease afterload and mobilize third-space fluids. I would start with small daily doses of a loop diuretic to achieve an even daily fluid balance. I will need to minimize the total crystalloid volume administered, including that required to deliver IV medications and infusions. Evaluation of patient response to diuretic therapy includes urine output, hemodynamic parameters, acid–base status, and serum electrolyte levels. It is important to avoid overly aggressive diuresis because hypokalemia, hypomagnesemia, and metabolic alkalosis may result.

Splenectomy results in a lifelong risk of overwhelming postsplenectomy sepsis, which occurs in 1 to 2% of trauma patients after splenectomy and carries a mortality rate of 40 to 70%. Now that the patient is well-resuscitated, I would order Pneumovax, H. influenzae, and meningococcal vaccines to protect against commonly implicated organisms.

An epidural catheter was inserted and good pain control was achieved using an infusion of bupivicaine and morphine. His post-splenectomy vaccines were given on postoperative day #3. After receiving daily doses of furosemide (20 mg) for 5 days, the patient's pulmonary edema resolved. He underwent percutaneous tracheostomy placement on postoperative day #7 to facilitate pulmonary hygiene and ventilator weaning. The patient remained in the ICU on inotropic therapy for 6 days and his repeat 12-lead ECG showed Q waves in leads II, III, and aVF. Repeat echocardiogram after the dobutamine was discontinued showed mild right ventricular dysfunction, ejection fraction 41%, and normal valve function. He was ultimately weaned from mechanical ventilation on postoperative day #14. On transfer to a rehabilitation hospital 3 weeks after his motor vehicle crash, the patient's cardiac status was stable on his usual dose of metroprolol and enteric coated aspirin.

Discussion

The complex clinical reasoning required for the management of critically ill, severely injured trauma patients can challenge even the most experienced clinician. Multiple medical and surgical problems create multiple priorities, each affecting the others. Successful early ICU management requires a systematic approach, with the flexibility to reset diagnostic and treatment priorities based on injury identification, complications, and medical comorbidities.

The multi-injured elderly patient warrants special consideration. In addition to numerous physiologic changes that occur with aging, the high occurrence of significant disease states may further influence an elderly person's response to injury and stress. Elderly patients often have substantial physiological deficits that markedly increase cardiovascular risk. Exposure to the severe cardiovascular stress associated with trauma, hemorrhage, and anesthesia increases myocardial oxygen consumption, intensifying the risk of myocardial ischemia. Even in the absence of preexisting cardiac disease, multi-injured elderly patients with uncorrected perfusion deficits can look "hemodynamically stable" and then proceed to develop sudden cardiovascular collapse. For this reason, invasive monitoring using a pulmonary artery catheter is important in multi-injured elderly blunt trauma patients for the early detection of occult shock (Scalea, Simon, Duncan, et al. 1990).

Hypotension after blunt trauma implicates an extensive list of differential diagnoses. Hypovolemia is the most likely cause, which may be *relative,* from vasodilation or autonomic dysfunction, or *absolute,* resulting from acute blood loss. Because the most common cause of hypotension in this setting is hemorrhage, complete evaluation for sources of blood loss must be performed. Importantly, the cause of hypotension in elderly blunt trauma patients may be multifactorial. Dysrhythmias, myocardial ischemia or infarction, valvular dysfunction (aortic insufficiency or stenosis), pericardial tamponade, tension pneumothorax, pulmonary embolus, and hypoxemia can lead to pump failure and cardiogenic shock. An orderly, complete diagnostic approach is critical. The reader is referred to an excellent reference on the differential diagnosis of hypotension in hospitalized adult patients (Hravnik & Boujoukos, 1997). In this patient, hypotension was caused by hypovolemia resulting from hemorrhage, and cardiogenic shock resulting from acute right ventricular infarction.

The diagnosis of hypovolemia was not difficult in this patient despite the influence of the beta-blockade therapy, which masked an early compensatory tachycardia. The patient's mechanism of injury and clinical presentation prompted CT scanning of the abdomen and pelvis, which identified injuries to two highly vascular organs as well as a large amount of blood in the peritoneal cavity. Volume resuscitation was initiated immediately. The subsequent laparotomy was both diagnostic, in terms of ruling out associated intraabdominal injury, and therapeutic, for splenectomy and control of hemorrhage. The significant postoperative fluid resuscitation that was required was not uncommon for his injury complex.

Contrarily, myocardial injury was more difficult to recognize because of the patient's atypical clinical presentation, impaired communication, and the normal CK-MB relative index. The ECG provided the earliest clues, but in many ICU patients, ECG changes are nonspecific, and there may be difficulty determining whether elevated levels of CK-MB are from cardiac or noncardiac causes (Guest et al., 1995). Elevated levels of troponin-I, a myocardial regulatory protein which is only expressed in heart tissue, are correlated with the development of new areas of regional dysfunction determined by echocardiography. Troponin-I has been shown to be a more sensitive marker than CK-MB mass for early detection of myocardial injury, even in patients with "minor" myocardial damage (D'Costa, Fleming, & Patterson, 1997; Apple, Falahati, Paulsen, et al, 1997).

The troponin-I assay is ideally suited for the detection of ischemic myocardial injury in complex clinical situations because of its high cardiospecificity and its high sensitivity for the delayed diagnosis of myocardial injury. This enzyme peaks within 1 day and remains increased for 4 to 5 days. Because elevated levels, once present, persist for 4 to 7 days, troponin-I levels can be monitored once a day (Bertinchant et al., 1996; Martins et al., 1996).

Coagulopathy was a major confounding factor in this case. Prompt recognition and treatment prevented this complication from causing further hemorrhage and exacerbating the acute volume deficit. Fortunately, the patient's pulmonary contusion did not lead to overwhelming difficulties with oxygenation and ventilation. Finally, recognition that his injury severity placed him at high risk for the development of hypothermia assured that appropriate monitoring and preventive measures were instituted.

REFERENCES

Apple, F. S. Falahati, A., Paulsen, P. R., et al. (1997). Improved detection of minor ischemic myocardial injury with measurement of serum cardiac troponin-I. *Clinical Chemistry 43*(11), 2047–2051.

Bertinchant, J. P., Larue, C., Pernel, I., et al. (1996). Release kinetics of serum cardiac troponin I in ischemic myocardial injury. *Clinical Biochemistry 29*(6), 87–594.

D'Costa, M., Fleming, E. G., Patterson, M. C. (1997). Cardiac troponin I for the diagnosis of acute myocardial infarction in the emergency department. *American Journal of Clinical Pathology 108*(5), 550–555.

Guest, T. M., Ramanathan, A. V., Tuteur, P. G., et al. (1995). Myocardial injury in critically ill patients: A frequently unrecognized complication. *Journal of the American Medical Association 273*(4), 1945–1949.

Hravnak, M., & Boujoukos, A. (1997). Hypotension. *AACN Clinical Issues: Advanced Practice in Acute and Critical Care 8*(3), 303–318.

Martins, J. T., Li, D. J., Baskin, L. B., et al. (1996). Comparison of cardiac troponin-I and lacate dehydrogenase isoenzymes for the late diagnosis of myocardial injury. *American Journal of Clinical Pathology 106*(6), 705–708.

Peitzman, A. B., Rhodes, M., Schwab, C. W., & Yealy, D. M. (1998). *The trauma manual.* Philadelphia: Lippincott-Raven.

Scalea, T. M., Simon, H. M., Duncan, et al. (1990). Geriatric blunt multiple trauma: Improved survival with early invasive monitoring. *Journal of Trauma 30*(2), 129–136.

Vandivier, R. W. & Cunnion, R. E. (1997). Hypotension complicating anterior chest trauma. In G. R. Park & M. R. Pinsky (Eds.). *Critical care management case studies: Tricks and traps* (pp. 34–40). London: W. B. Saunders.

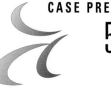

CASE PRESENTATION

5B

The Proof Is in the Planning

Celeste G. Villanueva

A 67-year-old white male was scheduled for an elective sigmoid colon resection for a malignant adenocarcinoma. He was admitted to the hospital 3 hours prior to his scheduled surgery and brought to the ambulatory surgery unit for preoperative evaluation. His past medical history revealed a history of chronic, stable angina, hypertension, type II diabetes mellitus, and hypercholesterolemia. Four months prior to the scheduled surgery, a percutaneous transluminal coronary angioplasty (PTCA) was performed successfully for a 90% stenotic lesion of the patient's proximal left anterior descending coronary artery.

The patient denied a recent history of chest pain, shortness of breath, orthopnea, or dyspnea on exertion except for one anginal episode 2-weeks post-PTCA, which was short-lived and relieved by taking 1 sublingual nitroglycerin (NTG) tablet. He was able to walk up the steps to the second floor of his home without difficulty and to take his daily 1 mile walk, but he admitted to being more tired after his normal activity than he was prior to his recent cardiac problems. The patient's post-PTCA echocardiogram revealed a left ventricular ejection fraction (LVEF) of 48%, no significant valvular disease, and mild concentric left ventricular hypertrophy (LVH). Any evidence of pleural effusion or infiltrates was absent from the preoperative chest radiograph. Examination of his neck did not reveal jugular venous distention, and chest auscultation indicated normal heart sounds and clear lung fields. There was no edema of the lower extremities.

The patient's preoperative ECG revealed a normal sinus rhythm with a heart rate (HR) of 70 beats per minute (BPM), nonspecific ST-segment and T wave changes in the anterolateral leads, and LVH. His blood pressure (BP) ranged from 110 to 130/70 to 80 millimeters of mercury (mm Hg) without orthostatic changes. His cardiac medication regimen included lisinopril, aspirin, and sublingual NTG as needed, which he had not used since 2 weeks after the PTCA. The patient had taken his usual morning dose of lisinopril the day of surgery and, as instructed, had discontinued the aspirin 1 week prior to his surgery date.

The patient stated that his diabetes was fairly well controlled with diet and an oral agent (glyburide, which was not taken the morning of surgery) and that he had never used insulin. There was no documented history of renal insufficiency, retinopathy, or peripheral vascular disease.

As the certified registered nurse anesthetist (CRNA) performing the preanesthetic evaluation and intraoperative management of this patient with known coronary artery disease (CAD) undergoing a noncardiac surgery, I need to determine his degree of cardiac risk. I would definitely check the most recent cardiac test results, specifically the patient's initial cardiac catheterization and a post-PTCA echocardiogram. I would also review the recommendations of the patient's cardiologist with respect to the cardiac medications best used as adjuncts to my anesthetic, seeking consultation if necessary. I would also confirm with the surgical team that it is in the patient's best interest to undergo this major intraabdominal procedure at this time. Any information the primary surgeon had regarding the tumor size or problems anticipated with the planned resection would also be useful in developing an anesthetic plan.

My initial focus would be determining the patient's functional capacity and the status of his left ventricle four months after his angioplasty. The patient's exercise tolerance allowed him to walk 1 mile without cardiac symptoms, which indicated moderate functional capacity. Furthermore, he exhibited reasonable resting ventricular function as evidenced by a LVEF significantly higher than 35%, the value under which the greatest risk of perioperative complications have been observed (Eagle et al., 1996). The absence of congestive heart failure (CHF) indicated by a clear chest radiograph in association with physical findings provide further assurance that his left ventricular function is stable enough to undergo the physiologic stress of anesthesia and surgery. I am a little concerned about his one brief episode of chest pain postangioplasty, as to whether it represented reocclusion of the revascularized vessel or coronary artery vasopasm. I will be sure to reaffirm that he has indeed been free of chest pain for more than 3 months and that he continues to maintain a moderate degree of exercise tolerance. The preoperative ECG conformed the absence of any current acute myocardial ischemia, a good indication that the revascularization was indeed successful, and it documented LVH, the result of hypertensive disease. The patient's blood pressure appeared to be well controlled with the ACE inhibitor. Reaffirming with the patient that he did continue his antihypertensive medication regimen until the day of surgery will be important in minimizing the potential for intraoperative rebound hypertension. The fatigue that the patient experienced is consistent with his diagnosis of carcinoma of the colon, but it is also a flag to check for the presence of significant anemia.

Based on the criteria delineated in the American College of Cardiology (ACC)/American Heart Association (AHA) Practice Guidelines for the perioperative cardiovascular evaluation for noncardiac surgery (Eagle et al., 1996), the patient had intermediate predictors of clinical risk, demonstrated moderate functional capacity, and was undergoing an intermediate-risk surgery. According to these guidelines, this combination of risk factors has been correlated to little likelihood of perioperative death or myocardial infarction. Nonetheless, I would still plan an anesthetic with the primary goal of minimizing the physiologic stress on the patient's myocardium.

A history of hypertension in a diabetic patient predicts a 50% likelihood of coexisting autonomic neuropathy (Morgan & Mikhail, 1996), which predisposes the patient to cardiovascular instability, even sudden cardiac death. This patient does not exhibit the cardinal signs of autonomic neuropathy, namely resting tachycardia and orthostatic hypotension. However, painless myocardial ischemia is particularly worrisome given this patient's recent cardiac history. This concern reinforces the need for a "cardiac friendly" anesthetic.

There were no known drug allergies. He weighed 84 kilograms (kg) and was 70 inches tall. The past surgical history included an appendectomy 10 years prior to admission, with no reported surgical or anesthetic complications. A prior anesthetic record indicated that there was no history of airway management problems. An airway evaluation revealed a Mallampati classification of II, thyromental distance of

5 cm and a mouth opening of 4 cm. A normal neck ROM was demonstrated and there was no evidence of temporomandibular joint dysfunction (TMJ).

The patient had been NPO for approximately 10 hours and had completed a preoperative bowel preparation. A recent prothombin time (PT) and international normalized ratio (INR) indicated a normal coagulation status. He denied a history of chronic lower back pain or neurologic deficits of his lower extremities.

In view of these normal airway findings, I would plan to use a general endotracheal anesthetic (GETA) in combination with a continuous lumbar epidural (CLE) for postoperative pain management, if the patient consented to have the CLE inserted. His normal coagulation status and the absence of preexisting back or lower peripheral neurologic problems rule out major contraindications to the placement of an epidural. This combined technique allows me to capitalize on the benefits of each of the two techniques while decreasing their respective risks. Epidural analgesia and/or anesthesia has been associated with lower opiate dosages, better ablation of the catecholamine response to stress, and a less hypercoagulable state (Eagle et al., 1996). I could use the CLE as a primary neuraxial technique; however, a colon resection requires a dermatomal level (T4–T5) that may cause adverse hemodynamic effects. General anesthesia ensures an adequate anesthetic level for this major abdominal procedure, and it will allow me to carefully titrate the anesthetic agents in order to control the patient's intraoperative hemodynamics. One major advantage of combining GETA with a CLE is that it establishes a method of instituting postoperative pain management during the intraoperative period. I would administer a local anesthetic (0.25% bupivacaine) and a narcotic (fentanyl) via the CLE catheter because it has been found that significant synergy and therefore excellent analgesia is produced with this combination. I would begin dosing the epidural during the early emergence phase of my anesthetic as I gradually decrease the depth of general anesthesia, thus facilitating a hemodynamically stable, pain-free emergence and minimizing myocardial stress.

The next logical decision to make is the choice of intraoperative monitors. The key issue is deciding the best method of detecting intraoperative myocardial ischemia. A multiple lead (II and V5) ECG monitoring with computerized ST-segment analysis is clearly indicated in this patient. Although the predictive value of intraoperative (as opposed to postoperative) ST-segment changes for adverse perioperative cardiac events has not been fully proven, there is general agreement in the current literature that ST-segment monitoring, properly used, is a sensitive and reliable monitor for intraoperative myocardial ischemia (Yao, 1998). I would not place a pulmonary artery catheter (PAC) in this patient because he did not have a history of a myocardial infarction or CHF, or does a colon resection usually involve the magnitude of fluid shifts that would indicate placement of a PAC. Moreover, PAC is reportedly an insensitive monitor for myocardial ischemia (Yao, 1998). Although transesophageal echocardiography (TEE) has been advocated as the most sensitive and arguably the most cost-effective method of myocardial ischemia detection, it has not been proven to have predictive value for perioperative cardiac events in patients with CAD having noncardiac surgery (Fleisher, 1996). In institutions where TEE is readily available and the anesthesia practitioners are skilled in the interpretation of TEE images, this might be a reasonable choice as a monitor for this patient; however, in this case, I would opt not to use it.

In addition to those monitors that constitute the standard of anesthesia care[1] and the aforementioned methods of ischemia monitoring, I would monitor intraarterial BP, central venous pressure (CVP), and the twitch response of peripheral nerves via a peripheral

---

[1]The American Society of Anesthesiologists (ASA) Standards for Basic Intraoperative Monitoring include inspired oxygen analysis, pulse oximetry, end-tidal CO_2 analysis, ECG, noninvasive BP monitor, and a temperature monitor.

nerve stimulator (PNS). The beat-to-beat monitoring of the BP will guide my titration of multiple anesthetic and adjunct drugs, as well as provide convenient access for blood sampling. The CVP monitoring will facilitate judicious fluid management, and the use of the PNS will be helpful in determining dosing strategies for muscle relaxants.

Prior to the placement of monitoring lines and the CLE in the preoperative holding area, I would administer small doses (0.5 to 1.0 mg) of a benzodiazepine (midazolam) along with supplemental oxygen. My goal is to provide adequate anxiolysis for the patient in order to minimize anxiety-induced hypertension and tachycardia. I would insert the CLE at approximately the L3–L4 level of the spine and test in the usual manner to rule out improper placement in either the subarachnoid space or in an epidural vessel. Prior to inducing the general anesthetic, I think it is important to gain reasonable assurance of the efficacy of the CLE. Injecting approximately 8 to 10 cc of 1% Lidocaine (without epinephrine) should result in a very low segmental block, which would demonstrate proper epidural placement without the risk of hypotension secondary to a sympathectomy. Having established a plan for the placement and confirmation of a functional CLE, I would proceed with the planning of the general anesthetic.

This patient is a good candidate for perioperative beta blockade because he would clearly benefit from an attenuated heart rate response to sympathetic stimulation, and he does not possess any contraindications to beta blockers (e.g., CHF, third-degree heart block, or bronchospastic disease). My choice would be intravenous atenolol, 5 to 10 mg given slowly in a monitored environment at least 30 minutes prior to the induction of anesthesia if his resting heart rate was greater than or equal to 55 bpm and his systolic blood pressure was greater than or equal to 100 mmHg. The same dose would be given in the immediate postoperative period, with the same parameters. The decision as to whether or not the atenolol would continue to be administered on subsequent postoperative days should be decided by the providers managing the patient's postoperative care.

Priorities during induction of general anesthesia on this patient are to avoid hypertension, hypotension, and/or tachycardia, which are conditions that precipitate myocardial ischemia. This is often a challenge because patients with hypertensive disease, regardless of the degree of preoperative BP control maintained with medication, experience extreme hemodynamic lability while undergoing anesthesia. Based on the patient's normal airway examination, it would be reasonable to proceed with an intravenous induction followed by neuromuscular paralysis in order to provide optimal conditions for intubation.

Another pertinent airway issue to consider is the high risk of gastroparesis caused by diabetic autonomic neuropathy. Although this patient does not exhibit symptoms of severe autonomic neuropathy or gastroesophageal reflux disease, the prudent thing to do is administer a gastrokinetic (metaclopromide, 10 mg IV) to enhance the emptying of gastric contents, as well as prophylaxis for aspiration pneumonitis (cimetidine, 300 mg IV). A rapid sequence induction (RSI) with cricoid pressure is also a precautionary measure taken in persons with diabetes to minimize the risk of aspiration. However, the disadvantage of an RSI in this patient is that it omits a period of mask ventilation after the patient has been rendered unconscious. This postinduction period is a time during which our patient's anesthetic level could be deepened (via inhalation or intravenous agents) thereby blunting the sympathetic response to laryngoscopy and intubation. In this situation, the benefit of performing a slower, smoother induction outweighs the benefit of a standard RSI. I would perform the induction with cricoid pressure, but would titrate the induction agents slowly, watching the vital signs as the drugs take effect. My goal would be to keep both the HR and BP within 20% of the patient's baseline values.

Because of the patient's history of chronic hypertension, 10-hour NPO status, and his bowel preparation, I would anticipate that he would be volume-depleted. He would definitely require prehydration with a crystalloid (Lactated Ringers) prior to administering induction agents. This would be done to minimize a hypotensive response to the vasodilatory and myocardial depressing effects of the agents. A standard bolus is at least 500 milliliters (ml) of crystalloid, but because his NPO deficit[2] is more than 1 liter, and the bowel prep usually contributes another liter of deficit, a larger bolus is indicated. The specific amount of fluid should be dictated by the baseline BP, HR and CVP reading. I would aim to maintain the preoperative CVP within 4–8 mmHg.

I would begin the formal induction period in this patient with preoxygenation. In addition to the aforementioned doses of midazolam and atenolol, I would give a narcotic [fentanyl, 5 to 8 micrograms per kilogram (mcg/kg) in divided doses (50 to 100 mcg)] throughout the induction period. Fentanyl provides some degree of preemptive analgesia, lowers the dose requirement of the induction agent, affords cardiovascular stability, and helps blunt the sympathetic response to laryngoscopy. Thiopental, a barbiturate, would be given in 50-mg doses to an approximate total of 3 mg/kg or until the patient loses consciousness and is rendered apneic. Thiopental can cause myocardial depression; however, with adequate prehydration and careful, slow titration of all of the induction agents, hypotension can be avoided. Once unconscious, the patient should be kept well oxygenated via gentle mask ventilations (with cricoid pressure). I would watch the BP and HR, continue to titrate fentanyl and thiopental, and perhaps administer an inhalation agent (isoflurane) via the mask to further deepen the anesthetic level. When the hemodynamics indicate an adequate anesthetic depth, I would give a depolarizing muscle relaxant (succinylcholine, 1.5 mg/kg) in preparation for airway instrumentation. When the patient is fully relaxed, I would accomplish intubation as expeditiously as possible.

My choice for the maintenance phase of the anesthetic for this patient would be moderate doses (0.8 to 1.0 MAC[3]) of the inhalation agent isoflurane given with relatively high inspired concentrations of oxygen (FiO_2 of 0.6 to 1.0) and air, and the intermediate acting nondepolarizing muscle relaxant vercuronium (.04 mg/kg per dose). I like to initiate the use of epidural opioids relatively early in the case. Administering 100 mcg of fentanyl via the CLE after the airway has been secured and prior to the surgical incision would provide further preemptive analgesia, and will enable me to decrease my total dose of parenteral narcotics. I want to avoid high doses of intravenous narcotics to decrease the potential need for postoperative ventilation and a period of weaning the patient off the ventilator in an intensive care setting. This weaning period has been associated with the development of myocardial ischemia (Eagle et al., 1996), which is what makes an inhalation-based maintenance phase with early extubation in the operating room a very reasonable option.

The preoperative hemoglobin (Hgb) and hematocrit (Hct) were 11.2 grams per deciliter (g/dL) and 33.4% respectively, and the platelet count was 220,000 per mm[3]. Two units of packed red blood cells (PRBCs) were available in the blood bank for the patient in a type and screen status. The electrolyte panel was normal, the serum BUN and creatinine were 11 and 1.1 mg/dL respectively, and the serum glucose was 150 mg/dL.

A hemoglobin of 11.2 in an elderly male is clearly considered anemic, and from the patient's history, it is apparent that it is a chronic condition. A key issue is determining reasonable parameters for the transfusion of PRBCs in this patient whose oxygen-carrying capacity must be optimized. The goal is to prevent myocardial complications owing to acute intraoperative anemia and still comply with current practice standards aimed at conserving blood, preventing bloodborne diseases, and minimizing the risk of other transfusion-related complications. A sigmoid colon resection is not usually associated with significant

---

[2]NPO deficit = (hourly maintenance fluid) × (# of NPO hrs). Hourly maintenance fluid (mls) = (weight in kg) × (1.5 ml/kg/hr). For this patient, NPO deficit = 84 kg × 1.5 ml/kg/hr × 10 hrs = 1260 ml.
[3]MAC = Minimum alveolar concentration, the unit dose by which inhalation agents are titrated.

blood loss especially if hemostasis is meticulously maintained by the surgical team. I would estimate the allowable blood loss (ABL) that would bring the Hct to approximately 30% (598 ml),[4] and as this ABL approached, I would begin closely monitoring the intraoperative Hct. Ultimately, I would make the clinical judgement to transfuse PRBCs based upon the patient's Hct, his intravascular volume, the presence of hypotension and/or tachycardia, and information gained from the surgeon regarding the probability of continued bleeding into the postoperative period.

The normal BUN-to-creatinine ratio indicated adequate renal function, but it is always prudent to implement measures that will provide adequate renal perfusion. These measures include maintaining intravascular volume and keeping the cardiac output and mean arterial pressure within the range that will most ensure urinary flow. The standard intraoperative criteria for minimum urine output is 0.5 ml/kg/hr. An intraoperative fluid management plan would incorporate his hourly maintenance rate of 125 ml/hr, his unreplaced NPO deficit, and an hourly replacement for anticipated third-space loss[5] of approximately 500 ml/hr. Estimated blood loss (EBL) would be replaced either with crystalloid in a 3:1 ratio, or with colloid in a 1:1 ratio. There are standard guidelines that delineate an hourly apportionment in these fluid needs; however, for this patient, I would titrate the fluids according to CVP trends because the readings will be more reflective of the patient's true volume status.

The essential goal in the intraoperative management of glucose in a person with diabetes is to avoid hypoglycemia. The brain is dependent on glucose as its energy source; therefore, any degree of hypoglycemia intraoperatively worsens the neurologic sequelae of cerebral ischemia. In addition, it is necessary to avoid ketoacidosis and hyperosmolar states. Because this patient has type II diabetes, I would reaffirm that he had not taken his oral hypoglycemic the morning of surgery, refrain from giving glucose-containing intravenous solutions, and monitor his blood glucose levels at a minimum of 2-hour intervals. I would not consider insulin administration until the blood glucose indicated a persistent level of approximately 250 mg/dL.

A combined GETA/CLE technique was discussed with the patient, including a delineation of the risks and benefits incurred by each technique. His questions were answered, and informed consent for anesthesia care was obtained. The patient was transported to the preoperative holding area where, according to the preinduction anesthetic plan, peripheral intravenous access was attained, monitoring lines were placed, and the CLE was inserted uneventfully.

The patient was then brought to the operating room where general anesthesia was induced smoothly, the airway secured without incident, and the surgical incision was made without any significant hemodynamic response. During a subsequent period of vigorous visceral retraction for tumor mobilization, the patient's HR increased from 65 to 108 bpm, and the BP increased from 110/65 to 150/90 mm Hg. Concomitant 2-mm horizontal ST-segment depression was noted in lead V5; no changes were noted in lead II.

High on the list of possible causes for these myocardial ischemic changes is the acute onset of hypertension and tachycardia caused by autonomic sympathetic response to an acutely increased level of surgical stimulation. Tachycardia increases myocardial oxygen demand (as does the elevated BP) as well as decreases the myocardial oxygen supply because

---

[4]Formula for calculating ABL = [(baseline Hct − desired Hct)/baseline Hct] × Total Blood Volume (TBV). Estimated TBV = (weight in kg) × (70 ml). For this patient, TBV = 5880 ml and ABL = [(0.334 − 0.300)/0.334] × 5880 = 598 ml.

[5]Hourly replacement for fluid for third-space loss for major abdominal procedures is approximately 6 ml/kg/hr. For this patient, third-space fluid replacement = 84 Kg × 6 ml/kg/hr = 504 ml/hr.

it shortens the diastolic period. I would immediately ensure that a FiO_2 of 1.0 be administered, ask the surgeon to temporarily stop surgical stimulation (if possible), and would deepen the level of anesthesia by either increasing the dose of isoflurane or administering an intravenous bolus dose of fentanyl. If this first intervention was not successful in resolving the ST-segment depression, and the increased HR and BP persisted, I would use bolus doses of the short-acting beta-blocker esmolol to treat the hemodynamic response. Other causes for the ST-segment depression to consider would be hypoxemia or acutely severe anemia, which I would also attempt to rule out by monitoring pulse oximetry, drawing blood samples for arterial blood gas, and conducting hemoglobin analysis.

The HR and BP subsequently decreased to previous levels, and the ST segments returned to baseline, where they remained throughout the duration of the case. No other intraoperative events transpired, and the surgical procedure was completed without complications. The bupivacaine and fentanyl was administered via the CLE during the latter phase of the anesthetic, which resulted in excellent analgesia; the patient emerged smoothly and was extubated in the operating room. An immediate postoperative 12-lead ECG done in the postanesthetic care unit (PACU) did not exhibit any significant change from the preoperative tracing.
The patient was closely monitored in a telemetry unit for 2 days postoperatively during which time he did not manifest any clinical symptoms of myocardial ischemia, nor did his subsequent ECGs demonstrate ischemic changes. The patient experienced an uncomplicated postoperative course and was discharged on the sixth postoperative day.

Discussion and Commentary

This case study illustrates several key issues in the anesthetic management of patients with cardiac disease undergoing noncardiac surgery that require clinical decision making. These issues are 1) preoperative risk assessment of the patient, 2) choice of anesthetic technique, 3) choice of anesthetic agents, 4) the use of perioperative beta blockade, 5) intraoperative monitoring strategies, and 6) determination of criteria for the transfusion of red blood cells.

The report by the Task Force on Practice Guidelines of the American College of Cardiology (ACC)/American Heart Association (AHA) (Eagle et al., 1996) contains the cardiac risk stratification scheme that I used with this patient. This particular scheme is gaining favor in clinical anesthesia practice over older schemes because it incorporates factors such as the prior medical or surgical treatment of CAD (e.g., PTCA) or the type of surgical procedure being performed. Furthermore, the ACC/AHA scheme involves a stepwise, algorithmic approach to risk assessment, which decreases the degree of ambiguity involved in the risk stratification process.

The question as to whether regional or general anesthesia is inherently better for a patient with a cardiac history is still the focus of many academic discussions. Similarly, the notion that one type of anesthetic drug (i.e., inhalation agents versus narcotics) confers better myocardial protection continues to be debated. From a clinical point of view, there is no one best myocardial protective agent or technique. The choice should always be made based on the overall risk-to-benefit ratio determined for each individual patient and surgical scenario. The ACC/AHA task force report (Eagle et al., 1996) contains a summary of the scientific evidence that supports this conclusion. The report also contains a comprehensive review of the data supporting the monitoring strategy I outlined for this patient.

Although the use of perioperative beta blockade in higher-risk cardiac patients is not yet routine, intraoperative use of beta-blocking agents have been shown in three well-known studies to be associated with improved outcome (Pasternak et al., 1987, 1989; Stone, Foex,

& Sear, 1988). A recent review by Fleisher (1996) of management strategies for cardiac patients undergoing noncardiac surgery also supports the appropriate use of beta blockade.

The American Society of Anesthesiologists Task Force on Blood Component Therapy (Stehling et al.,1996) states that a single hemoglobin "trigger" for all patients, and other approaches that fail to consider all important physiologic and surgical factors affecting oxygenation are not recommended. These days, many clinicians in fact do refrain from routinely transfusing even a patient with a cardiac history when the Hct decreases to 30%. However, two studies (Christopherson, Frank, & Norris, 1991; Nelson, Fleischer, & Rosenbaum, 1993) have documented adverse clinical sequelae from postoperative, iatrogenic acute anemia in cardiac patients. The threshold Hct values in these studies under which morbid cardiac events occurred were 28 to 29%. These findings support the notion that, the current transfusion guidelines notwithstanding, there is evidence to maintain the cardiac patient's Hct as close to 30% as possible.

Planning and implementing anesthesia and analgesia for a patient with a cardiac history undergoing noncardiac surgery is all about assessing that patient's risk of a perioperative cardiac event, and constantly reassessing the risk-to-benefit ratio of each step of the plan throughout each perioperative phase. Such considerations will lead to decreased perioperative morbidity and improved patient outcomes.

REFERENCES

Christopherson, R., Frank, S., & Norris, E. (1991). Low postoperative hematocrit is associated with cardiac ischemia in high-risk patients. *Anesthesiology 75:A99,* 1202–1203.

Eagle, K. A., Brundage, B. H., Chaitman, B. R., et al. (1996). Guidelines for perioperative cardiovascular evaluation for noncardiac surgery. A report of the American College of Cardiology/American Heart Association Task Force on Practice Guidelines. *Circulation 93,* 1278–1317.

Fleischer, L. A., (1996). Perioperative management of the cardiac patient undergoing noncardiac surgery. In P. G. Barash (Ed.). *American Society of Anesthesiologists Annual Refresher Courses: Vol. 24* (pp. 71–84). Philadelphia, Lippincott-Raven.

Morgan, G. E., & Mikhail, M. S. (1996). *Clinical Anesthesiology* (2nd ed.). Stamford, CT: Appleton & Lange.

Nelson, A. H., Fleisher, L. A. & Rosenbaum, S. H. (1993). Relationship between postoperative anemia and cardiac morbidity in high-risk vascular patients in the intensive care unit. *Critical Care Medicine 21,* 860–864.

Pasternack, P. F., Grossi, E. A., Bauman, F. G., et al. (1989). Beta blockade to decrease silent myocardial ischemia during peripheral vascular surgery. *American Journal of Surgery 158,* 113–116.

Pasternack, P. F., Imparato, A. M., Bauman, F. G., et al. (1987). The hemodynamics of beta-blockage in patients undergoing abdominal aortic aneurysm repair. *Circulation 76,* III-1–III-7.

Stehling, L. C., Doherty, D. C., Faust, R. J., et al. (1996). Practice Guidelines for blood component therapy. A report by the American Society of Anesthesiologists Task Force on Blood Component Therapy. *Anesthesiology 84* (3), 732–747.

Stone, J. G., Foex, P., & Sear, J. W. (1988). Myocardial ischemia in untreated hypertensive patients: Effect of a single, small oral dose of a beta-adrenergic blocking agent. *Anestheisology 68,* 495–500.

Yao, F. F. (1998). Ischemic heart disease and noncardiac surgery. In F. F. Yao (Ed.). *Yao & Artusio's anesthesiology: Problem-oriented patient management* (4th ed) (pp. 385–404). Philadelphia: Lippincott-Raven.

A Confounding Diagnosis in a Postoperative Neonate with Congenital Heart Disease

Lori D. Johnson

A 1-day-old male, weighing 2930 grams at birth, was admitted to the pediatric intensive care unit (PICU) of a tertiary care medical center for the surgical treatment of congenital heart disease. Pertinent maternal history included an uncomplicated twin pregnancy followed by a spontaneous vaginal delivery at 37 weeks gestation. Pertinent medical history included apgar scores of 6 and 8 at 1 and 5 minutes after birth, respectively. At 12 hours of age, he had developed peripheral and central cyanosis without respiratory distress. An oxygen challenge test was subsequently performed, which revealed an arterial oxygen tension (PaO_2) of 44 mmHg on both 60% and 90% oxygen. An infusion of prostaglandin E_1 (PGE_1) was initiated to maintain patency of the ductus arteriosus, which resulted in apnea requiring intubation, mechanical ventilation, and decreasing of the PGE_1 dose. A two-dimensional, color flow, surface echocardiogram revealed D-transposition of the great arteries (D-TGA) with an intact ventricular septum, a patent foramen ovale, and a patent ductus arteriosus. The left coronary artery arose from the left-facing sinus, giving rise to the anterior descending and circumflex coronary arteries, and a right coronary artery originated from the right-facing sinus.

On admission to the PICU his preoperative physical examination revealed a well-developed, well-perfused, and nondysmorphic neonate who was intubated and mechanically ventilated. His color was pink with mild central cyanosis. Preductal and postductal oxygen saturations by pulse oximetry (SpO_2) were 88% on 21% oxygen. Over the next 4 days, he demonstrated good hemodynamics with adequate oxygen saturation on a continuous PGE_1 infusion. He achieved an excellent diuresis and received nutritional supplementation.

On his fifth day of life, the neonate was taken to the operating room for an elective arterial switch operation. This was performed through a midline sternotomy using deep hypothermic cardiopulmonary bypass and general anesthesia. The surgical procedure was performed without any complications. Prior to the separation of cardiopulmonary bypass (CPB), a dopamine infusion of 5 μg/kg/min was initiated per standard protocol. The CPB time was 167 minutes, and the aortic cross clamp time was 82 minutes. Separation from CPB occurred without incident. Intraoperative transesophogeal echocardiography (TEE) following CPB separation showed good biventricular function, normal valve function, absence of any outflow obstruction, and no residual cardiac defects. Left atrial (LA), right atrial (RA), and pulmonary artery (PA) transthoracic intracardiac catheters, as well as atrial and ventricular pacing wires were placed. Sternal closure was delayed secondary to mediastinal bleeding. Observation of the suture lines showed no discrete bleeding sites and the cause of bleeding was believed to be due to a coagulopathy. Platelets, cryoprecipitate, and whole blood were administered; however, the prothrombin time (PT) remained at 27 seconds. Fresh frozen plasma was administered whereupon the bleeding stopped. Subsequent laboratory values revealed the following: PT 13.9 seconds, partial thromboplastin time (PTT) 42.0 seconds, platelet count 182 mm^3, fibrinogen 442 mg/dl, hematocrit (Hct) 32%, and ionized calcium 1.1 mmol/L. The dopamine infusion was increased to 7 µg/kg/min owing to hypotension. The sternum was closed over two mediastinal chest tubes.

The neonate was readmitted to the PICU at 1715. His mechanical ventilator settings were as follows: FiO$_2$ 1.00, SIMV 25 breaths per minute, tidal volume 80 cc, and peak end expiratory pressure 4 cmH$_2$O. His skin color was pink, extremities were pale and slightly cool, peripheral pulses were weak, and the distal extremity capillary refill was 3 seconds. No spontaneous motor movement was evident. His pupils were equal (2 mm) and briskly reactive. Mediastinal chest tubes were placed to 20 cm wall suction and were draining a small amount of blood; the sternal dressing was dry. Vital signs were as follows: heart rate (HR) 170 beats per minute (BPM), blood pressure (BP) 50/37 mmHg, RA pressure 4 mmHg, LA pressure 6 mmHg, PA pressure 20/11 mmHg, and rectal temperature 36.0° C. His electrocardiogram (ECG) demonstrated a sinus tachycardia and his atrial pressure waveforms were normal. A urinary catheter was present and draining a small amount of clear urine. The dopamine infusion was at 7 µg/kg/minute. The initial arterial blood gas (ABG) in the PICU revealed pH 7.41, PaCO$_2$ 44 mmHg, PaO$_2$ 250 mmHg, HCO$_3$ 27.8 meq/L, and base excess of (BE) 4.9 mmol/L on an FiO$_2$ of 1.00. Hemoglobin was 11.6 grams per deciliter, and a transfusion of packed red blood cells was initiated. Blood for analysis of electrolytes, coagulation studies, and complete blood count were sent to the laboratory. A 12-lead ECG revealed sinus tachycardia, normal ST-segment position and normal T waves. A chest radiograph revealed a normal heart size and normal pulmonary findings. A fentanyl infusion was initiated at 5 µg/kg/min to extend the effects of anesthesia and avoid adverse responses in hemodynamics to stimulation.

As the clinical nurse specialist caring for this postoperative neonate, I am immediately concerned with the abnormal findings of tachycardia, hypotension, and poor peripheral perfusion, which lead me to believe he has inadequate cardiac output. His pulmonary status is fairly stable although his ABG reveals a large alveolar-arterial oxygen gradient and a mild metabolic alkalosis. Major considerations in the differential diagnosis of inadequate cardiac output are inadequate preload, myocardial dysfunction, dysrhythmias, residual cardiac defects, elevated systemic vascular resistance (SVR), and pulmonary hypertension. Residual cardiac defects were not seen in his postoperative TEE and current monitoring rules out pulmonary hypertension and dysrhythmias. Although he appears to have an elevated SVR, this is unlikely the cause of his low cardiac output, and rather a consequence of sympathetic nervous system compensation for inadequate tissue perfusion. At this point in time, I think the most likely cause of his inadequate cardiac output is inadequate preload or myocardial dysfunction.

Inadequate preload could be caused by inadequate replacement of his previous blood loss, and expanding vascular bed secondary to vasodilation associated with peripheral warming, ongoing bleeding, or cardiac tamponade. Cardiac tamponade seems unlikely given his normal atrial pressures and normal pulse pressure. His chest tubes are not draining a large amount of blood, which suggests there is not ongoing overt blood loss. At this point, the most likely cause of inadequate preload would be the inadequate replacement of intraoperative blood loss and/or vasodilation secondary to peripheral rewarming. Although his core (rectal) temperature was normal, peripheral rewarming typically exists for a period of 6 to 8 hours following surgery resulting in peripheral vasodilation.

Coagulopathy following cardiac surgery occurs due to the activation of coagulation and fibrinolytic cascades during CPB resulting in consumption of coagulation factors and fibrinolysis. In addition, the exposure of patient blood to the artificial extracorporeal circuit causes platelet dysfunction that contributes to postoperative bleeding. Neonates have greater risk of bleeding following CPB than adults, secondary to extensive hemodilution and an exaggerated inflammatory response. The disproportionate size of the extracorporeal circuit relative to neonates' blood volume results in an increased reduction in fibrinogen, clotting factors and platelets. The inflammatory response to CPB alters vascular permeability, activating platelets and inducing fibrinolysis. Hepatic immaturity in neonates may result in decreased synthesis of prothrombin and delayed clearance of heparin, both of which may contribute to postoperative bleeding. A coagulopathy following a neonatal arterial switch operation is a serious problem because of the extensive circumferential suture lines on the aorta and pulmonary artery where bleeding can occur. Although there is no evidence of current bleeding in this neonate, particular attention must be given in the PICU to avoid hypertensive states and to closely monitor coagulation studies and provide necessary factor replacement in order to prevent further bleeding.

Poor myocardial contractility, as the cause of inadequate cardiac output, could be secondary to electrolyte and/or acid–base disturbances, worsening myocardial dysfunction from CPB and aortic cross clamp, or unrecognized myocardial ischemia. With the absence of an acidosis, hypocalcemia would be the most likely electrolyte disturbance to impair myocardial contractility and cause hypotension. Low serum ionized calcium levels could have resulted from the administration of citrate-anticoagulated blood products in the operating room with inadequate replacement of calcium. If this is the case, administration of calcium chloride and maintaining the ionized calcium at the high end of normal would improve systolic cardiac function and improve this neonate's hemodynamics.

Although his CPB and aortic cross clamp times were not prolonged, I do expect this neonate to have transient myocardial dysfunction. Neonates who undergo an arterial switch operation develop a predictable decline in cardiac output following CPB with a nadir occurring approximately 9 to 12 hours postoperatively. Although I do not believe this is a factor yet, I would anticipate a need to increase his inotropic support later this evening.

Another potential source for myocardial dysfunction is myocardial ischemia. This neonate's normal 12-lead ECG findings, along with the absence of dysrhythmias, makes myocardial ischemia unlikely. Late presentation of myocardial ischemia following an arterial switch operation is rare, but may occur secondary to complications from air emboli or thrombus. Therefore, continuous monitoring of his ECG and perfusion status are warranted.

By 1830 a total of 20 ml of packed red blood cells had infused and two doses of calcium chloride were administered. The hourly chest tube output was 16 ml and urine output was 3 ml. HR was 176 BPM and BP was 60/40 mmHg. Additional hemodynamics values are listed in (Table 5C-1). The laboratory studies from 1715 were: Hct 32.7%, PT 16.1 seconds, PTT 52.7 seconds, platelet count 170 mm³, fibrinogen 186 mg/dl, and normal serum electrolytes. Repeat ABG values (Table 5C-2) were stable. The patient's color remained pale pink and peripheral perfusion poor. The cardiac rhythm remained a sinus tachycardia.

Despite the improvement in BP following blood administration, I am worried about his ongoing tachycardia. The presence of a persistent tachycardia following fluid resuscitation leads me to consider ongoing fluid losses or cardiac tamponade as causes of his poor perfusion status. His atrial pressures were higher at this time point; however, they were not

TABLE 5C-1 *Hemodynamic Parameters in the Postoperative Period*

Time	HR (BPM)	BP (mmHg)	RAP (mmHg)	LAP (mmHg)	PAP (mmHg)
1715	170	50/37	4	6	20/11
1800	172	58/38	6	7	22/11
1830	176	60/40	7	8	22/12
1900	180	62/43	9	11	24/11
1930	184	60/46	10	11	22/10
1940	188	60/49	12	14	20/11
1955	76	58/48	17	16	16/10
1958	206	93/85	17	16	28/14
2003	202	99/86	8	10	24/12
2030	164	75/53	4	5	20/12

HR, heart rate; BP, blood pressure; RAP, right atrial pressure; LAP, left atrial pressure; PAP, pulmonary artery pressure; BPM, beats per minute; mmHg, millimeters of mercury.

excessively elevated. His chest tubes are patent and the output is not excessive. Although I am not concerned at this stage that his myocardial function is worsening, I would keep this diagnostic possibility in the back of my mind. The administration of additional intravenous fluids would be warranted with close subsequent evaluation of his hemodynamic and oxygenation parameters.

The reoccurrence of his coagulopathy may be a result of ongoing bleeding and subsequent dilutional coagulopathy from administration of packed red blood cells. Although his platelet count was normal, platelet dysfunction from CPB could still exist. In addition, neonatal hepatic immaturity could result in inadequate synthesis of prothrombin. The combination of these factors could precipitate bleeding around the aortic and pulmonary artery anastomoses.

By 1940 the neonate had received an additional 20 ml of packed red blood cells and one dose of calcium chloride. His HR was 188 BPM, BP 60/49 mmHg, RA pressure 12 mmHg and LA pressure 14 mmHg. His distal extremities were cold, and his capillary refill was 5 seconds. His ABG on an FiO_2 of 0.50 revealed a PaO_2 of 44 mmHg (Table 5C-2). His lung sounds were normal, there was good chest expansion with hand ventilation and no evidence of endotracheal tube obstruction. He was placed on an FiO_2 of 1.00 and a CXR was ordered. The mediastinal chest tubes were stripped and hand-suctioned, which produced no further subsequent drainage. A rapid intravenous push of packed red blood cells was initiated and a dose of calcium chloride was administered. During the next 10 minutes, the neonate's pulse pressure continued to narrow and atrial pressures remained elevated. The cardiac rhythm remained sinus tachycardia. An ABG at 1955 revealed continued severe arterial hypoxemia and a significant drop in base deficit as compared to his base deficit on PICU admission (Table 5C-2).

Given there is no good explanation for severe myocardial dysfunction and in lieu of his bleeding history, I am seriously suspicious of the possibility of mediastinal bleeding with the development of cardiac tamponade being the cause of his inadequate cardiac output. This would explain his elevated atrial pressures, his narrow pulse pressure (rise in diastolic

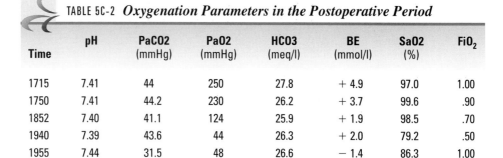

TABLE 5C-2 *Oxygenation Parameters in the Postoperative Period*

Time	pH	PaCO2 (mmHg)	PaO2 (mmHg)	HCO3 (meq/l)	BE (mmol/l)	SaO2 (%)	FiO₂
1715	7.41	44	250	27.8	+ 4.9	97.0	1.00
1750	7.41	44.2	230	26.2	+ 3.7	99.6	.90
1852	7.40	41.1	124	25.9	+ 1.9	98.5	.70
1940	7.39	43.6	44	26.3	+ 2.0	79.2	.50
1955	7.44	31.5	48	26.6	− 1.4	86.3	1.00
2030	7.41	40.9	358	26.4	+ 1.1	99.7	1.00

$PaCO_2$, arterial carbon dioxide tension; PaO_2, arterial oxygen tension; HCO_3, bicarbonate; BE, base excess; SaO_2, arterial oxygen saturation; FiO_2, fraction of inspired oxygen; mmHg, millimeters of mercury; meq/l, milliequivalents per liter; mM/l, millimoles per liter.

pressure), and worsening tachycardia. Cardiac tamponade impedes ventricular filling and could manifest itself in the manner in which this neonate is presenting. I am suspicious that this may have been the origin of the problem since his PICU postoperative admission. His failure to respond to rapid administration of intravenous fluids also corroborates the diagnosis of hemorrhage and cardiac tamponade.

Although his chest tubes were stripped and suctioned, I am highly suspicious that they are not functioning appropriately to drain any accumulated mediastinal blood. His severe arterial hypoxemia could be evidence of compression of the lung parenchyma from accumulating blood in the mediastinum and/or a hemothorax secondary to a communication between the mediastinal and pleural spaces, both of which would impair oxygenation. Although his hemodynamics suggest cardiac tamponade, severe hypoxemia and impaired cardiac output could be caused by a tension pneumothorax; this is unlikely though, given his normal lung sounds. His drop in base deficit is further evidence of developing metabolic acidosis due to serious impairment of cardiac output and/or oxygen saturation, ultimately resulting in inadequate oxygen delivery.

At 1955 this neonate developed sinus bradycardia with a HR of 76 BPM. A bolus dose of 30 µg of intravenous epinephrine was administered, the dopamine infusion was increased to 10 µg/kg/min, and chest compressions and hand ventilation with 100% oxygen were initiated. Rapid administration of packed red blood cells was continued. At 2000, emergency sternotomy revealed large amounts of blood in the pericardial and pleural spaces. Hemodynamics subsequently improved at 2003 and his SpO_2 increased to 99%. After the evacuation of 100 ml of blood from the chest, mediastinal exploration revealed no discrete bleeding sites. The chest tubes were repositioned to provide optimal drainage and the mediastinum was closed with a Silastic patch.

The development of bradycardia is evidence that this neonate could no longer maintain compensatory responses to low cardiac output and occurs when the myocardial oxygen delivery becomes inadequate. The emergency administration of epinephrine along with the chest compressions and rapid volume administration were only temporary treatment measures until emergency sternotomy could be performed. The emergency sternotomy provided visual evidence of mediastinal blood, which clearly confirmed the diagnosis of cardiac tamponade in this neonate. Sternotomy results in rapid decompression of the mediastinum allowing ventricular preload, cardiac output and oxygen delivery to be quickly restored. In addition, compression of the lungs was also relieved, which rapidly improved oxygenation. The rapid recovery of this neonate's hemodynamic and oxygenation parameters in association with rapid sternotomy decompression provided further evidence for the diagnosis of cardiac tamponade.

At 2030, the neonate's hemodynamics following the resuscitation were: HR 164 BPM, BP 75/53 mmHg, RA pressure 4 mmHg, left atrial pressure 5 mmHg, and PA pressure 20/12 mmHg. SpO_2 was 100% on an FiO2 of 1.00. Over the next 12 hours, the dopamine infusion was weaned to 5 µg/kg/min; the fentanyl infusion was discontinued and replaced with intravenous bolus morphine, and parenteral nutrition was initiated. The sternum was closed on postoperative day (POD) 1 without complication. The neonate was weaned from mechanical ventilation and extubated on POD #3. On POD #4, his dopamine infusion was discontinued, his intracardiac catheters were removed. The neonate was transferred to the neonatal intensive care unit on POD #5 where he continued to recover until discharge to home on POD #10. Hospital length of stay was 16 days; no evidence of organ system dysfucntion was present at the time of discharge.

Commentary

Cardiac tamponade following cardiac surgery is a life-threatening condition that requires prompt diagnosis and treatment to reverse the process. Cardiac tamponade exerts mechanical pressure on the heart, which reduces preload and stroke volume, and decreases ventricular compliance which consequently decreases cardiac output (Roth, 1998). It is usually caused by postoperative mediastinal bleeding with inadequate drainage; however, postoperative myocardial swelling may also result in cardiac tamponade and impair cardiac function (Schleien, Setzer, McLaughlin & Rogers, 1992).

Clinical signs of postoperative cardiac tamponade in neonates include hypotension, narrowed pulse pressure or pulsus paradoxus, elevated right and left atrial pressures, tachycardia and poor peripheral perfusion (Smith, Baker, Moynihan, et al, 1996). In particular, hypotension that is unresponsive to volume resuscitation often assists in the diagnosis of cardiac tamponade. Narrow pulse pressure is reflective of a rising systemic arterial diastolic blood pressure secondary to a compensatory rise in systemic vascular resistance. Neck vein distension is rarely seen in neonates because of their short, fat necks. Muffled heart sounds are rarely auscultated in neonates with cardiac tamponade since their thin chest wall readily transmits heart sounds. Sinus tachycardia is more exaggerated in neonates because their immature hearts limit their ability to increase stroke volume to compensate for low cardiac output. A chest radiograph and/or echocardiogram may assist with the diagnosis but these tests either may not be immediately available, or their results or interpretation may not be available promptly enough to effect the diagnosis. Thus, the diagnosis of cardiac tamponade in neonates relies heavily on the astute observation of changing clinical signs and symptoms.

Typically, clinical signs of postoperative cardiac tamponade present acutely in association with an abrupt cessation of chest tube output. In the case of this neonate, however, the clinical demise was slow and progressive. The slow development and worsening of shock in a postoperative cardiac neonate confounds the diagnosis since many causes for low cardiac output reside in the mind of the clinician. This neonate's clinical presentation of bleeding, progressive clinical findings of an elevated diastolic blood pressure and elevated atrial pressures, and progressive unresponsiveness to volume administration clearly confirmed the diagnosis of cardiac tamponade. The diagnosis in this neonate's case was based on integrating subtle changes in clinical status, which required astute observational skills and frequent refinement of the differential diagnosis.

REFERENCES

Roth, S. J. (1998). Postoperative Care. In A. C. Chang, F. L. Hanley, G. Wernovsky, & D. L. Wessel (Eds.). *Pediatric cardiac intensive care* (pp. 163–187). Baltimore: Williams & Wilkins.

Schleien, C. L., Setzer, N. A., McLaughlin, G. E., & Rogers, M. C. (1992). Postoperative Management of the Cardiac Surgical Patient. In M. C. Rogers (Ed.), *Textbook of pediatric intensive care* (pp. 467–531). Baltimore: Williams & Wilkins.

Smith, J. B., Baker, A. L., Moynihan, P. J., et al. (1996). Cardiovascular critical care problems. In M.A.Q. Curley, J. B. Smith, & P. A. Moloney-Harmon (Eds.), *Critical care nursing of infants and children* (pp. 557–618). Philadelphia: W. B. Saunders Company.

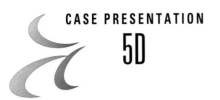

Fetal Growth Restriction

Jan M. Kriebs

The patient, an 18-year-old single white female having her second child (para 1001), presented to the midwife's office for her first obstetric visit. Her last regular menstrual period was 10 weeks ago. Her medical/surgical history was benign. She had no known allergies. She smoked about one pack of cigarettes per day, with a history of 4 pack years. She denied the use of alcohol or street drugs. Her genetics, teratology, and infection history was negative. However, her first pregnancy was complicated by severe fetal growth restriction, preeclampsia, and induction of labor, with vaginal delivery of a 3 pound, 1 ounce baby at 37 weeks.

When an obstetric history is taken, details such as duration of smoking or accuracy of previous pregnancy dating are useful in determining what degree of risk may persist in the current pregnancy. In this case, smoking, inadequate care, or preeclampsia may have affected fetal growth in the first pregnancy; the pregnancy may have been inaccurately dated. Inaccurate dating of a pregnancy can led to iatrogenic prematurity with a lower than expected birth weight. I find that a conversational tone allows women to recall and share details that they may not include when closed questions are used.

During this visit, she had a physical examination and laboratory tests performed. She asked about having a sonogram "to know what sex the baby is." On examination, her uterus was anteverted, just at the pelvic brim, and appropriately sized for 10 weeks gestation. The fetal heart was easily audible with handheld doppler at 150 bpm. The rest of her physical examination was benign. Blood pressure (BP) was 110/60 mmHg; weight, 123 pounds; height, 5 feet 2 inches. A record request was signed for her previous care.

An obstetric examination during the first 3 months of pregnancy is ideal, because a baseline weight and blood pressure can be established before pregnancy changes are significant. Later in pregnancy, weight gain and rate of gain can provide support for assessing nutritional status and offer clues about fluid shifts. The expected gain for a teenager at normal weight for height is 25 to 35 pounds. Blood pressure decreases during pregnancy until late second trimester, then returns to the baseline by delivery. When a prepregnant or early pregnancy BP can be obtained, it is easier to assess for elevated BP at term. Much of the benefit of prenatal care derives from the teaching and counseling that supports the mother in making healthy life choices. I would include teaching at this visit about normal pregnancy progress, nutrition and normal weight gain, what will be done at prenatal visits, and lab tests and procedures that can be done. Informed consent for testing should be obtained. I would also offer smoking cessation materials and reinforce the risks of smoking in pregnancy.

Ultrasound examination will add nothing to the quality of dating this pregnancy. At this point, an ultrasound by a competent obstetric sonographer will be accurate to within 1 week; however, this patient had clear dates which correlate with both her uterine sizing and the auscultation of fetal heart tones. There was no evidence of early pregnancy complications. Therefore, the test would be an added expense with little benefit. When ultrasound is indicated, but not needed for diagnostic purposes in the first trimester, I generally schedule an anatomy scan for 18 to 20 weeks of pregnancy.

Patient education will continue throughout the pregnancy, with targeted teaching for best effect. One message that needs to be reinforced to this woman at every contact is smoking cessation.

At 10 weeks, the patient had normal laboratory results, except for a urinary tract infection (E. coli), which was treated with Macrodantin. Test of cure at 14 weeks was negative. Uterine assessment had equaled the expected growth. The rest of the examination was benign at both 14 and 16 weeks. The patient was still smoking and "didn't want to try" to quit.

The usual pattern of prenatal visits is every 4 weeks until 28 weeks. In this case, the visit at 16 weeks had been scheduled to take advantage of triple screen (hcg, estradiol, and alpha fetoprotein [AFP]) testing. Fetal screening tests require the informed consent of the patient, including an explanation of screening versus diagnostic tests. I would explain that the tests are intended to help identify fetuses with a greater than average risk of neural tube defects and Down syndrome, that other follow-up tests are necessary to identify specific problems. While triple screen testing offers a valuable opportunity for assessing risk to the pregnancy, it also carries some risk itself. Because normal values vary with fetal age, maternal race, and medical status, abnormal findings always dictate reassessment of gestational age, fetal number, and maternal history. Decisions about follow-up testing, which includes an ultrasound and possibly an amniocentesis, require parents to consider what they will do if their baby has a major anomaly. Additionally, abnormal results on triple screen tests are associated with poor pregnancy outcomes, even when no anomaly is discovered.

At this visit I also offer an ultrasound, to be scheduled at 18 to 20 weeks gestation. Ultrasound has become one of the most pervasive and desired technologies associated with pregnancy. Even among women planning to minimize medical intervention in pregnancy, frequent requests to "see" the fetus are heard. Usually, sonography is considered a reassuring event. Advances in technique and equipment enable competent obstetric sonographers to produce detailed assessments of fetal well-being. Having said this, it must be also said that the general scans offered in many clinician's offices do not meet the criteria put forth by professional organizations for ultrasound indications and clinical training. Ultrasound done at this point in pregnancy is still early enough to assist in verifying dating (to within 10 to 14 days); an anatomy scan can be requested which will evaluate the fetus for developmental anomalies (Gegor and Kriebs, 1997). Helping patients understand the value and risk of pregnancy interventions is a building block for a trusting relationship. In turn, that relationship can promote self-care and involvement in informed decision making.

At 18 weeks, after the office received the report of this patient's triple screen, she was asked to return to the office 2 weeks before her next scheduled appointment. Her medical records from the previous pregnancy were not available. Fetal growth was ap-

propriate; maternal signs were all normal, with a total weight gain of 8 pounds (131 lb.), BP 106/58 mmHg. Her triple screen value was reported as 6.5 multiples of the median (normal is less than 2.0), indicating a 1:10 risk of open neural tube defects, but her sonogram had confirmed her pregnancy dating and not demonstrated any physical abnormalities. The fetus was at the 55th percentile for gestational age. After discussion of the test results, the patient declined genetic counseling or testing.

Many times, false-positive or indeterminate test results can produce stress, which has a negative effect on pregnancy. Informed decision making and careful explanation of results can help patients feel more secure. Even though this pregnancy has been proceeding normally, the unusual findings on triple screen act as a red flag that warns the clinician to be particularly conscious of "soft" findings. At this point, I would consult with a perinatologist to confirm a plan. This can involve a review of the records and discussion between clinicians, or a visit by the patient.

Discussion with my consultant about this patient centered around the patient's poor previous pregnancy history, the nonavailability of her previous chart, and her abnormal lab results. The plan includes careful monitoring of fetal growth both clinically and with sonography, screening for antiphospholipid antibodies (APA), and fetal testing for placental sufficiency and fetal well-being with biophysical profiles (BPP) beginning at 34 weeks (Cunningham et al., 1997).

Many midwives care for women with risk factors which may affect pregnancy outcomes. A collaborative model of care provides the opportunity for women to stay with her known care providers and receive the style of care she prefers. This consultation has established a framework in which, if complications develop, she will have easy access to high risk services.

At 28 weeks, the patient had a total weight gain of only 13 pounds (136 lbs). There was "plenty of food" in her home; her reported dietary intake was acceptable. She continued to smoke although she cut intake to one half pack per day. She denied symptoms of preterm labor and preeclampsia. Her BP was 100/56 mmHg. Urine protein and glucose were negative. She had pedal edema. Her reflexes were 2+. Her first serial ultrasound reported normal growth, normal amniotic fluid volume. Doppler studies of the uterine, umbilical, and middle cerebral arteries were within normal limits. Her laboratory tests, including routine blood glucose screening, hematocrit, and APA were within normal limits. She expressed concern that she wanted a "normal" baby this time.

Although the patient's ultrasound examination was benign at this time, her weight gain was lagging and she continued to smoke daily. Her examination reveals no evidence of preeclampsia. She needed to be counseled at every visit regarding health risks that were in her control (i.e., smoking cessation and increasing calories and protein intake). Clinical care cannot substitute for self-care in the domain of lifestyle and personal behaviors.

Serial ultrasounds are ordered when a pattern of fetal growth or other parameters of intrauterine life need to be assessed in an ongoing fashion. By taking repetitive body measurements for which growth pattern criteria exist, an individual fetus can be compared to the averages, giving both size and growth velocity information (Owen & Khan, 1998). The addition of Doppler flow measurements of placenta and fetal brain blood flow helps to monitor for fetal hypoxia (Marsal, 1994). Single measurements cannot predict future events; they need to be confirmed in relationship to other data.

At 32 weeks, she had gained only 2 more pounds (138 lbs). She said she had "been real busy." Clinical assessment showed normal maternal parameters—urine protein trace, BP 100/52 mmHg—and an active fetus, but the fundal height was now lagging, at 30 cm. Her sonogram showed the fetus at the 29th percentile for growth. Third trimester laboratory test results were all within normal limits. Repeat screens for infectious diseases were negative.

At this time, I would counsel the woman again about the importance of proper nutrition and smoking cessation for fetal development, describing the fetal and neonatal problems which can result from fetal growth restriction. In order to decrease physical stress, I would give her a disability release note from her part-time job, placing her on modified bedrest at home. She needs to return weekly for visits and begin twice weekly modified BPP testing at 34 weeks gestation (Nageotte, Towers, Asrat, & Freeman, 1994). Fetal movement counting can be taught.

Although this fetus is still within the normal range for growth, there has been a decrease from the normal curve. Poor nutrition or smoking are the most likely causes. Relative sparing of the head measurements, normal amniotic fluid volume, and normal doppler flow all suggest that the best course is observation, decreased activity, and continued reinforcement of health messages. More frequent office visits are planned as a way to monitor clinical presentation. The addition of twice weekly fetal testing will evaluate fetal tolerance of the intrauterine environment by assessing neurological status and adequacy of amniotic fluid.

At 36 weeks, all of the modified BP results had been normal. The patient's weight jumped 5 pounds in the first 2 weeks of bedrest, and 4 pounds this week (now 147 lbs). Her BP was 105/60 mmHg, reflexes 2+, urine protein trace, edema 1+ in calves only. She denied headache, visual changes, epigastric pain, preterm contractions, or pressure. Fundal height was only 32 cm. Her sonogram placed the fetus at the 25th percentile for growth. She was restless, worried about her baby's health, and "just wanted this over."

A sudden jump in weight can be a marker for the onset of preeclampsia; and in the case of severe disease in the previous pregnancy, it is a particular concern. No other clinical evidence for this diagnosis exists. She has had decreased energy usage while on bedrest, and possibly increased her nutritional intake, which would explain her weight gain in another way. For these reasons, preeclampsia is an unlikely cause of the continued lagging fetal growth. Patient education regarding normal fetal growth, and ways the mother can affect this, has been emphasized throughout this pregnancy. Now, the mother needs reassurance that our observation of her pregnancy can guide us. Clinicians send mixed messages when parents are told your baby is not growing, but you need to stay pregnant anyway. Taking time to explain findings at her level of comprehension is essential. She needs reasons to cooperate in maintaining the pregnancy as long as the fetus is tolerating it well.

At 38 weeks, she still denied symptoms of preeclampsia; her blood pressure was 112/58 mmHg. Weight was now 142 lbs, urine trace protein, 1 + edema in the lower calves, reflexes 2+ bilaterally. Her BP testing and Doppler scans were all appropriate. However, the ultrasound placed the fetus well below the 10th percentile for growth although absolute weight gain had occurred.

Because there was no evidence for fetal compromise other than lagging weight, it is appropriate to continue the pregnancy. Patient education should include fetal movement counting, an explanation of each test, and reassurance. At this point, the patient was willing to wait for labor. In the absence of fetal compromise, I would have no justification for intervening urgently in this pregnancy. Maternal fears alone are not a rationale for intervention either. However, each clinician needs to be sure that her patient not only understands what the tests results say, but is confident of her ability to recognize changes in the baby's movement pattern, signs of labor, and signs of preeclampsia.

Three days later. The patient came to the hospital in early labor, 1 cm dilated, 75% effaced, −1 station, membranes intact. Her vital signs and physical examination were benign. Her monitor tracing on arrival was reassuring but nonreactive, and showed no evidence of fetal distress. She was contracting every 3 to 5 minutes for 45 seconds. In view of her prior pregnancy history and current fetal growth restriction, the patient was admitted for continuous monitoring of labor. Eight hours later, she delivered a healthy 5 pound, 12 ounce baby boy.

In general, I do not admit women to the hospital in labor until they have demonstrated active progress. Many midwives would prefer to keep women at home until active labor occurs, and, once admitted, use ambulation, water therapy (showers or tubs), or other supportive measures, while monitoring fetal heart rates intermittently, to promote progress in a natural fashion. For a patient with well-documented fetal growth restriction the need to monitor a fetus for signs of distress outweighs this. Labor interventions such as position changes, being up to move around the birth room, and the like, can still be implemented during continuous monitoring. Creative support is a hallmark of midwifery practice; it requires adaptation to the birth at hand.

Commentary

The differential diagnosis of fetal growth restriction is very broad (Table 5D-1). In this case, the patient's initial history and laboratory testing excluded many of these, leaving preeclampsia or poor maternal lifestyle and nutrition as the most likely causes for her previous low birth weight infant. Fetal growth restriction is defined in relation to the gestational age. Thus, after 37 weeks gestation, 5 lb 8 oz (2500 grams) is considered the lower limit of normal; at 34 weeks, this would be a well-grown infant. For this reason, women with a history of low birth weight infants need to be carefully dated; an inaccurate gestational age could lead to the delivery of an iatrogenically premature infant. If dates and examination confirm gestational age in the first trimester, this is an acceptable technique.

Because preeclampsia is primarily a complication of first pregnancies, it is less likely to be associated with recurrent growth restriction. Monitoring pregnancy for hypertensive complications is a part of routine care; in the absence of signs of active disease, this can be excluded as a cause of this patient's progressive lag in fetal growth.

Maternal nutrition and smoking play a role in fetal growth by affecting the quality and quantity of resources for fetal growth. Poor maternal weight gain in the midtrimester indicates lack of nutrient availability at the time of most rapid growth. Tobacco use produces ischemic changes in the placenta and decreased oxygen flow to the fetus. Patient counseling for lifestyle changes is an integral part of prenatal care. Many of the most effective interventions in pregnancy are under the sole control of the mother.

Women with history or current findings suggesting fetal growth restriction need careful monitoring during pregnancy. Screening for pregnancy abnormalities with triple screen and/or ultrasound, close attention to clinical findings, and assessment of fetal growth and well being are all essential. Identifying women with congenitally small, healthy fetuses and those whose body height or weight disguise a well-grown fetus, as well as those fetuses whose intrauterine position masks normal growth, provides reassurance for clinicians and mothers alike. Fetal growth restriction in the current pregnancy suggested the need to use serial ultrasound and doppler studies to conform clinical findings.

TABLE 5D-1 *Differential Diagnosis of Fetal Growth Restriction*

Maternal	Fetal
small maternal size	intrauterine infections
poor maternal weight gain	genetic abnormalities
poor maternal nutrition	teratogen exposure
history of growth-restricted fetus	developmental abnormalities
tobacco use	placental/cord abnormalities
alcohol use	multiple pregnancy
substance abuse	chronic hypoxia
physical abuse	
chronic disease	
vascular	
renal	
anemia	
cyanotic heart disease	
diabetes (Class C or above)	

Adapted from: Parker, B., McFarlane, J., & Soeken, K., 1994; Varney, H., & Reedy, N. J., 1997.

Morbidity associated with fetal growth restriction can include birth asphyxia, meconium aspiration, hypoglycemia, and hypothermia. Fetal losses are also increased. Cunningham and colleagues (1997) and Minior and Divon (1998) studied infants born at term, controlling for medical risk factors that could influence infant health, and matching small for gestational age infants born of normal pregnancies with those of average birth weight. They found a higher incidence of neonatal morbidity in those infants whose growth had been restricted in utero. Newnham (1998) discussed findings regarding consequences in adult life that have been linked to fetal growth restriction, for example, hypertension. This evidence that fetal nutrition and growth can program one's health for life should emphasize the importance of close follow-up during the prenatal period.

Timing and route of delivery are determined by fetal response. If the fetus is tolerating pregnancy and labor, it is clearly preferable to deliver a term infant vaginally. Supportive care and education of the mother enable her to participate knowledgeably in decisions about pregnancy management.

Finally, it is worth considering the role of midwives in managing pregnancies at risk. None of the interventions required to monitor this patient's pregnancy required the presence of a perinatologist other than to evaluate the ultrasounds. Indeed, few primary obstetrical providers, physician or nurse, are trained to offer targeted ultrasound testing. What was useful in this case was the availability of collegial consultation to verify that the management plan was accurate and complete, and ensure later access to tertiary care if needed. Midwifery education includes emphasis on nutrition, lifestyle counseling, and patient teaching, which contribute to improved outcomes by promoting self care. Choice of provider for women with risk factors should include consideration of access to consultation services, patient preferences, and the nature of any interventions needed.

REFERENCES

Cunningham, F. G., MacDonald, P. C., Gant N. F. (1997). Fetal growth restriction. In F. G. Cunningham, MacDonald, P. C., Gant, N. F., et al. (Eds.). *Williams obstetrics* (20th ed). Stamford, CT: Appleton & Lange.

Gegor, C. L., & Kriebs, J. M. (1997). Fetal Assessment. In H. Varney (Ed.) *Varney's midwifery* (pp. 283–316). Sudbury, MA: Jones and Bartlett.

Marsal, K. (1994). Role of Doppler sonography in fetal/maternal medicine. *Current Opinion in Obstetrics and Gynecology 6,* 36–44.

Minior, V. K., & Divon, M. Y. (1998). Fetal growth restriction at term: Myth or reality. *Obstetrics and Gynecology 92,* 57–60.

Nageotte, M. P., Towers, C. V., Asrat, T., & Freeman, R. K. (1994). Perinatal outcome with the modified biophysical profile. *American Journal of Obstetrics and Gynecology 170,* 1672–1676.

Newnham, J. (1998). Consequences of fetal growth restriction. *Current Opinion in Obstetrics and Gynecology 10,* 145–149.

Owen, P., & Khan, K. S. (1998). Fetal growth velocity in the prediction of intrauterine growth retardation in a low risk population. *British Journal of Obstetrics and Gynecology 105,* 536–540.

Parker, B., McFarlane, J., & Soeken, K. (1994). Abuse during pregnancy: Effects on maternal complications and birth weight in adult and teenage women. *Obstetrics and Gynecology 84,* 232–328.

Varney H., & Reedy, N. J. (1997). Screening for and collaborative management of antepartal complications. In H. Varney. *Varney's midwifery* (pp. 317–377). Sudbury, MA: Jones and Bartlett.

Changing Environments and Patient Diversity in Healthcare Delivery

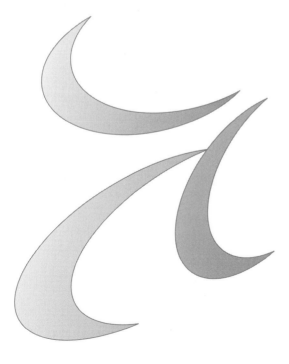

CHAPTER 6

Healthcare Delivery Systems and Environments of Care

Sandra L. Venegoni

Imagine standing at the brink of a new century, looking back to the past and forward to the future. Everywhere you look, in everything you hear and read regarding the health and healthcare of the people, as you know it in this present moment, you experience words indicating action, movement. Words such as "reforming" and "changing" healthcare, "emerging" trends, "shaping" the future, "gearing up" for a new age. There is, indeed, the obvious perception of a transition from what was known to something new and unknown.

And yet, one may ask the question "Which century is beginning and which is ending?" Is it the 20th or 21st century? For regarding the beginning of both centuries, historians will record numerous movements, actions, similarities, and differences in the changing perspectives of healthcare. No one can deny the remarkable advances that have occurred during the 20th century in diagnosing and treating diseases, in researching and developing medications and advanced technologies, as well as promoting health and preventing illness. In the 100 years occurring between the centuries, one constant occurs—Change! But the speed at which change occurs is accelerated at the beginning of the 21st century at a rate probably not even dreamt about 100 years ago.

Each moment of the beginning millennium is a composite of the past and what happened before. The Buddhist monk Thich Nhat Hanh (1998) stated that "the present moment contains the past and the future. The secret of transformation at the base lies in our very handling of this very moment." This is true at the turn of the 21st century. Massive regulatory and marketplace changes and demands have occurred as a reaction to the past and will be the stimuli for future changes. Perhaps one might compare the changes to the waves of the ocean as they hit the shoreline, one wave after another. After one wave hits, others will follow, rolling in on the previous one, which, like an undertow, proceeds out to open water under other incoming waves. Each change in our healthcare delivery system is followed by other waves that build on the previous change wave. And each wave will produce and be followed by both positive and negative effects.

As unsettling as change is for most people, for our lives and professional careers, we are forced to "unfreeze, experience the change, and refreeze" in different patterns and ways of behaving (Lewin, 1947). Change in our healthcare delivery system happens and will continue to happen; of that we can be certain. The focus of this chapter is to discuss the healthcare delivery system in the United States as we begin the third millennium. It will include the major driving forces that created the changes and how these changes have shaped both the environment of care and the practice of advanced practice nurses (APNs) (see Table 6-1).

 ## Major Forces Driving the Healthcare Delivery System

The Chinese have a saying that is considered both a blessing and a curse: "May you live in interesting times." One might apply this to the healthcare delivery system at the dawn of the 21st century. For some people, it may be a curse. For others, a blessing. For all, it is interesting. Just as most other types of industry and organizations, the healthcare industry in the United States has experienced major changes during the century. Basic to all regulatory and marketplace changes in healthcare reform during the post–World War II era

 TABLE 6-1 *The Changing World of Health Care Delivery Systems, Environments of Care, and APNs' Models of Practice*

MAJOR DRIVING FORCES

1. Cost of health care
2. Federal regulatory impact
3. Movement to capitated, managed care and integrated delivery systems
4. Home to hospital/institutional to home care
5. Chronic to acute to chronic care
6. Aging of health care recipients
7. Telecommunications and informatics

Health Care Environments and Settings for Care Effected by Major Factors

1. Acute care hospitals and ambulatory care
2. Long-term care:
   —Nursing facilities
   —Subacute units
   —Assisted living facilities
3. Home health care
4. Others:
   —Hospice, renal-dialysis units, mental health/mental retardation units, rehabilitation hospitals, long-term hospitals

APNs' Models of Practice

1. Emerging practice issues
2. Collaborative
3. Interdisciplinary
4. Independent
5. Faculty practice
6. Specialty practice models

---

were the advancement of one or more of the following key topics: (1) access to care, (2) cost-effectiveness of care, (3) quality of care, and (4) consumer satisfaction. At any given time, one topic may predominate over others and be the precipitating impetus for change. After that wave of change has passed, another focus may come into place to overtake the results of the previous wave. For example, when the costs of healthcare became excessive, changes in the method of reimbursement were made, resulting in a decreased use of services that will affect access to care.

The following sections will briefly review the major driving forces that are largely responsible for most changes in the healthcare delivery system.

COST OF HEALTHCARE

One of the most significant driving forces for the reorganization of healthcare has been the increasing costs to both government and private employers. Healthcare is a large industry throughout the global marketplace. Brian D. Wong, MD, MPH, partner and worldwide director of healthcare strategy for the accounting firm Arthur Andersen, states that "as a $1.3 trillion industry, healthcare is the fourth-largest economy in the world" (as cited in Mycek, 1998, p. 27). The U.S. healthcare system is one of the leading systems in the world. With its innovative technology for the diagnosis and treatment of illness and its increasing efficiency, it has saved many lives. Employing one in seven Americans, it is the "country's largest industry" (Fox, 1998, p. 314). And, yet, that prestigious position comes with an enormous price tag. Trends during the century showed that what the United States spends for personal healthcare exceeds that of any other industrialized nation (Levitt, Lazenby, Braden, & the National Health Accounts Team, 1998). During the last 3 decades of the century, the health sector's share of the economy, as reflected as a percent of the gross domestic product (GDP), has rapidly increased. During the last part of the 1980s and early 1990s, health costs and spending increased rapidly when compared to national heath care expenditures for 1960 (5.1%) and 1970 (7.1%). In 1980, healthcare accounted for 8.9% of the GDP, then increased to 13.4% by 1992. A considerable slowing period followed in the latter years of the decade. The percentage reached 13.6% in 1996 and remained approximately the same for the next several years (Medicare Payment Advisory Commission, 1998). Currently, healthcare accounts for almost one-seventh of all U.S. output. In their projection for the decade between years 1998–2007, Smith, Freland, Hefler, McKusick, and the Health Expenditures Projection Team (1998) anticipated that by the year 2007 heath spending will rise to an estimated 16.16% of the GDP ($2.1 trillion).

Escalating costs of healthcare during the last three decades of this century had a negative impact on the nation, resulting in: (1) higher insurance premiums, most of which are paid by employers, and (2) a larger portion of the federal budget required to finance government-sponsored health insurance.

FEDERAL REGULATORY IMPACT

The Congress of the United States, along with state legislatures, has played a major role in reforming healthcare during the 20th century. Through passage of laws such as the Social Security Act (1935), the amendments to the Social Security Act that established Medicare and Medicaid (1965), and later laws, Congress demonstrated its efforts to provide for the needs of the elderly, the indigent, persons with disabilities, and younger persons with specific chronic conditions. The federal government is also the major purchaser of healthcare and, for this reason, Congress demonstrated its need to control the rising healthcare costs of the nation. Members of Congress passed laws, funded studies, and established committees that either directly or indirectly affected the health of the citizens and carried their impact well into the new millennium (for a select list of such laws, see Table 6-2).

TABLE 6-2 *Select Congressional Acts Affecting Health Care*

1946 Hospital Survey and Construction Act (Hill-Burton)—increased construction of hospitals

1954 Medical Facilities Survey and Construction Act (Amendment of Hill-Burton Act)—amended act to include nursing homes, rehabilitation facilities, chronic disease hospitals, and diagnostic or treatment centers

1965 Amendment of Social Security Act—provides medical care for the elderly (Title 18—Medicare) and grants to the states for indigent (Title 19—Medicaid)

1973 Health Maintenance Organizations (HMO) Act—provided financial assistance to establish and expand HMOs; required employers to offer HMOs as an alternative to regular health insurance; market established for growth of cost-effective care

1980 Omnibus Budget Reconciliation Act (OBRA)—significant amendments to Medicare and Medicaid

1982 Tax Equity and Fiscal Responsiblility Act (TEFRA)—hospice services authorized Medicare reimbursement

1983 Amendments to Social Security Act—established Medicare hospital prospective payment (reimbursement) system based on diagnosis-related groups (DRGs)

1985 Consolidated Omnibus Budget Reconciliation Act (COBRA)—increase in rates for hospice (under both Medicare and Medicaid)

1987 Omnibus Budget Reconciliation Act (OBRA 87)—several significant changes in Medicaid, reform to Medicaid nursing home law (Nursing Home Reform Act), authorized home/community based care for persons 65+ years of age

1990 American with Disabilities Act (ADA)—provided for specific employment and "reasonable accommodation" rights for persons with disabilities

1993 Omnibus Budget Reconciliation Act (OBRA 93)—5-year cut in Medicare funding, reductions in reimbursement rates for hospice care and laboratory fees

1996 Health Insurance Portability and Accountability Act (HIPAA)—Insurance reform legislation; goal to increase number of persons who have and maintain accessiblity to "affordable" health insurance when changing jobs or becoming unemployed

1996 Welfare reform bill—states received more latitude in how they use welfare money; replace Aid to Families with Dependent Children (AFDC) with Temporary Assistance for Needy Families (TANF) a block grant program; a person does not automatically qualify for Medicaid by being eligible for TANF

1997 Child Health Insurance Reform (CHIP)—expands health insurance to children whose families earn too much for traditional Medicaid, yet not enough to afford private health insurance

1997 Balanced Budget Act (see discussion in text)

1998 Patients Bill of Rights (unfinished Congressional business at this time but meant to provide protection to persons under managed care)

One of the most consequential laws of the last two decades of the century was the 1983 passage of the amendment to the Social Security Act (PL98–21). Its intent was to make the Medicare system more cost-efficient and, to accomplish this, it changed the method by which hospitals received reimbursement for care to Medicare inpatients. The law resulted in a prospective, as opposed to the existing retrospective, form of payment. Simply stated, prior to the new regulation, hospitals received payment for Medicare recipients after they left the hospital and, depending on their needs, while hospitalized. With the new system, the number of days a Medicare recipient could be hospitalized was prospectively based on the diagnostic related groups (DRGs), the individual's diagnosis. If the number of hospitalized days exceeded the preestablished number, the hospital suffered a financial loss and would have to absorb the cost. This new system resulted in hospitals finding it "harder to shift the costs of treating the uninsured to Medicare" (Thompson, 1997, p. 172). It also resulted in Medicare recipients, especially the elderly, being discharged "quicker and sicker," thus increasing the number of discharges to nursing homes and the growth spurt of out-of-hospital delivery services and home health services (Guterman, Eggers, Riley, Green & Terrell, 1988; Russell & Manning, 1988). Fourteen years later, in 1997, a similar prospective payment system (PPS) was imposed on outpatient services, skilled nursing facilities, and home health.

In the early part of the 1990s, the Congressional Budget Office (CBO) (1992) sent a clear warning to the nation. Unless some change occurred in benefits or financing, the CBO projected that the increasing federal deficit in the late 1990s would primarily result from federal health spending. According to a later report by the same agency (CBO, 1994), a plan for reining-in entitlement spending was mandatory to control the federal deficit. "More than half of the current federal budget goes to entitlement programs, among which Social Security, Medicare, and Medicaid represent the largest share" (Battistella & Ostrick, 1997, p. 3). After years of fragmented attempts to balance the budget, Congress reached a solution. A united, bipartisan 105th Congress passed and President Clinton signed HR 2015, the 1997 Balanced Budget Reconciliation Act (BBA 97). Although it contained numerous welfare-related and health provisions, some of the major ones are the following:

1. Created the Medicare+Choice program which fundamentally changed the way Medicare had operated for the previous 30 years. It offered eight types of health plans, including fee-for-service plans, HMOs, medical savings accounts (MSA), and provider-sponsored organizations. These plans would receive a fixed amount (capitation) for services to each enrollee.

2. A prospective payment system (PPS), similar to the one established for hospitals in 1983, was imposed on outpatient services, beginning in 1999, and on Medicare skilled nursing facilities (SNFs) with a 4-year phase-in for cost reporting periods beginning on or after July 1, 1998. Per diem rates in SNFs was based on case mix, which will be determined by Resource Utilization Groups, Version III (RUGs-III). The groups are based on the amount of nursing and rehabilitation staff time required to provide necessary services.

3. Mandated various ways to save money spent on Medicare, which according to the Executive Director of the American Association of Retired Persons (AARP), "added nearly a decade to Medicare's solvency" (Detts, 1998, p. 3). There were reductions to provider payment updates through the year 2002, and growth of Medicare payment rates for hospital services; limits on care for outpatient physical, speech-language-pathology, and occupational therapy; and limits on growth in Medicare home health costs.

4. Permitted Medicare officials to negotiate "best price" with multiple suppliers such as oxygen, hospital beds, and other types of durable medical equipment.

5. Lowered Medicare's indirect medical education adjustment to teaching hospitals, which is based on ratio of medical residents to hospital beds.

6. Provided Medicare reimbursement for Telehealth services.

7. Authorized nationwide establishment of Program-for-All-Inclusive Care for the Elderly (PACE) sites.

8. Authorized coverage of selected preventive services.

9. Most importantly for advanced practice nurses (APNs), the BBA 97 increased Medicare reimbursement for nurse practitioners (NPs) and clinical nurse specialists (CNS) irrespective of geographic setting, increased the fee schedule amount, and provided direct payment for both groups. Reimbursement will vary depending on whether the NP is acting in an independent practice (the 85% option) or employed by a physician (the 100%, 85%, or 0% options). When the NP is employed by a physician, two factors will determine the percent of reimbursement: the physician's presence or whether the NP operates in a state with "friendly" or "restrictive" collaboration requirements (ACNP, 1998).

THE "NEW" HEALTHCARE INDUSTRY

However and in whichever way one chooses to describe the healthcare industry at the end of the 20th century, it is "new"—different from what preceded it. True to the statement by Euripides, the 5th century BC Greek playwright, who stated that the "only thing permanent in life is change," the healthcare industry underwent a complete overhaul, especially during the last two decades of the century. Sometimes, it is difficult to know which "wave" hit the shoreline first, which was cause and which was effect. Overall, the industry changed from:

- a fee-for-service to a capitated, managed care system;
- an individual or multisystem hospital to an integrated delivery system;
- home care to hospital/institutional care and back to home care again; and
- chronic care (treatment of epidemics) in the beginning of the century to acute care and back to chronic care.

Each of these topics will be briefly discussed in the following sections (see Chapters 7, 8, 9, and 16 for in-depth discussions).

Movement to Capitated, Managed Care, and Integrated Delivery Systems

A person looking back at the end of the 20th century might question, "Why were Congress and state legislatures discussing patient protection laws in 1998?" and "What wave(s) came before this date to necessitate federally mandated, managed care reform legislation— a Patients' Bill of Rights?" Although a variety of congressional bills existed, the central discussion in all of them dealt with "rights" for 125 million Americans who are enrolled in plans regulated by the Employment Retirement Income Security Act (ERISA): rights to sue HMOs; rights to appeal HMO decisions to an independent third-party review board and to get a timely, legally binding response; and rights to access a specialist when necessary and obtain certain healthcare services, such as use of emergency services.

As expected, there were differences in the "rights" bills proposed by congressional Democrats, Republicans, and the president. Based on recommendations from President Clinton's Advisory Commission on Consumer Protection and Quality in the Healthcare Industry, the proposed bills were a culmination of years of concerns regarding managed care and the point it had reached by the late 1990s. Senator Tom Daschle (D-SD), who introduced the Patients Bill of Rights Act of 1998 (S 1890/HR 3605), made the statement that 48% of Americans experienced problems with HMOs (Daschle, 1998). Although strongly supported by the American Nurses Association, the American Medical Association, and 170 other organizations, his bill was defeated in the House and replaced by the Republican bill sponsored by House Speaker Newt Gingrich (R-GA). In the meantime, a 1998 federal appeals court case in San Francisco granted the nearly 6 million Medicare beneficiaries enrolled in HMOs the right to fair and speedy appeals if denied care (McLeod, 1998).

But still the haunting question, "Why must Congress and states step in to curb actions of managed care plans and enact rules to protect citizens?" How did our nation arrive at this point? During most of the post–World War II period, the major type of payment for healthcare was the traditional fee-for-service. It gave any licensed physician the authority to "control both the number and kind of services offered as well as the prices charged for the services" (Harrington & Estes, 1997, p. 202). As the cost of healthcare continued to escalate, the policymakers fostered more cost-containment efforts. Managed care, although it had existed in some regions of the country for decades during the early part of the century, thrived and increased especially after the 1973 Health Maintenance Organization (HMO) Act. This act encouraged the formation and expansion of prepaid healthcare plans, especially the health maintenance organization. Although there are different types of managed care plans, from the group model or staff model to the relatively open independent practice association (IPA) model, the HMO serves as the prototype for all. Basic to all managed care is capitation—a fixed, upfront payment for each enrollee.

Fox (1998) referred to managed care as the "third reorganization of healthcare" when he tracked the changes in authority, resources, and division of labor that determine how physicians, other workers, and patients experience healthcare. The first reorganization, which began in the late 1800s and lasted until the 1980s, advanced the "new authority of science" (p. 314) with its science-based medicine, and improvement in its individual practitioners, specialists, and researchers. The authority of the physician became unquestioned and flowed from medical science.

During the second reorganization of healthcare, which occurred during and for two decades after World War II, priority was focused on supply—increased supply of services, specialists, and training for specialists. Following World War II, a large number of physicians left the armed forces and used their G.I. Bill for speciality residency training. Healthcare services were increased to older adults, poor persons, persons with disabilities, and persons with end-stage renal disease through enactment of Medicare and Medicaid. Services were extended to long-term care and hospice care. Stimulated by wartime experiences and expectations, increased supply prompted increased demand, which became very expensive. Veterans' rights and fringe benefits in the workplace increased along with insurance plans for physician and health services. Health insurance was linked to employment and there was growth in the number of Americans insured by an increasing number of privately held insurance companies and the nonprofit Blue Cross and Blue Shield. Lastly, there were increased subsidies for medical schools, teaching hospitals, and research. The basic philosophy of this period was "more is better" and with it came the unacceptable increase in cost of care.

The third reorganization of healthcare, beginning in the 1980s, focused on decreasing the growth of healthcare costs. This was accomplished through many regulations that decreased the oversupply of healthcare services, funding for graduate medical education, and research grants. Collective purchasers of healthcare, including federal, state, and local governments, as well as private employers, "made policy to eliminate what they described as wasteful oversupply in the health industry" (Fox, 1998, p. 314). The era of generalists physicians erupted as the country was faced with an oversupply of specialists, outnumbering the generalists "three to one" (Fox, 1998, p. 314) (see Chapter 8).

Enrollment in managed care plans tripled from 10 million to 30 million persons during the period from 1981 to 1987 (Kraus, Potter, & Ball, 1991). This trend of increasing numbers continued, stimulated by the presidential campaign of the early 1990s in which President Clinton promised healthcare "security." His failed health reform policy, the Health Security Act, promised universal coverage without higher costs. By the end of 1995, 66.1 million persons were enrolled in some form of managed care (Zelman, 1996). Depending on the source, by 1998, there was somewhere between 123 million (Daschle, 1998) to 160 million (Shapiro, 1998) enrollees. Eighty-six percent of workers and their families were enrolled (Shapiro, 1998) and it became "increasingly common for employers, especially smaller employers, to offer only a managed care plan" (Luft, 1997, p. 43).

But throughout this same period, while the number of enrollees was increasing, people gradually began to lose confidence in their physicians and their healthcare; they became discontent with their managed care plans. In 1987, Jim Taylor, then head of the research/consulting firm Yankelovich Partners, conducted a study for *Time Magazine* about consumer's confidence in American institutions. He found that confidence decreased both for confidence in physicians (less than the 50% level) and in the belief that healthcare and Social Security systems would be available when needed (to 5%) (Mycek, 1998). The source of the "backlash" against managed care was not always clear (Blendon, 1998), some held negative opinions about restrictions on care and others were dissatisfied because of a lack of insurance choice (Gawande et al., 1998).

During the period of increased enrollment, two other waves of change followed. The market continued to be more competitive, and words such as downsizing, reengineering, restructuring, and reorganization became commonplace. Also, large multihospital systems were changing in order to "adjust to the new realities of both the marketplace and health reform" (Shortell, Gillies, Anderson, et al., 1996, p. ix). During this change, it was typical to hear about mergers, joint ventures, agreements of affiliations, acquisitions, takeovers, and alliances as healthcare organizations came together to deliver care. Eventually, many emerged as networks, multihospital systems, or "integrated" delivery systems (IDS). Shortell and his colleagues (1998) refer to them as "organized" delivery systems (they believe "integration is an end state that few, if any, current systems have achieved") (p. xiv). By definition, an IDS is "a network of organizations that provides or arranges to provide a coordinated continuum of services to a defined population and is willing to be held clinically and fiscally accountable for the outcomes and the health status of the population served" (Shortell et al., 1996, p. 7). An IDS may be integrated horizontally (with like entities), vertically (coordinates activities within the same organization), clinically (manages patients across the continuum of care), and/or functionally (coordinates support functions) (Satinsky, 1998).

At this point in time, when the present converges with the past and the future, one wonders what the next step(s) will be in the evolution of healthcare delivery systems. Can there and will there be only so many giants, such as the "1,700 bed colossus" (Rauber, 1998, p. 56) formed by the merger of Barnes and Jewish Hospitals in St. Louis, Missouri? Will Congress be dealing in the future not only with patients' rights, but deregulation of healthcare monopolies? Fox predicts that "policies of government and business will emerge during the next decade as a result of current events . . . [and] . . . the consequences of these policies, those that are foreseen and others not anticipated, will eventually cause the fourth reorganization to begin" (1998, p. 317). Change will occur . . . of that we can be certain.

Home Care to Hospital/Institutional Care and Back to Home Care

In tracing the sites of healthcare delivery in the United States during the 20th century, a historian might be tempted to paraphrase the old adage "what goes around, comes around."

In the early period of the 20th century, most healthcare services were provided in the home setting, including those for the two most important events: birth and death. Early institutions for illness care were predominantly those involved with epidemics and infectious diseases, such as tuberculosis sanitariums. Following the world wars, but especially after World War II, the hospital increased in importance as the delivery site for acute healthcare. Several major factors led to this situation. The construction and renovation of hospitals, as well as the addition of equipment to hospitals, escalated in the mid-1940s when the government provided funding of these projects through the Hill Burton Act of 1946. Along with the increased capacity for care, hospitals were assured a guaranteed source of payment with two new forms of reimbursement: the "Blues" and Medicare. Blue Cross and Blue Shield, a healthcare benefit offered in rapidly increasing numbers to employees, soon became a bargaining chip between labor and corporate management in our industrialized society. Acute care quickly began to be delivered in a hospital setting and employees abruptly forgot that, in essence, they were the bill payers for such healthcare. In a personal interview, one of the nation's foremost health economists, Uwe Reinhardt (cited in Rovner, 1994), stated that one of the biggest misconceptions Americans have about our healthcare systems is "that someone else, their employer, is paying their health bill" (p. 64). Employees, who forgot that the cost of healthcare benefits actually comes out of their paycheck, demanded more hospital care because it was covered through their benefits. True to the laws of supply and demand, the more and better hospitals that were available (supply), the greater the demand by employees. Along with increased supply and demand came escalated hospitalization costs.

Use of hospitals for healthcare by older people also escalated with the passage of Medicare, the Title XVIII Amendment to the Social Security Act, in 1965. Medicare was the largest addition to the Social Security legislation since the 1930s. Of its two parts, Part A, which covers hospital insurance benefits for aged people, and Part B, which is the supplementary medical insurance benefits for aged people, Part A had the most effect on hospital care. In his 1965 State of the Union Address and Economic Report to Congress, President Johnson defined Medicare as the "biggest single increase budgeted—a $2 billion annual rise in Social Security benefits for the aged" (*Facts on File Yearbook*, 1965, p. 277). In 1966, 18.9 million older people (almost all of those potentially entitled) were enrolled in hospital insurance and more than 6000 hospitals and 1200 home health agencies had been certified for participation in the program (Breslow, 1973, p. 17).

By the mid1970s, spurious effects of the new policy were that hospitals and healthcare services "were able to receive compensation for services previously provided gratis, and at the same time to purchase new equipment and meet labor demands more readily. Costs . . . increased 10% annually between 1966 and 1973" (Smith & Hollander, 1973, p. 2). Physicians, likewise, increased their prices and reduced bad debts through Medicare. "Between 1966 and 1973, their fees increased 5–8% per year and their incomes increased nearly 11% per year" (Smith & Hollander, 1973, p. 1). Although extremely necessary, the passage of Medicare in 1965, with its later additional coverage of people with endstage renal disease, has negatively affected the national budget throughout its 35-year history.

As the United States rapidly approaches the beginning of a new century, healthcare delivery sites have again begun to change dramatically. As healthcare reform continues to become included in state and federal laws, it has escalated the switch of care delivery from inpatient hospital settings to outpatient ambulatory settings. To curb the rising healthcare costs, three effective healthcare system changes occurred. One dealt with how Medicare's retrospective payment system would pay for hospital care for senior citizens; the second dealt with the "gatekeeper" effect of managed care, competition, and capitation; and the third addressed the amazing advances in medical technology that have permitted an increasing number of procedures to be conducted in ambulatory outpatient settings. Thus, the stage was set for more healthcare services to be delivered by community care delivery systems. This action has only escalated during the continued cost-containment efforts and downsizing of hospitals and acute care during the 1990s.

Epidemics (Chronic Care) to Acute Care to Chronic Care

At the turn of the 20th century, healthcare was primarily delivered to individuals who experienced illness as a result of epidemics and unsanitary living conditions. Later, individual, acute conditions predominated. Through advances in research and development of modern technology and life-saving medications, an increase in both the number of persons with chronic conditions and the demand for chronic care occurred toward the end of the century. The number of Americans with chronic conditions that cause a major limitation of their activity has steadily increased. In 1987, there were 22 million Americans, increasing to 27 million (20% of population) by 1993, and projected by the year 2020 to be 134 million persons with chronic conditions and 39 million with a limitation in major activity (Robert Wood Johnson Foundation, 1996). Many of the conditions, but certainly not all, are associated with an individual's lifestyle and behavior. Richard J. Bringewatt (1998, p. 15), President and CEO of the National Chronic Care Consortium, states the following about chronic conditions in the United States:

- they account for about 80% of all deaths and 90% of all morbidity
- almost 100 million Americans have one or more chronic ailments
- 70% of all medical costs relate to people with chronic conditions
- one-half trillion dollars a year is spent on chronic illness
- people with cancer, diabetes, respiratory disease, congestive heart failure, Alzheimer's disease, arthritis, and other chronic diseases are the highest-cost, fastest-growing, most complex group in healthcare.

According to the U.S. Census Bureau (1996), the three major causes of death (heart disease, cancer, and stroke) among the elderly in the early 1990s were the same as they were the previous decade. These three conditions were responsible for 7 of 10 elderly deaths. Two other important leading causes of death in this age group were influenza/pneumonia and chronic obstructive pulmonary disease. In 1994, the most frequently occurring conditions per 100 noninstitutionalized, older persons were: arthritis (50), hypertension (36), heart disease (32), hearing impairments (29), cataracts (17), orthopedic impairments (16), sinusitis (15), and diabetes (10) (AARP, 1997). The number of chronic illnesses increases with age, and are higher in older women than in men. "Eighty percent of the senior population have one or more chronic diseases, 50 percent have two or more chronic conditions, and 24 percent have severe chronic conditions that limit their ability to perform one or more activities of daily living" (HCFA, 1998, p. 1).

Chronic illness, likewise, affects every other age group including infants, adolescents and young adults. It has been estimated that the prevalence of chronic health conditions in children is between 10 and 30% (Jackson & Vessey, 1992; Newacheck, McManus & Fox, 1991; Newacheck, & Taylor, 1992). The four most common chronic conditions for infants through teenagers of 18 years of age are hay fever, sinusitis, chronic bronchitis, and asthma (National Health Survey, 1993). HIV infections and AIDS in the young population are two other conditions causing alarm for the health community. Fifty percent of the 14 million individuals worldwide who are infected with HIV acquired the virus between the ages of 15 and 24 years. In 1990, for persons aged 25 to 44, AIDS accounted for 16.5% of all death in men and 4.8% in women (Hein, 1993).

The cost for chronic care is—and will continue to be—staggering. Nearly 70% ($425 billion) of the nation's 190 expenditures spent on personal care were for people with chronic conditions. The future healthcare system will be faced with more people with more chronic conditions that affect their day-to-day lives, causing disability in some. Focus will have to be redirected to improving their functional status as opposed to curing the disease, which so frequently happens in the current healthcare arena.

AGING OF HEALTHCARE RECIPIENTS

The American population continues to age. Since the beginning of the 20th century, the number and percentage of Americans 65 years of age and older has significantly increased. In 1900, 3.1 million persons (4.1% of the population) were in this age group. By 1996, the pool had increased to 33.9 million persons (12.8%). The 1998 pool of 34 million seniors is projected to double to 68 million by the year 2030 (HCFA, 1998). Life expectancy has also increased. A child born in 1900 could expect to live to age 47. With improved health and living conditions, the death rates for children and young adults decreased. A child born in 1996 could exceed the previous life expectancy by 29 years, to age 76. For persons reaching age 65 in 1996, the average life expectancy was 82.7 years (an additional 17.7 years). For females, the average number of additional years was 19.2, and for males, 15.5 years (AARP, 1997).

A second aspect of the gerontological explosion is those in the "oldest old" group, which is comprised of persons 85 years of age and older. Within the elderly population, persons between 85 and 100 years of age comprise the second-fastest-growing segment (Perls, 1998). In coming decades, persons 85 years old and older will continue to comprise an increasing proportion of the elderly population. It has been projected that this age group will more than double from 3 million in 1990 to 7 million in 2020 and to 14 million by 2040 (U.S. Bureau of the Census, 1993). A subset of the "oldest old" are those persons who have celebrated their 100th birthday—the fastest-growing cohort in America (Perls, 1998). It has been estimated that more than 52,000 persons are in this age group, almost three times the number in 1980. Dr. Thomas T. Perls (1998), a geriatrician who heads the New England Centenarian Study at Harvard Medical School, Division of Aging, presents facts he knows about this age group:

- estimates that 30% have acute minds;
- 20% or more may have short-term memory problems but still are "getting by just fine";
- half of all centenarians live in nursing homes, for reasons that range from failing bodies and minds to lack of support system of family or friends;
- they have better overall health than those 10 or 20 years younger.

Another major aging factor that will dramatically influence the first half of the third millennium is the 76 million Americans, commonly referred to as "Baby Boomers," who were born between the years 1946 and 1964. Their births accounted for 70% more people than born during the two preceding decades (U.S. Bureau of the Census, 1996). In 1998, the oldest of this group turn age 50, while the youngest were 30 years of age. By sheer numbers alone, they have impacted every aspect of American life during their lifetime—the public school system, the healthcare delivery system, and the employment market. In the year 2006, the first cohort of Baby Boomers will turn 60 years of age, with a massive increase in numbers during the years 2010 to 2030 when they reach age 65. They have been characterized as a group "who grew up in an age of affluence, fought in Vietnam, and spent midlife in an era of downsizing" (Morgan, 1998, p. 7). At the 1998 convention of the American Association of Retired Persons (AARP), outgoing president Margaret A. Dixon defined the Baby Boomers as "boisterous, rebellious youthfulness" (Levine, 1998, p. A1). There is absolutely no doubt that as they age they will continue to effect the healthcare system and the availability of resources. As part of his testimony to the National Bipartisan Committee on the Future of Medicare, Federal Reserve Board Chairman Alan Greenspan stated "the mere aging of the population will increase healthcare spending by as much as 20% over the next 30 years" (Greenspan, 1998).

TELECOMMUNICATIONS AND INFORMATICS

We live in an ever rapidly changing world of technology and information. It has been said that "if you were to take all that was known in human history from 3000 BC to 1990 and store it as one unit of knowledge, and then take all the information known from 1990 to 1996, the figure would double. Between 1996 and 2001, it would double again. And between 2001 and 2005, it would double yet again" (Mycek, 1998). With information doubling so fast, it is difficult to keep up and maintain a sense of equilibrium. It is no wonder that futurists such as William Knoke (1996)—an economist, international investment banker, and president of the Harvard Capital Group—claim that everything in today's society causes people to become "placeless." He believes we have entered an "Age of Everything, Everywhere," a period of time in which place does not matter. So, too, with the new technology in healthcare which has been "the primary determinant of the evolution of the U.S. healthcare system over the past thirty years" (Shortell et al., 1996, p. 281). During the last quarter century, we have expanded the world of healthcare technology to its present state of telehealth—a "placeless" health community. What was initially very simple technology (i.e., a finger probe connected to a telephone line to record an EKG in another state or a telephonic triage or healthcare check) changed drastically to today's sophisticated global diagnosis, surgical procedures, and the possibilities of tomorrow's future technological advances.

Consider, for example, the advances that computer technology, including both software and hardware, has brought to healthcare. Sophisticated information systems now exist that are an integral part of the data retrieval system used in the management of patients' medical records. It is now possible to maintain patients' records in a central database, to be tied together with all members of a healthcare system by way of voice systems and computerized telecommunications networks. A step beyond that includes the electronic information superhighways and community health information networks. These networks provide the potential to integrate multiple systems: hospitals, care providers in their offices and on clinical sites, payers, researchers, laboratories, and suppliers. Large central databases, such as FAMUS, the primary care project in Quebec, are collecting longitudinal data on 2000 patient visits per month. This information will be used to identify a risk register for cardiovascular disease and to determine the success of interventions based on clinical guidelines (Grant, Niyonsenga, & Bernier, 1994).

Some of the advanced technology used in healthcare was initiated by the military in its ongoing preparation for the battlefield. Individual, handheld computers, with 6-inch touch-type video screens, were expected to improve communications and information available to the soldier of the future. This equipment was researched and tested by members of the U.S. Army, which planned to fully computerize at least part of an armored brigade by 1996 (Matthews, 1994). Such computers have unlimited potential for the advanced practice nurses (APNs) of the future as a means of communication linkage and storage of updated healthcare information.

As part of the Balanced Budget Act of 1997 (BBA 97), Congress provided Medicare reimbursement for telehealth services (HR 2015, Sec 4206). Starting January 1, 1999 approximately $100 to $200 million should become available for telemedicine consultations to providers working in rural areas designated as Health Personnel Shortage Areas (HPSAs). Payments are to be shared between the referring and consulting physician or practitioner. Individual states also passed telemedicine bills. The federal bill provides for the expectation that telemedicine and telehealth systems will expand access to quality healthcare services, provide clinical efficacy, and be cost-effective.

The BBA 97 also provided for a single, 4-year Informatics and Telemedicine Educational Demonstration Project (HR 2015, Sec. 4207). Earmarked primarily for Medicare beneficiaries with diabetes mellitus who reside in medically underserved rural or inner-city areas, the project provided for direct telecommunications link with information networks in order to improve patient quality of life and reduce overall healthcare costs. Two additional objectives were to develop a curriculum to train health professionals in the use of medical informatics and telecommunications and to apply advanced technologies such as video-conferencing from a patient's home.

As required by the Telecommunications Act of 1996, the Federal Communications Commission (FCC) adopted the Universal Service Order. With a cap of $400 million per year, this order became effective in May, 1997. It required that public and nonprofit rural healthcare providers have access to telecommunications services necessary for the provision of healthcare services at rates comparable to those paid for similar services in urban areas.

The future of telehealth is unlimited as to how it can be used and what can be accomplished. As had been so aptly stated in the past, "man can achieve what the mind can conceive." Imagine the convenience for people in the future of being directly linked to their healthcare provider's office via two-way, interactive, network video from their homes. No more having to bring a frail, elderly, or disabled person out in bad weather, to transfer in and out of a vehicle, or to travel long distances to see a practitioner. It will be possible to hold a hand-screen device over their area of concern to visualize their problem or over their lung fields to hear the problem. Impossible! say the naysayers. This and more will be accomplished in the 21st century. And, along with the new world of healthcare will come waves of other legal and regulatory changes: telelaw, legal liability, new regulations for distant providers, and standards of care for virtual home visits. The future will become the present, and we will witness emergent settings and models of practice.

Healthcare Environments and Settings for Care

Based on the driving forces of healthcare discussed in the previous section, different and varied healthcare environments and settings continue to emerge. Some may surface for a time and then disappear. Others will continue to evolve, take on a different focus, and survive future changes. The following section briefly addresses current and potential settings and the changes occurring in them.

ACUTE CARE HOSPITALS AND AMBULATORY CARE

During the past several decades, more and more healthcare began to be delivered in "out of hospital" settings. Stimulating the trends away from inpatient hospital care have been the changes in reimbursement for care, the era of managed care, the development of outpatient diagnostic and therapeutic procedures, and advances in technology that can be used in outpatient settings. The American Hospital Association (1993) reported that between 1980 and 1992, outpatient visits grew by 73%, and ambulatory surgeries (as a percentage of all surgeries) approximated 70% (American Hospital Association, 1993b). Today, patients are being encouraged to receive care as outpatients whenever possible and when it is not medically contraindicated. The overall effect on hospitals has been a gradual decrease in their number and an increase in the development of multihospital systems, especially networks and integrated delivery systems (IDSs). The largest number of hospitals (7174 with a total of 1,513,000 beds) was reached in 1974 (Paone, 1996). By 1993, the number decreased to 5600 acute care hospitals with approximately 900,000 beds (Jonas, 1998). What happened in the nation affected every large city. Between the years 1975 and 1983, northern Manhattan and the Bronx witnessed a closing of 7 hospitals with a total of 1,100 beds (Totten, Lenz, & Mundinger, 1997, p. 11). The percentage of hospitals that became members of multihospital systems increased from approximately 30% in 1979 to more than 50% in 1991 (Paone, 1996).

During the last two decades of the century, hospitals began to expand their outpatient, primary care, and community services. They began to provide more long-term care services, especially for older adults. Some of these services were driven by extended posthospital care needs that were the result of earlier discharges and shorter lengths of stay. These occurred as a result of the new patient management systems to decrease cost and length of stay. The prospective payment system (PPS) was mandated on hospitals through federal regulations. A few of the most common expanded services included home healthcare; outpatient rehabilitation programs for people with functional limitations, disabilities, and cardiac and joint replacement rehabilitation; comprehensive geriatric assessment clinics; hospice; and senior membership programs. Through a variety of restructured delivery systems and more cooperation between IDS players, hospitals became more involved with long-term care facilities such as assisted living/elderly housing, geriatric day care centers, nursing homes, rehabilitation hospitals, and hospital-based skilled nursing facilities (HB/SNF). In the American Hospital Association (1993a) surveys conducted in the early 1990s, the results showed that of the reporting member hospitals, 51% were licensed for skilled nursing care, and 85% reported some type of organized rehabilitation service.

LONG-TERM CARE

By definition, "long-term care is a range of health, personal care, social, and housing services provided to people who have lost or have never developed the capacity to care for themselves independently as a result of chronic illness or mental or physical disability"

(Richardson, 1995, p. 194). The focus of long-term care (LTC) is on providing care for persons with functional disabilities, as opposed to a specific disease or condition. Overall, 12.6 million Americans need LTC or help with their activities of daily living (ADLs) or instrumental activities of daily living (IADLs). This represents one-fourth of all people with disabilities and 5% of the U.S. population (Stone, 1995). The following sections will discuss the major components of the LTC continuum. It must be remembered, however, that the majority (80 to 90%) of LTC in this country is provided by family and friends (Doty, Liu, & Wierner, 1985).

Nursing Facilities

Nursing facilities (previously called nursing homes) have been the landmark facility and mainstay of the long-term care industry from their initial focus as almshouses and homes for the poor, through the "mom and pop" growth spurt in the early to middle part of the century, to the present day large-scale industry. The 1991 National Center for Health Statistics survey reported that there were 14,744 nursing homes in the United States with 1,559,394 available beds. Approximately 1.4 million persons reside in the homes at any given time, which collectively have a 91.5%, occupancy rate (Sirrocco, 1994). Medicare-certified SNFs can be either hospital-based, free-standing or rural hospital swing-beds (can be used for either acute or skilled nursing care). Since 1990, the total number of SNFs has grown 6% annually to a total of 16,161 facilities in 1997. According to the Pepper Commission report, private, out-of-pocket payment by nursing home residents and their families is the largest bill payer (48%) for nursing home care, followed by Medicaid (45%), Medicare (2%), and other federal and state programs (5%) (U.S. Bipartisan Commission on Comprehensive Healthcare, 1990). In 1998, the average annual cost of nursing home care was $46,000 per person. Although not the largest SNF bill payer, Medicare covers SNF stays for the first 100 days for beneficiaries who were admitted after a minimum of a 3-day hospital stay and who entered the SNF within 30 days of hospital discharge. "SNF payments have been among the fastest growing components of Medicare spending, increasing 33% annually, on average, since 1986" (Medicare Payment Advisory Commission, 1998, p. 90).

As part of the Balanced Budget Act of 1997, SNFs entered the "age of computers." Effective as of July 1998, SNFs were required to electronically transmit to HCFA, at designated intervals, the Minimum Data Set (MDS), the multidimensional assessment component of each resident's care plan. The MDS is a part of the Resident Assessment Instrument (RAI), the standardized, comprehensive, functional assessment instrument. In 1987, as part of OBRA '87 (the Nursing Home Reform Act), the RAI became mandatory in all nursing facilities that receive Medicare reimbursement. The fixed daily rate for each facility's prospective payment system (PPS) will be generated based on the residents' acuity levels as calculated from the MDS. And, although the PPS will be implemented over a 4-year schedule, there are those who believe it is the "step to move everyone to managed care" (Fisher, 1998a). The future of many nursing facilities seems dependent on what happens with PPS, the "frenzied pace of merger and acquisition activity" (Fisher, 1998a, p. 41), the presence of major financial investors, and the federal and state governments' continued focus on improving quality of care.

Two other relatively new posthospital care programs, in addition to existing long-term care facilities such as nursing homes, accept and care for patients who are not yet ready for discharge to their homes. These programs include the rapidly multiplying subacute units, also called transitional units by some authors (Evanshick, 1996), and the assisted-living facilities.

Subacute Units

As a newly created step in the integrated delivery systems, subacute units initially became a part of the free-standing nursing homes but eventually were also created as hospital-based subacute units. They were created to provide a link between acute care and long-term care and, as such, focus on more of a medical model. By 1995, these units, which numbered 700 (Ting, 1995), were especially able to care for individuals recovering from acute conditions; for a growing number of chronically ill elderly people (Griffin, 1994; McDowell & Brown, 1994); and for other people with special needs, such as ventilator-dependent residents (Griffin, 1994; McDowell & Brown, 1994).

As the number of subacute units increased, associations such as the American Subacute Care Association developed and standards for accreditation were written by JCAHO and CARF (Congress of American Rehabilitation Facilities). Most subacute units fall under one of two major umbrellas: either a medically complex unit for chronically or seriously ill patients or a subacute rehabilitation unit. In a letter to HCFA, the executive vice president of the American Healthcare Association (AHCA) stated "there is no question that subacute care, as provided in skilled nursing facilities, offers lower-cost care at a comparable level of quality when compared to treatment in an acute care setting" (Hawryluk, 1998, p. 25). Both freestanding and hospital-based subacute units receive a growing funding source from a variety of managed care contracts, including Medicare Managed Care (10%), Medicaid Managed Care (3%), and Managed Care contracts (10%).

The future of subacute units, however, will be dependent on the BBA of 1997 which changed hospitals' payment plan for early discharges of patients to postacute providers. Called the "10 transfer-and-discharge rule DRGs" (Hawryluk, 1998), HCFA will treat the discharge of patients with 10 specific DRGs as transfers and reduce established payments to discharging hospitals. Scheduled to begin January 1, 1999, a long-term implication may be that rather than accept a reduced payment, hospitals will retain patients longer, thus decreasing the number of persons admitted to subacute units. It could also create a system where patients are moved quickly to a lower cost setting. For instance, within a very short period of time, a person who survived a cerebrovascular accident may be discharged into several sections of an IDS: from hospital to acute rehabilitation for intensive therapy to a skilled nursing facility, and then to home care (Hawryluk, 1998). One can only wait and see how this secondary wave of change will affect the industry.

Assisted Living Facilities

If subacute units were created to fill the gap between hospitals and nursing homes, assisted living facilities (ALFs) were created to fill the gap between nursing homes and home care. The number of assisted living facilities, estimated between 30,000 and 40,000, "combines housing with a variety of personalized healthcare and supportive services, normally for frail elderly persons aged 82 and over" (Cerne, 1994, p. 72). Their mission statements usually stress independence, autonomy, dignity, privacy, and decision making for the residents while providing assistance with some ADLs and other daily activities (e.g., medication administration). Since their inception, the number of ALFs has mushroomed, and by 1998, it was estimated that 1 million elderly Americans resided in them. Initial reports from the National Study of Assisted Living for Frail Elderly (Manard & Cameron, 1998) from the DHHS, Assistant Secretary for Planning and Evaluation, Office of Disability, Aging and LTC Policy showed that 81% of the Continuing Care Retirement Communities (CCRC) included an assisted living facility on their campuses.

Although ALFs were primarily developed as an option for upper-income elders, more and more states have become involved in regulatory policy, setting minimum acceptable standards, and establishing Medicaid reimbursement policies for a low-income and Medicaid-eligible population. Even though the assisted living industry is experiencing tremendous growth, the future will be largely dependent on the residents' rising acuity levels, which are expected to impact their design and fundamental concept. As people "age in place," they will have increased needs for assistance in ADLs and IADLs. With an already established annual turnover rate of 50% and a length of stay of only approximately 2 years (O'Connor, 1998), assisted living facilities could find themselves challenged in maintaining a high occupancy rate.

Home Healthcare

The last category of long-term care to be discussed is that of home healthcare. What was originally designed as a short-term measure has developed into a long-term healthcare component. Incrementally, more and more categories of persons and clinical conditions were added to the list of home care recipients, including the elderly, the poor, persons with end-stage renal disease, persons with disabilities, and terminally ill elders. The National Association of Home Care reports an increase in the number of home care agencies, from 1100 in 1963 to 12,000 by 1993 (Halamandaris, 1993). The rapid increase is the result of three major trends: (1) increase in number of older persons; (2) improved and sophisticated technology permitting a variety of types of care (skilled, high-tech, and low-tech) to be administered in the home; and (3) popular demand (a change in people's preferences to wanting to stay in their own homes rather than in institutions for care). The type of ownership of the agencies and the percent of the total number are as follows: freestanding (more than 50% of all agencies, the majority of which are proprietary); part of another facility (more than 25%) were based in either skilled nursing or rehabilitation facilities, or acute care hospitals; government agency (13%); and visiting nurse associations (5%) (Medicare Payment Advisory Commission, 1998).

Hughes stated that "home care expenditures have been the fastest growing component of healthcare expenditures over the past 30 years" (1996, p. 63). Payments for Medicare Part A benefits for home care increased from $0.8 billion in 1980 to $17.5 billion in 1996 (Medicare Payment Advisory Commission, July, 1998). It is expected that backlash from the Balanced Budget Act of 1997 and its prospective payment system for home care will dramatically effect home health utilization. One may question then, if this happens, what secondary wave of change will follow? Will persons who may not be able to receive services at home be admitted to other components of the long-term care continuum (e.g., skilled nursing facilities, rehabilitation facilities, etc.), thus impacting their numbers and cost? Only time will tell.

The preceding examples are but a few of the LTC methods utilized to contain costs of hospitalizations and healthcare delivery. There are many other long-term care providers. (See Table 6-3). Although they all play a unique role, space limits discussion of each type of provider. More future nontraditional delivery programs will likely be created based on consumer needs. This trend has already begun with the customer focus of quality care initiatives. In the future, more healthcare will be delivered at convenient sites, such as schools, churches, exercise gyms, and shopping malls—perhaps even at fast-food restaurants. And as previously stated, more diagnostic and therapeutic healthcare will be delivered in people's homes via the computer. "Healthcare where the people are" will become more and more a way of our daily life. Instead of automatic teller machines for delivery of cash, perhaps one may stop at the local automatic health machine for a simple diagnostic or treatment intervention.

 TABLE 6-3 *Other Participants in Long-term Care Continuum*

Adult day care

Adult day health centers

Dialysis units

Hospice care

Long-term care hospitals

Mental health/mental retardation care

Rehabilitation facilities

Respite care

Special care units

Emerging Practice Issues and Models of Practice

Advanced practice nurses are a reputable, strong, and vital part of the American healthcare system. Even with a current force of all practicing APNs numbering 52,900, it has been estimated by the DHHS that, by the year 2000, there will be a need for an additional 19,000 (Abdellah, 1997). Their roots and success stories throughout their 30-plus years of existence are well documented in this nation's history (Yedidia, 1981; Chard, Dunn, & Mandelbaum, 1983; Freund, 1986; Towers, 1989; Venegoni, 1991) Of that fact, the profession can stand proud and APNs can all "toot their horn" as loudly as they can! As this nation begins the 21st century, one knows that in the rapidly changing, turbulent world of healthcare, there will be more changes, more storms to weather, more hurdles to cross. The major driving waves of change, discussed previously in this chapter, will continue and, in all probability, accelerate. The nation will continue to deal with the ever-increasing cost of care and promotion of cost-effective measures, the effects of federal and state regulations, the capitated, managed care of integrated delivery systems, the changing sites of healthcare delivery, the increasing number of aging recipients of care, the impact of chronicity, and the escalating opportunities in the evolving world of telecommunications and informatics. The driving forces plus the changes in healthcare environments and settings will continue to impact the practice of the APN.

But the question is *how* will we deal with the changes? What will our future look like? How will we adapt to meet the new reality? And how can we work to make our future what we want it to be? A discussion of the answers to these questions follows. As you ponder these questions, the words of the Pew Health Professions Commission should come to mind. What the members of that commission recommended to the leadership of the academic health professions must become a part of each and every APN. Their work must "begin and end on the fundamental values that define and shape their calling" (O'Neil, 1993, p. 13). APNs' fundamental values, skills, and attitudes must be grounded in the very reason for our professional existence—to provide quality healthcare. When that is kept in mind, success will happen, whatever the future challenges may be.

EMERGING PRACTICE ISSUES

The current and future education and practice of APNs will continue to be shaped largely by the driving forces of healthcare—especially, federal and state legislation, federal funding for the Professional Nurse Traineeship Program (under section 830 and 831a of the Public Health Service Act), role definitions and regulations, licensure laws, governing boards, third-party reimbursement, admitting privileges, and malpractice reform. (In-depth discussion of these topics can be found in various chapters throughout this book).

One additional action, which will impact future practice of APNs, is the proposed measure of the National Council of State Boards of Nursing (NCSBN) to implement "multi-state license recognition." This action would allow registered nurses to hold one nursing license in the state in which they live yet practice in different states without having to obtain another license. Utah became the first state to adopt the law, which becomes effective January 1, 2000.

MODELS OF PRACTICE

What will the practice of the 21st-century APN be like? How and with whom will the APN share clinical and collegial responsibility? The following section discusses the three major practice models that will exist in the 21st century—collaboration, interdisciplinary teams, and independent practice. Innovative and different models may be developed in the future, but for now, these three seem to be the basic foundation of any future variation.

Collaboration

Collaborative practice is a phrase not new in healthcare. In their historical review of nurse–physician collaboration, Hughes and Turner (1996) stated that it has been in existence for at least two decades. Steele (1986) quoted "collaborative practice" through the words of the 1972 National Joint Practice Commission (p. 3). With the complexity of today's changes in the healthcare delivery system, the focus on highly managed capitated healthcare, with its push toward quality and cost-effective primary care, collaborative practice is widely espoused as the preferred approach to healthcare delivery (Sullivan, 1998; Buchanan, 1996; Norsen, Opladen, & Quinn, 1995; and Steel, 1986). Fagin (1992) claims that nurses and physicians need to work together; it is no longer a choice. Sullivan (1998) calls collaboration a "healthcare imperative" for the future (p. 621). Not only is it preferred and required, but in some states, it is legislatively mandated. For example, in 1996, after years of negotiation by members of a Joint Committee with representatives from the State Board of Nursing, Board of Healing Arts (Medicine), Board of Pharmacy, and members of state professional associations and state policy development, the state of Missouri legislated the Collaborative Practice Rule (HB 564). A form of "induced collaboration," the bill presented collaborative practice guidelines but was limited to "specifying geographic areas to be covered, the methods of treatment that may be covered by collaborative practice arrangements and the requirements of review of services provided pursuant to collaborative practice arrangements" (Sullivan, Morgan, Heimerichs, & Scott, 1998, p. 333).

By definition, collaborative practice appears relatively simple, but it becomes more complicated when conditions, responsibilities, and behavior are detailed. Sullivan (1998) defines collaboration as "working together for a common goal [which] requires of its practitioners the acquisition and application of a complex constellation of values and abilities" (p. xiii). Whether the collaborative arrangements are intradisciplinary, interdisciplinary, or multidisciplinary, the participants are expected to share values, agree on plans and actions, and work toward a mutually satisfying and productive relationship. In his 7-year evaluation of joint or collaborative practices between NPs and MDs delivering primary care, Campbell (1998) found that ". . . collaborative practice rests on preconditions of cooperation such as mutual respect and acceptance of the validity of different approaches to patient care" (p. 169). The author identified the fact that NPs and MDs exhibited different diagnostic, therapeutic, and interaction styles. Whether or not these differences became a problem depended on what 44% of the sample respondents identified as the most important ingredients for a successful collaboration practice: competence, cooperation, flexibility, compassion, confidence, and good communication skills (p. 189). Clark-Collier (1998) elaborated additional requirements for a successful collaborative practice: "a nonhierarchial relationship between the professions with an equitable distribution of work, authority, responsibility, and credit for success" (p. 2).

As if providing a warning for the future, Campbell (1998) reminded his readers that "regarding the nurse practitioner as physician substitute prevents a full exploration of the nursing presence in collaborative practice" (p. 168). Nursing brings a unique and different set of priorities and underlying philosophy to the relationship, which are distinct from that of medicine. As in any collaborative process, whether it is between two persons, institutions, or nations, each must recognize, accept, and value what the other brings to the relationship. Recognizing these differences will result in a practice that will bring out the best in each participant and, over time, develop an integration of their practices.

Regardless of what the professionals bring to the collaborative relationship, the federal government, through the Healthcare Financing Administration (HCFA), will play a significant role. As the agency that oversees Medicare reimbursement, HCFA published the proposed rules implementing the direct Medicare reimbursement provisions of the Balanced Budget Act of 1997. These rules in the Federal Register (42 C.F.R. 410.75[c][2]) have major implications for NPs' practice. One of the major concerns was that HCFA attempted to redefine NPs and how they should collaborate with physicians. The federal rules, which mandated collaboration with a physician, preempted many state statutes and regulations that do not require collaboration as a condition of licensure. Thus, creating an atmosphere of potential confusion between state and federal guidelines and the possibility that access to care, especially in rural areas, would again be limited. As of the early part of 1998, there were 26 states, including the District of Columbia, which explicitly have no requirements for physician collaboration or supervision (Pearson, 1998). A second concern was that according to the rules, NPs were not listed among the designated providers who could order outpatient physical and speech–language–pathology therapy.

On the other hand, in December 1997, HCFA issued proposed rules with major implications for certified registered nurse anesthetists (CRNAs) that seem contradictory to those for NPs. The 1997 rules revised Medicare Conditions of Participation for Hospitals and Conditions of Coverage for Ambulatory Surgical Centers (ASCs). They included a "provision removing the federal requirement requiring physician supervision of nurse anesthetists and deferring to state law" (Sharp, 1998, p. 128).

Future collaborative practice models will vary depending on the clinical roles, the practice sites, and the type of care being delivered. Some APNs may be involved with single patient populations, but others may cover a diverse group of patients in a variety of settings that are part of an integrated delivery system. The structure of the practice will continue to be challenging.

Interdisciplinary

As with collaborative practice, interdisciplinary practice has a long history in U.S. healthcare. In their historical review, Singleton and Green-Hernandez (1998) traced the initial primary care interdisciplinary team to a physician, Martin Cherkasky, at Montefiore Hospital in New York City. In 1948 he used interdisciplinary teams to provide home healthcare. Later, interdisciplinary teams were employed with family health, faculty interaction and role modeling, student experiences, and the federal government's "War on Poverty" project, which funded community health centers. A change in practice occurred when federal funding for interdisciplinary teams ended in the late 1970s. Since that time, the Department of Veterans Affairs, Area Health Education Centers (AHEC), and private foundations have continued to support interdisciplinary education and training but not to the same large-scale efforts of the early funding era by the federal government.

In striving for a working definition of "interdisciplinary teams," one can first define the individual words. Covey (1991) in his work on leadership, defined three levels of personal maturity—dependence, independence, interdependence—and how an individual functions in each level. These categories are analogous to the APN's professional growth and maturation. As a student and new graduate, an APN is more dependent. After becoming more proficient through clinical experience, one can work in a more independent or interdependent fashion, depending on criteria previously discussed such as state statutes, reimbursement, etc. To function interdependently is to function in the "paradigm of *we—we* can do it; *we* can cooperate; *we* can combine our talents and abilities and create something greater together" (p. 49). Scholtes (1998) defines a team and its benefits in the following manner: "A group of people pooling their skills, talents and knowledge . . . [which often results in] major gains in quality and productivity." "An additional advantage of a team is the "mutual support that arises between team members" (pp. 2–7). An interdisciplinary team (IDT), then, is a group of healthcare professionals who function in a collaborative and interdependent manner, in a paradigm of "WE," who pool their individual clinical skills, talents, and knowledge to provide the best possible holistic healthcare for their clients and patients.

In addition to the benefit for the professionals of mutually supporting one another, other benefits and outcomes of an IDT are specific to the care recipient and the healthcare delivery system. These include improved quality care and quality of life, improved functional outcomes, enhanced preventive measures, coordinated care with less duplication of services, increased efficiency, and decreased costs and time involvement for all members of the team. With the complexity of today's healthcare issues and delivery, it seems ideal to bring together a team of healthcare experts, each of whom brings their expertise to the table. In the emerging models of healthcare delivery, APNs will find themselves on various types of IDTs, in both acute and chronic care situations. Some may be more involved with a specific population with highly complex needs. Others will follow clients across the continuum of care in an integrated delivery system and be members of several teams (e.g., a geriatric nurse pracitioner following an elderly person admitted to an ICU, stroke rehabiliation unit, skilled nursing home unit, adult day healthcare, and adult day care when each of these facilities belong to the same IDS). It will be the APN in this example who will cut across the system and follow the older person over time in each setting, thus providing much more continuity of care and increased customer satisfaction.

One of the most critical issues for the APNs' success as future members of interdisciplinary teams is that as students they must learn how to function as members of teams and gain respect for other professionals on the team. This can be accomplished through sharing courses with other health profession students, which are taught by faculty from various disciplines. In their discussion of interdisciplinary education and practice, Singleton and Green-Hernandez (1998) identified the following barriers to such education: "faculty attitudes, students' perceptions, physical facilities, administration, technology, evaluation, and the placement within nursing and medical education" (p. 4). A collegial relationship should not be expected to start *after* graduation. It is imperative that the attitudes and skills needed for commitment and collaboration as a member of an IDT start early in one's professional development. All too frequently, a spirit of conflict and antagonism—an "us versus them" attitude—permeates education as opposed to the needed spirit of cooperation and respect.

Independent Practice

As healthcare moves into the third millenium, fewer and fewer APNs will be involved in independent practice, but there will be a small number who will choose to remain independent, whether it be in a solo or group practice. Depending on current and future changes in reimbursement, more APNs may find that, depending on federal and state regulations and mandates, they can contract with managed care organizations to provide care, especially in the arena of primary care. It has been documented that "NPs can handle 80% of primary-care doctor's services" (Abdellah, 1997, p. 453). The Department of Veterans Affairs Undersecretary, Kenneth Kizer, MD, stated that in the VA medical centers "nurse practitioners and clinical nurse specialists can handle up to 80 percent of patient care needs" (American Nurses Association, 1997) (see Chapter 17, Exemplar C for discussion regarding APNs in Veteran Hospitals). The following section will briefly discuss independent practitioners who are a part of that 80% in primary care and other settings.

Nurse-managed clinics, though small in number, are not new in our country. Wachs (1997) described the work of Lillian Wald, Mary Breckenridge, and Margaret Sanger at the beginning of the 20th century when they established nurse–managed centers. More recent models are unique in certain elements. For example, in the fall of 1997, the Columbia Advanced Practice Nurse Associates (CAPNA) opened a practice in Manhattan, New York, after negotiating contracts with three HMOs. What was unique about this arrangement was that the APNs who serve as the primary care providers are reimbursed at the same rates as the HMO's physicians. The APNs use a " nursing model [which] emphasizes individualized health promotion and disease prevention, patient empowerment and participation in care" (CAPNA, 1998, p. 1). The establishment of the community-based practice followed a $3 million demonstration project that had been in effect since 1994 (Totten,

Lenz, & Mundinger, 1997). As part of this project, 20 faculty members from Columbia University School of Nursing, who were also NPs, were assigned primary care provider status. As such, they had prescriptive authority (already a part of New York State's Nurse Practice Act) and hospital-admitting privileges. Their practice at Columbia-Presbyterian/Eastside is a collaborative practice with the on-site physicians who are a part of the referral network. The NPs are not under the physician's direct supervision—a large area of contention with the proposed rules written by HCFA for BBA 97.

Future opportunities will abound for APN entrepreneurs, especially in rural and underserved areas, with people who are indigent and have chronic illness, and in all areas of gerontological nursing (acute care for elders [ACE] units, senior apartments, senior centers, and especially nursing homes). From results of the National Physician Professional Activities Census, Katz, Karuza, Koassa, and Hutson (1997) studied medical practice with nursing home residents. Of the 21,578 physicians involved in the study, the majority (77.4%) reported spending no measurable time caring for nursing home patients during a typical week. Of the physicians who had nursing home practices, the median time spent was 2 hours per week with all of their patients. Studies such as this, which attempt to demonstrate the need for more physician involvement with the frail elderly in nursing homes, also emphasize a significant role for geriatric nurse practitioners who with future third-party reimbursement can develop a full-time, independent practice. Success and survival of these practices will require use of accurate business plans, a broad vision of community and how their clientele are a part of the whole community, and finally, being associated with delivery systems that will support their needs for referral services.

The Future

Without a crystal ball, it is difficult to predict the future. One can study the past and consider the major waves of change driving our healthcare delivery system, environments, and settings and still not be able to accurately predict what lies in store for the future. At this point, perhaps the best that can be done is to heed and carry out the wise words of others. In his forward to the book *You Can Make It Happen: A Nine-step Plan for Success,* Covey stated "the best way to predict your future is to create it" (1997). Korniewicz and Palmer defined the "preferable future for nursing" (1997). Building on the work of others, they identified this type of future as "the future that one wants to happen." They discussed the requirements for making a preferable future happen: (1) "vision, especially long-term vision, to articulate shared goals of an organization, profession, or society; (2) a proactive stance; (3) address the issues and make the necessary changes" (p. 108). Individually and collectively, this must be done so that the future of APNs is the preferable future!

REFERENCES

Abbey, F. B., Carneal, G., Fox. P. D., et al. (1998). What might the future hold? In P. R. Kongstvedt (Ed.). *The managed healthcare handbook* (3rd. ed.) (pp. 976–985). Gaithersburg, MD: Aspen Publication.

Abdellah, F. G. (1997). Managing the challenges of role diversification in an interdisciplinary environment. *Military Medicine 162*(7), 453–458.

American Association of Retired Persons. (AARP). (1997). *A profile of older Americans.* Washington, DC: Author.

American College of Nurse Practitioners. (ACNP). (1998). *Summary of reimbursement options under new Medicare law.* http://www.nurse.org/acnp/medicare/incident.html.

American Hospital Association. (1993a). *Guide to the healthcare field.* Chicago: Author.

American Hospital Association. (1993b). *Transforming healthcare delivery: Toward community care networks.* Chicago: Author.

American Nurses Association. (1997). ANA joins VA inpatient safely effort. *The American Nurse November/December,* 10.

Battistella, R. M. (1997). The political economy of health services: A review and assessment of major ideological influences and the impact of new economic realities. In T. J. Litman & L. S. Robins (Eds.), *Health politics and policy* (pp. 75–108). Albany, NY: Delmar Publishers.

Blendon, R. J. (1998). Understanding the managed care backlash. *Health Affairs 17*(4), 80–94.

Bringewatt, R. J. (1998). The metamorphosis of chronic care: Healthcare's next big hurdle. *Healthcare Forum Journal 41*(5), 15–21.

Buchanan, L. (1996). The acute care nurse practitioner in collaborative practice. *Journal of the American Academy of Nurse Practitioners 8*(1), 13–19.

Campbell, J. D. (1998). Collaborative practice in the 1980s. In T. J. Sullivan (Ed.). *Collaboration: A healthcare imperative* (pp. 167–205). New York: McGraw-Hill.

CAPNA. (1998). Frequently asked questions about advanced practice nurses. Columbia University School of Nursing. URL http://cpmcnet.columbia.edu/dept/nursing/capnafaq.html.

Cerne, F. (1994). Consumer choice could give big boost to assisted living. *Hospitals & Health Networks June 5,* 72.

Chard, M. A., Dunn, B., & Mandelbaum, J. (Eds.). (1983). *Nurse practitioners: A review of literature (1965–1985).* Kansas City: American Nurses' Association.

Clark-Coller, T. (1998). Collaborative practice: Beyond the bureaucratic shadow [Editorial]. *Journal of Nurse-Midwifery 43*(1), 1–2.

Congressional Budget Office (CBO). (1992). *Projections of national health expenditures.* Washington, DC: U.S. Government Printing Office.

Congressional Budget Office (CBO). (1994). *Reducing entitlement spending.* Washington, DC: U.S. Government Printing Office.

Covey, S. R. (1991). *The 7 habits of highly effective people.* New York: Simon & Schuster.

Covey, S.R. (1997). Foreward. In S. Graham. *You can make it happen: A nine-step plan for success* (pp. 11–13). New York: Fireside.

Daschle, T. (1998). Defending patients' rights. *Washington Post,* August 21, A23.

Deets, H. B. (1998). Now Congress must turn to unfinished business. *AARP Bulletin 39*(8), 3.

Doty, P., Liu, K., & Wiener, J. (1985). An overview of long-term care. *Healthcare Financing Review 6*(3), 69–78.

Fagin, C. (1992). Collaboration between nurses and MDs: No longer a choice. *Academic Medicine 67*(5), 295–303.

Fisher, C. (1998a). Crossing over to PPS. *Provider 24*(1), 29–34.

Fisher, C. (1998b). Subacute providers seek safe landing under PPS. *Provider 24*(8), 28–39.

Freund, C. M. (1986). Nurse practitioners in primary care. In M. D. Mezey & D. O. McGivern (Eds.). *Nurses, nurse practitioners* (pp. 305–334). Boston: Little, Brown and Co.

Fox, D. M. (1998). Managed care: The third reorganization of healthcare. *Journal of the American Geriatrics Society 46*(3), 314–317.

Gawande, A. A., Blendon, R. J., Brodie, M., et al. (1998). Does dissatisfaction with health plans stem from having no choices? *Health Affairs 17*(5), 184–193.

Goka, R. (1994). President's message. *ASCA Quarterly 1*(2), 4.

Grant, A., Niyonsenga, T., & Bernier, R. (1994). The role of medical informatics in health promotion and disease prevention. *Generations 18*(1), 74–77.

Greenspan, A. (1998). Testimony to the National Bipartisan Committee on the Future of Medicare, April 20.

Gutterman, S., Egger, P.W., Riley, G., et al. (1988). The first 3 years of Medicare prospective payment: An overview. Special Report. *Healthcare Financing Review 9*(3), 67–77.

Halamandaris, V. J. (1993). *Basic statistics about home care, 1994.* Washington, DC: National Association of Home Care.

Harrington, C., & Estes, C. L. (Eds.) (1997). *Health policy and nursing.* Boston: Jones and Bartlett Publishers.

Hawryluk, M. (1998). Discharge rule first to recognize subacute. *Provider 24*(8), 25–26.

HCFA (1998). Healthy aging project. Fact Sheet, October 14, p.1–2. HCFA Press Office. URL http://www.hhs.gov/news/press/1998pres/981014.html.

Hein, K. (1993). HIV in teens exploding: We need rapport badly [Editorial]. *Medical Tribune 8,* 12.

Hughes, A. M., & Turner, L. C. (1996). Nurse–physician collaboration: Historical review and impact today. *CACCN 7*(3), 24–28.

Hughes, S. (1996). Home health. In C. J. Evashwick (Ed.). *The continuum of long-term care: An integrated systems approach* (pp. 61–81). Albany, NY: Delmar Publishers.

Jackson, P., & Vessey, J. (1992). *Primary care of the child with a chronic condition.* St. Louis: Mosby Year Book.

Jonas, S. (1998). *An introduction to the U.S. healthcare system* (4th ed.). New York: Springer Publishing Co., Inc.

Katz, P. R., Karuza, J., Kolassa, J., & Hutson, A. (1997). Medical practice with nursing home residents: Results from the national physician professional activities census. *Journal of the American Geriatrics Society 45,* 911–917.

Kongstvedt, P. R. (1996). *The managed healthcare handbook* (3rd. ed.). Gaithersburg, MD: Aspen Publication.

Knoke, W. (1996). *Bold new world: The essential guide to surviving and prospering in the twenty-first century.* New York: Kodansha International.

Korniewicz, D. M., & Palmer, M. H. (1997). The preferable future of nursing. *Nursing Outlook 45*(3), 108–113.

Kraus, N., Porter, M., & Ball, P. (1991). *The InterStudy edge—Managed care: A decade in review 1980–1990.* Excelsior, MN: InterStudy, 1991.

Levine, S. (1998). "AARP hopes boom times are ahead." *Washington Post,* June 2, 1998, p. A1.

Levit, K. R., Lazenby, H. C., Braden, B. R., & the National Health Accounts Team. (1998). National health spending trends in 1996. *Health Affairs 17*(1), 35–51.

Lewin, K. (1947). Frontiers in group dynamics: Concept, method, and reality in social science; social equilibria and social change. *Human Relations 1*(1), 5–41.

Luft, H. S. (1997). Perspectives and evidence on efficiency in managed care organizations. In J.D. Wilkerson, K. J. Devers, & R. S. Given (Eds.). *Competitive managed care: The emerging healthcare system* (pp. 30–54). San Francisco: Jossey-Bass Publishers.

Manard, B., & Cameron, R. (1998). *A national study of assisted living for the frail elderly: Report on in-depth interviews with developers.* URL http://aspe.os.dhhs.gov/daltcp.reports/indepth/htm.

McLeod, D. (1998). A win for Medicare patients. *AARP Bulletin 39*(9), 3.

Medicare Payment Advisory Commission. (June, 1998). *Report to the Congress: Context for a Changing Medicare Program.* Washington, DC: Author.

Medicare Payment Advisory Commission. (July, 1998). *Healthcare spending and the Medicare program: A data book.* Washington, DC: Author.

Morgan, D. L. (1998). Introduction: The aging of the baby boom. In: The baby boom at midlife and beyond. *Generations XXII*(1), 5–9.

Mycek, S. (1998). Leadership for a health 21st century. *Healthcare Forum Journal 41*(4), 26–30.

National Health Survey. (1993). *Vital and health statistics: Health promotion and disease prevention, United States, 1990.* (DHHS Pub. No. (PHS) 93–1513). Washington, DC: Department of Health and Human Services.

Newacheck, P. W., McManus, M. A., & Fox, H. B. (1991). Prevalence and impact of chronic illness among adolescents. *American Journal of Disabled Children* 145, 1367–1373.

Newacheck, P. W., & Taylor, W. R. (1992). Childhood chronic illness: Prevalence, severity, and impact. *American Journal of Public Health* 82, 364–371.

Norse, L., Opladen, J., & Quinn, J. (1995). Practice model: Collaborative practice. *Critical Care Nursing Clinics of North America 7*(1), 43–52.

O'Connor, J. (1998). The hot option that could burn out? *Aging Today 19*(4), 7–8.

O'Neil, E. H. (1993). *Health professions education for the future: Schools in service to the nation.* San Francisco: Pew Health Professions Commission, 1993.

Paone, D. (1996). Hospitals. In C. J. Evashwich (Ed.). *The continuum of long-term care: An integrated systems approach.* Albany, NY: Delmar Publishers, Inc.

Patterson, D. (1995). The subacute Saratoga story. *Nursing Homes: Long Term Care Management 44*(4), 13–15.

Pearson, L. J. (1998). Annual update of how each state stands on legislative issues affecting advanced nursing practice. *The Nurse Practitioner 23*(1), 14–19, 62.

Perls, T. T. (1998). The New England Centenarian Study. URL http://www.harvard.edu/programs/necs/background.htm.

Rauber, C. (1998). Emerging leaders. *Healthcare Forum Journal 41*(4), 54–57.

Richardson, H. (1995). Long term care. In A. Kovner (Ed.). *Jonas' healthcare delivery in the United States* (5th ed.). New York: Springer Publishing Co.

Robert Wood Johnson Foundation (1996). Chronic care in America: The health system that isn't. *Advances [Online] Issue 4,* 1–5. URL http://www.rwjf.org/library/cveris4.htm.

Russell, L. B., & Manning, C. L. (1988). The effect of prospective payment on Medicare expenditures. *The New England Journal of Medicine 320*(7), 439–444.

Satinsky, M. A. (1998). *The foundations of integrated care: Facing the challenges of change.* Chicago: American Hospital Publishing, Inc.

Scholtes, P. R. (1988). *The team handbook: How to use teams to improve quality.* Madison, WI: Joiner Associates.

Shapiro, J. P. (1998). Managed care finds itself in the hot seat. *U.S. News & World Report (July 20) 124*(3), 20.

Sharp, N. (1998). Our colleagues: The CRNAs. *The Nurse Practitioner 23*(4), 128–131.

Shortell, S. M., Gillies, R. R., Anderson, D. A., et al. (1996). *Remaking healthcare in America.* San Francisco: Jossey-Bass Publishers.

Singleton, J. K., & Green-Hernandez, C. (1998). Interdisciplinary education and practice: Has its time come? *Journal of Nurse–Midwifery 43*(1), 3–11.

Sirrocco, A. (1994). Nursing homes and board and care homes (Data from 1991 National Health Provider Inventory). *Advance Data From Vital and Health Statistics (Feb. 23)* 244.

Smith, S., Freeland, M., Heffler, S., McKusick, D, & the Health Expendiures Projection Team (1998). *Health Affairs 17*(5), 128–140.

Steel, J. E. (Ed.). (1986). *Issues in collaborative practice.* Orlando, FL: Grune & Stratton.

Stone, R. I. (1995, June 27–28). *Long-term care policy in the United States.* Paper presented at the U.S.–Italy Conference on Long-Term Care.

Sullivan, T. J. (1998). *Collaboration: A healthcare imperative.* New York: McGraw-Hill.

Sullivan, T. J., Morgan, S., Heimrichs, B., & Scott, J. (1998). When collaboration is legislatively mandated. In T. J. Sullivan (Ed.). *Collaboration: A healthcare imperative* (pp. 325–373). New York: McGraw-Hill.

Thich Nhat Hanh (1998). *Heart of the Buddha's teaching: Transforming suffering into peace, joy, & liberation: The four noble truths, the noble eightfold path, & other basic Buddhist teachings.* Berkeley, CA: Parallax Press.

Ting, H. M. (1995). What's ahead for subacute care market? *Nursing Homes: Long Term Care Management 44*(4), 16, 18, 21.

Thompson, F. J. (1997). The evolving challenge of health policy implementation. In T. J. Litman & L. S. Robins (Eds.). *Health politics and policy* (pp. 155–175). Albany, NY: Delmar Publishers.

Totten, A. M., Lenz, E. R., & Mundinger, M. O. (1997). Differentiated primary care and evidence-based practice: The Columbia nursing experiment. *Advanced Practice Nursing Quarterly 3*(3), 9–18.

Towers, J. (1989). Part I: Report of the American Academy of Nurse Practitioners national nurse practitioner's survey. *Journal of the American Academy of Nurse Practitioners 1*(3), 91–94.

U.S. Bipartisan Commission on Comprehensive Healthcare (The Pepper Commission). (1990). *A call for action, Final report 1990.* Washington, DC: U. S. Government Printing Office.

U.S. Bureau of the Census. (1996). *Current population reports, Special Studies, P23–190, 65+ in the United States.* Washington, DC: U. S. Government Printing Office.

U. S. Bureau of the Census. (1993). *Current population reports, P25–1104, Population projections of the United States by age, sex, race and Hispanic origin: 1993 to 2050.* Washington, DC: U. S. Government Printing Office.

Venegoni, S. L. (1991). *Geriatric nurse practitioner's health promotive behaviors: A test of the theory of reasoned action.* Doctoral dissertation, Virginia Commonwealth University, 1991.

Ventura, M. J. (1998). NPs vs. MDs. *RN February,* 27–29.

Wachs, J. E. (1997). Nurse managed occupational health centers: An overview. *AAOHN-Journal 45* (10), 477–483.

Yedidia, M. J. (1981). *Delivering primary healthcare: Nurse practitioners at work.* Boston: Auburn House Publishing Co.

Zelman, W. A. (1996). *The changing healthcare marketplace: Private ventures, public interests.* San Francisco: Jossey-Bass.

CHAPTER 7

The Renaissance of Primary Care: An Opportunity for Nursing

Jean Goeppinger
Rosalie Hammond

Primary care is both a familiar phrase and one with multiple meanings. It has become a common term because of recent debates over national proposals for healthcare reform. These proposals have sought to increase access to healthcare for more than 40 million Americans while controlling costs and, irrespective of the proposal, assumed that increased access and decreased cost required an expansion of primary care (Franks, Nutting, & Clancy, 1993). Although the proposal made by the federal government has been defeated, debates among policymakers, healthcare professionals, and the public continue. Controversy concerns how best to improve access to healthcare while also controlling escalating costs and maintaining quality. Healthcare professionals have also raised questions about the contributions of primary care to healthcare reform and of advanced practice nurses (APNs) to primary care (Capriotti, 1994; Ford, 1997; Kassirer, 1994; Mundinger, 1994; Zuger, 1994). The term primary care has been used consistently throughout the debates but with considerable confusion about its meaning.

This chapter provides a conceptual foundation for today's debates, a foundation that strengthens the abilities of APNs to respond thoughtfully and proactively to new opportunities for recognition and reimbursement as primary care providers. The chapter begins with an historical overview of three primary care practice models—*community-oriented primary care, primary care,* and *primary healthcare*—continues with a discussion of the differences and similarities among the models, and concludes with a futuristic view of a "new" or revitalized primary care.

Practice Models

Practice models represent a perspective or broad approach within which the activities of health professionals and their clients can be described. As used here, they are neither prototypes of the practice world nor specific and detailed guidelines for practice. Rather, they are frameworks within which practice can be examined. In the following, each of the three practice models is described. The models are compared using a modified version of the ty-pology first presented by Rothman (1979) in a seminal paper on social work practice. Rothman delineated a set of characteristics, or practice parameters, including the goal of practice, the roles of the practitioner and client, and the most common change strategy employed by social workers in each model—to differentiate individual, organization, and community-centered social work practice. These characteristics are also salient descriptors of primary care practice.

COMMUNITY-ORIENTED PRIMARY CARE

The term community-oriented primary care (COPC) was adopted initially to reflect emerging collaborative relationships between epidemiology, a population-based science, and community medicine, the population-oriented but clinical practice of medicine (Kark, 1974). The five defining characteristics of the original COPC model included: (1) a specified user or target population for which physicians assumed responsibility and against which they measured the impact of their services[1]; (2) programs designed to address identified health problems within the target population; (3) participation by the target population in determining the need for health programs; (4) clinical practice that emphasized a community-based and family-centered approach to patient care, encompassing health promotion and disease prevention and treatment; and (5) accessibility that included not only geographic accessibility but also the absence of fiscal, social, cultural, and communication barriers (Kark, 1974).

COPC began in the 1950s in South Africa, Israel, and the United Kingdom, countries with national programs of socialized medicine and capitated healthcare systems. It was subsequently adapted in the United States to reflect our multipayer system. Some well-known early examples of COPC in the United States include the Kaiser-Permanente Medical Care Program of Oregon; the federally funded Montefiore Family Health Center in the Bronx; the Checkerboard Area Health System in rural New Mexico, supported by the Presbyterian Medical Services; the Tarboro-Edgecombe Health Services System of rural North Carolina, a coalition of a private, fee-for-service, multispecialty medical group practice and the county health department (Nutting; 1985; Nutting, Wood, & Conner, 1985); and more recently, the Oregon Basic Services Health Act (Dougherty, 1991).

The Montefiore-sponsored Care for the Homeless Team is a contemporary example of a COPC program that illustrates the multiple roles of APNs (Plescia, Watts, Neibacher, & Strelnick, 1997). In the Montefiore progam, an outreach team comprised of two groups of APNs (nurse practitioners [NPs] and psychiatric clinical nurse specialists), a social worker, and a family physician, provide integrated medical, social, and mental health services to a homeless population at community sites in the Bronx—a soup kitchen, several homeless shelters, and Montefiore's own Family Health Center. In 1995, 66% of patients seen by the Team were seen by NPs, and 93% of all medical encounters were with NPs (Plescia, Watts, Nelbacher, & Strelnick, 1997, pp. 61–62). The roles of nurses include community outreach to the homeless population and case management and direct patient care of homeless individuals.

PRIMARY CARE

In March of 1982, the Institute of Medicine convened a national conference in the United States on "Community Oriented Primary Care" (Connor & Mullen, 1982). Although conference participants endorsed Kark's description of COPC, a more restricted interpreta-

---

[1]The target population was originally considered a geographic community or neighborhood and later defined as any aggregate or group of patients who were users of healthcare.

tion, generally labeled primary care (PC), had become popular (Institute of Medicine, 1978). This interpretation represents primary care as most Americans experience it today.

> Primary care provides basic services, including those of an emergency nature, in a holistic fashion. It provides continuing management and coordination of all medical care services with appropriate retention and referral to other levels. It places emphasis, when feasible, on the preventive end of the preventive-curative spectrum of healthcare. Its services are provided equitably in a dignified, personalized, and caring manner. (Parker, Walsh, & Coon, 1976)

In the PC model, care is delivered and success assessed on individual clinical parameters. The community denominator for evaluating the impact of clinical practice on the populations individual patients represent, characteristic of COPC, has been eliminated. This has occurred because of the relative political strength of clinical medicine over public health, the increased specialization of medical practice, and the rapid proliferation of discipline-specific health professional educational programs. The emphasis is less on COPC provided to members of specifically targeted populations, the healthcare underserved and at-risk, and more on the provision of first-contact and person-centered medical services. Professional healthcare provided within the PC model is largely responsive to patient-initiated care seeking, not to community or population health needs. Persons present themselves, with self-identified healthcare needs, to professional healthcare providers who, in turn, respond with medical care.

The PC model has continued to describe a basic level of medical care, most of which is provided in an outpatient setting, that emphasizes a patient's general health needs (Office of Technology Assessment, 1990; Starfield, 1992). The most common aspects remain first-contact professional care that is accessible, comprehensive, coordinated, continuous, and accountable. Primary care advocates continue to argue that by improving the quality of the initial or "primary" contact between a care seeker and professional provider, health is enhanced, disease controlled, illness minimized, and cost-effective health and illness care increased. Despite a growing awareness that these expectations are not necessarily realistic (Franks, Nutting, & Clancy, 1993) and many calls for changes in healthcare delivery, primary care in the United States has continued to emphasize clinical care provided by medical care professionals who are often referred to as the "usual source of care." The new definition of primary care adopted in 1996 by the IOM Committee on the Future of Primary Care reflects this continued emphasis.

> Primary care is the provision of *integrated, accessible healthcare services* by clinicians who are *accountable* for addressing a large *majority of personal healthcare needs*, developing a *sustained partnership* with *patients,* and practicing in the *context of family and community* (Institute of Medicine, 1996).

The Abbottsford Community Health Center is a contemporary example of nurse-managed and nurse-delivered primary care (Kerekes, Jenkins, & Torrisi, 1996). The center serves residents of the 600 households in the urban housing community of Abbottsford Homes. Although the Center is situated in a community and targets its services to a defined population (community residents), it best reflects the comprehensive and coordinated primary care described by the Institute of Medicine in 1996. NPs provide direct clinical care to needy Abbottsford residents who seek their services. The nurse manager, also a nurse practitioner, coordinates the fiscal and clinical aspects of the center. Success is measured largely by decreases in patients' emergency department visits, hospital days, and client care costs, and not by improvements in the health status of all Abbotsfords residents.

PRIMARY HEALTH CARE

At approximately the same time that the COPC model was evolving into PC in the United States, it was evolving internationally into Primary Health Care (PHC). The PHC model has a community focus and uses a multilevel, multisectoral approach. The landmark Alma-Ata Conference Joint Report for WHO and UNICEF defined primary health care as:

essential health care based on practical, scientifically sound and socially acceptable methods and technology made universally accessible to individuals and families in the community by means acceptable to them, through their full participation and at a cost that the community and country can afford. It forms an integral part both of the country's health system, of which it is the nucleus, and of the overall social and economic development of the community. . . . It is the first level of contact of individuals, the family and the community with the national health system, bringing health care as close as possible to where people live and work, and constitutes the first element of a continuing health care process. (WHO and UNICEF, 1978)

Today, 20 years after Alma-Ata and despite uneven progress toward "Health for All" (WHO, 1981, pp. 18–19), the seven basic tenets of PHC remain.

1. PHC is shaped by the life patterns and responds to the needs of the community it serves.
2. PHC is supported by the national health system.
3. PHC is fully integrated with the activities of other sectors involved in health and development (agriculture, education, housing, transportation, and communication).
4. The local population is actively involved in the design, prioritization, and implementation of healthcare services.
5. The healthcare offered places maximum reliance on the available community resources.
6. PHC involves a melding of preventive, promotive, curative, and rehabilitative services for the individual, family, and community.
7. Interventions for health are undertaken at the most peripheral level practicable, i.e., the community (WHO, 1975, p. 116).

Health workers from multiple disciplines and traditional practitioners are expected to collaborate, as well as to work with the individuals, families, and communities they serve. The development of self-responsibility for health, at individual, family and community levels, is expected to encourage the development of strong healthcare systems, including, but not limited to, professional providers (Alarcon, 1994; Goeppinger, 1984).

In response to rapid changes around the world in health problems, determinants of health, and national healthcare systems, WHO has recently launched an initiative to update the Health for All policy (WHO, 1997). The update will reflect the centrality of health to development, and the need for sustainable healthcare systems able to meet the challenges of the 21st century. Delineation of desired outcomes that are achievable, epidemiologically sound, and measurable has been identified as the main challenge.

The current interest in healthy cities internationally (Duhl, 1996; Flynn, 1996; Tsouros, 1995) and healthy communities in the United States (IOM, 1996) reflects the basic tenets of PHC. Healthy cities and healthy communities have often been misrepresented, however, as overall public health, especially in the United States (Citrin, 1998; Schwab & Syme, 1997). PHC, with its emphasis on partnering with communities and community organizations, includes but is not limited to public health. PHC encompasses a wide range of formal and informal healthcare systems.

Examples of current U.S. nursing practice representing the PHC model are the Open Gates Health Center in inner-city Baltimore (Hatcher, Scarinzi, & Kreider, 1998) and the Mountain City Extended Hours Health Center in rural northeastern Tennessee (Edwards, Kaplan, Barnett, & Logan, 1998). The Open Gates Health Center serves uninsured residents of "Pigtown," an inner-city community in South Baltimore. NPs, certified nurse–midwives, community health nurses, a substance abuse counselor, a social worker, medical assistants, and a psychiatrist provide clinic care for minor episodic illnesses, women's health promotion, chronic disease management, and psychological disorders. Community participation in directing the center is sought, and community input is respected. The center also works actively with state and federally sponsored health and welfare programs, the school system, a local literacy program, and the Village Council of the Empowerment Zone encompassing Pigtown. These multisectoral efforts reflect the community and societal levels of PHC action.

Mountain City Extended Hours Health Center targets an isolated and underserved rural community in the mountains of northeastern Tennessee. NPs, registered nurses, a nurse–manager, and clinic and community support staff operate the center. They provide extensive community-based services, ranging from community wellness and screening programs and the diagnosis and treatment of common health problems to active participation in the redesign of Mountain City's health services. The Mountain City Center seeks explicitly both to improve population and clinically focused outcomes and to build the community's capacity for healthful change.

MODEL CHARACTERISTICS

The existence of multiple practice models, together with the similarity of their labels and the liberal mixing of labels and descriptions, is a source of considerable confusion for novice APNs and their teachers. Though the models overlap to some extent, clarity can be achieved by comparing them using a modified version of Rothman's typology (1979). COPC, PC, and PHC have somewhat different views of the: (1) goal and (2) scope of healthcare practice, (3) client roles, (4) health professional roles, (5) nurse roles, (6) medium of change or intervention, (7) practice environment or setting, and (8) locus of responsibility for costs. In the next section, the characteristics are described and the COPC, PC, and PHC models are compared across each characteristic. The characteristics, that is, practice model variables, are depicted in Table 7-1.

GOALS OF PRACTICE

Health Promotion and Disease Prevention

The major goals for healthful change are health promotion and disease prevention. Traditionally, health promotion and disease prevention have been distinguished by level of specificity, target of action, and time orientation. Health promotion involves activities designed to improve the physical, social, and mental well-being of individuals, families, and communities, whereas classical disease prevention involves the following: (1) altering specific behavior patterns that increase the risk of a particular disease state among identified aggregates (primary prevention), (2) detecting disease early and treating it promptly (secondary prevention), and (3) rehabilitation to prevent disease progression and disability (tertiary prevention) (Leavall & Clark, 1958). Secondary prevention in particular is oriented to the present; health promotion and primary and tertiary prevention activities are more typically undertaken with long-term goals in mind. Patients with self-limiting acute conditions, for instance, seek disease treatment and immediate recovery. Disabled clients, in contrast, often consider that returning to work after prolonged rehabilitation is reasonable; young adults from at-risk populations aim to prevent the occurrence of chronic disease in later adulthood.

The Ottawa Charter for Health Promotion, formulated at a WHO meeting in Ottawa, Canada, broadened the definition of health promotion from well-being (Leavall & Clark, 1958) to include the "process of enabling people to increase control over, and to improve their health" (WHO, 1986, p. 1). It emphasized partnerships between formal and informal, professional and indigenous community leaders; shared power between lay and professional participants; social interaction aimed at enhancing problem-solving skills in culturally acceptable ways; and multilevel, multimethod interventions. The narrow definition of health promotion as changes in individual lifestyles and health behaviors to improve

TABLE 7-1 *Defining Characteristics of Primary Care Practice Models*

	Practice Models		
Characteristics	*COPC*	*PC*	*PHC*
1. Healthcare Goals	Disease prevention (primary and secondary); health promotion	Disease prevention (secondary); problem resolution	Health promotion, capacity building
2. Scope of Practice	Individuals and aggregates within community settings	Individuals within family and community contexts	Community, populations, aggregates
3. Client Roles	Data sources, participants, targets, patients	Patients, consumers, recipients, victims	Partners
4. Professional Roles	Investigators, collaborators	Provider, program implementor, content expert	Enabler, catalyst, teacher of problem-solving skills
5. Nurse Roles	Often APNs	APNs especially NPs, CNMs	Nurses as one type of community worker. Includes, but not restricted to, APNs
6. Change Medium	Small, multidisciplinary groups; individuals	Data	Small, multisectoral group, health policy
7. Change Environment	Community-based	Healthcare institution	Public arena
8. Cost Locus	National, federal government	Patient and third-party payer	Community

well-being was broadened to include community development, capacity building, health policymaking, and empowerment of individuals and communities.

Primary Care Practice Goals

In the COPC model, practice goals have been described in traditional terms. Care encompasses individual-level and family-level health promotion and disease prevention activities. Disease prevention, particularly primary and secondary prevention, has been emphasized. Examples include the CHAD Program in Israel, a program whose acronym represents the "community syndrome of hypertension, atherosclerosis and diabetes," a set of diseases and disease risk factors (Abramson et al., 1994). CHAD was established in 1969 to target adults with cardiovascular disease risks who lived in an urban neighborhood served by a multidisciplinary family practice group of a local health center. Family conferences, clinic sessions, and health education were used to decrease the behaviors placing community members at risk. The work of the North Carolina Comprehensive Breast and Cervical Cancer Control Coalition to educate healthcare providers about detecting and treating breast and cervical cancer, which are among the highest causes of mortality for North Carolina women, represents COPC within the United States (North Carolina Comprehensive Breast and Cervical Cancer Control Coalition, 1995a & 1995b).

The goals of the PC model emphasize secondary and tertiary disease prevention although primary prevention is also deemed important. Vision and hearing screening of elementary school classes by public health department nurses, and mammograms and follow-up provided to low-income women at risk through a federally sponsored program are examples of secondary prevention. Tertiary prevention, the amelioration of complications from treated diseases, is represented by the growing number of self-management programs for chronic diseases (Lorig et al., 1999). Lorig and her colleagues found, for instance, that educating persons with four different chronic diseases (arthritis, heart disease, lung disease, and stroke) is effective. The intervention was led by trained community members and occurred in community settings. It aimed to empower patients, that is, program participants with a physician-confirmed diagnosis, to self-manage their symptoms. Intervention participants increased healthful behaviors, maintained or improved health status, and lowered their hospitalization (Lorig et al., 1999). This evidence-based intervention has now been adopted by the Health Care for the Aged Program of the California State Health Department (K. Lorig [personal communication], May 11, 1998).

In contrast, the goals of PHC practice relate to health promotion as envisioned by the Ottawa Charter, that is, capacity building and enhanced problem solving at all levels. Some of the clearest examples of healthcare practice directed toward health promotion broadly understood come from activities in developing countries 20 years ago, such as those in Tanzania and Ghana (Bennett, 1979). More recently, the Healthy Cities movement has reflected use of the PHC model in industrialized countries such as Canada, England, and the United States, countries where PHC is often referred to as the "New Public Health" (Ashton, Gray, & Barnard, 1986). Programs in Healthy Cities Indiana, for example, have aimed at building citizen commitment and developing civic leadership to address community-level problems related to physical activity and fitness; use of tobacco, alcohol and other drugs; family planning; violence and abuse; oral health; maternal and infant health; and mental health (Flynn, Rider, & Ray, 1991).

SCOPE OF PRACTICE

Health professionals have targeted their care to individuals, families, aggregates, communities, and the public at large. In the United States, public health professionals have usually provided care directed to the common good, that is, the public's health, whereas most professionals in the private healthcare sector have provided care to individuals. As the public health system assumed increased responsibility for providing personal health services to the indigent, uninsured, and underserved, the traditional distinction between public and private blurred. The privatization of the public health system occurring today has further obscured the distinction (Lairson et al., 1997). The public health system remains unique, however, in its orientation toward the common good and populations-at-risk and in its use of case-finding strategies. Environmental protection, assurance of quality medical care, and case finding remain hallmarks of the public health system.

Both COPC and PHC practice models have identified communities and aggregates as their practice focus. Success is assessed using the population as the denominator; rates and percentages are calculated to express, for instance, the prevalence of cigarette smoking among adolescent boys and girls living in an urban neighborhood (Abramson et al., 1994). COPC also addresses clinical practice objectives and evaluates success in terms of individual patient outcomes. The PC model is focused at the level of the active patient, i.e., care seeker, although the patient is usually viewed within his or her family and community environments, and interventions include both professional and self-care approaches. This represents a contextualized approach to primary care.

CLIENT ROLES

In COPC, clients are viewed as important data sources for healthcare providers. They may also be seen as targets of change efforts although the change process is recognized and respected as a collaborative one that requires client input. The client's perspective is always sought, irrespective of whether the client is a single individual or a geographic community. Health surveys, screening programs, and morbidity and mortality rates compiled from the clinical records of a medical practice are epidemiological approaches to gaining this perspective (Abramson et al., 1994). Comprehensive health histories, physical assessments of individuals and their work and home environments, and diagnostic reasoning are common approaches when the individual patient is seen within a family and population-focused care system.

In the PC model, clients are usually termed "patients," "consumers," or "recipients" of care. Occasionally, clients are seen as victims of catastrophic events beyond their control, such as in the case of stroke and cancer "victims." Always the client role is more passive than in COPC. Health professional care is given to, rather than for or with, clients.

Clients in PHC are seen as partners in a common venture, partners whose active, informed contributions are essential to success. Everyone—client and health professional—participates; everyone is responsible for the outcomes. The Healthy Cities movement, for instance, emphasizes city commitment, formation of Healthy Cities committees, and development of community leadership. Broad-based participatory leadership is seen as critical to goal achievement; health promotion is understood as capacity building. But, although Healthy Cities have expanded worldwide, the evidence demonstrating their effectiveness is limited (Flynn, 1996).

HEALTH PROFESSIONAL ROLES

Health professional roles reflect those of clients. In the COPC model, where clients are healthcare data sources and targets of care, health professional roles are investigative and collaborative. Professional expertise is recognized, particularly the diagnostic and epidemiological skills necessary to frame a problem, to access the "hard to reach," and to case find. In PC practice, professional roles are more clearly defined on the basis of substantive expertise; the majority of contemporary health professional education, regardless of the discipline, is focused on the attainment of this substantive expertise. Professionals are often termed "providers" of healthcare to "consumers." They respond to care-seeking behaviors on the part of patients by gathering data, formulating a diagnosis, and intervening. They may also triage patients using a computerized protocol (Lincoln et al., 1991) and implement a standardized program of care.

The expertise of a health professional working within the rubric of the PHC model is less dependent on disease-specific knowledge than skillful interaction. Health professional roles within PHC include those of enabler, mediator, catalyst, and teacher of problem-solving skills. Professionals cooperate in coalition-building, advocacy, identification of common interests and reconciliation of differences, and nurturing productive interpersonal relationships. PHC has legitimized activities linking the client and the professional. These links are frequently made by persons identified as informal community leaders—lay health advisors, community health advisors, natural helpers, and community outreach workers (Eng & Young, 1992). They both identify with the target community and agree to represent and extend a professional healthcare system that has been challenged to serve individuals and communities labeled "hard to reach" (Eng, Parker, & Harlan, 1997). The need for health professionals to learn to work in participatory relationships, not as the chief actor but partner, is increasingly recognized (Courtney et al., 1996).

Arnstein's typology of citizen participation (see Figure 7-1), depicted as eight rungs on a ladder ranging from citizen manipulation by the professional, the lowest rung, to citizen control of the professional, the highest rung, has become a classic in the field of community organization (Arnstein, 1970). It offers a simple way to summarize client and professional roles in the primary care practice models.

PC would be placed near the bottom of the ladder because it engages clients in therapy and treats their illnesses (rung 2), informs them about alternatives (rung 3), and consults with them about their problems and makes referrals (rung 4). PHC would be placed near the top of the ladder as it strives for full partnership (rung 6), delegated power, and

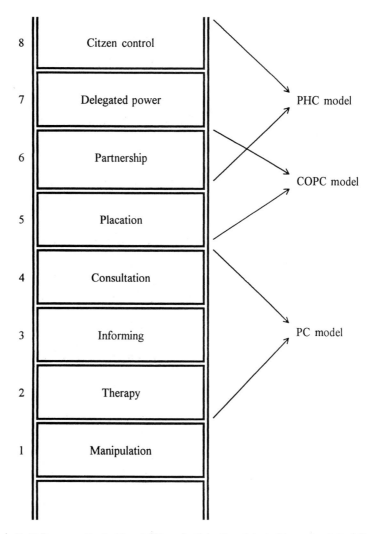

FIGURE 7-1 Eight Rungs on the Ladder of Citizen Participation. Adapted from: Arnstein, S.R. (1970). Eight rungs on the ladder of citizen participation. In E.S. Chen & B.A. Passett (Eds.). *Citizen participation: A casebook in democracy* (p. 336) New Jersey: Community Action Training Institute.

equitable decision-making (rung 7), and ultimately, citizen control (rung 8). This figure focuses on professional roles that emphasize self-help, involvement of a broad and representative cross-section of people, technical assistance, consensus building, and the deliberate involvement of informal community leaders. COPC practitioners would be standing on the middle rungs, usually involving clients in participating relationships (rungs 5 and 6).

NURSE ROLES

Nurse roles in these models often mirror those of other health professionals. In CHAD, the example of COPC presented earlier, nurses were involved in the planning group and are responsible for community outreach activities as well as physical examinations of individual patients, family assessments, counseling patients and families, and case management (Abramson et al., 1994). Their principal roles are in intervention, not program design or evaluation. The roles of APNs on the Montefiore Outreach Team are similar, with nurses planning, coordinating, supervising, and providing much of the care (Plescia, Watts, Nelbacher, & Strelnick, 1997).

Nurses practicing in the PC model are traditional "midlevel providers," NPs and certified nurse–midwives who provide primary and secondary prevention and health promotion services to care seekers defined by age (most nurse practitioners) and gender (certified nurse–midwives and women's healthcare nurse practitioners). The range of services given by midlevel providers depends on their geographic location, federal and state legislation regarding practice scope and reimbursement, patient population, and the patient–provider ratio.

Nurses, as a specific professional group, are seldom mentioned in descriptions of the PHC intervention strategies used in developed countries. In developing countries, nurses (who may be APNs) often link the lay and professional healthcare systems. In both developed and developing countries, nurses are but one type of community health worker. In programs such as the Open Gates Health Center (Hatcher, Scarinzi, & Kreider, 1998), nurses play prominent roles in the delivery of direct patient care and the establishment of connections between professional healthcare providers and the communities they serve.

MEDIUM OF CHANGE

The Ottawa Charter for Health Promotion delineated five strategies for health promotion: (1) building healthy public policy, (2) creating physical and social environments supportive of individual change, (3) strengthening community action, (4) developing personal skills such as increased self-efficacy and feelings of empowerment, and (5) reorienting healthcare systems to the population and partnership with clients (WHO, 1986, pp. 1–2). This is the broadest approach to health promoting change and fully represents the orientation of PHC. PHC change strategies are aimed at individual, family, and community levels, as well as at organizations and public policy. Changes are sought in behaviors, lifestyles, social norms, environments, policies, and resources. Small task-oriented and multisectoral groups, mass organizations, and political processes are all viewed as ways of introducing and stabilizing change at individual and community levels. Empowerment theory supports this view of change; its utility is now being subjected to empirical testing in health education and community psychology (Fetterman, Kaftarian, & Wandersman, 1996; Israel, Checkoway, Schulz, & Zimmerman, 1994; Rappaport, 1987).

In PC change is sought primarily at the individual or care seeker level. Individuals' learning about their diseases and effective disease management strategies are assumed to be primarily responsible for changes in their attitudes, beliefs, and behaviors. The COPC model uses a blend of change media, primarily individuals and small groups, including interdisciplinary teams of physicians and nurses, epidemiologists, biostatisticians, health educators, and public health nutritionists. Change media typically used in COPC differ from those used in PHC by the composition of the small group and the target of change. Group members in COPC represent health professionals from a variety of disciplines, rather than lay and professional workers from multiple sectors of the community (e.g., religion, housing, and education). COPC practice is also more likely to simultaneously view the individual who is the target of change as a medium of change.

CHANGE ENVIRONMENT OR SETTING

None of the practice models is setting-specific. The PC model is used in family health centers, health maintenance organizations, physicians' offices, and increasingly in the work place and community-based hospitals and homes. Care is provided in community clinics but remains oriented to the individual care seeker. PHC is not associated with a setting. It occurs, however, before the public—in community action groups, at foundation board meetings, and at hearings sponsored by town councils. The practice sites of COPC include any institution that is located in the community where people work (occupational health clinics and the factory floor), play, worship, attend school, and live out their lives.

LOCUS OF COST

The responsibility for healthcare costs, the final practice variable, has only recently gained visibility. Its importance continues to vary considerably with the predominant national healthcare system. In the United States, costs for COPC have been assumed, to some extent, by the federal government via programs targeted at specific population groups, such as Medicaid and Medicare, and at-risk populations, such as military veterans served by the Veterans' Administration and the homeless served by Montefiore's Outreach Team. In the PC model, costs are assumed by the care recipient and now the third-party payer. The previously documented cost-effectiveness of midlevel providers such as NPs is sometimes referenced (Safriet, 1992). Interestingly, in the PHC model, the issue of costs has not yet been addressed, perhaps because the emphasis of PHC has not been on disease treatment where cost-accounting procedures can be applied.

Comparison of Model Characteristics

We have examined the practice models by comparing them across eight defining characteristics. We have seen how the COPC model, an early blend of clinical and community-oriented medical care, has served as the base from which more specialized development occurred nationally and internationally. The PC model, which emphasizes the individual care seeker as the client and professionally given problem-focused care, represents a clinical perspective, and the PHC model emphasizes the community as the client, health promotion as the practice goal, and broad community involvement as imperative.

All models seek to improve the acceptability of care. COPC has also been found effective in increasing geographic and fiscal accessibility (Connor & Mullen, 1982). Evidence indicates that access to primary care is linked with improved health outcomes and that clients are satisfied with their primary care (Franks, Nutting, & Clancy 1993; Safriet, 1992). COPC offers more comprehensive care than PC, integrating the clinical and population perspectives and responding to health needs identified by both professionals and clients. Clients often are included as participants in healthcare, although their roles range from passive data sources, e.g., via chart reviews of patients in medical practices, to full participation in problem identification, intervention design and implementation, and outcome evaluation.

It is important for clinicians immersed in the practice world to be able to respond to the questions posed by the practice model variables. What are the appropriate goals, scope, and setting of primary care practice? What is the nature of client and professional roles in healthcare? What are some of the barriers to the cost-effective provision of care? What are appropriate change/intervention strategies? And, who should bear the financial responsibility for care? In this way, the practitioner acts thoughtfully and systematically. Practitioners must also understand the situational utility of each practice model and respond flexibly, as well as thoughtfully, to the challenges of particular clients and healthcare environments. It is equally important for practitioners in today's chaotic world of healthcare reform to help shape a "new" primary care.

The "New" Primary Care

Much recent attention has centered on ways of simultaneously improving access to healthcare while controlling costs and preserving quality. Essential to these efforts, although often overlooked in debates increasingly restricted to cost issues, are needs to redefine the client of care, the goals of the healthcare system, and the relationship between the public and private healthcare sectors (Lairson et al., 1997). A "new" primary care is needed that integrates managed care and community-oriented care and that serves vulnerable and underinsured populations as well as HMO subscribers and public health program recipients. As the 1991 and 1993 reports of the Pew Health Commission make clear (O'Neil, 1993; Shugars, O'Neil, & Bader, 1991), redefinition requires changes in health professional education and the healthcare system. "Reforming the education of health professionals combined with policies that address their availability, distribution, and utilization is one of the foundations of long-term reform in healthcare" (O'Neil, 1993, p. 5).

In *Health Professions Education for the Future: Schools in Service to the Nation* (O'Neil, 1993), the Pew Commission describes the "emerging health care system" (p. 6), termed here the "new" primary care, as one characterized by its orientation toward health, population perspective, intensive use of information, focus on the consumer, knowledge of treatment outcomes, constrained resources, coordination of services, reconsideration of human values, expectations of accountability, and growing interdependence with other community systems. The emphasis on care directed to improving a population's health, irrespective of the care delivery setting, coupled with the reorientation toward health and a consumer focus, suggest that the "new" primary care must take a broad view of both the client and goal of healthcare. Disease prevention, health promotion, injury prevention, and environmental hazards reduction are all goals; responsibility for achieving these goals involves the participation of individuals, groups, and communities, and changes in public policy. A multidisciplinary approach, involving professionals with knowledge of behavioral change, environmental restructuring, disease diagnosis and treatment, and social ecology, will be essential (Stokols, 1996). "Patient partnerships in decisions " (O'Neil, 1993, p. 6) and links between public health and primary care (Lasker, 1997; Starfield, 1996; Welton, Kantner, & Katz, 1997) need to be stressed. By the year 2005, practitioners will be expected to care for the community's health, practice prevention and promote healthy lifestyles, involve patients and families in healthcare decision making, and influence the development of healthy public policy (Shugars, O'Neill, & Bader, 1991, pp. 17–20).

One illustration of the "new" primary care (Garr, Rhyne, & Kukulka, 1993; Rhyne, Bogne, Kukulka, & Fulmer, 1998) reflects these changes in the definitions of the client and the goal of care. Garr, Rhyne, and Kukulka define the client or target population as "the [physician's] practice population as a whole" (Garr, Rhyne, & Kukulka, 1993, p. 1699), and the goal of care as one of meeting identified needs of active clients in the practice. These emphases are similar to elements of the COPC model, but the target population is defined more by access to care—that is, the possession of health insurance—than by geographic residence.

The Pew Commission reports also call for an emphasis on coordinated care, interdisciplinary teamwork, and cost-effective care (O'Neil, 1993; Shugars, O'Neill, & Bader, 1991). As we have seen in the review of existing models of primary care, these variables and particularly the links between coordination, interdisciplinary teamwork and cost-effective care have not yet been addressed. The most recent presentations of COPC (Garr, Rhyne, & Kukulka, 1993; Nutting, Nagle, & Dudley, 1991) fail to reflect the new opportunities for service coordination, teamwork, and improved efficiency and effectiveness. This omission has occurred despite recognition that APNs have assumed "new responsibilities in the delivery and management of care, particularly in primary care settings" (O'Neil, 1993, p. 83), and that nurse midwives and NPs "are proving to be important sources for primary healthcare" (O'Neil, 1993, p. 85). Safriet notes that the "empowerment" of NPs and nurse–midwives "would have the greatest immediate impact on access while preserving quality and reducing costs" (Safriet, 1992, p. 421). Collaborative practice arrangements between mid-level and physician providers are, however, emerging slowly, perhaps because of traditional boundaries among healthcare professionals and increased competition for reimbursement (Payne & King, 1998).

There are, however, promising examples of educational innovations designed to foster collaboration. They focus on the education of healthcare providers and provide a first step towards testing the cost-effectiveness of an interdisciplinary approach to healthcare. The Pew Charitable Trusts and the Rockefeller Foundation funded the "Health of the Public" program in 1986 to stimulate academic health centers to emphasize a population perspective through curricular reform (Showstack et al., 1992). Partnerships with communities and collaboration among health professional schools were required. By 1997 when grants ended, the program had grown from 6 to 33 participating schools, and grants were directed by faculty in Schools of Medicine, Pharmacy, Nursing, Dentistry, and Public Health (Inui & Showstack, 1994).

Changes in the ways participating schools educated their students and defined their roles in the community included student-initiated development of a comprehensive statewide approach to prenatal and postnatal care for pregnant drug abusers; student analysis of outcome data for HMO patients with hypertension and the feedback of their findings to participating physicians; several collaborative teaching and learning activities among faculty and students from the multiple health professional schools in academic health centers; and the teaching of population-level provider roles through partnerships with community-based AIDS service providers.

A collaborative family-oriented model of providing healthcare to homeless persons has been developed in New York City, illustrating the promise of interdisciplinary faculty and student collaboration in the practice setting (Morrow et al., 1992). The model involves alliances among the nurse-managed clinics of a school of nursing, the family practice department of a medical center, a community hospital, a county health department, and a network of social services for homeless persons. The alliances ensure homeless persons flexible, responsive community-oriented healthcare beyond the expertise and resources of any single partner. Faculty members have the opportunity to provide interdisciplinary professional education and training in a population-focused project. And, the family-oriented care model has a stable (relatively) base of institutional and fiscal support (Morrow et al., 1992, p. 315).

The development of partnerships among health professional faculty and students and between health professional schools and the communities they serve is an essential step toward demonstration of the cost-effectiveness of the "new" primary care. Once such partnerships are developed, they can be tested to determine the extent to which they represent cost-effective use of healthcare resources. Findings from these studies will help answer questions about the contributions of primary care to healthcare reform and of APNs to primary care. APNs have new opportunities to collaborate in the redefinition of healthcare goals and the targeting of healthcare clients, to examine the usefulness of new approaches, and to disseminate their findings to the public and policymakers. Aggressive participation in today's healthcare reform debates and experiments is imperative, as healthcare system reform remains a top priority.

REFERENCES

Abramson, J. H., Gofin, J., Hopp, C., et al. (1994). The CHAD program for the control of cardiovascular risk factors in a Jerusalem community: A 24-year retrospect. *Israeli Journal of Medical Science 30,* 108–119.

Alarcon, N. G. (1994). The role of healthcare professionals in increasing access to primary healthcare. *Family and Community Health 17,* 15–21.

Arnstein, S. R. (1970). Eight rungs on the ladder of citizen participation. In E.S.. Chen, & B. A. Passett (Eds.), *Citizen participation: A casebook in democracy* (pp. 335–357). New Jersey: Community Action Training Institute.

Ashton, J., Grey, P., & Barnard, K. (1986). Healthy Cities—WHO's new public health initiative. *Health Promotion 1,* 319–324.

Bennett, F. J. (1979). Primary health care and developing countries. *Social Science and Medicine 13A,* 505–514.

Capriotti, T. (1994, May). [Letter to the editor]. *New England Journal of Medicine* 1538.

Citrin, T. (1998). Public health—community or co-modity? Reflections on Healthy Communities. *American Journal of Public Health 88,* 351–352.

Connor, E., & Mullen, F. (Eds.) (1982). *Conference proceedings, community-oriented primary care.* Washington, DC: National Academy Press.

Courtney, R., Ballard, E., Fauver, S., et al. (1996). The partnership model: Working with individuals, families, and communities toward a new vision of health. *Public Health Nursing 13,* 177–186.

Dougherty, C. J. (1991). Setting health priorities, Oregon's next steps. *Hastings Center Report May–June,* 1–10.

Duhl, L. J. (1996). An ecohistory of health: The role of "Healthy Cities." *American Journal of Health Promotion 10,* 258–261.

Edwards, J. E., Kaplan, A., Barnett, J. T., & Logan, C. L. (1998). Nurse-managed primary care in a rural community. *Nursing and Health Care Perspectives 19,* 20–25.

Eng, E., Parker, E., & Harlan, C. (1997). Lay health advisor intervention strategies: A continuum from natural helping to paraprofessional helping. *Health Education and Behavior 24,* 413–417.

Eng., E., & Young, R. (1992). Lay health advisors as community change agents. *Journal of Family and Community Health, 15,* 4–40.

Fetterman, D. M., Kaftarian, S., & Wandersman, A. (Eds.) (1996). *Empowerment evaluation, knowledge and tools for self-assessment and accountability.* Newbury Park, CA: Sage Publications, Inc.

Flynn, B. C. (1996). HEALTHY CITIES: Toward worldwide health promotion. In Omenn, G. A., Fielding, J. E., & Lave, L. B. (Eds.), *Annual review of public health 17* (pp. 299–309). Palo Alto, CA: Annual Reviews Inc.

Flynn, B. C., Rider, M., & Ray, D. W. (1991). Healthy cities: The Indiana model of community development in public health. *Health Education Quarterly 18,* 331–347.

Ford, L. C. (1997). Advanced practice nursing: A deviant comes of age. *Heart and Lung 26,* 87–91.

Franks, P., Nutting, P. A., & Clancy, C. M. (1993). Health care reform, primary care, and the need for research. *Journal of the American Medical Association 270,* 1449–1453.

Garr, D., Rhyne, R., & Kukulka, G. (1993). Incorporating a community-oriented approach in primary care. *American Family Physician 47,* 1699–1701.

Goeppinger, J. (1984). Primary health care: An answer to the dilemmas of community nursing. *Public Health Nursing 1,* 129–140.

Hatcher, P. A., Scarinzi, G. D., & Kreider, M. S. (1998). Meeting the need: A primary health care model for a community-based/nurse-managed health center. *Nursing and Health Care Perspectives 19,* 12–19.

Institute of Medicine. (1978). *A manpower policy for primary health care: Report of a Study 1.* Washington, DC: National Academy Press.

Institute of Medicine. (1996). *Primary Care: America's health in a new era.* Washington, DC: National Academy Press.

Inui, T. S., & Showstack, J. (1994). *Health of the public: An academic challenge.* San Francisco: National Program Office, Health of the Public.

Israel, B. A., Checkoway, B., Schulz, A., & Zimmerman, M. (1994). Health education and community empowerment: Conceptualizing and measuring perceptions of individual, organizational, and community control. *Health Education Quarterly 21,* 149–170.

Kark, S. L. (1974). *Epidemiology and community medicine.* New York: Appleton-Century Crofts.

Kassirer, J. P. (1994). What role for nurse practitioners in primary care? *New England Journal of Medicine 330,* 204–205.

Kerekes, J. J., Jenkins, M. L., & Torrisi, D. (1996). Nurse-managed primary care. *Nursing Management 27,* 44–48.

Lairson, D. R., Schulmeier, G., Begley, C. E., et al. (1997). Managed care and community-oriented care: Conflict or complement? *Journal of Health Care for the Poor and Underserved 8,* 36–55.

Lasker, R. D., & Committee on Medicine and Public Health. (1997). *Medicine and public health: The power of collaboration.* New York: The New York Academy of Medicine.

Leavall, H. R., & Clark, E. G. (1958). *Preventive medicine for the doctor in his community.* New York: McGraw-Hill.

Lincoln, M. J., Turner, C. W., Haug, P., et al. (1991). Iliad training enhances medical students diagnostic skills. *Journal of Medical Systems 15,* 93–110.

Lorig, K., Sobel, D. D., Stewart, A. L., et al. (In press). Evidence suggesting that a chronic disease self-management program can improve health status while reducing hospitalization: A randomized trial. *Medical Care.*

Morrow, R., Halbach, J. L., Hopkins, C., et al. (1992). A family practice model of health care for homeless people: Collaboration with Family Nurse Practitioners. *Family Medicine 24,* 312–316.

Mundinger, M. O. (1994). Advanced-practice nursing: Good medicine for physicians? *New England Journal of Medicine 330,* 211–214.

North Carolina Comprehensive Breast and Cervical Cancer Control Coalition. (1995a). *Breast cancer in North Carolina: A handbook for health care providers.* Raleigh: North Carolina Department of Environment, Health, and Natural Resources.

North Carolina Comprehensive Breast and Cervical Cancer Control Coalition. (1995b). *Cervical cancer in North Carolina: A handbook for health care providers.* Raleigh: North Carolina Department of Environment, Health, and Natural Resources.

Nutting, P. (1985). Community-oriented primary care: A promising innovation in primary care. *Public Health Reports 100,* 3–4.

Nutting, P. A., Nagle, J., & Dudley, T. (1991). Epidemiology and practice management: An example of community-oriented primary care. *Family Medicine March/April,* 218–226.

Nutting, P., Wood, M., & Conner, E. M. (1985). Community-oriented primary care in the United States, a status report. *Journal of the American Medical Association 253,* 1763–1766.

Office of Technology Assessment, U.S. Congress. (1990). *Health care in rural America 483* (OTA-H-434). Washington, DC: U.S. Government Printing Office.

O'Neil, E. H. (1993). *Health Professions Education for the Future: Schools in Service to the Nation.* San Francisco, CA: Pew Health Professions Commission.

Parker, A. W., Walsh, J. M., & Coon, M. (1976). A normative approach to the definition of primary health care. *Milbank Memorial Fund Quarterly 54,* 416–438.

Payne, P. A., & King, V. J. (1998). A model of nurse–midwife and family physician collaborative care in a combined academic and community setting. *Journal of Nurse-Midwifery 43,* 19–26.

Plescia, M., Watts, G. R., Nelbacher, S., & Strelnick, H. (1997). A multidisciplinary health care outreach team approach to the homeless: The 10-year exerience of the Montefiore Care for the Homeless Team. *Family and Community Health 20,* 58–69.

Rappaport, J. (1987) Terms of empowerment/exemplars of prevention: Toward a theory for community psychology. *American Journal of Community Psychology 15,* 121–144.

Rhyne, R., Bogue, R., Kukulka, G., & Fulmer, H. (1998). *Community-oriented primary care: Health care for the 21st century.* Washington, DC: America Public Health Association.

Rothman, J. (1979). Three models of community organization: Their mixing and phasing. In F. M. Cox, J. L. Erlich., J. Rothman, & J. E. Tropman (Eds.), *Strategies of community organization* (pp. 25–45). Itasca, Illinois: F. E. Peacock Publishers, Inc.

Safriet, B. J. (1992). Health care dollars and regulatory sense: The role of advanced practice nursing. *Yale Journal of Regulation 9,* (2).

Schwab, M., & Syme, S. L. (1997). [Editorial—On the other hand: On paradigms, community participation, and the future of public health.] *American Journal of Public Health 87,* 2049–2051.

Showstack, J., Fein, L., Ford, D., et al. (1992). Health of the Public: The academic response. *Journal of the American Medical Association 267* (18), 2497–2502.

Shugars, D. A., O'Neill, E. H., & Bader, J. D. (Eds.). (1991). *Health America: Practitioners for 2005, an agenda for action for U. S. health professional schools.* Durham, NC: The PEW Health Professions Commission.

Stokols, D. (1996). Translating social ecological theory into guidelines for community health promotion. *American Journal of Health Promotion 10,* 282–298.

Starfield, B. (1992). *Primary care: Concept, evaluation, and policy.* New York: Oxford University Press.

Starfield, B. (1996). Public health and primary care: A framework for proposed linkages. *American Journal of Public Health 86,* 1365–1369.

Tsouros, A. D. (1995). The WHO Healthy Cities Project: State of the art and future plans. *Health Promotion International 10,* 133–141.

Welton, W. E., Kantner, T. A., & Katz, S. M. (1997). Developing tomorrow's integrated community health systems: A leadership challenge for public health and primary care. *The Milbank Quarterly 75,* 261–288.

WHO. (1981). Global strategies for health for all by the Year 2000. Geneva: WHO.

WHO. (1997, Summer). *Health for All in the 21st Century Newsletter* [On-line]. Available: http://www.who.ch/programmes/ppe/index.htm

WHO. (1975). *Official Records No. 226: Twenty-eighth World Health Assembly, part 1.* Geneva: WHO.

WHO. (1986). *Ottawa charter for health promotion.* Copenhagen: WHO Regional Office for Europe.

WHO & UNICEF. (1978). *Primary health care.* Joint Report of the Director General of WHO and the Executive Director of UNICEF. Geneva, New York: WHO, UNICEF on the International Conference on Primary Health Care, Alma Ata, U.S.S.R., September.

Zuger, A. (1994, May). [Letter to the editor]. *New England Journal of Medicine 11,* 197.

CHAPTER 8

Marjorie A. Satinsky

The Advanced Practice Nurse in a Managed Care Environment

The financing and delivery of healthcare has changed dramatically within the past decade, bringing communities in most parts of the United States into a managed care environment. Although state, regional, and local variations exist, almost everyone will be affected in some way by managed care.

As advanced practice nurses (APNs) determine their place and plan their career paths in this new environment, it is important that they understand the concepts and assumptions that are the essence of managed care. This chapter explains why managed care is so prevalent, who manages care, varieties of managed care plans in the private and public sectors, integrated healthcare systems, transitional strategies, the characteristics of a mature managed care market, and opportunities for APNs.

 ## Why Managed Care?

Managed care has existed in the United States for many years although the common use of the term is relatively recent. For example, California visionaries created the Kaiser Health Plan and many of the foundations for medical care long before the 1970s, the decade when the term *heath maintenance organization (HMO)* was coined and federal legislation enacted. Managed care in the 1990s is related to, but not the same as, many of the earlier efforts. Why the current explosion?

Traditionally, the provisions of care and reimbursement have been unrelated. Physicians and hospitals provided as much care as they chose, and payers reimbursed providers on a fee-for-service basis. Payers devoted minimal attention to the level and appropriateness of services, quality, and efficiency.

Technological advances in medicine have been a mixed blessing. As new techniques have become available, providers have been eager to use them, regardless of the cost to the healthcare system. So long as payers were willing to reimburse the healthcare providers, consumers were eager to take advantage of new treatment modalities; they, too, welcomed state-of-the-art care.

For people fortunate enough to be insured by commercial health insurance or by public entitlement programs such as Medicare and Medicaid, expectations grew. Oregon was a pioneer in limiting the availability and accessibility of healthcare, but most states have been unwilling to confront the rationing issue.

Under the scenario described, the healthcare industry flourished. By 1996, it represented 14% of the gross domestic product (GDP). That same year, the United States spent $1 trillion on healthcare, making the American healthcare delivery system the most expensive in the world (Levit, Lazenby, & Braden, 1998). Although healthcare represented a disproportionately large share of the national economy, the growth rate between 1995 and 1996 was actually lower than it had been in 37 years.

The high cost but lower growth rate of healthcare was no accident. It reflected the market's response to the industry. Healthcare costs for some companies had become so prohibitive that these employers began to lose their competitive edge over companies based in other countries. Furthermore, the concept of cost shifting, in which not all payers pay the same price for healthcare, was having an increasingly negative impact on the private sector as the government sought to limit federal healthcare spending in entitlement programs. In the public sector as well, the amount and growth rate of healthcare costs became unacceptable.

At some point, both private and public sectors insisted on limits in healthcare spending that would not compromise the excellence in quality that technological advancement had brought. When the Clinton administration's healthcare reform proposal captured national attention in 1993, fear of national healthcare reform mobilized many states, insurers, and providers to make changes on their own. The market demanded not only limits to spending and growth of spending, but quality and accountability as well. Today, managed care implies healthcare dollars well spent. As the U.S. healthcare system moves toward the 21st century, there is growing emphasis on care that meets quality standards as defined by consumers and providers, and legislative and regulatory bodies.

Overview of Managed Care

When experts predict that the country is moving toward a scenario in which most population groups, including those covered by commercial insurance, Medicare, and Medicaid, will be covered primarily by managed care health insurance, they are not all speaking the same language. In a narrow sense, managed care means a type of heath insurance plan. In a broader sense, managed care means a "wide range of heath care delivery and payment strategies designed to hold down costs while assuring quality of care" (Lewin-VHI, Inc., 1993).

Managed care encompasses more than types of plans and global strategies. A point that is often overlooked is the obligation to manage. Whose responsibility is it? The obligation to manage is shared among providers, consumers, payers, and more recently, the government.

PROVIDERS

Physicians, facilities, and other *health care providers* have historically played the most important role in determining when, if, and how patients will receive care. As the relationships between insurers, providers, and health plan enrollees change, however, providers have taken on a new role. They no longer dictate what care will be rendered regardless of price. Instead, they agree with payers to provide care within budgetary constraints. When providers assume partial or total financial risk for a specific population of enrollees assigned to them, they develop internally driven but externally sensitive standards for delivering high-quality, cost-effective care.

Consumers also have a responsibility to managed care. Compared with the 1970s and 1980s, employees covered by commercial health insurance already have fewer choices of health plan coverage and more financial responsibility (e.g., copayments and deductibles). In many states, both Medicare and Medicaid populations are required or have the option to select managed care insurance; therefore, these groups, too, must seek care according to the rules and regulations of particular health plans. For consumers, accessing the healthcare system is no longer the free-for-all that it once was when indemnity insurance dominated. Consumers must manage both their health and ways of seeking care when they need it.

Payers—health plans, employers, and third-party administrators—also manage care. They no longer reimburse whatever care is ordered by physicians. They have become smarter shoppers, and they have learned to manage their healthcare dollars through benefit design, selective contracting, shifting financial risk to providers, and by using a variety of tools to manage cost and utilization.

The role of *government* in managing care has evolved somewhat differently than might have been predicted during endless legislative debates over national healthcare reform. In response to consumer and provider concerns about potential abuses of managed care, state legislatures and the federal government have become protectors of the public interest. Furthermore, embedded in managed care is the notion of improving the health of individuals and populations, a principle that public health has embraced for many years.

EXAMPLES OF MANAGED CARE PLANS

Health plans that are subcategories of the generic heading "managed care" can be distinguished by organizational structure, freedom of access to providers, risk sharing, and utilization and quality management activities (Table 8-1). The most common types of managed care plans are health maintenance organizations (HMOs), preferred provider organizations (PPOs), point-of-service plans (POSs), and managed fee-for-service plans. There is significant variation within each type of managed care plan. Insurers blur distinctions even more by packaging two or more products together so purchasers can buy from a single source.

Unfortunately, no standard managed care plan exists. Plans that provide care to Medicare and Medicaid enrollees must meet criteria set by the federal government. Many plans seek certification from the National Committee on Quality Assurance (NCQA) and from the Joint Commission for Accreditation of Healthcare Organizations (JCAHO). Requirements for state licensure vary, as does the aggressiveness/passivity of enforcement. Table 8-2 lists some of the ways in which legislatures allow managed care plans to operate while also holding them accountable.

Health Maintenance Organizations (HMOs)

HMOs are the most common type of managed care plan. By 1997, national HMO enrollment had reached 83.7 million, representing 31.2% of the population (Hoechst Marion Roussel Inc., 1998). About one-third of the total HMO enrollment was in 25 large plans (Table 8-3). HMO benefit packages include preventive care as well as inpatient and outpatient care after the onset of symptoms or illness.

All HMOs offer a set of benefit packages defined in advance. The HMO price tag is driven by the market; what payers can afford to pay determines the premiums. HMOs contract with providers (e.g., community and tertiary hospitals, physicians, and other health providers) to provide care to consumers who are *enrollees* in the plan. Providers are at financial risk for some or all of the care provided and therefore have a financial incentive to deliver cost-effective, high quality care.

In most but not all HMOs, each enrollee selects a primary care physician (PCP) who

TABLE 8-1 *Characteristics of Managed Care Plans*

	Managed Fee-for-Service	Preferred Provider Organization (PPO)	Point-of-Service (POS)	Health Maintenance Organization (HMO)
Organizational structure	Separation between healthcare delivery and financing of care	Separation between healthcare delivery and financing of care	Relationship between delivery and financing of care depends on whether option is HMO-related or PPO-related	Delivery and financing of healthcare are linked
Choice of providers	Broad	Broad network with option to go outside	Broad network with option to opt in or out	Limited network
Assumption of financial risk	Insurer	Insurer	Insurer	Shared by insurer and providers
Utilization and quality management activities	Minimal	Some—likely to be prior authorization	Some—likely to be prior authorization	Must meet federal, state, and certifying agency comprehensive requirements
Licensing certification	Must meet state insurance department requirements	Some state requirements. 1997 legislation will require federal license if serving Medicare enrollees	Depends on whether option is HMO-related or PPO-related	Federal licensing if serving Medicare and Medicaid enrollees; state licensing varies; certification available from NCQA, JCAHO

manages that person's care by authorizing visits to specialists, hospitalization, and other services. Many plans call these PCP managers "gatekeepers," and some plans pay them an administrative fee for the management and coordination of patient care. Although the gatekeeper concept makes good sense to many consumers and providers, the managed care industry itself and some state governments have questioned the approach and advocated alternative ways to manage care (Walker, 1998). Within the industry, United HealthCare Corporation, headquartered in Minneapolis, Minnesota, has long supported the concept of open access to physicians. The company started by providing management services to physician-owned HMOs. Initially, the company was operated by specialists who did not support primary care coordination of patient care. As United HealthCare Corporation has grown over the years, it has found little evidence to justify a change in strategy. Its recent entry into Medicare risk sharing, however, has required a modification of its traditional approach.

PacifiCare, a large HMO based in California, is another HMO that has altered its gatekeeper approach. In 1996, this plan streamlined its referral process without eliminating the role of PCPs. Its Express Referral Program allows PCPs the option of referring enrollees to participating physicians in sixteen specialties without further authorization. Not all PacifiCare physicians have chosen the option, and those who have usually practice in large groups and have managed care experience.

HMOs are categorized as staff model, group model, and open panel (independent

TABLE 8-2 *Legislative Responses to Managed Care*

Type of Law	Issues Addressed
Anti–managed care laws	Any-willing-provider laws
	Freedom-of-choice laws
	Direct access laws
	Constraining incentives
	Constraining exclusive provider networks
Quality-of-care legislative incentives	Length-of-stay laws
	Mandated coverage
	Direct-access laws
	Regulation of utilization management
	Mandating point-of-service plans
	Anti–gag rule laws
Insurance regulations and statutes	Prohibition of false, misleading, or deceptive materials
	Adequate access to facilities and providers
	Quality assurance programs and follow-up
	Grievance procedures
	Reporting to state on enrollment, utilization, number of grievances
	Informing enrollees on coverage, exclusions, complaints, obtaining service, enrollee financial responsibilities
	Involvement of enrollees in governance
	Ensuring solvency and holding enrollees harmless
	Requiring maximum provider:patient ratios
	Requiring maximum travel times/distances
National Association of Insurance Commissioners Model Acts	Quality assessment and improvement
	Provider credentialing
	Utilization review
	Data collection
	Confidentiality
Federal licensure	Required for plans that enroll Medicare and Medicaid enrollees
Legislation supporting managed care	State-specific legislation allowing managed care to operate

Source: McLaughlin, C. (1998). Managed care and its relationship to public health: Barriers and opportunities. In P. K. Halverson, A. D. Kaluzny, & C. P. McLaughlin (Eds.). *Managed care and public health*. Gaithersburg, MD: Aspen Publishers, Inc.

TABLE 8-3 *25 Largest HMOs in the U.S., 1997*

Plan	1997 Enrollment
Kaiser Foundation Health Plan/N CA[1]	2,819,031
Kaiser Foundation Health Plan/S CA[2]	2,481,987
PacifiCare of California/Cypress, CA	2,130,094
HealthNet/Woodland Hills, CA	1,392,862
CaliforniaCare/Woodland Hills, CA	1,390,270
Oxford Health Plans/New York, NY	1,323,100
HMO Blue-Boston/Boston, MA	932,069
Tufts Associated Health Plans/Waltham, MA	924,218
HMO Blue-New Jersey/Newark, NJ	923,898
Physicians Health Services/Shelton, CT	836,345
HMO Illinois/Chicago, IL	816,622
Blue Plus/St. Paul, MN	807,533
HIP Health Plan of New York/New York, NY	801,686
Keystone Health Plan East/Philadelphia, PA	799,788
Medica Choice/Minneapolis, MN	760,996
Health Options (Statewide)/Jacksonville, FL	760,417
Aetna US Healthcare-NY/Uniondale, NY	727,627
Aetna US Healthcare-SE PA/Blue Bell, PA	682,594
Blue Shield of California/San Francisco, CA	619,069
HealthPartners/Minneapolis, MN	616,579
Kaiser Foundation Health Plan/Northeast	592,416
Health Maintenance Plan/Cincinnati, OH	581,931
Blue Choice/Rochester, NY	571,237
Kaiser Foundation Health Plan/Mid-Atlantic[3]	560,197
Harvard Community Health Plan/Brookline, MA	528,033
Total	25,380,599

[1]Kaiser Foundation Health Plan/Northern California region
[2]Kaiser Foundation Health Plan/Southern California Region
[3]Kaiser Foundation Health Plan/Mid-Atlantic Region
Source: Hoechst Marion Roussel Managed Care Digest Series/HMO-PPO Medicare - Medicaid Digest, 1998.

practice association [IPA]) plans (Table 8-4). In *staff model plans,* physicians are employed by the plan. Most of the income that they generate belongs to the plan although some staff models have developed methods for providing incentives to their physicians or giving them some share of equity. The staff physicians provide most of the healthcare services, and thus these plans are often described as *closed panel plans.* Some services may be provided on a contracted basis. Physicians provide outpatient care at ambulatory care sites owned by the health plan; these locations are commonly called health centers. Some staff models own their own hospitals and other facilities; others have divested themselves of sites. Because staff model plans own both physicians and often hospital facilities, the opportunity to control unnecessary costs has historically been great. During the early development of HMOs, they were generally able to provide care at the lowest cost. More recently, other types of HMOs have also demonstrated their abilities to manage care and lower their premiums.

In *group model plans,* care is provided by a group of primary (and often specialty) physicians who provide outpatient care in their own offices. The group(s) and health plan have a contractual relationship. The group practice model has at least three variations. Sometimes, the physician group is organized as a separate but legal entity but provides care only to members of the HMO with which it is affiliated. The Kaiser-Permanente groups are an example. Or, the physician group may have existed prior to its decision to affiliate with the HMO and provide care not only to the HMOs enrollees but also to enrollees in other plans and fee-for-service patients. The third kind of group arrangement is not mutually exclusive with the first two; two or more groups may be part of a network that contracts selectively with hospitals and other nonphysician providers.

Open-panel plans offer enrollees more provider choice than staff or group model plans. Providers deliver outpatient care in their own offices. They are financially at risk for some or all of the care that they provide. In some open panel plans, physicians are legally organized into an IPA; the IPA as well as individual physicians are then at financial risk. Hospital and other institutional care is provided by selected providers with whom the health plan contracts.

Both open-panel and closed-panel HMOs reimburse physicians and hospitals by a variety of methods, depending on the degree of risk that is shifted and/or shared. For example, physician reimbursement ranges from discounted fee-for-service to capitation. The plan may also *withhold* a percentage of the physicians' fees, keeping it in a separate pool until the end

TABLE 8-4 *Examples of Health Maintenance Organizations (HMOs)*

Type	Plan	1997 Enrollment	Age (Years)
Staff	Group Health Cooperative of Puget Sound (Seattle, WA)	717,574	51
Group	Kaiser Foundation Health Plan, Northern CA Region (Oakland, CA)	2,819,031	53
	HealthNet (Woodland Hills, CA)	1,392,862	19
IPA	Medica Choice (Minneapolis, MN)	760,996	23
	Tufts Associated HealthPlans (Waltham, MA)	924,218	17
Network	HMO Ilinois (Chicago, IL)	816,622	21
	HIP Health Plan of NY (NY, NY)	801,686	51

Source: Hoechst Marion Roussel Managed Care Digest Series/HMO-PPO/Medicaid Digest, 1998.

of the year. If the physicians deliver care within budget, the withheld money (or a portion of it) is returned. Hospital reimbursement methods include discount from charges, per diem payments, per diem rates, case rates, global case rates that include the physician component, and capitation. Many HMOs are gradually moving toward capitation. In most cases, however, HMOs are using a variety of methods of reimbursement. These methods may be inconsistent with each other and create conflicting incentives within a healthcare community.

Enrollees in all types of HMOs have many advantages over individuals with other types of insurance coverage. The benefit package is comprehensive compared to that of indemnity plans. It includes prevention and screening as well as care after the onset of illness. Enrollees have minimal out-of-pocket costs because most HMOs have small copayments for office visits and other services. Another advantage to HMO enrollees is the lack of paperwork. The HMO premium, paid in advance, pays for covered services, and enrollees do not submit bills for payment.

Theoretically, all types of HMOs should spend less but "buy smarter" than other types of healthcare plans. Control mechanisms, such as coordination of care by PCP gatekeepers, provision of preventive care, utilization management, and quality assurance programs, can enable HMOs to save dollars and pass the savings on to plan members (or stockholders if they are publicly traded).

Preferred Provider Organizations (PPOs)

PPOs are a managed care option that is considered to be between indemnity and HMO insurance. There is no standard PPO plan; the term refers to a variety of arrangements between insurers, providers, and third-party administrators. In general, PPOs use financial incentives to influence consumer and provider behavior. Many, but not all PPOs have some type of utilization management. Most PPO owners develop or rent provider networks, compensate providers on a discount fee-for-service basis, and perform administrative tasks such as marketing and claims administration. In some PPO arrangements, a corporate entity may also organize a network of insurers.

PPOs, like HMOs, have the option of meeting qualification standards set by professional organizations. The American Accreditation Program Inc., established in 1989, is a PPO accreditation organization (Kongstvedt, 1993). Until Medicare made PPOs available in 1997, there were no federal PPO requirements. State licensing requirements vary. In 1997, 1,035 operating PPOs in the United States covered medical care for 89.1 million eligible employees (Hoechst Marion Roussel Inc., 1998). More than half of these PPOs were owned by insurance companies. HMOs and independent investors were also PPO owners.

PPOs have historically been available to the employed commercial population. The Balanced Budget Act of 1997 made them available to the Medicare population as well. Eligible patients are encouraged to use participating hospitals and physicians, but they have the option to use out-of-network providers for an additional out-of-pocket cost. As in open panel HMOs, physicians provide care in their offices. PPOs contract with hospitals and other providers. Although PPOs have less comprehensive utilization management than HMOs, almost three-fourths of all PPOs used pharmacy benefit management in 1997.

The premium for PPO insurance usually is between that of indemnity and HMO plans. Out-of-pocket costs vary, depending on whether or not the eligible patient chooses to use in-network or out-of-network providers and pay a copayment or deductible. Unlike HMOs, PPOs do require paperwork; eligible subscribers do submit bills, particularly when they use out-of-network services.

Point-of-Service (POS) Plans

In response to both employer and employee demands, some plans have modified either their HMO or PPO products and added a feature that enables consumers to decide at the "point of service" whether to use the provider network or seek care outside of the network.

If the POS plan is a variation of an HMO, enrollees usually use PCPs to coordinate all care. If the POS plan is a variation of a PPO plan, eligible patients have the option to opt *into* the provider network at a lower cost to themselves.

Given the attractiveness of flexibility and choice to the American public, it is no surprise that licensed POS plans are growing rapidly. By 1997, enrollment in these POS plans accounted for 21.1% of all national HMO enrollment (Hoechst Marion Roussel, Inc., 1998).

Managed Fee-for-Service Plans

Managed fee-for-service plans are the least managed of the managed care options. These plans neither shift financial risk to providers nor control member access to care by building selective provider networks. Utilization management is minimal and is often limited to prior authorization for hospitalizations or specific procedures. The value of managed fee-for-service to both insurer and provider is that it may enable them to enter a relationship that in time might evolve into one of the other managed care options.

Carve-Outs

As purchasers have become more sophisticated about the design of their benefit plans, some have "carved out" specific problem areas and purchased insurance coverage and medical management from companies with particular expertise. For example, mental health and substance abuse care has been costly and difficult to manage; many payers have decided to deal directly with companies that specialize in the insurance and management of these services. The three largest behavioral health plans in the country are Magellan Health Services (including its component plans Human Affairs International, Green Spring Health Services, and Merit Behavioral Care Corp.), Value Behavioral Health, and United Behavioral Health (Roskey, 1998).

Another example of a carve-out is pharmacy benefits; these, too, are often separated from the total health benefit package. In fact, by 1997, 92% of HMOs and 77.7% of PPOs used managed pharmacy programs or pharmacy benefit managers (PBMs) (Hoechst Marion Roussel Inc., 1998). Techniques to manage pharmacy costs/quality include the following: use of formularies, practice guidelines, and drug utilization management. One of the more controversial aspects of pharmacy benefit management is the ownership of them by pharmaceutical companies themselves.

There are advantages and disadvantages to the carve-out approach. Specialist physicians often champion the carve-out of their particular areas of expertise because it preserves a way of providing care that is comfortable for them. Payers may select the carve-out approach to avoid high costs in problem areas like mental health and substance abuse. However, when carve-outs exist and specific benefits are insured and managed separately, information on and treatment for a single patient may not be coordinated.

Centers of Excellence

Particularly for high-cost tertiary care, some payers develop special arrangements with provider networks that can provide care across a large geographic area. The providers agree to accept a particular level of reimbursement, with the understanding that the payer will direct patients to them in a preferred relationship. Among the services for which centers of excellence are commonly developed are cardiovascular care and transplantation (e.g., bone marrow and solid organ). An example of a center of excellence is the Medicare network for coronary artery bypass graft surgery established in 1991. The federal government selected seven hospitals to participate in the demonstration program (American College of Cardiology, 1993).

PUBLIC SECTOR MANAGED CARE

The public sector, like the private sector, has been faced with dramatic increases in healthcare costs and growth in spending. The Federal Employees Health Benefits Program (FEHBP), Medicare, and Medicaid programs, the Department of Defense, and the Veterans Health Administration are all committed to using managed care as a way to not only control costs but also to improve the coordination and quality of care.

Federal Employees Health Benefits Program

In 1996, FEHBP offered HMO coverage to 2 million workers (Hoechst Marion Roussel Inc., 1997). Most of the government enrollees in HMOs were in group model and IPA plans.

Medicare

Over the years, Medicare beneficiaries have had the opportunity to select a managed care option as a total Medicare replacement or as a Medicare wraparound or supplement (Kongstvedt, 1993). The number of Medicare risk plans has fluctuated widely over the years. County-specific reimbursement within the federal formula has had different impacts throughout the country. Although some plans have experienced financial and operational problems, others have been very successful in caring for Medicare enrollees. Some of the demonstration plans and pilot programs have also been successful with subpopulations like the frail elderly. By 1997, 5.6 million (14.9% of all Medicare beneficiaries) Medicare enrollees had selected HMO coverage (Hoechst Marion Roussel Inc., 1998).

The Balanced Budget Act of 1997 created major changes in Medicare managed care that will occur in a rolling timetable over a 5-year period. Medicare beneficiaries have more managed care options than they previously had, including HMOs, PPOs, POS plans, and Provider-Sponsored Organizations (PSOs). The POS option allows Medicare to contract directly with providers who meet specific standards. In 1998, medical savings accounts (MSAs) were introduced. By 1999, there will be annual coordinated election periods and PSOs will become an option. Restrictions on enrollment and plan switches will take effect by 2002. Successful demonstration programs will be retained.

Medicaid

Medicaid recipients can also participate in managed care, primarily in HMOs. Many states have obtained from the Healthcare Financing Administration (HCFA) the waivers necessary to develop programs. Some states mandate managed care participation for particular categories of Medicaid recipients, and other states offer recipients the option of selecting HMO or traditional coverage. Another state-specific variation is the development of Medicaid-specific managed care plans or, alternatively, the addition of a Medicaid program within an existing commercial plan. Table 8-5 shows some of the state leaders in Medicaid managed care.

Department of Defense: CHAMPUS

Healthcare programs for members of the armed forces, dependents, and others entitled to Department of Defense (DOD) medical care have also moved toward managed care (Kongstvedt, 1993). The medical benefits provided under the Civilian Health and Medical Program of the Uniformed Services (CHAMPUS) traditionally have been generous and costly. In the early 1990s, the DOD tested a variety of managed care mechanisms through demonstration programs. The demonstrations achieved good results. Consequently, in 1992, the DOD introduced TRICARE on a national level with a 3-year phase in period (Bartling, 1995). The system created 12 health services regions and designated major military centers as lead agents. A new triple option benefit included TRICARE Prime (HMO with POS option), TRICARE Extra (PPO), and TRICARE Standard (indemnity

TABLE 8-5 *States Leading in Medicaid Managed Care, 1997*

	IPA	Network	Group	Staff	Other	Total
Tennessee	601,575	332,489	11,052	0	243,454	1,188,570
Washington	60,919	76,272	10,039	48,883	474,125	670,238
Alabama	19,300	31,624	0	0	376,927	427,851
Arizona	144,664	0	0	32,556	189,432	366,652
Hawaii	0	0	48,371	21,000	65,354	134,725
Delaware	64,147	0	0	0	914	65,061
Michigan	269,354	31,952	40,024	0	524,104	865,434
Maryland	17,209	26,966	1,597	21,760	280,108	347,640
South Dakota	0	0	0	0	41,542	41,542
Florida	136,780	36,444	0	75,280	702,924	951,428

Source: Hoechst Marion Roussel Managed Care Digest Series (1998). HMO-PPO Medicare-Medicaid Digest, p. 63.

insurance). Medical treatment commanders were given the tools, authority, and flexibility to focus on the delivery of care, organization, accountability, and control and measurement of costs.

VETERANS HEALTH ADMINISTRATION

The Veterans Health Administration (VHA) has a 5-year plan to reorganize itself so that it can continue to provide its comprehensive package of services with a lower level of federal financial support (Wilder, 1998). More than 1000 sites of care, including hospitals, nursing homes, clinics, domicilaries, counseling centers, home health programs, and contract treatment centers, have already been consolidated into 22 Veterans Integrated Service Networks (VISNs) that have become the systems' budgetary and operating units. Emphasis is on outpatient care that is more convenient to veterans than large inpatient centers located many miles apart. With VA funding expected to remain the same for 5 years, the system is seeking to emulate many of the managed care techniques that have worked in the private sector. These include case management, practice guidelines, telephone triage, telemedicine, and customer service standards.

Integrated Healthcare Systems

In a managed care environment, market forces encourage the coming together of disparate elements of healthcare delivery and financing. The result is "integrated healthcare systems." By the end of 1996, there were 570 integrated systems in the United States. Astute observers of the healthcare scene were predicting that, by the year 2000, the number would increase to 1200 (Sokolov, 1996). The participants in integration include healthcare providers, heath insurers, pharmaceutical companies, and other vendors.

In spite of these predictions, there is a dark side to integration. The process of conceptualizing, developing, and maintaining integrated healthcare is so challenging that many systems give up before they are very far along (Hallam, 1998). Some fail. Others make major midcourse strategic adjustments. Skeptics believe that buyers may not want what the supply side is creating (Satinsky, 1997) and that integrated systems exist because their components "will them into being" (Shortell, 1993). By 1997, the Advisory Board Company (1998) had rethought its earlier predictions on integrated systems and was emphasizing excellence within specific product lines.

Regardless of the uncertainty about the future expansion or demise of integrated healthcare systems, healthcare professionals need to understand what they are. In general, most systems strive to develop the following five characteristics:

1. *Market:* Focus is on the health needs of both individuals and populations. Collaboration between the system and other organizations is expected to improve access to care.
2. *Scope of care:* Providers offer the entire continuum of care either directly and/or through contractual relationships.
3. *Information:* Information is used to understand the health needs of individuals and populations and the financial and qualitative outcomes of different options for care. Information enables systems to develop and/or purchase the capacity to link patients, providers, and payers across the continuum. Finally, systems use information to create accountability to both internal and external publics.
4. *Alignment of incentives:* Financial, governance, and management incentives are aligned to promote system goals.
5. *Ongoing improvement of care:* Focus on continuous improvement of care.

Integrated healthcare systems are more prevalent in some parts of the country than in others. They develop for different reasons. The literature suggests that those systems that develop in response to market pressures rather than in response to the needs of specific population groups (e.g., immigrants or religious groups) or to raise capital are best-positioned to meet the needs of the future (Jones & Mayerhofer, 1994).

The development of integrated healthcare systems is a *process,* not an act. Not all systems are at the same place in this process (Table 8-6). Although systems development does not follow a prescribed track, all systems must deal with market forces, organization, and internal operations as they move toward their goals. They address these three factors over and over again as they move through at least seven stages of growth, including at least: preliminary planning, creation of a system, assimilation, competitive contracting, refocus of market forces, acceptance of system components, system redesign, and advocating community health.

Throughout the integration progress, the meaning of "integration" may shift. There are seven variations on the theme.

1. Is there *horizontal integration* among like entities?
2. Does *vertical integration* link production functions of individual organizations that precede or follow other organizations' core business?
3. Are key support activities, such as human resource, purchasing, financial services, planning, and marketing, *functionally integrated*?
4. Does *clinical integration* link care that is delivered at different sites so that the patients are the focus?
5. Does *public/private integration* support collaborative efforts directed toward improvement of the health of individuals and populations?
6. Does informal *virtual integration* support formal ownership and contractual arrangements?
7. Do recipients of care, payers, and vendors *visualize and experience* the system as integrated?

Because most integrated healthcare systems are relatively new entities, drawing conclusions about their impact or future is difficult. Nonetheless, there is sufficient experience to understand common factors that contribute toward success or failure. These are summarized in Tables 8-7 and 8-8. The consensus of professionals who work within systems and observers who measure them from the outside is that the single most important factor is clinical integration (Conrad, 1993).

TABLE 8-6

Investing in System Infrastructure (Still Largely Fee-For-Service)	Managing Risk and Lives (Still Largely Reducing Costs)	Integrating Care Delivery (The Work Never Ends)
Leading Health Systems	*Leading Health Systems*	*Leading Health Systems*
Adventist Health System-West	Allina Health System	Geisinger Healthcare System
Allegheny Health Education and Research	BJC Health System	Group Health Cooperative of Puget Sound
Alliant Health System	Florida Hospital Healthcare System	Henry Ford Health System
Baptist Health System (Birmingham)	Harris Methodist Health System	Intermountain Healthcare, Inc.
Carilion Health System	Helix Health, Inc.	Kaiser Foundation Health Plan, Inc.
Columbia North Texas Division	Legacy Health System	
INOVA Health System	Northwestern Healthcare Network	
Jefferson Health System	Orlando Regional Healthcare System	
Mercy Health Corporation, Southeastern	Promina Health System	
Mercy Health Services (Farmington Hills)	Sentara Health System	
SSM Health System	Scripps Health	
St. John Health System (Detroit)	Sharp HeathCare	
Tidewater Health Care, Inc.		
University Hospitals of Cleveland		

Source: The Advisory Board Company (1997). State of the union for America's health systems. Washington, DC: The Advisory Board Company.

TABLE 8-7 *Success Factors for Integrated Healthcare Systems*

- Philosophical commitment
- Clear purpose and vision
- Physician involvement in key leadership roles
- Alignment of incentives and rewards that recognizes system performance: risk, consistency, recognition of system goals
- Customer focus
- Information systems/technology that support goals and objectives
- Ongoing emphasis on quality initiatives
- Focus on creating market-driven value

TABLE 8-8 *Barriers to Successful Development of Integrated Healthcare Systems*

Failure to:
- Identify and communicate vision of end and interim states
- Identify population that system expects to serve and desired outcomes
- Plan for capital needs
- Address differences in philosophy and culture
- Take time to build trust
- Identify leadership skills and recruit and train talent
- Understand the importance of primary care
- Come to terms with governance
- Clarify lines of authority
- Orchestrate unique aspects of integrated systems
- Deal with ongoing change
- Work with partners, not subordinates

TRANSITIONAL STRATEGIES

Integrated healthcare systems have not yet come to most parts of the country. Most places are experimenting with a variety of transitional strategies that include, but are not limited to, the following options. The options are not mutually exclusive.

- *Management service organization (MSO):* an organization created to provide basic practice management services to physicians such as physician recruitment, office staff training, group purchasing, and computerized billing.
- *Comprehensive management service organization:* going one step beyond the MSO, the comprehensive version not only provides practice management services, but also purchases the hard assets of practices, manages the practices, and negotiates managed care contracts.
- *Group practice without walls:* individual physicians continue to practice in their separate offices but form a group-like practice to recognize economies of scale in marketing, purchasing, and negotiation with managed care plans.
- *Physician–hospital organization (PHO):* a legal entity that includes at least one hospital and physicians. The physicians may be organized into a physician organization (PO) like an IPA, or physicians may join the PHO without first organizing themselves. A PHO is generally empowered to negotiate or contract with managed care plans on behalf of both the hospital(s) and physicians (Satinsky, 1997).
- *Foundation:* the health system buys the tangible and intangible assets of physician practices; the foundation is a not-for-profit wholly owned subsidiary that signs professional services agreements with physicians who remain in a separate professional corporation.
- *Staff model:* the health system employs physicians, generally under a physician-managed clinic; it has more control over physicians than the foundation model.
- *Equity model:* a for-profit group practice owns the facilities of an integrated

system; physicians are employed, generally on a salaried basis and have the opportunity to share in the system's equity (The Advisory Board, 1993b).

Physician practice management organizations (PPMs) can also be described as transitional strategies. At present they are too new and unproven to be categorized as anything more permanent. As solo practices, single-specialty groups, multispecialty groups, and IPAs try to deal with the complexities of managed care contracting, management of financial risk, and measurement of the quality of care, many have decided that they can benefit from the leadership provided by large-scale for-profit companies that provide these services on a regional, statewide, or even national basis (Robinson, 1998). Unfortunately, many of the largest PPMs have failed to reach their goals and have experienced major financial downturns.

In general, all PPMs face three major challenges: growth in physician affiliations; improvement of economic efficiency, customer service, and clinical quality; and making necessary changes without undermining physician confidence and control at the local level. The recent failure of a number of large PPMs has placed their future in doubt.

Characteristics of a Mature Managed Care Environment

Organizations are only part of managed care. Even more important are three characteristics: market forces; reimbursement; and delivery of care. All three differ in a managed care environment and impact payers, providers, and consumers. Most parts of the country can be described as somewhere between non–managed care and managed care environments.

In examining the differences between managed care and non–managed care environments, it is important to understand that successful integrated healthcare systems respond to market forces. Attention to payers' wants and budgets helps systems and their components shift gears and provide evidence of value.

MARKET

The market in a mature managed care environment contrasts with that in a non–managed care market in at least two important ways: (1) competition is among integrated healthcare delivery systems, not individual components, and (2) health plans and employers use many strategies to contain healthcare costs while simultaneously ensuring quality of care.

Systems Competition
In a mature managed care environment, integrated systems vie for business, and competition is fierce. In non–managed care environments, competition is among such system components as hospitals, physicians, and health plans.

Health Plan and Employer Strategies
for Balancing Cost Containment and Quality of Care
Purchasers, both health plans and employers, wield considerable influence in a mature managed care environment. They use a variety of strategies to balance cost containment with assurance of quality care.

Health plans use strategies such as product diversification, plan consolidation, selective contracting, risk shifting, and demonstration of value. These techniques can keep costs under control and make sure that providers deliver high quality care.

Product Diversification
Many managed care plans encourage employers to replace existing multiple health insurance offerings with a single product. To encourage the total replacement decision, these plans adopt a multiple option strategy, offering HMOs, PPOs, and often exclusive provider

networks (EPOs) options under a single umbrella. For example, in New England, Harvard Community Health Plan began as a staff model plan. Mergers with Multi-Group and Rhode Island Group Health Association and a linkage with the Lahey Clinic and Mary-Hitchcock Clinic organizations added a group model to its portfolio. An agreement with John Hancock added a PPO option. The merger of Harvard Community Health Plan and Pilgrim Healthcare added more options to the offering package.

Linking workers' compensation coverage to health insurance benefits is another diversification strategy. The Tufts Associated Health Plan in Massachusetts created the Managed Comp product to fill this niche. CIGNA developed a system of bonuses and penalties designed to capture workers' comp business on a nationwide basis.

Health Plan Consolidation

The number of managed care health plans has fluctuated over time. Some plans have indeed gone out of business, but new plans continue to develop. Within the past few years, large-scale mergers have created megaplans that can compete for business on a regional level. Examples of large-scale mergers are CIGNA and HealthSource (a move that followed a HealthSource/Provident relationship), and Aetna/U.S. Healthcare. As already mentioned, 25 HMOs represented 31.2% of the total HMO enrollment in 1997 (Hoeschst, Marion Roussel Inc., 1998).

Selective Contracting

Many health plans have taken the selective approach to contracting with healthcare providers, working to establish partnerships in lieu of contractual relationships. The partnership approach facilitates a joint focus on problem areas. An obstacle to the selective approach has been the emergence in some states of *any willing provider laws* that require plans to contract with all qualified providers who are willing to accept their payments.

Risk Shifting

Financial risk shifting is another strategy health plans use to control costs. Plans move from discounted fee-for-service arrangements to alternative methods of reimbursement that hold providers more accountable for the cost and utilization of care. Examples of risk shifting are (1) per case payment, (2) global rate payment covering both technical and professional components, and (3) capitation.

Demonstration of Health Plan Value

Managed care plans have always had financial targets and worked toward achieving their own budgets by managing utilization of care. With the growth of managed care, meeting external standards set by certifying, licensing, and regulating agencies has become important. More recently, the focus has been on consumer satisfaction (Satinsky, 1997).

Within the past few years, health plans have increasingly sought recognition of their value from the National Committee for Quality Assurance (NCQA) and the Joint Commission on Accreditation of Healthcare Organizations (JCAHO). NCQA is a nonprofit organization founded in 1990 to develop ways to define and measure quality and then share that information with purchasers and the public. Large employers such as AT&T, PepsiCo, US Airways, and Proctor & Gamble consider only NCQA-accredited plans. Accreditation is difficult to achieve; only 42% of plans evaluated as of July 31, 1996 received full accreditation (Burns, Mandelker, & Northrup, 1996).

NCQA has worked with employer representatives to develop the Health Plan Employer Data and Information Set (HEDIS) criteria. These criteria have undergone numerous updates. The public sector, like the private sector, now uses them. Although critics of HEDIS have complained about its process orientation, in general, employers and consumers are happy to have the tool. The 1996 HEDIS 3.0 version had 75 performance indicators, including new ones on health prevention and the quality of clinical care. It also focused on major disease states.

JCAHO has traditionally evaluated inpatient institutions. Because so many of those organizations have developed relationships with insurance providers and/or become a part of integrated healthcare systems, JCAHO has expanded its scope to include health plans, PPOs, and integrated systems. In 1997, JCAHO launched its new Oryx system, which made performance measurement an integral part of evaluations. By the end of the year, hospitals were expected to select at least one approved system from the approved list and identify and use at least two clinical measures that together addressed at least 20% of the patient population (Morrisey, 1997).

The consumer perspective has broadened the definition of health plan "value." Consumers are interested in many of the same factors as payers. They are also concerned about some of the features of managed care that they believe can have a negative impact on them. These include the following:

- *Gag rule* language in physician contracts that allows plans to limit the providers' ability to discuss with patients limitations of a health plan's benefits and processes for referral, authorization, and payment of claims. In many states, anti–gag rule legislation has addressed this problem.
- *Consumer desire for choice* has been expressed in many ways, including the popularity of point-of-service and other open access plans; consumer pressure has also convinced some plans to remove or modify the gatekeeper feature.
- *Incentive pools* that reward physicians for meeting predetermined financial and utilization targets are often perceived as inappropriate interferences in the provision of high-quality care. Some states require that health plans disclose such language and be more open about limitations and prohibitions.
- Limiting stays for procedures such as hysterectomies and mastectomies has raised objections among consumers as well as providers. Some states have taken an aggressive stand on such limitations and have legislated *minimum benefit coverage.*
- *Objections to changing provider networks* are yet another consumer complaint. Enrollees who sign up for a particular primary care physician within a health plan network expect that the provider network will remain intact and that the plan will not downsize the list of available providers without adequate notice.

Employer strategies for cost containment and maintenance of quality include, but are not limited to, the following: limited choice of health insurance options; methodological evaluation of health insurance options; formation of purchasing coalitions; increase of employee cost-sharing; creation of carve-out products; contracting directly with providers; and, more recently, developing their own healthcare systems (Satinsky, 1995).

Limiting Choice of Health Insurance Options

As their healthcare costs have soared, many employers have taken draconian steps to control them. A common strategy is the reduction of health insurance options available for employees and provision of financial incentives for selection of plans that incorporate cost controls into their structure and organization. Some large national employers have cast their lots with specific plans and have entered multiyear relationships. Examples are the innovative Allied Signal–CIGNA partnership and the General Electric Corporation preferred provider arrangement strategy.

Methodological Evaluation of Heath Insurance Options

Employers who once delegated decisions on health insurance to a midlevel staff person are frequently relying on people with a new area of expertise: healthcare cost containment. Many companies have hired individuals and/or created departments to manage the evaluation of health insurance options and the management of care. Others use outside benefits consultants.

Although the federal government is the last organization many people would expect to emulate for efficient, cost-effective management, the Federal Employees Health Benefits Program (FEHBP) indeed sets a good example for other health benefit administrators. FEHBP provides health insurance to civilian government workers, retirees, and families. The Office of Personnel Management (OPM) covers 8 million people and contracts with 350 insurance carriers. OPM methodologically evaluates health plan options and is particularly clear in the comparison information provided to employees (Minton, 1998). Table 8-9 lists some of the facts that FEHBP furnishes to employees in its annual report card.

In both private and public sectors, employer evaluation of health insurance options and performance has been aided by the development of state-of-the-art methods for management (Satinsky, 1997). By 1996, employers had access to three new methods for assessing quality and cost: CONQUEST 1.0 (Computerized Needs-Oriented Quality Measurement), developed by the Agency for Healthcare Policy and Research (AHCPR) and two proprietary methods, the Mercer Value Process and the Med-Score Value Purchasing Initiative. Both proprietary products can be tailored to measure the particular factors that an employer wants to monitor ("New Quality Measures Abound," 1995).

Formation of Purchasing Coalitions

Purchasers at national, regional, and local levels have joined together to analyze healthcare costs, maintain data, and negotiate with providers.

Two important national developments occurred in 1995. A small group of major employers banded together to form the National HMO Purchasing Coalition. The new group included American Express, Merrill Lynch, Pfizer, Inc., Marriott International, Nabisco Brands, Inc., IBM, ITT, Sears, and two other companies that preferred anonymity ("Presenting the First Nationwide Health Coalition," 1995). The coalition represented 600,000 covered lives and was expected to purchase $1 billion of health care services throughout the country. Within a year after its formation, the coalition released information on the methodology used to select health plans: 30% of the equation was related to cost and 70% was related to quality (How the Big Guys Rank HMOs, 1996).

In the other national development, the Foundation for Accountability, known as FACCT, was formed by leading purchasers (Winslow, 1995). The new group represented major public and private purchasers, including HCFA. It identified five major diseases for which it would define quality of care delivered by HMOs: asthma, coronary artery disease, breast cancer, diabetes, and low back pain. To achieve its goal, FACCT developed a process to review current medical literature, identify quality indicators, endorse quality measurement sets, and encourage use by purchasers and customers (Burns, Mandelker, & Northrup, 1996).

TABLE 8-9 *Sample Factors from Federal Employees Health Benefit Plan Report Card*

- Quality of care
- Access to care, including emergency coverage
- Overall coverage
- Information, customer service, paperwork
- Thoroughness, competence, and provider availability
- Outcomes
- Explanation of care
- Choice of PCP and specialist physicians

Source: Minton, E. (1998, February). Purchasing lessons from the feds. *Business and Health,* 21–28.

Regional coalition activity has been strong. SMG Marketing Group has identified 138 local employer coalitions representing 22 million employees ("Employer Coalitions Exert Clout, Affect Some HMO Premium Rates," 1998). An example is the Buyers HealthCare Action Group (BHCAG) in Minneapolis/St. Paul, which was formed by influential employers following an unsuccessful attempt to influence the passage of favorable legislation. By 1998, the coalition represented 38 employers, including General Mills, Pillsbury, 3M, and the State of Minnesota (What's Squeezing Out Capitation in the Land of HMOs?).

BHCAG's strategy has evolved. At first, members developed a common self-insured health plan and a POS option. The group then contracted with a small number of systems and with 50 medical groups. Employers and providers jointly supported the creation of the Institute for Clinical Systems Integration to encourage health plans to demonstrate commitment to cost and quality management. BHCAG was able to reduce healthcare costs and to increase employee satisfaction with both medical services and health plan administration (Kemnitz, 1996). Yet BHCAG was still not satisfied with the level of competition. Beginning in January 1997, the group implemented its innovative consumer choice model in which teams of caregivers competed for consumers, based on price and quality of care provided (Health Care, 1996). Consumers had access to information on particular clinics, individual physicians, specialist referral and hospital relations, system-level comparisons of quality of care, and customer service satisfaction. BHCAG expected its new strategy to foster more competition than dealing with large managed care plans, most of which had overlapping provider participation.

Employers organized into purchasing coalitions have influenced not only provider performance but also health plan performance and pricing. For example, in San Francisco, an 11-member coalition that was part of the larger Bay Area Business Group on Health obtained rate concessions from more than a dozen HMOs (Kenkel, 1994). It also linked premium payment to health plan ability to meet criteria for customer service, quality of care, and data reporting. Other coalitions that have directly influenced health plans are the Central Florida Healthcare Coalition, the Memphis Business Group on Health, the Colorado Health Purchasing Alliance, and the Health Action Council of Northeast Ohio (Hausner, 1995).

Introducing Employee Cost Sharing

It is no surprise that the employee who pays has more of an interest in cost than the employee who gets a free ride. Once somewhat reluctant to shift a portion of healthcare costs to employees, many companies are now willing to increase employees' financial risk by introducing copayments and deductibles, and on a more positive note, by offering financial incentives for "good behavior" (e.g., participation in exercise and health education programs).

The carve-out approach described earlier is another popular employer strategy for cost containment. In fact, as integrated health systems struggle to develop and mature, many payers have asked them to consider specialty-specific packaging. The 1997 introduction of the Provider Sponsored Organization (PSO) alternative for Medicare managed care is likely to encourage carve-outs.

Using Direct Contracting

Employers may use the direct contracting approach to control healthcare costs and maintain high-quality care. Historically, self-insured companies have carried the banner for direct relationships with providers. Recent legislative developments in 1996 and 1997 have encouraged interest by others. The 1996 legislation dealt with EPOs, and the Balanced Budget Act of 1997 opened up the possibility for PSOs to contract directly with Medicare.

The health plan industry and other skeptics believe that providers have enough difficulty operating their own core businesses and should not enter the insurance arena. Aside from legal issues, some providers believe that they will jeopardize their existing relationships with health plans if they, too, take on the responsibilities that have traditionally belonged to the insurance industry.

Developing Healthcare Services

Some large employers have decided to produce as well as purchase healthcare services (Solovy, 1994). Delta Airlines, for example, built a primary care center near Hartsfield International Airport in Atlanta. The John Deere Family Healthplan in Des Moines developed primary care centers that provide services not only to company employees, but to local employers as well.

Reimbursement

In an aggressive managed care environment, providers (i.e., both physicians and hospitals) agree to accept financial risk for the care they provide to a specific population of enrollees. They are paid on a capitated basis. They receive capitation payments in advance, and the payment level reflects the expected use by the enrolled population for which they are responsible. To manage risk and live within the capitation budget, providers must control both volume and cost. They are usually rewarded for efficiency. For example, bonus payments may be related to operating within budget and to achieving specific goals for quality and efficiency. PCPs are key players when providers are at financial risk. They typically act as gatekeepers who steer enrollees to other providers, if and when necessary.

In contrast, in a non–managed care environment, providers are reimbursed when they actually provide care. Compensation for care offers incentives for performing high volumes of service. Physicians, for example, receive fee-for-service payments and have no financial incentive to monitor the amount and intensity of care they provide. Likewise, hospitals may be paid on a discount-from-charge basis and may be rewarded for every day that patients remain in the hospital. Specialty care is highly compensated, and PCPs do not become involved in determining which patients will need specialty care or other services.

In most of the country, provider reimbursement has elements of both managed care and non–managed care systems.

Service Delivery

Service delivery in a managed care environment differs from that in a non–managed care environment in at least three ways: emphasis on continuity of care, focus on nonhospital alternatives for care, and collaborative practice. In a managed care environment, benefits include preventive care that contributes to enrollee health and well-being. Providers and payers use many techniques to facilitate the integrated provision of care across the continuum and to monitor resource utilization. Both heath plans and healthcare providers may use case management to ensure that enrollees receive the care they need in the appropriate setting. Other useful tools are practice guidelines, clinical protocols, and care mapping.

In contrast, in a non–managed care environment, patients usually have more freedom to access providers without input from and coordination by PCPs or payers. Providers have a great deal of autonomy in ordering. Fragmented care may result. In addition, provider participation is inclusive, not selective, making the payers' job of monitoring cost and quality more difficult.

Market forces affect use of resources as well. Payers do not tolerate overuse of ancillary services, unlimited prescriptions, or provision of care in a costly setting that could have been rendered more appropriately. The scope of covered benefits and plan rules encourages providers to provide outpatient, not inpatient, care, provided the healthcare can be rendered in a medically safe way. Telephone triage services allow providers and/or enrollees to discuss options for care. In a managed care environment, there usually is a significant shift from inpatient to outpatient care.

Service delivery in a managed care environment is collaborative. The collaboration occurs both among providers and between provider and health plan staff. On the provider side, for example, enrollees are expected to move through a continuum of care, and there is need for healthcare professionals at different points along the continuum to work together. When providers develop close working relationships with insurers, the two must work together—again, with the patient and family as the focus.

Effects of Managed Care on Consumers

When managed care was in its early growth stages, measuring and describing its impact on consumers was difficult. Now that it is so prevalent, both positive and negative impacts are apparent. Managed care can offer consumers several advantages. Access to comprehensive care may improve. With managed care, their healthcare dollar can buy coordinated care, often with a PCP as a focal point. Health plan or provider staff may offer case management services to guide enrollees through the different components of care. Prevention and wellness are included in the benefits. Depending on the cost of their previous health insurance plan, many enrollees experience a decrease in their health insurance premiums and/or out-of-pocket costs.

However, consumers may also experience a negative impact from managed care. The transition from non–managed care to managed care is not always smooth. New participants in managed care plans may become confused by the benefits and operational rules and need clarification from caregivers, health plan member relations departments, or help lines. Another problem from the consumer perspective has been the "gag" clauses—language in agreements with managed care plans that prohibits providers from criticizing the plan, from trying to influence patients to change plans, and sometimes from discussing treatments disallowed by the plan.

Still another consumer problem concerns processes for resolving complaints. Medicare has a process for dispute resolution by an outside group. Many commercial plans do not have this function. Recent legislation proposed in California would change the situation.

Effect of Managed Care on Providers

The provider role in a managed care environment also changes (Satinsky, 1995). Hospitals are no longer the hub of all healthcare activity. Rather, they become revenue centers of a total system that also includes nonhospital providers such as home care agencies, long-term care facilities, and so forth.

As health plans exert pressure for more efficient care, significant changes occur in the balance of inpatient versus ambulatory care. Predictions have indicated that by 2000, 30% to 40% of traditional hospital admissions will shift to outpatient encounters as a result of changing demographics, technological advances, and payer pressure.

Internally, many hospitals have looked at *reengineering,* defined by Hammer (cited in Bergman, 1994), as "the radical redesign of the critical systems and processes used to produce, deliver, and support patient care in order to achieve dramatic improvements in organizational performance within a short period of time" (p. 28).

In a managed care environment, providers concentrate on *patient-focused care,* in which the enrollees, not providers, are the target for changes in service delivery. Some hospitals use physical redesign. For example, previously centralized ancillary services such as laboratory and radiology may be decentralized into satellites so that the diagnostic testing can occur within inpatient units.

Another critical component of patient-focused care is the ability to develop and link patient-specific information. The idea of a computerized patient-focused information system is the glue that can hold together service provision at multiple delivery points.

As their roles in the healthcare scenario change, hospitals and physicians often link closely together. As already mentioned, transitional strategies (e.g., physician–hospital organizations, management service organizations, and so forth) can bring these two groups together.

Another change on the provider side has been the recognition of provider responsibility to manage the health and wellness of a specific population. The American Hospital Association's vision for reform set forth in 1993 focuses on the community care network (American Hospital Association, 1993). The essence of the concept is that collaboration will improve a community's health status through the provision of a seamless continuum of services by healthcare providers operating within a fixed budget. The provider's accountability is to the community (Satinsky, 1995). To compete and survive in a managed care environment, providers and their staffs must learn to behave in new ways. The opportunities for APNs are challenging.

Effect of Managed Care on Advanced Practice Nurses

The managed care environment gives APNs significant opportunity for professional growth and contribution to the healthcare system. Advanced practice nurses have the training and experience that, combined with new skills, places them in an ideal position to assume a variety of important roles.

Skills for the Future

Two characteristics of healthcare organizations will directly impact APNs: (1) ongoing change and (2) physician leadership. With respect to change, it is safe to say that the majority of healthcare organizations will continue to change externally and internally. New external relationships will take the form of mergers, partnerships, and alliances. Internally, reorganization, downsizing, and reengineering will occur. With respect to physician leadership, many physicians are making the transition from practicing medicine to the assumption of executive responsibilities. For most of them, the shift is a difficult one that alters previous relationships with colleagues, including APNs. As physicians change their roles, they often experience isolation, strong fear of failure, and an acute lack of business skills (Rubin, 1991).

Some health professionals will grow with their organizations and contribute to the change; others will seek opportunities elsewhere by choice or necessity. In his book *The Fifth Discipline,* Senge (1990) suggests characteristics of leading, in the "learning organizations." These characteristics apply to individual employees as well as to organizations: personal mastery, mental models, shared vision, team learning, and systems thinking.

- *Personal mastery:* "the discipline of continually clarifying and deepening our personal vision, of focusing our energies, of developing patience, and of seeing reality objectively" (p. 7). Personal mastery in an organization contributes to that organization's strength.
- *Mental models:* "deeply ingrained assumptions, generalizations, or even pictures or images that influence how we understand the world and how we take action" (p. 8). In a learning organization, the staff is aware of these pictures and willing to challenge them.
- *Ability to build a shared vision:* perceiving a vision of the future that thrives on "commitment," not "compliance."
- *Team learning:* thinking together on an ongoing basis.
- *Systems thinking:* understanding the interconnectedness of the component parts.

In addition to skills that will enable them to contribute to the success of learning organizations, APNs need to master new professional and interpersonal skills, including, but not limited to: (1) understanding the managed care environment, (2) combining clinical and managerial skills, (3) functioning comfortably when roles remain ambiguous and negotiable, (4) interacting with multiple professionals both within and outside the organization, and (5) finding new solutions. Each of these skills is described in the following sections.

Understanding the Managed Care Environment

Managed care, that is, health plans themselves and techniques for managing, is continuously evolving. Advanced practice nurses need to understand not only what managed care is today, but what it is likely to be tomorrow as they work toward defining their own roles in the new environment.

To learn about managed care in its current stage, APNs can develop working relationships both inside and outside of the settings in which they work. Internally, most organizations have a managed care "guru" whose primary responsibility is managed care contracting and operations. That individual can be a good resource for both managers and staff. Educational programs sponsored by external organizations are also important. Some of the most enlightening are not directed specifically toward the nursing profession, but are geared toward other professionals who also need to learn about managed care.

Another way for APNs to learn about managed care is to talk and visit with colleagues in parts of the country that are already characterized as mature managed care markets.

Combining Clinical and Managerial Skills

Advanced practice nurses in a managed care environment need both clinical and managerial skills and the ability to combine them. For most, clinical skills are a given. They may be less proficient in other skills such as healthcare finance, accounting, and conflict resolution.

An effective way to learn some of these newer skills is to attend courses and conferences. Another approach is to talk with APNs who are already using some of these techniques: they can provide concrete examples of new skills that they learned and provide guidance on how to acquire and apply them. Some organizations have developed comprehensive continuing education programs by using in-house experts on finance, outcomes measurement, case management, and so forth, to educate each other. Conflict resolution programs are available from the Harvard School of Public Health in Massachusetts and CDR in Boulder, Colorado.

Functioning Comfortably When Roles Remain Ambiguous and Negotiable

Of all the characteristics of the managed care environment, the most difficult to comprehend is the ongoing change and evolution. With this change comes a never-ending ambiguity about the role of APNs and other professionals as well. An example from the case management literature illustrates the point (Satinsky, 1995). At the Malden Hospital in Malden, Massachusetts, a new case management program was developed to integrate the previously separate functions of utilization review, discharge planning, and social services. Although case management was initially envisioned as focusing on the inpatient population, it became clear that the case managers could go well beyond the walls of the hospital. The director of case management, an APN with experience in both provider and payer relationships, perceived an opportunity to expand the case manager role beyond the official job description. Other institutions with case management programs have similarly encouraged the function to evolve.

Similarly, case managers who are employed by managed healthcare plans, usually HMOs, have also experienced an evolution of roles. In many plans, case managers exercise a high degree of autonomy for managing clinical and financial aspects of care. Their roles expand and shrink as needed.

Interacting with Multiple Professionals Inside and Outside the Organization

Mature managed care markets are competitive. Each healthcare professional plays a major role in ensuring that relationships with health plans, with employers, and with patients and families are good.

Advanced practice nurses are in a particularly good position to perform this function. By virtue of their knowledge, experience, and formal place within an organization, they are well suited to facilitate both internal and external linkages. The more skilled they are at identifying and resolving problems of coordination and collaboration, the more they can contribute to their organization's functioning as a cooperative partner. For example, many academic medical centers and community hospitals have initiated comprehensive efforts to measure quality of care and to implement cost-containment programs. APNs frequently hold key jobs. They interpret external demands for information, collect and interpret data, and collaborate with other professionals to make improvements.

With many health plans, APNs perform similar roles to those in medical centers. Some are responsible for maintaining good relations with the plan enrollees. Others act as the liaison with the providers with which the plan contracts.

Finding New Solutions

Although the evolution from a non–managed care market to a mature managed care market will occur in many parts of the country, it will not occur in exactly the same way in multiple markets. The challenge to APNs in a case management role is a good one (Satinsky, 1995). Stanford University Hospital in California and the New England Medical Center in Massachusetts are both academic medical centers that developed case management programs. Their case management programs differed, however, according to institutional cultures and local market conditions. Similarly, in a systems context, Sharp HealthCare in California and Lutheran General HealthSystem in Illinois took different case management strategies. Each was successful in its own unique way.

Potential Roles for Advanced Practice Nurses

There are many roles for APNs in a managed care environment (Hicks, Stallmeyer, & Coleman, 1993). If care is indeed provided along a continuum, the provision and management of care at different levels is the shared responsibility of providers and insurers. Advanced practice nurses have the opportunity to function at any one or multiple points in the continuum. Combining clinical, financial, and administrative skills makes the field wide open.

Opportunities for APNs in a managed care environment include, but are not limited to, primary care, case management, utilization management, patient advocacy, member services, education, triage, quality assurance, and resource management. Each role is described in the following sections, and examples are provided.

Primary Care

Conceptually, the idea of primary care has multiple meanings. As Goeppinger and Hammond explain in Chapter 7, it may mean health promotion and disease prevention at the individual, family, and community levels. It may also mean secondary prevention, that is, the resolution of health problems in their early stages, such as screening for cervical cancer and vision and hearing testing. Primary care might also mean building capacity and enhanced problem solving in health promotion at the community level.

Within a managed care context, primary care has even broader implications. PCPs, often called gatekeepers, not only provide care, but also coordinate appropriate referrals and ensure that enrollees for whom they are responsible have access to a variety of wellness and preventive services. As care shifts away from the institutional setting, the ability of PCPs to manage enrollees' total care requires familiarity with a vast array of services, settings, and intervention techniques. Plans often pay a management fee to PCPs in recognition of their dual role as providers/coordinators.

Because primary care in a managed care environment is so comprehensive, many health plans and private practices employ APNs to work with physicians in the provision and collaboration of care. The collaborative role of APNs in a primary care setting can vary. In some instances, both the nurse and physician maintain independent practices of patients, collaborating when necessary. In other instances, the provision of all care is collaborative.

Case Management

As the financing and delivery of healthcare evolve, the popularity of the case management concept has grown. Although the term has many different meanings and applications, a good working definition includes the following three concepts (Satinsky, 1995):

1. Comprehensive application to a patient's entire episode of illness, regardless of the pay class or location in which the service is provided
2. Organization around a system of multidisciplinary services and resources needed to provide high-quality care in the most cost-effective way
3. Coordination by clinical and financial management of care by coordinators, not direct caregivers, who have a financial incentive to manage risk and maximize the quality of care

All case managers perform at least the following tasks: assessment, planning, intervention, monitoring, and evaluation. They perform their roles in a variety of settings. For example, managed healthcare plans use case managers to manage high-risk, high-cost, or other segments of the total enrollee population. Acute-care hospitals use case managers to manage the use of resources by patients. Large hospitals, particularly academic medical centers, often focus case management activities on patients with particular diseases, such as cardiovascular disease, cancer, or renal disease. Employers, too, may use case managers to work with particular segments of the employed populations. The list of possibilities is long.

In all settings in which case management has been implemented, APNs have proven to have the knowledge and skills for the job. Examples of innovative program development exist in single hospitals (e.g., Winchester Medical Center in Virginia); in integrated systems (e.g., Sharp HealthCare in California); and in separate ambulatory settings (e.g., Carondelet St. Mary's Hospital and Health Center in Arizona). Although each case management program is different, all offer unique opportunities for nurses to creatively coordinate the clinical and financial management of care.

Utilization Management

The concept of utilization management is a broad one, including prospective, concurrent, and retrospective review of care being rendered and resources being used. Many organizations have incorporated utilization review, discharge planning, social services, and sometimes quality assurance under a utilization management umbrella. In more advanced situations, case management may replace utilization management. In all of these situations, APNs can play an important role.

Patient Advocacy

The change from non–managed care to managed care insurance can be difficult for enrollees who may have been previously accustomed to relatively free access to the healthcare system. Although managed care benefits may be clearly explained in subscriber information packages, most people welcome assistance in interpreting the fine print. Many institutions, particularly hospitals, have expanded the roles of their existing patient advocates or ombudsmen to include health insurance–related questions. In one Massachusetts suburban health system, the patient ombudsman was initially responsible for responding to patient complaints. When managed care began to grow in popularity, she found that many patients' questions dealt with insurance coverage and plan rules and regulations. Patients tended to blame the hospital if the health plan limited acute care coverage and worked to move the patient to a less intense and more appropriate setting. The patient ombudsman worked closely with the hospital's director of managed care and with the different health plans to resolve clinical and financial problems.

Member Services

All managed healthcare plans have member services departments, and many use APNs in key roles. In these roles, APNs answer enrollee questions about covered benefits. In some plans, they do more than explain benefits; they actively assist enrollees to use the plan in the right way.

Education

Advanced practice nurses have many opportunities as educators in a managed care environment. Their targets may be patients, physicians, or institutions, and other staff. Enrollees, for example, may benefit from several different kinds of education. When they first enroll in a plan, they may need details on plan programs for health education and prevention. When they use services, they may need help in understanding the referral authorization process. If they are dissatisfied with some aspect of a plan's process, they need to understand the grievance process.

Physicians benefit from managed care education as well. Although all managed care plans have similarities, each plan has its own set of rules. Many plans use APNs in provider relations to recruit, educate, and maintain ongoing relationships with network physicians.

Institutions, like physicians, need education on health plan operations. Most organizations have many contracts, each with a different set of rules. Health plans often use APNs to explain the rules and to act as an ongoing problem solver.

In addition, there is an opportunity for education among professionals. In a managed care environment, care is collaborative, and it is important for all team members to share information with each other as well as with patients and their families.

Triage

Nurses have several opportunities to participate in the triage function that is intrinsic to managed care. Most health plans use telephone triage systems to answer enrollee inquiries during and after regular business hours and to direct people to the appropriate level of care.

Triage opportunities exist in provider settings as well. For example, managed care enrollees are discouraged from inappropriately using costly emergency room services in lieu of accessing their PCPs. Many hospital emergency departments have made staffing changes and designated triage nurses to assess and steer patients accordingly.

Quality Assurance

Quality of care in a managed care environment is of concern to both health plans and providers. Plans take pains to protect themselves against unjust accusations of poor quality because their structure emphasizes cost containment. Furthermore, payers have become adamant that plans be held accountable for the quality of the services they provide. For both of these reasons, health plans take careful steps to ensure that quality standards are set, measured, and communicated to participating enrollees, providers, and purchasers. The use of report cards as a tool has already been described. Providers, like the health plans, need to ensure that the quality of care meets certain standards—their own, those of regulatory agencies, and those of the health plans with which they have relationships. In both health plans and provider settings, APNs can play key roles in identifying problems, developing solutions, and communicating results.

Resource Management

Managed care emphasizes the provision of high-quality, cost-effective care. Both health plans and providers have learned that care may be costly because of inappropriate resource use, and each has taken steps to address the problems.

Health plans have the advantage of access to provider-specific information generated from claims data. Plan staff can use this information to work with individual providers. At the provider level, too, there is growing sophistication in physician profiling. Advanced practice nurses play an important role in both cases.

REFERENCES

The Advisory Board Company. (1993b). *The grand alliance: Vertial integration strategies for physicians and health systems.* Washington, DC: Author.

The Advisory Board Company. (1998). *Future revenues: Sustainable growth strategies for America's health systems.* Washington, DC: Author.

American College of Cardiology. (1993). *Managed care primer.* Bethesda, MD: Author.

American Hospital Association. (1993). *Transforming health care delivery: Toward community care networks.* Chicago: Author.

Bartling, A. (1995). Trends in managed care. *Healthcare Executive 10,* 3–11.

Bergman, R. (1994). Reengineering health care. *Hospitals and Health Networks 68,* 28–36.

Conrad, D. A. (1993). Coordinating patient care services in regional health systems: The challenge of clinical integration. *Journal of the Foundation of the American College of Healthcare Executives 38,* 491–507.

Burns, J., Mandelker, J., & Northrup, L. (1996). Buyers shift their focus to quality improvement. *Managed Healthcare 6,* 24–27.

Employer coalitions exert clout, affect some HMO premium rates (1998). *BNA's Managed Care Reporter 4,* 89–90.

Hallam, K. (1998). From out of the rubble. SC systems build a future of out their broken merger. *Modern Healthcare 28,* 18.

Hausner, T. (1995). Purchasing coalitions and managed care. *Managed Care Quarterly 3,* 76–88.

Hicks, L., Stallmeyer, J.M., & Coleman, J.R. (1993). *The role of the nurse in managed care.* Washington, DC: American Nurses Publishing.

Hoechst Marion Roussel Inc. (1998). *HMO-PPO/Medicare Digest.* Kansas City, MO: Author.

How the big guys rank HMOs. (1996). *Business and Health 14,* 16.

Jones, W. J. & Mayerhofer, J. J. (1994). Regional health care systems: Implications for health care reform. *Managed Care Quarterly 2,* 31–44.

Kemnitz, D. (1996). *What employers are looking for.* Paper presented at the 32nd Annual National Forum on Hospital and Health Affairs, at Duke University, Durham, NC.

Kongstvedt, P. R. (1993). *The managed care handbook* (2nd ed.). Gaithersburg, MD: Aspen Publishers.

Levit, K. R., Lazenby, H. C., & Braden, B. R. (1998). National health spending trends in 1996. National Health Accounts Team. *Health Affairs 17*(1), 35–51.

Lewin-VHI, Inc. (1993). *Managed care: Does it work?* (Report prepared by R. Atlans, D. Kennell, D. Sockel, & L. Lewin). Chicago: American Hospital Association.

Minton, E. (1998). Purchasing lessons from the feds. *Business and Health 2,* 21–28.

Morrisey, J. (1997). Quality measures hit prime time. *Modern Healthcare 27,* 66–76.

National Committee on Quality Assurance. (1993). *Health Plan Employer Data Information Set and users' manual. Version 2.0.*

New quality measures abound (1995). *Business and Health 13,* 12–17.

Presenting the first nationwide health coalition (1995). *Business and Health 13,* 13.

Robinson, J. (1998). Consolidation of medical groups into physician practice management organizations. *Journal of the American Medical Association 279,* 144–149.

Roskey, E. (1998). Managed care key to ensuring mental health parity, experts say. *BNA's Managed Care Reporter 4,* 131–133.

Rubin, I. (1991) Commentary: Organizations have to grow up. In I. Rubin & C.R. Fernandez (Eds.), *My pulse is not what it used to be.* Honolulu: The Temenos Foundation.

Satinsky, M. (1995). *An executive guide to case management strategies.* Chicago: American Hospital Publishing.

Satinsky, M. (1997). *The foundations of integrated care: Facing the challenges of change.* Chicago: American Hospital Publishing, Inc.

Senge, P. M. (1990). *The fifth discipline: The art and practice of the learning organization.* New York: Doubleday.

Shortell, S. M. (1993). Creating organized delivery systems: The barriers and facilitators. *Journal of the Foundation of the American College of Healthcare Executives 38,* 447–466.

Sokolov, J. (1996). Presentation at Private Sector Conference, Duke University Medical Center, Durham, NC.

Solovy, A. (1994). New power strategies (the battle for control). *Hospitals and Health Networks 68,* 24–34.

Walker, L. (1998). Is the gatekeeper becoming a dying breed? *Business and Health 16,* 30–36.

What's squeezing out capitation in the land of HMOs? (1998). *Executive Solutions for Healthcare Management 1,* 4–7.

Wilder, T. (1998). Veterans incorporating managed care to improve outpatient care, trim costs. *BNA's Managed Care Reporter, 4,* 89–90.

Winslow, R. (1995). "Care at HMOs to be rated by new system." *Wall Street Journal,* p. B14.

CHAPTER 9

Advance Practice Nursing in the Postacute Continuum for the Older Person

Mary Pat Rapp

The role of the advanced practice nurse (APN) in the postacute continuum has been expanded greatly with the congressional Balanced Budget Act of 1997. Effective January 1, 1998, this landmark legislation enhances the role of the APN in home care, personal care homes, assisted living and other senior congregate living arrangements, thus offering an even greater opportunity to improve management of chronic disease through interdisciplinary collaboration. The advance practice nurse (APN), with knowledge of medical management blended with expertise in nursing, augments both the traditional nursing care and medical services delivered in these settings.

This chapter will explore the role of the APN in the postacute continuum. It will describe the practical aspects of managing chronic disease conditions that can be adapted to a variety of collaborative practice models. The models themselves will demonstrate the diversity and opportunities awaiting the APN. An explanation of various payer sources will be offered in an effort to help understand how the rules and regulations affect clinical practice. Outcome studies evaluating the clinical effectiveness of the various practice models will be presented. Finally, the use of readily available data will be discussed in relation to clinical outcomes and productivity.

Defining Chronicity

American medical care carries a tradition of diagnosing acute illness early on, relieving symptoms, and developing a cure. Historically, physician reimbursement has been weighted toward procedures, giving less credit to the cognitive activities of diagnosis, planning, and follow-up needed to help the patient manage a disease process over time.

Nurses have been part of the medical intervention team with a focus on maximizing the environment to promote healing. Even with the holistic view characteristic of nursing care, the emphasis has been on recovery and healing in the acute phase of illness. Disease conditions such as hypertension, which are rarely cured, have been treated as episodic illnesses. The consequence has been costly to the entire healthcare system.

Curtin and Lubkin (1998) have described acute illness as the human experience of a disease with an abrupt onset, and when treated results in resolution of symptoms and recovery to baseline activity. The authors compare acute illness to the "unexpected visitor who leaves one's house after a short-term visit" (p. 3). In contrast, chronic illness lingers indefinitely, gradually becoming integrated into the personality of the individual and the surrounding environment.

The challenge of chronic disease is maintaining function and optimal health in the face of exacerbation and remission of signs and symptoms of the disease. Chronic disease will often complicate the management of episodic acute illness. Distinguishing the exacerbation of a chronic illness from a new, acute, unrelated problem can be difficult. The medical treatment of any long-term illness must be carefully monitored and evaluated while the individual wishes of the patient are honored. A prescribed course of a chronic disease in an individual may be difficult to predict. The American Diabetes Association (1995) has identified the sequelae of unmanaged diabetes mellitus type 1 and type 2 and is beginning to demonstrate the positive outcomes of maintaining vital parameters such as plasma glucose and plasma lipids within the range of the disease-free individual.

MANAGEMENT OF CHRONIC STABLE DISEASE

APNs may be the first provider to diagnose a new condition; however, in the older adult it is just as likely the patient will be returning for follow-up care of previously diagnosed medical problems. The discipline of nursing, with its emphasis on human response to health and disease and the expanded role of the advance practice nurse, has the potential to rein in the devastating consequences of diseases that have been diagnosed and poorly controlled.

The literature regarding clinical practice guidelines for follow-up of chronic stable disease is beginning to emerge and has been associated with a reduction in hospital days and improved functional status for patients with congestive heart failure (Collins, Butler, Gueldner, & Palmer, 1997; Kornowski, Zeeli, & Averbuch, 1995; Rich et al., 1995). Near-normal glycemic control in diabetes mellitus type 1, integrated with a behavioral plan for exercise and nutrition, has shown to delay and minimize long-term vascular effects (American Diabetes Association, 1995). The American Diabetes Association (1995) is hopeful that a chronic disease management plan for diabetes mellitus type 2 focusing on normalizing glycemic control may delay the onset of nephropathy, neuropathy, retinopathy, and cardiovascular effects in the older adult as well. These and other published guidelines suggest that middle-age and older adults who take part in longitudinal follow-up studies with a carefully designed management plan may maximize their chances of staying healthy and maintaining functional status longer. The evaluation aspects of chronic illness follow-up include inquiry regarding functional status and how the patient is handling the practical aspects of the disease such as diet, exercise, and medications. The goals of therapy should be reviewed, and if problems are identified, they should be addressed. It is important not to ignore the social and emotional impact on the patient and others in the social environment. An appropriate interim health history and a focused physical examination may uncover early complications of the disease while offering the APN another opportunity to provide anticipatory guidance and disease-specific education. Diagnostic studies to monitor aspects of the disease not accessible through the history and physical examination should follow a deliberate schedule. Drug levels and blood chemistry tests can substantiate the patient's perception of how they are managing the illness and offer an objective view of the stability of the disease. Special diagnostic tests such as electrocardiogram, echocardiogram, computerized tomography, or arterial Doppler to evaluate a new symptom can be ordered as necessary for symptom evaluation.

Medically complex patients with more than one disease may need more frequent follow-up examinations. The APN may want to encourage more frequent visits for those with questionable social and environmental supports and the inability to monitor significant changes (Box 9-1).

Box 9-1	*Stable Disease Management Plan: Diabetes Mellitus Type 2*

EVERY 2 TO 3 MONTHS:

▪ Focused interim history
  Ability to deal with illness, i.e., exercise, diet, home glucose monitoring
  Frequency, causes, and severity of hypoglycemia or hyperglycemia
  Signs and symptoms of late complications, i.e., angina, exercise intolerance, dizzi
      ness, changes in sensation, change in functional status
  Review home blood glucose monitoring results
  Adjustments made in the therapeutic plan
  Current medications and other health concerns
▪ Physical examination
  Blood pressure, pulse, and weight
  Any system with a previously abnormal examination should be repeated
  HEENT: fundi, periodically with dilation or referral to ophthalmology
  CV: murmurs, clicks, rhythm; lower extremity examination for peripheral vascular changes
  Skin: especially lower extremity and feet for sensation, and skin condition
  Neurological: Cranial nerves, cerebellar testing, reflexes

EVERY 3 MONTHS (OR AS NECESSARY FOR NON–INSULIN-TREATED PATIENTS)

▪ Diagnostics
  Glycosylated hemoglobin
  Fasting plasma glucose to test accuracy of home monitoring system
  Every 6 to 12 months
  Urinalysis
  Microalbuminuria test
  BUN
  Serum creatinine
  Total cholesterol, fasting triglycerides, HDL cholesterol, and LDL cholesterol
▪ If symptoms develop
  Electrocardiogram or exercise ECG
  Lower extremity arterial Doppler study

 ## Communication Across the Continuum of Care

APNs with expertise in nursing and educated in the medical model are in a unique position to interface with both nursing and medicine in the postacute environment. Nurses have a long tradition of serving the elderly both in the home and institutional living facilities. Nurses, with a holistic view of the patient and environment, are the most qualified professionals for integrating the complex needs of the frail elderly in the postacute continuum.

Primary care physicians—especially family practitioners and internal medicine specialists—comprise the bulk of physicians who manage the care of the frail elderly in the home and nursing facility (NF) settings. A survey of members of the American Medical Association reported by Katz, Karuza, Kolassa, and Huston (1997) found that only 23% of all physicians and 33.3% of primary care physicians cared for NF patients and that the time allotted for NF visits averaged 2 hours per week. Reasons cited for the lack of physician involvement in these environments have included the difficulty and hassle of communicating with nurses in the institutional and other postacute settings. Physicians cite 24-hour-per-day phone calls for events regardless of the severity of the condition, a lack of a system to triage telephone calls, resulting in multiple calls daily from one agency or facility, and insufficient assessment skills by the nurses making the calls (Kane, 1993). An examination of NF calls by Catogan, Franzi, and Osterweil (1998) found the facilities place approximately 2 to 4 calls per month per patient to the physician. An analysis of telephone calls from skilled NFs by Fowkes, Christenson, and McKay (1997) found that acute illness accounted for only 5% of all calls, and skilled NFs placed approximately five calls per month per patient. In a study by Kane, Dennik-Champion, and Willis (1993) involving two community-based NFs, nurses spent an average of 3.2 hours per day contacting physicians by telephone.

A comparison of the medical model and the nursing process used by RNs, contrasted with that used by licensed vocational/practical nurses (LVN/LPNs), seen in Table 9-1, helps explain the particular communication challenges encountered when information is imparted.

The medical model characteristically begins with the chief symptom, which initiates the process of weighing the probabilities of the particular diagnosis. The flow of the process stems from the presenting symptom to the affected system(s). Clinical reasoning is based on the presenting pathology, an impression of the constellation of signs and symptoms, and the probability of a particular diagnosis (Barondess & Carpenter, 1994).

In their approach to the patient, RNs use the medical diagnosis as one piece of data in the entire assessment. RNs gather data to assess the human response to health, using a global, holistic approach. Basic professional nursing education is designed to teach physical examination of body systems while incorporating the psychological, cultural, and social milieu of the patient. Advance practice nursing education introduces the concept of differential diagnosis through symptom analysis. The LVN/LPN is educated in the nursing model with a focus on data collection and communication to the RN or physician. As with the RN, the data gathering is usually holistic. In the nursing model, the RN synthesizes the assessment data to determine the nursing diagnosis.

Nurses and physicians speak the language of the patient in health and disease, but they do so with different dialects. These similar but very different approaches challenge communication across disciplines. When the nurse calls a physician about a change in condi-

TABLE 9-1 *The Dialects of Medicine and Nursing*

Medical Model Physician	Nursing Process Registered Nurse	Nursing Process Licensed Vocational/Practical Nurse
Chief symptom	Assessment	Data collection
History of present illness	Physical	Inspection
Past medical, surgical, family, and social history	Psychological	Auscultation
Review of systems	Social	Report findings to: registered nurse physician
Physical examination	Cultural	
Assessment	Nursing diagnosis	Delegated implementation
Plan	Plan	Supervised evaluation
	Implementation	
	Evaluation	

tion, assessment data may include information from the global domains of physiology, psychology, social environment, and culture. The physician will be asking for specific symptoms and a related history in order to understand the constellation of physical signs and symptoms that lead to the appropriate diagnosis, and thus order treatment. Nurses unfamiliar with the process of differential diagnosis may give information regarded as irrelevant by the physician, impart data not related to the symptom, or fail to assess for symptoms that may assist in diagnosing. Physicians have cited lack of assessment skills and poor communication of information regarding an acute change in condition as a reason for hospitalization of the NF patient (Kayser-Jones, Weiner, & Barbaccia, 1989). Clearly, there is room for closing the communication gap.

APNs are the bridge to communication in the postacute arena (see Figure 9-1). The APN is able to coalesce findings from the nursing assessment and the symptom-focused physical examination. In the event of minor acute illness or chronic stable disease, the APN may function autonomously and intervene without physician consultation. In the event of an unstable acute change in condition, the APN is prepared to perform a symptom-based assessment, formulate a differential diagnosis, and present the case to the collaborating physician in a concise, cogent fashion. The skill of the APN enhances the interface for both nursing and medicine.

Settings of Care in the Postacute Continuum

The goals of acute care for the elderly are to diagnose, treat, and prevent complications of hospitalization. With the exception of prevention of complications, these are primarily medical functions. In contrast, Kane, Ouslander, and Abrass (1994) have suggested that the goals in postacute care include providing a safe living environment, maximizing functional performance, preserving autonomy and quality of life, providing comfort measures at the end of life, stabilizing acute and chronic conditions, and finally, preventing hospitalization. The ability of APNs to blend the medical model with the nursing model uniquely qualifies them for the chronic care environment.

HOME CARE

Prior to January 1998, skilled nursing services provided by RNs and delegated to LVN/LPNs were the only nursing services covered by Medicare to the homebound elderly. APNs employed by a home health agency were not necessarily excluded, but their services for traditional medical management were covered only in rural areas. The Balanced Budget Act of 1997 specifies that services by the APN for medical management in the home and assisted living environments are covered, regardless of geographic location. This is a welcome change for APNs who recognize the opportunity to expand services to the homebound elderly and participate in wellness programs that are incorporated into the structure of many assisted living environments. The Physicians' Current Procedural Terminology Manual (1998) lists evaluation and management codes for home settings. Additional Care Plan Oversight codes allow the provider to congregate supervisory home care services in order to be paid for the time spent on care without the patient's presence. The patient must be eligible for home healthcare as defined in Medicare Part B services. Included in Care Plan Oversight is the review of care plans developed by home health agencies, subsequent reports of patient status, diagnostic study results, and communication with other healthcare professionals involved in the patient's care. The decision making required to integrate the information to formulate the plan of care or adjust medical therapy is included. The number of the minutes spent on non–face-to-face activities per month must be accurately documented in order to meet the requirements of these codes. The docu-

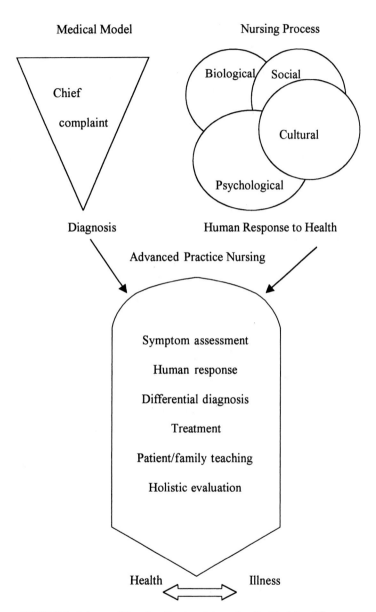

FIGURE 9-1 Advanced Practice Nursing: Integrating the Model and Process.

mentation requirements for Care Plan Oversight may be burdensome and inconvenient for some practitioners. The rules stipulate only one provider may report oversight services for a given period of time, thus making sharing of call responsibilities or a team approach difficult. Coverage of Care Plan Oversight may be carrier-specific; therefore, the APN will need to contact the local carrier to determine if services are covered.

ASSISTED LIVING

The American Association of Homes and Services for the Aging (AAHSA, 1998) defines assisted living as a "program that provides and/or arranges for the provision of daily meals, personal and other supportive services, healthcare and 24-hour oversight to persons residing in a group residential facility who need assistance with activities of daily living." The philosophy of most assisted living facilities is based on a social model that is consumer-driven, flexible, and individualized while maximizing consumer independence and dignity.

The profile of the assisted living resident is one who needs some assistance with the basic activities of daily living (ADLs), but who does not require 24-hour skilled nursing care and medical oversight. The settings are designed to be home-like, and resemble private apartments. Assisted living residences may be free-standing or part of a comprehensive continuum of care.

Services are provided to the resident through one of two models, direct services or contracted services. The facility staff members in the direct service model provide assistance with ADLs. States usually require licensure in this environment. In a contracted service model, the facility contracts with a home health agency to provide the personal care services. Personal care services for ADLs are not a covered service under Medicare; thus this would be an out-of-pocket expense for the individual. Because the facility is not providing any direct care to the resident, it does not have to be licensed in the contracted service model. Because the care attendants are not employees of the facility, supervision of them becomes a greater challenge in the contracted service model.

There are no federal regulations governing assisted living. State licensure laws typically address structural design, staffing requirements, and types of services delivered. The care emphasis in these environments is wellness and health promotion within a social model. Assisted living facilities have resisted attempts to introduce medical standards of care or require physician oversight, fearing the regulations may "overmedicalize" the environment at the expense of innovation and creativity.

The interface of the APN in this setting is similar to the home environment. There are no formal rules in assisted living facilities for maintenance of medical records; therefore, the APN will need to develop a system to document visits that is accessible and portable. As in the home, arranging for delivery of new prescriptions or changes to the plan of care may become the responsibility of patient and/or the family. Domiciliary, rest home, or custodial care service current procedural terminology (CPT) codes are appropriate here.

PROVIDING CARE IN THE NURSING FACILITIES

Nursing facilities (NFs) have the option of participating in Medicaid, Medicare, Veterans' Affairs contracts, and private pay—singly or in combination. All the facility beds or a designated number of beds may be allocated to each program. The regulations of each program differ in regards to APNs. Facilities participating in Medicaid follow the rules of the Health Care Financing Administration (HCFA) outlined in the Omnibus Budget Reconciliation Act 1987 (OBRA 87). Routine physician visits, covered by Medicare Part B, with Medicaid and private insurance supplemental, are required by OBRA 87 every 30 days for the first 90 days, and every 60 days thereafter. Under OBRA 87 rules, the APN may substitute for every other required physician visit. The federal rules offer individual states the option to waive the physician visit requirement and allow the APN to substitute for all physician visits in the Medicaid program. An unlimited number of medically necessary visits to evaluate an acute change in condition are covered when performed by either the physician or the APN. Medicare will cover 1.5 routine patient visits per month if one of the visits is performed by an APN who is a team member in a physician group practice. Skilled nursing facilities (SNF) participating in Medicare Part A are also regulated under OBRA 87. During the Medicare Part A stay, which is typically less than 100 days, APNs may substitute for every other required physician visit after the physician's initial visit. Individual states do not have the option of allowing the APN to substitute for all physician visits in the Medicare Part A skilled NF stay. In addition to substituting for every other routine visit, APNs can conduct medically necessary visits that will be covered by Medicare. HCFA requires that the initial physician visit must occur within 30 days of admission. Individual states and facilities participating in the Joint Commission for Accreditation of Health Care Organizations (JCAHO) may have a more strict standard for the initial visit. Physician visits are required every 30 days for the first 90 days, then every 60 days thereafter. The question is often asked whether or not the APN can perform the admission history and physical prior to the initial physician visit under the Medicare Part A SNF stay. The answer is "yes" because this would qualify as a medically necessary visit and thus qualify as a covered service. The physician's initial visit would incorporate the work of the APN.

Many skilled NFs are electing to become accredited through JCAHO. Fortunately, the rules of this organization also allow APN substitution for physician visits. The initial visit must be made within 72 hours, and the APN may perform the initial history and physical because it becomes part of the work incorporated into the physician's initial visit. In a JCAHO-accredited dementia-specific facility or long-term acute hospital (subacute), the initial visit must be made within 24 hours.

Veterans' Affairs (VA) may operate their own NFs or contract for services with community facilities. The physician must personally examine the patient within 72 hours of admission and then routinely every 30 days. The physician services are billed to the NF, which reimburses the physician on a fee-for-service basis. Coverage and recognition of the services of the APN will vary from location to location.

NFs electing to serve only private-pay patients are termed licensed-only facilities. They are not regulated by OBRA 87 but abide by state-specific licensing rules and regulations. Typically, the regulations are less stringent. Requirements for physician visits may vary, as does the recognition of the APN.

APNs have a valuable contribution to make in improving the care and outcomes of NF residents. Burl, Bonner, Rao, and Khan (1998) have documented the unique and valuable contribution of APNs to the interdisciplinary team in this environment. The nursing expertise of APNs and their ability to effectively solve problems, mentor other nurses, and act as liaison with medicine has been crucial to their success. The roles and responsibilities for the APN in this setting will be determined by federal and state regulations regarding physician requirements, the skills and career ambitions of the APN, and the role negotiated with the physician and the facility.

Clinical responsibilities of the APN outlined by Ouslander, Osterweil, and Morley (1997) in the NF may include primary care in collaboration with the attending physician and a consulting role as a resource to implement the Resident Assessment Instrument, which is a comprehensive interdisciplinary functional assessment required for all NF patients. Acting as a consultant to interdisciplinary team members and families, the APN is able to discuss medical care, to explain advance directives, and to assist in setting goals of care.

Ouslander, Osterweil, and Morley (1997) support the use of the APN to augment the role of the medical director. The APN can participate in quality assurance activities and facility committees, help develop policies and procedures, and assist in the employee health program. The APN is a valuable resource for educational programs involving in-service education for the staff, presentations to families and residents, and formal education programs for nursing and medical students. Hopefully, research activities to facilitate the implementation of studies, assist with data collection, and design and conduct independent clinical projects will be supported.

Understanding the clinical responsibilities in the NF and designing tools to maximize productivity will assist in organizing practice in the NF (Ouslander, Osterweil, & Morley, 1997). The reader is referred to the information in Boxes 9-2 and 9-3 for suggested formats for annual and routine visits designed to meet the expected visit requirements for NF patients.

Management of telephone calls is imperative in order for the APN to manage time and productivity effectively. As alluded to earlier, the facility nurses may lack the necessary skills to determine the appropriate timeliness of the calls, assess, and subsequently communicate an acute change in condition. Federal guidelines stipulate that the physician must be notified immediately if an acute change of condition occurs; however, facilities often notify physicians immediately of any change in condition, regardless of the urgency. The APN, along with the attending physician, can develop guidelines for physician notification as shown in Table 9-2 and discussed in Ouslander, Osterweil, and Morley (1997).

Development of such a policy requires agreement on the parameters by the medical director, other attending physicians, the APN, the facility director of nursing, and the facility administrator. Once a policy is developed, the APN can be expected to offer in-service education regarding the policy and procedure. The time devoted to support, mentoring, and gentle reminders when telephone calls are placed inappropriately will help ensure suc-

---

Box 9-2   *Sample SOAP Note for Nursing Facility Patients*

- Subjective
  New complaints
  Symptoms related to active medical problems
  Reports from nursing staff, i.e., behavior, functional status
  Progress in rehabilitative therapies if relevant
  Reports from consultants, other team members
- Objective
  General appearance
  Weight and vital signs
  Abnormal and relevant negative physical findings related to the new complaint and/or
    active medical problems
  Diagnostic data
- Assessment
  Presumptive diagnoses of new complaints
  Stability of active medical problems
  Response to interventions
- Plan
  Changes in medications
  Nursing interventions
  Consults by other disciplines
  Diagnostic studies
  Discharge planning

Adapted from: Ouslander & Osterweil (1994).

Box 9-3	*Format for Annual History and Physical: Nursing Facility Patient*

Active medical problem list
Description of acute medical conditions in the past year, and diagnostic tests done to monitor active problems, symptoms relevant to active medical problems
Symptom review
Physical examination, noting specific abnormal and relevant negative findings
Functional status
Social status
Health maintenance: review results of screening evaluations by other disciplines
Screening diagnostic tests
Advance directive, healthcare proxy
Plans

Adapted from: Ouslander & Osterweil (1994).

TABLE 9-2 *Physician Notification Summary: When to Call the Doctor*

Condition	Immediate	Nonimmediate (next office day)
Acute change in mental status	Sudden onset of change in mental status	Gradual change in responsiveness
Decreased oral fluid intake	Drinking less than 50% of fluids in previous 24 hours	Persistent symptoms for more than 24 hours in spite of nursing intervention
	More than one episode of vomiting in 24 hours	
Fall/Injury	Obvious deformity of extremity	No injury, or minor bruise, or skin tear
	Inability to bear weight	Increased frequency of falls in 24–72-hour period
	New onset abnormal neurological status	
	Laceration with uncontrolled bleeding	
Complete blood count	WBC > 12,000 with change of condition	WBC > 10,000 without symptoms or fever
	Hb < 8.0 mg/dl	
	Hct < 24	
	Platelets < 50,000	
Urinalysis	Abnormal results in someone with signs and symptoms; i.e., fever, burning, pain, altered mental status	Abnormal urinalysis results in someone without signs and symptoms
Weight loss		5% or more in 30 days
		10% or more in 6 months

Used with permission from: Texas Nurses Association/Foundation (1996).

Box 9-4	*Telephone Assessment Guide*

Name of patient
Vital signs, advance directives
Characteristics of the symptom
Course of the illness
    Ability to maintain posture
    Ability to drink fluids
    Ability to eat the usual diet
    Mental alertness
Onset
Location of the symptoms
Aggravating factors
Relieving factors
History
Allergies
Medications
Recent laboratory work

Adapted from: Rapp & Rapp (1996). Used with permission.

cess. Use of a telephone symptom assessment guide such as the one in Box 9-4 may be helpful as a reference to the nurse placing the call.

The use of a form (Box 9-5) for facsimile transmission of nonurgent communication is another tool to consider using. The advantage is that the nurse can report the nonurgent condition any time of day, thereby increasing the likelihood that the nurse noticing the change is also the one reporting it. Another advantage is that it can also eliminate calls from ancillary personnel, such as the consulting dietician and consulting pharmacist. Because the APN will have documentation from the facility regarding a change in condition, it may be appropriate to upgrade the subsequent visit to intermediate in follow-up. Voice mail is another time-conserving measure to consider. The majority of telephone calls from facilities are routine notification messages (Fowkes, Christenson, & McKay, 1997), with approximately 30% requiring a provider response. Voice mail messages can be accessed throughout the day, with the APN returning necessary telephone calls when convenient. For after-hours communication, arranging to have the on-call number forwarded to the cellular telephone of the person on call eliminates the time consumed in waiting for the nurse who placed the call to come to the telephone.

Standardized procedures or protocols have been shown to be effective in reducing telephone calls for nonurgent events and also standardizing care for commonly occurring events (Cadogan, Franzi, & Osterweil, 1998; Kane, 1993; Rapp, Rapp, & Kyba, 1998). The Texas Nurses Association/Foundation (TNA) (1996) has written 25 protocols designed to guide the RN as well as the LVN/LPN through the assessment and appropriate physician notification. See Box 9-6 for an example of the unexpected weight loss protocol.

Included in each protocol are standardized orders to address the problem. Rapp, Rapp, and Kybe (1998) and Cadogan, Franzi, and Osterweil (1998) have observed that this system requires a commitment from the medical director, administrator, the facility owner, and the director of nurses. The APN devoting time and energy to the nursing system in the facility can contribute to improving the care of its frail elderly residents.

Box 9-5	*Best Practices Nursing Facility Fax Form for Nonimmediate Communication*

Nursing Section

Return Fax to:

Name	Station	Date/Time
Blood pressure	Temperature	Pulse　　　Respirations

Physician/APN:

Concern and Nursing Assessment

Laboratory Notification: Include medications related to the test

What were the previous lab results for this test?

Allergies	Pertinent Medications

Physician/APN Response Requested　☐ Yes　☐ No, this is for notification only

Nurse Signature

Physician/APN Section

Physician/APN Order and Diagnosis

Physician/APN Signature/Date

Adapted from: Rapp & Rapp (1996). Used with permission.

Delivery Models for Long-term Care

INTERDISCIPLINARY TEAMS

As changes in the healthcare system have occurred, new models of care delivery for the community dwelling frail elderly have emerged. The long-term goals of these programs are to provide cost-effective care that maximizes community services, prevents avoidable exacerbation and complications of chronic disease, promotes health, and optimizes functioning. The HMO Workgroup on Care Management (1998) suggests the Medicare fee-for-service model of patient-initiated visits, symptom relief, and treatment to cure is becoming outmoded. Boult and colleagues (1998) recommend comprehensive geriatric assessment be accompanied by treatment from the evaluation team because of a high failure rate to follow recommendations for treatment if the encounter is restricted to evaluation. Summarized by Collins, Butler, Gueldner, and Palmer (1997) and identified by the HMO Workgroup

Box 9-6	*Unexpected Weight Loss*

Unexpected Weight Loss

Definition: Unexpected weight loss of 5% or greater in the past 1 month, or 10% or greater in 6 months

Assessment: CIRCLE positive findings, add additional findings as indicated

Does the resident complain of any?
- Taste alterations, nausea, indigestion, vomiting, diarrhea, hunger, absence of hunger, oral pain, ill-fitting dentures

Are there any contributing factors?
- Therapeutic diet: _____ Tube feeding: Formula _____ Rate _____
- Medications to alter taste; chemotherapy, digoxin, diuretics, antidepressants
- Chronic obstructive pulmonary disease, shortness of breath with increased calorie need, fear of choking
- Recent hospitalization

Inspect:
- Oral examination for ill-fitting dentures, poor dentition, mouth lesions
- Swallowing: coughs, chokes, no difficulty, tube fed
- Summary of dietary record for the past month _____
- ADLS: new inability to feed self, inattentiveness, wandering during meals, increased amount of time needed to eat a meal
- Change in mental status, new onset: confusion, sleepiness, inability to maintain posture, agitation
- Other conditions: pressure ulcer(s), edema, constipation, infection

Measure: Finger stick blood sugar --

Plan/Goal: Weight gain as appropriate and practical within resident's plan of care

Implementation

Notify the physician, NP, PA, or CNS immediately by phone or beeper of: Time of notification _____ Initials _____ • Finger stick blood sugar over 430 with sliding scale or machine reads HI; over 300 and no sliding scale; less than 70 in diabetic; or less than 50 in anyone _____ *unless values are consistently at this level	**Notify physician, NP, PA, or CNS on or by next working day of: (may use fax, e-mail, voice mail, etc.)** • Weight loss of greater than 5% in 1 month, and greater than 10% in 6 months • To request albumin, transferrin level if not done in 10 days • Dietary evaluation and recommendation • Pharmacy evaluation and recommendation

Proceed with Physician Orders

Action
- Supervise all meals and snacks
- Add nutritional supplement
- Offer nourishment every 2 hours while awake until weight is achieved or weight stabilized
- Offer juice or nutritional supplement with medications unless contraindicated

Monitor
- Calorie count for 3 days
- Weight every week until weight stabilizes
- If diabetic, finger stick blood sugar 30 minutes before meals and at hours of sleep; if tube fed, do every 6 hours.

Consult
- Dietary for calorie count, evaluation, recommendation
- Pharmacist (within 30 days) for anorexic side effects of medications
- Add weight loss to care plan
- Family or responsible party for change in condition

Evaluation: Resolved when: 1. Dietary intake has increased and 2. Weight stabilized at appropriate level

Documentation: Record assessment, implementation, evaluation

TNA Long Term Care Protocols 1996. Used with permission.

on Care Management (1998), the components of innovative comprehensive care delivery systems for the elderly include liberal wellness programs, provision of care at home, and targeting the impoverished or underserved. Long-term goals emphasize maximizing functioning and quality of life. One community-based program, On Lok Program of All-Inclusive Care for the Elderly (PACE) (Kunz & Shannon, 1996), has demonstrated success in care management for the frail and vulnerable adult. PACE has reduced overall costs through medication reduction, fewer hospitalizations, and financial support of family caregivers. The PACE model of care pools Medicare and Medicaid funds to provide comprehensive services through interdisciplinary teams (Eng et al., 1997). Frail older adults who are at risk for hospitalization and institutionalization are specifically targeted for services. Originally allowed as waiver programs, PACE models were granted Medicare provider status with the Balanced Budget Act of 1997. States have the individual option to include PACE as a benefit.

The APN is uniquely prepared to contribute to these teams in a variety of roles because of expertise in clinical practice, ability to function in the case manager role, and individual experience in program administration. Responsibilities that the interdisciplinary team has to educate the members of the team and surrounding service community as well as patients and families can be borne by the APN.

NURSING FACILITY MODELS

Traditional Physician/Advance Practice Collaboration Model

In the traditional model of care, the physician or physician practice employs the APN and enters a collaborative relationship for medical management of patients. The APN may develop a patient base in the office setting or choose to treat patients only under "incident to" service. The APN and physician share the NF responsibilities and usually negotiate a call schedule to cover the NF. Responsibilities for hospital care, i.e., admission history and physical, daily progress notes, discharge planning, and the discharge summary, may be included in the job description.

A Nursing Facility As an Employer

With the advent of prospective pay in Medicare SNFs, there may be a desire for greater nursing expertise in patient assessments. The comprehensive functional assessment based on the Minimum Data Set (Norris, Hawes, Murphy, & Nonemaker, 1993) will be linked to a prospective payment system for reimbursement for Medicare Part A SNF stays. Nurses skilled in performing the assessments accurately will be in demand. If the attending physicians approve, the APN employed by the facility can make medically necessary visits to evaluate and manage acute changes in condition. The facility is able to bill for these services under Medicare Part B, thus partially covering the cost of the APN salary. As a facility employee, the APN may not act as a substitute for any regulatory physician required visits. Additional responsibilities may include taking first call for off-hours patient concerns. Relief from nursing home calls would most likely be attractive to the attending physicians in the facility.

Physician Practice/Facility Collaboration Model

NFs with a goal to maintain census and improve care may want to consider a model that combines the traditional physician/APN practice style with the NF as employer model. In this model, the APN is employed by the physician or a physician practice but is assigned to one or two facilities to visit on a daily basis. The primary care responsibilities for the practice remain, but with negotiation with other attendings, the APN may complete medically necessary visits as well as regulatory required visits for the physician. Because the practice bills for the visits and not the facility, the APN is able to alternate required visits with the attending physician. The model naturally necessitates establishing a trusting relationship with other attending physicians, the patient, and the families. Once again, the attraction to the primary care physicians may be the relief of call. Families will likely appreciate the ready availability of an assessment of an acute change in condition. By detecting changes in condition early, hospitalization may be reduced.

Health Maintenance Organizations

Health Maintenance Organizations (HMOs) targeting the Medicare population are developing systems to maximize the use of the APN to meet goals of promoting health, preventing illness, and reducing hospitalization. HMOs have three levels of involvement to consider in a relationship with Medicare. First, they can elect to accept full risk and receive a capitated rate for the enrollee. Second, they can be paid allocated costs for all Medicare services or only those from Medicare Part B. Third, Medigap policies are available to supplement Medicare through the HMO.

HMOs assuming full risk are highly motivated to reduce hospitalization days, the most expensive component of care. Provider groups (Fama & Fox, 1997) have demonstrated a reduction in hospitalization using a physician/APN model for service delivery. The model adopted by The Fallon Clinic (Burl, Bonner, Rao, & Khan 1998) typifies the relationship of the APN/physician team in the NF. The APN has a patient census of 100 to 150 in 1 to 3 facilities and is responsible for the initial and annual history and physical examination, episodic examinations, family conferences, and formal and informal education of facility staff. The physician and APN visit jointly within 7 to 10 days to review the findings, discuss the care plan, and if possible, meet with the family. The physician is responsible for routine visits every 60 days. The APN and physician often share call responsibilities.

Paying for Healthcare

The primary sources of payment for healthcare for the elderly are federally funded and state-funded sources, private insurance, and out-of-pocket expenses. Rarely considered in the expenditures are the vast array of nonfunded resources such as family caregivers and informal support networks in religious organizations and neighborhood watches.

FEDERAL PROGRAMS FOR THE ELDERLY

Medicare and Medicaid in combination are the largest payers for healthcare for the elderly (Ouslander, Osterweil, & Morley , 1994). Medicare Part A, which pays full coverage for in-patient hospital care after a deductible, is available for all persons eligible for Social Security and others with chronic disabilities, such as end-stage renal failure. Medicare has shifted from a cost-based system to a prospective payment system in which the payment for the hospitalization is based on the patient's hospital diagnosis. Since July 1998, a per diem rate has been initiated to pay for Medicare Part A skilled nursing facility (SNF) care, including hospital-based units and those located in community NFs. The payment will be based on the minimum data set assessment and the rate for hospital SNFs will be the same as community facilities. Services provided by the physician and/or APN is specifically excluded in this per diem rate.

Medicare Part B is an elective supplemental insurance available to those covered under Part A. Participants pay a monthly premium for physician services, supplies and services related to physician services, rehabilitation therapies, diagnostic tests and procedures, radiographs, prosthetics, and ambulance services. Unless specified in the individual policy, medications are not covered under Medicare Part B. Participants pay an annual deductible and a 20% copayment. The service of the APN is reimbursed through Medicare Part B if that service is one traditionally covered as a physician service.

Medicaid is federal funding for healthcare that is administered by the states individually. Eligibility criteria vary from state to state, but Medicaid is usually available to the poor and/or chronically disabled. The patient spends assets until eligible, and there are no copayments. Medicaid must provide inpatient hospital services, SNF care, a limited amount of home healthcare, and laboratory tests and radiographs. A majority of NF care is funded through the Medicaid program. States can limit the amount and duration of services for dental care, medications, home healthcare, NF care, eyeglasses, prosthetics, and medical transportation. Reimbursement for services provided by the APN is state-specific.

Title III of the Older Americans Act is available to all persons 60 years of age and older; targeted populations are low-income, minority, and isolated older adults. Some payment may be requested based on income. Services include homemaker services, home-delivered meals, transportation, legal services, counseling, information and referral, and an array of other services.

OUT-OF-POCKET EXPENSES

Many elderly persons purchase supplemental insurance, or "Medigap policies," to cover the costs of healthcare not paid for under Medicare. By covering deductibles, copayments, and often prescription drugs, these policies reduce the financial risk associated with healthcare. Additional out-of-pocket expenses include dental care, vision services, over-the-counter medications, and some assistive devices.

MEDICARE REIMBURSEMENT FOR THE ADVANCE PRACTICE NURSE

Medicare Part B will reimburse the APN for covered services, provided certain conditions are met. The services must be considered traditional physician services, be performed by a person who meets the definition of an APN, be performed in collaboration with a physician, be a service that is not otherwise excluded from coverage by law, and be allowed to be performed by an APN. Advance practice nursing services are covered regardless of the place or setting. Collaboration is defined as APN services rendered within the scope of practice of the APN and provided in combination with medical direction and supervision as required by state law (Moore, 1998).

To bill for Medicare services, the APN applies to the Medicare carrier for a performing provider number. APNs may bill Medicare directly under their own provider number or reassign their billing to their employer. The APN must reassign billing rights to the physician practice that hires or contracts with them for services. All APN services are reimbursed at 80% of the billed amount or 85% of the allowable charge, whichever is lower. "Incident to" services are reimbursed at 100% of the physician fee schedule, using the physician's provider number. To meet the "incident to" criteria, the physician must physically be in the same office suite or NF wing as the APN at the time the service is rendered. The APN must be employed by a physician or a physicians' group and not be an independent contractor. Finally, the physician must have initiated the course of treatment for the condition the APN is monitoring, and the physician must be involved in the course of treatment on an ongoing basis. Deciding to bill separately or "incident to" is a matter to discuss with the physician. If the APN and physician meet the criteria for "incident to," there is no reason to unnecessarily discount the services.

In the event the service is provided as part of a team in the NF, the practitioner will use a modifier to identify which member of the team performed the visit. Nurse practitioners use the "AL" modifier for the urban setting and "AK" to designate rural settings. Clinical nurse specialists use an "AY" modifier.

MEDICARE BILLING

The introduction of the resource-based relative value scale (RBRVS) has increased the value of nonprocedural services that typify primary care. Published and updated annually by the American Medical Association (AMA), the explanation of evaluation and management (E&M) and other procedural codes are found in the Physicians' Current Procedural Terminology (CPT) Manual (1998). The codes were developed for Medicare claims; however, Medicaid and private insurance companies have adopted these billing codes. Although APNs may perform some procedures, i.e., cerumen removal, suturing of lacerations, simple cystometrogram, the majority of services will be for evaluation and management. The E&M codes recognize seven components of a patient encounter: history, examination, medical decision making, counseling, coordination of care, nature of the presenting problem, and time. The history, examination, and decision making are considered the key components and most often used to determine the level of service. The history includes the chief symptom, history of present illness, review of systems, and past, family, and social history. Eleven systems are recognized for the physical examination. Examination guidelines include a general multisystem examination most often used in primary care and additional in-depth examinations of a single system. Decision making depends on several factors including the number of diagnoses and management options, amount or complexity of data, and risk of complications. To use the comprehensive examination codes, all three components—history, examination, and decision making—must be addressed. Follow-up visits and subsequent care require only two of the three components. Documentation must substantiate the level of visit coded. Specific codes are used, depending on the place of service, i.e., office, NF, assisted living, or home. Table 9-4 references the documentation requirements for the level of service provided.

New documentation guidelines for the E&M codes developed by the HCFA and the AMA were published in January 1998, with an implementation date of July 1998. Because of physician concerns regarding the complexity of the documentation required, the new documentation guidelines were put on hold indefinitely in June 1998. Practitioners are to continue to use the guidelines published in 1994 (Owen & Moore, 1995; Edsall & Moore, 1995a,b,c).

✺ *Outcome Evaluation Studies in the Postacute Continuum*

APNs share common goals of compassion for the patient and effectiveness in practice. Quality, variously defined as adherence to standards of practice that result in fewer hospital admissions or a reduction in complications of disease, is threatened as programs for the chronically ill are restructured, downsized, or unregulated (Mezey & Fulmer, 1997). Several studies based on a variety of care delivery models have evaluated their effectiveness. Evans, Yurkow, and Siegler (1995) describe an innovative nurse-managed collaborative model to improve function of frail older adults. The model is interdisciplinary with goals to maximize independence, promote health, and enhance quality of life. Medicare and other third-party payers provide funding to support the program. An APN functions as the clinical services and operations manager. For each patient, a geriatric advance practice nurse serves as care manager, coordinating, monitoring, and providing care in collaboration with the interdisciplinary team. Following physician referral, the APN does the initial screening history and physical examination, assesses healthcare status, and serves as care manager.

Medical care issues specific to the patient are discussed with the collaborating physician. Using the Functional Independence Measure (Forer & Granger, 1987) to measure progress in rehabilitation, the program has had a positive outcome on the functional status of the participants.

Medicare HMOs have been criticized for cost-saving measures that compromise health and quality of life. Hospitalization of the frail elderly is not without hazards; thus, programs designed to reduce hospital transfers from NFs would not only save costs but also enhance quality of life.

In describing the experience of a multispecialty physician group, Burl, Bonner, Rao, and Khan (1998) report favorably on the use of a collaborative practice model with APNs. In this study of 1077 NF residents, the APN–physician teams cared for 414 patients. A patient admitted to a NF was seen by the APN within 24 to 48 hours for the admission history and physical. The initial plan was developed with the physician and discussed with the patient and family. Additional areas known to have an effect on health were addressed, i.e., functional status and psychosocial issues, polypharmacy, advance directives, healthcare proxy, and health maintenance. A cost-benefit analysis revealed costs associated with emergency department (ED) transfer and/or hospitalization were 45% lower with the APN–physician teams than with physician-only care. A small loss of $2.00 per patient per month was realized with the model. By increasing the number of patients covered by APN–physician teams and developing teams dedicated to the NF environment, this may be resolved. The assumption is that physicians and APNs whose practices are dedicated to a specialty will provide better care with lower costs.

Homebound patients may benefit from house calls. Fried, Wachtel, and Tinetti (1998) describe a program designed to target the homebound elderly who have difficulty leaving home for traditional medical care. Routine visits by physicians or APNs were scheduled every 3 to 4 months and periodic visits were made based on medical necessity. Home health agencies, families, and patients themselves called the office site to report a change in condition thought to require medical attention. Interventions aimed at curing illness and palliative care services were provided for the patients, depending on their specific wishes. An analysis of the practice demonstrated that some ED visits were eliminated as a result of the availability of the home visit. The authors concluded that the house calls program was feasible economically with reimbursement from Medicare Part B for episodic visits and Care Plan Oversight (see Exemplar 18B).

The effectiveness of the APN in a NF can be evaluated using tools that currently exist. The Resident Assessment Instrument, comprised of the Minimum Data Set and Resident Assessment Protocols, characterizes each resident's functional status while guiding the interdisciplinary care plan. The core areas assessed include activities of daily living, cognition, continence, mood, behaviors, nutritional status, vision and communication, activities, and psychosocial well-being. The Resident Assessment Protocols are comprised of 18 problem-focused, in-depth assessments used to identify treatable causes of common problems. Software programs that generate the MDS data and allow for evaluation of congregate data will allow the APN to evaluate the success of programs designed to address common problem areas such as continence and behavioral symptoms of dementia.

APNs would be remiss if they failed to evaluate productivity outcomes. In a chronic care environment, with home and institutional care, the number of visits generated daily may not accurately reflect time spent in patient encounters. A software program described by Kearnes (1992) that uses a standard spreadsheet format may be helpful in making a more accurate determination. This productivity formula compares the assigned time, according to CPT codes, to actual time devoted to patient care, thus generating a percentage for clinical productivity. High and low productivity ratings generate a practice evaluation of travel time, scheduled clinic visits, inadequate staffing, and facility-based inefficiencies.

TABLE 9-4 *Documentation Guideline Worksheet*

History

Component:	Level:	Problem-focused	Expanded problem-focused	Detailed	Comprehensive
Chief complaint Acute illness F/U past illness Fam/nurs request Regulatory requirement		Any	one	component	required
HPI		Brief	Brief	Extended	Extended
Location — Timing Quality — Severity Duration — Context Modifiers — S/S		1–3 items discussed	1–3 items discussed	4+ items or 3 chronic Stable conditions	4+ items or 3 chronic Stable conditions
ROS		NA	Problem pertinent	Extended	Complete
General — GU Eyes — MSK ENT — Neuro Resp — Psych CV — Endo GI — Skin All/Imm — Heme/ Lymph			Positives and negatives related to HPI	2–9 additional systems discussed	10+ systems addressed
Past/Fm/Soc		HxNA	NA	Pertinent 1 of 3 99343, 99349	Complete 2 of 3 (3 of 3 for initial)
Meets 1 of the criteria for:		99311, 99321, 99341, 99347	99312, 99322, 99342, 99348	99301, 99302,99313, 99323, 99331, 99332,	99303, 99333 99344, 99345, 99350

Physical

Component:	Level:	Problem-focused	Expanded problem-focused	Detailed	Comprehensive
General — GU Eyes — ENT Neck — MSK Skin — Neck Resp — Neuro GI/Abd — Psych Lymphatic Chest/Breast		1–5 affected systems addressed	6+ affected or other symptomatic systems addressed	6+ with 2 components of each affected or other symptomatic systems addressed or 12 systems with single components addressed	12 with 2 components of each system addressed 99331, 99332, 99333
Meets 1 of the criteria for:		99311, 99321, 99341, 99347	99312, 99322, 99342, 99348	99313, 99323, 99343, 99349,	99301, 99302, 99303 99344, 99345, 99350

Complexity

Component:	Level:	Straightforward	Low	Moderate	High
Presenting problem		1 self-limited illness	2+ self-limited one stable chronic or acute uncomplicated illness	1 or more chronic with exacerbation 2+ stable chronic acute c systemic S/S or acute complicated	1 or more chronic with severe exacerbation acute life-threatening or abrupt change in neuro status
Dx procedures		Venepuncture or CXR or EKG or UA, or Ultrasound	PFTs or superficial Bx/s, atrial punctures, non-CV imaging	CV stress/imaging deep Bx or –centesis endoscopies	CV imagining with contrast, endoscopies with ID'd risk
Mgt. Options		Rest, gargles, bandages, dressing	OTC, minor/s/, PT/OT, IV fluids without additives	Prescription RX, minor s/s elective major Sx, IV fluids with additives, closed red of Fx	Elective major Sx emergency major Sx decision of DNR 2nd to poor prognosis
Meets 1 of the: criteria for:		99311, 99321, 99341, 99347	99301 or 99311, 99331 99321, 99342	99302, 303, 99312, 13 99322, 23, 99332, 33, 99343, 349	99302, 99303, 99313 99332, 333, 323, 99344, 345, 350

Final Coding

99301–3, 99321–3, 99341–45	Must	Meet	3 of 3	Criteria
99311–3, 99331–3, 99347–50	Must	Meet	2 of 3	Criteria

APNs will continue to contribute to the health and welfare of chronically ill and frail older adults. Innovative models representing research-based practice will inspire others to refine the models and create others. Barriers to practice such as physician acceptance and lack of adequate reimbursement will continue to disappear as APNs document positive outcomes affecting health and the economics of practice.

CASE STUDY

Mrs. Smith, age 67, was diagnosed with type 2 diabetes mellitus 6 years ago. She does a finger stick blood glucose 2 days per week in the morning before breakfast and in the evening before dinner. Her fasting blood glucose ranges from 98 to 135 mg/dL, and her evening blood glucose is a bit higher, ranging from 130 to 170 mg/dL. The record she brings to the office shows she occasionally does a 2-hour postprandial test that has been as high as 280 mg/dL. Six months ago, her fasting plasma cholesterol was 250 mg/dL; her fasting plasma triglyceride was 220 mg/dL. During the past year, her hemoglobin AZC has risen gradually from 7.8% to 8.5%. The APN recognizes Mrs. Smith has only modest control of her disease and is at risk of vascular complications if this trend continues.

She is 5 feet 5 inches tall and weighs 160 pounds, with a central body fat distribution. She has been unsuccessful in losing weight in the past 6 years, but she has not gained weight in the past year since she began walking 2 miles 5 to 6 times per week. She is taking glyburide 5 mg daily and has not reported any hypoglycemic episodes. She and her husband of 45 years have an active retirement, traveling in their recreational vehicle 3 to 4 months of the year.

The APN has been having Mrs. Smith come in for a routine visit every 3 months, encouraging her to schedule the appointments around her busy travel schedule. She inquires into Mrs. Smith's ability to follow her diet during travel times, and she asks about missed doses of medications and monitoring of blood glucose when she is away from home. She is interested in her energy level, especially when away from home and off a predictable schedule. The APN further questions Mrs. Smith about any signs or symptoms signaling late complications, i.e., angina, dizziness, slow-healing wounds, and change in vision. On each visit the APN performs a physical examination focusing on detection of end-organ damage. The office assistant measures the blood pressure and pulse, and if abnormal, the APN rechecks them. She inspects the retinas, listens to the heart and lungs, performs a neurological examination, and pays special attention to the lower extremities and feet looking for signs of peripheral vascular disease, corns, and calluses. She tests lower extremity sensation with a 10-gram monofilament. A review of the record indicates Mrs. Smith has been seen by an ophthalmologist annually for the past 5 years.

Mrs. Smith admits to the APN she has difficulty adhering to her diet at home and during her travels owing to persistent hunger and her interest in sampling a variety of foods. She admits to feeling guilty and frustrated with her inability to adhere to a structured diet. She maintains she exercises faithfully, regardless of her location. The APN knows that weight reduction would probably offer better control but chooses to focus on the strengths Mrs. Smith displays in her adherence to an exercise program and self-monitoring of her blood glucose. She recommends increasing her walking to 4 miles per day over the next 3 months. If improved glycemic control is achieved by exercise, Ms. Smith will begin to see the difference in the checking of finger stick blood glucose she performs.

This case illustrates the challenge the APN faces in the management of chronic, stable disease. In this case, the patient feels well and understands the implications of poor metabolic control. She is motivated, but has been unsuccessful in making dietary changes to improve glycemic control. She has demonstrated the ability to make some behavioral changes by persisting with an exercise program even while travelling. The APN recognizes the strengths of the patient, evaluates her past success, and engages the patient in planning a change in her exercise program. The follow-up plan is disease-specific, yet individualized for this patient.

REFERENCES

American Association of Homes and Services to the Aging (AAHSA). (1998). Assisted living. Washington, DC: Author.

American Diabetes Association. (1995). Standards of medical care for patients with diabetes mellitus. *Diabetes Care 18* (Suppl. 1), 8–15.

American Medical Association. (1998). Physicians' Current Procedural Terminology. Chicago.

American Medical Association. (May, 1997). Documentation guidelines for evaluation and management services [On-line]. Available: *http://www.hcfa.gov/medicare/mcarpti.htm.*

Boult, C., Boult L., Morishita, L., et al. (1998). Outpatient geriatric evaluation and management. *Journal of the American Geriatrics Society 46*(3):296–302.

Burl, J. B., Bonner, A., Rao, M., & Khan, A. M. (1998). Geriatric nurse practitioners in long-term care: Demonstration of effectiveness in managed care. In M. Mezey & T. Fulmer (Eds.), *Journal of the American Geriatrics Society 46*(4), 506–510.

Cadogan, M. P., Franzi, C., & Osterweil, D. (1998). Utilization of standardized procedures in skilled NFs: The California experience. *Annals of Long Term Care 6*(4). 130–139.

Collins, C. E., Butler, F. R., Gueldner, S. H., & Palmer, M. H. (1997). Models for community-based long-term care for the elderly in a changing health system. *Nursing Outlook 45*(2), 59–63.

Curtin, M., & Lubkin, I. (1998). What is chronicity? In I. M. Lubkin & P. D. Larsen (Eds.), *Chronic illness: Impact and interventions* (pp. 3–25). Toronto: Jones and Bartlett.

Edsall, R. L., & Moore, K. J. (1995a). A documentation toolbox. *Family Practice Management May,* 35–43.

Edsall, R. L., & Moore, K. J. (1995b). Exam documentation: Charting within the guidelines. *Family Practice Management March,* 53–59.

Edsall, R. L., & Moore, K. J. (1995c). Thinking on paper: Guidelines for documenting medical decision making. *Family Practice Management March,* 49–60.

Eng, C., Pedulla, J., Eleazer, G. P., et al. (1997). Program of all-inclusive care for the elderly (PACE): An innovative model of integrated geriatric care and financing. *The Journal of the American Geriatrics Society 45*(2), 223–32.

Evans, L. K., Yurkow, J., & Siegler, E. L. (1995). The CARE program: A nurse-managed collaborative outpatient program to improve function of frail older people. In D. B Ruben (Ed.), *The Journal of the American Geriatrics Society 43*(10), 1155–1160.

Fama, T., & Fox, P. D. (1997). Efforts to improve primary care delivery to nursing home residents. *Journal of the American Geriatrics Society, 45*(5), 627–632.

Forer, S., & Granger, C. (1987). Functional independence measure. Buffalo, NY: The Buffalo General Hospital, SUNY-Buffalo.

Fowkes, W., Christenson, D., & McKay, D. (1997). An analysis of the use of the telephone in the management of patients in skilled NFs. *Journal of the American Geriatrics Society 45*(1), 67–70.

Fried, T. R., Wachtel, T. J., & Tinetti, M. E. (1998). When the patient cannot come to the doctor: A medical housecalls program. In D. B. Reuben (Ed.), *Journal of the American Geriatrics Society 46*(2), 226–231.

Health Care Financing Administration. (1987). Guidance to surveyors: Long-term care facilities. Washington, DC: Author.

The HMO Workgroup on Care Management. (1998). In K. V. Brummel-Smith (Ed.), Essential components of geriatric care provided through health maintenance organizations. *Journal of the American Geriatrics Society 46*(3), 303–308.

Kane, R. L., Ouslander, J. C., & Abrass, I. B. (1994). *Essentials of clinical geriatrics.* New York: McGraw-Hill.

Kane, R.S. (1993). Physician's attitudes toward nursing home practice in Milwaukee. *Wisconsin Medical Journal 92*(4), 2208–2211.

Katz, P. R., Karuza, J., Kolassa, J., & Hutson, A. (1997). Medical practice with nursing home residents: Results from the national physician professional activities census. *Journal of the American Geriatrics Society 45*(8), 911–917.

Kayser-Jones, J. S., Wiener, C.L., & Barbaccia, J. C. (1989). Factors contributing to the hospitalization of nursing home residents. *The Gerontologist 29*(4), 502–510.

Kearnes, D. R. (1992). A productivity tool to evaluate NP practice: Monitoring clinical time spent in reimbursable, patient-related activities. *Nurse Practitioner 17*(4), 50–55.

Kornowski, R. K., Zeeli, D., Averbuch, M., et al. (1995). Intensive home-care surveillance prevents hospitalization and improves morbidity rates among elderly patients with sever congestive heart failure. *American Heart Journal 129*(4), 762–765.

Moore, K. J. (1998). Billing for NP services: What you need to know. *Family Practice Management 5*(5), 12–15.

Norris, J. N., Hawes, C., Murphy, K., & Nonemaker, S. (1993). MDS+ reference manual. In C. Boulter (Ed.). Natick, MA: Eliot Press.

Ouslander, J. G., Osterweil, D., & Morley, J. (1997). *Medical care in the nursing home* (2nd ed.). New York: McGraw-Hill.

Ouslander, J. G., & Osterweil, D. (1994). Physician evaluation and management of nursing home residents. *Annals of Internal Medicine 120*(7), 584–592.

Owen, A., & Moore, K. J. (1995). Don't read this article! *Family Practice Management Feb.,* 47–53.

Rapp, M. P., & Rapp, K. L. (1996). *Symptom assessment for the long term care nurse.* Unpublished manuscript.

Rapp, M. P., Rapp, K., & Kybe, F. (1998). Use of standardized procedures in long-term care. *Annals of Long-Term Care 6*(4), 147–148.

Rich, M. W., Beckman, V. B., Wittenberg, C., et al. (1995). A multidisciplinary intervention to prevent the readmission of elderly patients with congestive heart failure. *The New England Journal of Medicine 333*(18), 1190–1195.

Texas Nurses Association/Foundation. (1996). *Long term care protocols* (2nd ed.). Austin: Texas Nurses Association.

CHAPTER 10

Carol A. Romano

Nursing Informatics

The delivery of healthcare service is a complex endeavor that depends extensively on information. Information processing is integral to nursing care. Information systems—old or new, paper-based or computer-based—affect nursing practice. Information systems exist wherever nursing is practiced, and they directly affect the quality and effectiveness of patient care. Inadequate or ineffective information seriously hampers the clinical decisions of providers, the safety of consumers, and the ability of a healthcare agency to deliver services (National Center for Nursing Research, 1993). Nursing informatics is concerned with the information-handling work of nursing. The purpose of this chapter is to explore the definition and context of nursing informatics, to review the requirements for information management, and to address informatics issues from the perspective of the advanced practice nurse (APN).

Definition and Context

Nursing informatics is defined in the American Nurses Association (ANA) *Scope of Practice for Informatics Nursing* (1994). It is the specialty that integrates nursing science, computer science, and information science in identifying, collecting, processing, and managing data and information to support nursing practice, administration, education, research, and the expansion of nursing knowledge. It is defined as the specialty that serves nursing by supporting the information-handling work of other nursing specialties. The core product of informatics nursing is the provision of information to the patient care process. The core phenomena are all the data, information, and knowledge involved in nursing. These data, information, and knowledge are the symbolic representation of nursing care. The core operations of informatics nursing include identification, acquisition, aggregation, analysis, storage, retrieval, management, and transmission of the data, information, and knowledge of nursing. These activities are directed so as to create meaningful and useful data to nurses. All nurses use information and the product of informatics. The focus of this specialty, however, includes the methods and the technologies of information handling, not the content or context of the information (ANA, 1994). It is this focus that differentiates nursing informatics from other nursing specialties. The focus on nursing information requirements, as opposed to the information needs of other disciplines, is what differentiates nursing informatics from other nonnursing disciplines.

Since 1985, several authors have offered definitions of nursing informatics, each focusing to some extent on one or more of three themes (Turley, 1996). The first theme focuses on the use and position of the computer and computer science and suggests that informatics is derived from changes in computer technology. The second theme focuses on conceptional issues and concepts that organize and represent nursing knowledge. The third theme emphasizes functional performance, in which the focus is not on the computer but on how the computer helps nurses enter, organize, and retrieve information. Although these themes are useful, no one alone captures the entire scope. Turley offers a useful model that proposes that the domain of informatics is formed by the area bounded by the disciplines of cognitive science, information science, and computer science. It is assumed that informatics is multidisciplinary. Nursing informatics, then, is the interaction between the discipline-specific science, that is, nursing science, and the area of informatics, as noted previously. It is recognized that research is still needed at each intersection of this proposed model. Graves and Corcoran (1989) define nursing informatics as the combination of computer science, information science, and nursing science designed to assist in the management and processing of nursing data, information, and knowledge to support the practice of nursing and the delivery of nursing care. This definition is consistent with the ANA scope of practice and Turley's model. As knowledge expands in all aspects of informatics, it is clear that this science and the definition of nursing informatics will continue to evolve and will respond to the sharing of data, information, and knowledge by various health disciplines in the healthcare delivery system.

SPECIALIZATION

Criteria

The ANA defined nursing informatics as a specialty area of nursing practice in 1992. Criteria for defining a specialty were developed by the ANA Congress of Nursing Practice and endorsed by the American Nurses Credentialing Center (ANCC) Board of Directors in 1991. These criteria assert that a nursing specialty would be recognized as such if it first defines itself as nursing and subscribes to the overall purpose and functions of nursing and adheres to the overall licensure requirements of the profession. Next it needs to be national in scope and identify a need and demand for itself. A nursing specialty also needs to be clearly defined and distinct from other nursing specialties and be organized and represented by a nursing specialty association or a branch of a parent organization that sets standards for it. In addition, a specialty needs to have standards that reflect a well-defined base of knowledge and be concerned with phenomena within the discipline and practice of nursing. It needs existing mechanisms for supporting, reviewing, and disseminating research to support its knowledge base with educational programs that prepare nurses in the specialty. Finally, a specialty needs to provide for peer review of its members through a specialty certification program (ANCC, 1998b).

It is of note that nursing informatics meets these criteria. Informatics nursing has been organized as a special interest area within the American Medical Informatics Association, the Informatics Council of the National League for Nursing, and within the Nursing Systems Council of the ANA. In addition, national priorities for federal research funding were also established and published by the National Center for Nursing Research at the National Institutes of Health in 1993. Educational programs to prepare nurses for this specialty have also been developed and reported (Mills, Romano, & Heller, 1996). A scope of practice for nursing informatics was published by the ANA in 1994 and standards of practice were defined in 1995. The first certification examination for this specialty was offered in 1995 by the ANCC (1998a).

Standards

ANA standards are defined as statements of authority by which the nursing profession describes the responsibilities for which its practitioners are accountable. Standards of practice are divided into two types: (1) standards of care that address the competent delivery of nursing care demonstrated via the nursing process and (2) standards of professional performance that address the competent level of behavior in the professional role. There are six standards of practice for nursing informatics. These standards focus on the requirements of the informatics nurse to analyze, design, develop, modify, implement, evaluate, or maintain information technologies. The scope and function of such information technologies are those that collect patient data, support decision making, identify patient outcomes, develop plans of care, document implementation, and provide for evaluation of outcomes. Performance standards of informatics nursing address the following areas: quality of practice, evaluation, appraisal of performance, education, collegiality, ethics, collaboration, research, and resource utilization. The content domain of informatics nursing is addressed by domain standards reported in the standards of practice (ANA, 1995b). These domain standards encompass the areas of information life cycle, principles and theory, information technology, communication, and databases. These standards help to circumscribe the content area around which competencies and certification examinations can be developed.

Certification

Certification is the process by which an association validates, based on standards, a nurse's qualifications and knowledge to practice in a defined area of nursing. Certification meets the public expectation that nursing will regulate itself (ANCC, 1998b). The ANCC is the only organization that offers certification in informatics nursing. Certification is usually granted for a 5-year period. The ANCC has defined competencies, eligibility criteria, and a process for applying for informatics nursing certification. Eight competencies have been defined for informatics nursing. These competencies parallel the domain standards that are addressed in the standards of practice. The competencies provide the framework around which certification test questions are developed. These competencies include information systems analysis and design, system implementation and support, system testing and evaluation, human factors, computer technology, information and database management, professional practice trends and issues, and theories related to and about informatics nursing (ANA, 1995b; ANCC, 1998a).

INFORMATICS COMPETENCIES

Although competencies have been defined for those wishing to specialize in informatics nursing, there is consensus that all nurses need basic informatics competencies to practice in the future healthcare delivery system. The ANA scope of informatics nursing proposes that all nurses should be competent in the following four areas. First, nurses need to identify, collect, and record data related to nursing. Second, they need to analyze and interpret patient and nursing information to plan services and provide care. Third, they need to use information technology applications, and finally they need to implement policies related to privacy, confidentiality, and security.

These competencies imply that nurses need to be familiar with the information technologies that are increasingly becoming a standard part of society and of the healthcare delivery system. Computer literacy includes an *awareness* of the importance and versatility of information technologies, *knowledge* of what computers are and how they work, including familiarity with basic technical jargon, and the *ability to interact* with computers for simple applications. Familiarity with a basic tool kit of task-oriented software, sometimes called "productivity software," can make the information work of nurses easier and faster. The major categories of productivity software include word processing, spreadsheets (electronic matrix of rows and columns), database management (collection and manipulation of interrelated files), graphics, and communications software (Capron, 1998). All nurses, but especially APNs, need basic skills in using this software because their information tasks are complex and their need to structure and manipulate data from multiple sources is pervasive.

In addition to these basic competencies, informatics nurse specialists and APNs are called on to design and implement automated information systems and applications. This requires skills in analyzing and evaluating the information requirements of nursing. It also requires one to appraise technology for its applicability and appropriateness to nursing, for its effectiveness in addressing specific problems, for its impact on efficiency and productivity, and for the social and ethical impact of its use. These informatics competencies are important because they allow one to better manage information.

Information Management

Because health services are provided by many individuals, disciplines, and specialists, the information related to these services must be integrated, coordinated, and managed. The management of information is a central component of the ongoing operations and strategic decisions made within organizations. It plays a significant role in the changing and evolving healthcare delivery system. Information management is a function that focuses on meeting an individual's or organization's need for meaningful data or information. This function includes a set of processes and activities directed at acquiring needed information and at transmitting, storing, representing, assimilating, and using information in an economical, efficient, and productive way. Information as a concept consists of three aspects: data, information, and knowledge. Data are defined as discrete entities objectively described, without interpretation or context. Data that are interpreted, organized, structured, and given meaning are referred to as information. Information that has been synthesized in such a way as to create formalized, identifiable relationships is referred to as knowledge. Knowledge is used in supporting the multiple clinical and administrative decisions of nurses (Graves & Corcoran, 1989).

Information in the generic sense, then, needs to be managed (aggregated, organized, transmitted, etc.) so that it can be processed to support decision making. The goal of information management is to improve the effectiveness of the assimilation, interpretation, and representation of data so that informed decisions are made. Mills, Romano, and Heller (1996) propose that the study of information management in nursing encompasses five dimensions: (1) the databases required; (2) the strategies to manage the transformation of data and the processes in systems that channel them; (3) the clinical content of data and the purpose for which they are collected; (4) the administrative systems that support the purposes of use; and (5) the social, political, legal, and professional environments in which the information management process occurs. Because the databases—or content format of information—are critical, they are discussed in more detail in the next section.

NURSING DATABASES

The study of information management includes issues related to the development and use of a consistent language that represents the domain of the healthcare profession. A common, uniform, comprehensive approach to the representation of nursing and medical information is needed to express observations, problems and diagnoses, interventions, and outcomes of patient care management. A uniform language allows one to index, sort, retrieve, and classify nursing data in patient records, health information systems, and nursing and medical literature. Use of a consistent language allows one to evaluate and aggregate data across different healthcare settings and across different patients and facilitates the use of clinical data for research (Mills, Romano, & Heller, 1996). The description of nursing diagnoses, interventions, and outcomes in consistent language also allows the development of a national computerized database that can be used to measure, evaluate, and validate the impact of nursing on national health policy (ANA, 1995a). The content of a national database directly relates to standards of practice and clinical guidelines. The incorporation of standards and guidelines into practice requires identification of data elements and thus influences what content is required in practice databases. Duff and Casey (1998) also assert that informatics can provide strategies that support the access, communication, and evaluation of clinical guidelines. Informatics, then, can be used to access information from a knowledge base, to exchange information among databases, and to generate and analyze data about the impact of guidelines on practice and quality of care. To develop a nursing database, definition of a minimum set of data elements for that database is needed.

Nursing Minimum Data Set

The nursing minimum data set (NMDS) was designed to reflect the common core of data that describes nursing practice. Its development and implication have been discussed since 1987. The NMDS was built on the concept of the Uniform Minimum Health Data Set defined in 1983 by the U.S. Health Information Policy Council. It was developed to reflect the criteria for development of minimum health data sets. These criteria assert that data items in a minimum data set need to be useful to most, if not all, potential interdisciplinary users; items selected must be able to be collected readily with reasonable accuracy; items must not duplicate available data sources; and confidentiality should be protected (ANA, 1995a). The purposes of the NMDS have been defined (ANA, 1995a, p.21). These purposes are to

1. Establish comparability of nursing data across clinical populations, settings, geographic areas, and time;
2. Describe the nursing care of patients or clients and their families in a variety of settings, both institutional and noninstitutional;
3. Demonstrate or project trends regarding nursing care that is provided and nursing resources that are allocated to patients or clients according to their health problems and nursing diagnosis;
4. Stimulate nursing research through links to the detailed data existing in nursing and other healthcare information systems; and
5. Produce data about nursing care to facilitate and influence clinical, administrative, and health policy decision making.

The NMDS was designed so that a core of data elements can be collected for all clients receiving care. The three types of elements in the NMDS are nursing care elements, elements related to patient/client demographics, and service elements. A total of 16 elements are defined, 10 of which are already collected in other uniform health data sets. These do not need to be re-collected. The four nursing elements are unique and do not appear in other data sets and include nursing diagnosis, nursing intervention, nursing outcome, and intensity of nursing care. The five demographic elements are patient identification, date of birth, sex, race and ethnicity, and residence. The seven service elements are the unique facility or service agency number, episode admission or encounter date, discharge or termination date, disposition of the patient, expected payer, unique number of the principal registered nurse provider, and unique health record number of the patient or client. These last two items also do not appear in any other health data sets.

To use the NMDS, a common language for nursing practice is required. In 1989 the ANA Cabinet on Nursing Practice appointed a Steering Committee on Databases to Support Clinical Nursing Practice to propose policy regarding nursing classification schemes and nursing data sets and their inclusion in national databases. This charge included the challenge to develop a Unified Nursing Language System to facilitate linkages across various nursing systems and to identify data elements for inclusion in computer-based patient records. This steering committee adopted the NMDS and formally recognized four nursing vocabularies or classification systems for nursing: the North American Nursing Diagnosis Association's (NANDA) Nursing Diagnosis Taxonomy, the Omaha System, the Home Health Care Classification (HHCC), and the Nursing Intervention Classification (NIC). These vocabularies or classification schemes for practice were selected for the following reasons: they were found to be clinically useful; terms were precisely defined (they were tested for reliability of the vocabulary terms); they were validated as to their clinical purposes; they were accompanied by documentation of a systematic method for development; they were accompanied by evidence of a process for periodic review and revision; and they had terms that were associated with unique identifiers or codes. However, it is recognized that no single vocabulary or classification scheme is consistently used in nursing, and no scheme is fully developed or consistent with the multiple purposes for which it is needed. A brief overview of the four approved schemes is provided in the following sections.

North American Nursing Diagnosis Association's Nursing Diagnosis Taxonomy

The history of the development of the NANDA Nursing Diagnosis Taxonomy spans a period of 40 years. In 1950, interest in the idea of a taxonomy was reported. Later, in the 1970s, development of diagnoses, education, and implementation of the concept proliferated. In the 1990s, emphasis has been on the development of nursing diagnosticians and the articulation of the taxonomy with other disciplines. The process of development of a diagnosis includes a phase of submission of the diagnosis to a peer review group, establishment of content validity, and research and reexamination at defined time intervals. Nursing diagnosis is defined as the human responses to problems or processes in individuals, families, or communities. There are three types of diagnoses in the taxonomy. *Actual diagnoses* are those with defined signs and symptoms, causes, and defining characteristics. *At-risk diagnoses* are those for which risk factors are present. *Wellness diagnoses* are those that reflect the potential to develop a higher level of health. NANDA's diagnoses are classified into nine patterns. These patterns include exchanging, communicating, relating, valuing, choosing, moving, perceiving, knowing, and feeling. These patterns reflect the human responses involved in mutual giving and receiving, sending messages, establishing bonds, assigning relative worth, selecting alternatives, involving activities, receiving information, being associated with information, and the subjective awareness of information, respectively. The patterns are used to categorize the diagnoses and to develop an identification coding system for the diagnostic labels. Also, in this taxonomy, qualifier terminology is used to describe the diagnosis. Examples of these qualifiers include the terms acute, chronic, deficient, depleted, excessive, impaired, and ineffective. When a diagnostic label is proposed, it is usually proposed with the qualifier term. Examples of NANDA Nursing Diagnoses include altered nutrition—more than body requirements, ineffective denial, risk for impaired skin integrity, fatigue, hopelessness, and pain.

The Omaha System

The Omaha System is a practice-based initiative to name nursing practice. It consists of three components that address nursing diagnoses, interventions, and clinical outcomes. The system has evolved during the past 20 years under the leadership of Karen Martin and has developed with the support of 11 years of federally funded research. This system has been used extensively in home care, public health, school health, clinic, ambulatory care, parish, migrant, jail, and nursing education programs (ANA, 1995a).

The first component of the Omaha System is the problem classification component, which addresses nursing diagnoses and provides a consistent language to reflect client concerns. In this scheme, 44 problems are organized into the four domains of environment, psychosocial, physiological, and health-related behavior. Each problem can be defined as actual or potential and can refer to an individual or a family. For example, the problem of role change is categorized in the psychosocial domain and can refer to the actual situation of a woman adjusting to motherhood. The intervention scheme of the Omaha System reflects a systematic arrangement of nursing activities into one of four categories—health teaching/counseling, treatment/procedures, case management, and surveillance. In addition, 62 targets or objects of nursing intervention are defined and used to delineate an activity in terms of the four categories just mentioned. For example, the target "bladder care" can be identified as the object of surveillance, health teaching, or treatment/procedure, depending on the patient care situation. This system also allows for the designation of client-specific descriptive information.

The problem rating scale for the outcome component of this system is used to evaluate change over time and to judge the effectiveness of a plan of care. The problem rating scale consists of three 5-point Likert-type ordinal subscales. One subscale is for the concept of knowledge and rates the ability of the client to interpret information. The behavior subscale rates the appropriateness of a client's behavior. The status subscale rates the degree of manifestation of a client's signs and symptoms. These scales are used to make relative comparison's of a patients progress and are not scored or summed quantitatively. This system can be easily automated and used for clinical documentation as well as administrative management.

Home Health Care Classification

The HHCC was developed at Georgetown University in 1991 by Virginia Saba through a research project designed to assess and classify patients to determine required resources for Medicare patients with home care needs. The HHCC consists of two classification schemes: one for nursing diagnoses and one for nursing interventions. It uses 20 nursing components to provide a framework for classification (ANA, 1995a). The nursing diagnosis classification scheme consists of 145 home healthcare diagnoses (104 of these were derived from the NANDA-approved labels). These are classified into the 20 nursing components. Of the 145 labels, 50 are major diagnoses and 95 are subcategories. For example, fluid volume deficit and fluid volume excess are subcategories of the major diagnosis fluid volume alteration. These are categorized under the fluid volume component of the nursing framework. The specific outcome measure is considered a facet of the nursing diagnosis label. The expected outcome or goal of home healthcare is defined by one of three measures or conditions for each diagnosis. These conditions can be defined as improved, stabilized, or deteriorated.

The home healthcare nursing intervention component of the HHCC comprises 160 interventions that are organized into the same 20 nursing component frameworks as the nursing diagnoses. Sixty major interventions are defined with 100 subcategories. The scheme provides the opportunity to select one of four types of nursing actions that relate to each intervention. The four types of intervention actions include assessment, direct care, teaching, and management of nursing services. For example, range of motion is a subcategory of the major intervention of rehabilitative care. These are categorized into the activity component of the nursing framework. The action could be to teach range of motion, to assess the patient's range of motion, or to manage a referral for this activity, depending on the patient care situation.

Nursing Intervention Classification

The initial development of the NIC began at the University of Iowa in 1987 under the leadership of Gloria Bulechek and Joanne McCloskey. It was initially published as the Iowa Intervention Project, supported by federal nursing research funds. This classification and the ongoing efforts at Iowa reflect the initiative to develop a standardized language to describe nursing treatments. The NIC consists of a comprehensive list of 336 nursing interventions, each with a label, definition, references, and set of activities critical to its performance (ANA, 1995a). The interventions are classified into six domains: physiologic (basic), physiologic (complex), behavioral, safety, family, and health systems. Each domain is further subdivided into classes. For example, pain management is an intervention classified in the physiologic (basic) domain and the physical comfort promotion class. The most recent publication of the NIC links the NIC to NANDA diagnoses.

Research to develop a nursing-sensitive outcome classification was also initiated at the University of Iowa, Iowa City, in 1991. This classification initiative contains patient outcomes, indicators, and measurement activities at three to four levels of abstraction. A *nursing-sensitive patient outcome* is defined as a variable patient or family caregiver state, condition, or perception responsive to nursing intervention. This research has major implications for practice because it will provide the first standardized language and measurement for nursing-sensitive patient outcomes.

Informatics Issues

Despite the critical role that informatics plays and will continue to play in the many areas of nursing, several theoretical, empirical, and practical information management issues have been identified and need to be addressed (Hays, Norris, & Androvich, 1994). Theoretical issues relate to the current lack of standardized nomenclature in nursing. Although efforts to address this have been pursued since the 1970s, consensus on this issue is difficult because of the broad scope of nursing's phenomena of concern and the diversity of clients, settings, and disciplines contributing to nursing knowledge. Despite efforts toward an NMDS, multiple taxonomies are used for the elements of the data set. This creates problems of standardization, comprehensiveness, validity, and reliability of data.

Empirical issues of information management relate to the accuracy, reliability, and validity of data. Accuracy is important if documentation of patent care is to be useful for either clinical or research purposes. Reliability refers to consistency of data. Measurement error can occur when a patient observation is made, when it is documented, and when it is retrieved. Comprehensiveness, timeliness, distortion, and omissions are concerns that relate to the reliability of information and how it is managed in clinical situations. The validity of data can be affected by the labels we use to represent clinical phenomena. The classification of clinical information into categories is never perfect and is continuously evolving. These empirical issues directly relate to how we manage and handle information and use it to make decisions in our practice.

Practice issues of information management encompass controversies over how the information content should be formatted, accessed, and structured in terms of the level of detail. Questions about who controls clinical data and who has access, ownership, and disclosure rights are also practice concerns not always easily answered. Consideration about the confidentiality of patient information is also a critical issue in any discussion about automation of clinical records. The development of policies related to patient privacy and security practices related to use of information systems are frequent areas overlooked in the clinical environment. Computer security training programs are needed to address appropriate practices to protect electronic information. A prototype of one such education program, developed at the National Institutes of Health, is available on the Internet at http://www-oirm.nih.gov to help address the void in the area. National guidelines for a security educational program have also been developed (Computer-Based Patient Record Institute, 1995).

PRIVACY AND CONFIDENTIALITY

In our information-oriented society, new technologies have made possible the accumulation of an unlimited quantity of health data. This has created a resurgence of the traditional controversies surrounding the issues of privacy and confidentiality. Privacy is the control over exposure of self, property, and information about oneself so that it is inaccessible to others unless access is authorized for particular reasons. It is related to the human vulnerability to harm as well as to the human need to retain a sense of control over one's life. Privacy denotes the right of an individual to decide how much personal information to share. It is valued because it is the condition within which relationships of trust, love, friendship, and respect occur. Any threat to privacy potentially threatens one's ability to maintain significant relationships that define one's individuality. Privacy is necessary to the development of trust and mutual respect between patient and provider. The moral obligation to hold in confidence patient information is explicit in both the ANA's Code for Nurses and the American Medical Association's Principles of Medical Ethics.

Although privacy refers to self-concerns, confidentiality presupposes a relationship between one who discloses personal information and another who receives that information. Confidentiality, then, concerns redisclosure of information. Unlike privacy, which is controlled by an individual, confidentiality is controlled by the person to whom one confides or relinquishes privacy. Although privacy is viewed as a right, confidentiality is seen as the health professional's duty to safeguard the secrecy of information collected, stored, transmitted, and retrieved in a manual or automated health information system. Confidentiality has utilitarian value because it enhances the goal of healthcare. The expectation that physicians and nurses maintain confidentiality is necessary because it enables individuals to seek help without fear of public knowledge or exposure. If patients can expect that information about them will be held in confidence by the healthcare provider, then they will be more willing to fully reveal their health problems. This disclosure allows for enhanced treatment, resulting in more efficient and effective healthcare outcomes.

Confidentiality also enhances a patient's right to make healthcare choices free from the influence of others. When patient information is held in confidence, patients retain the moral authority to determine what will be known about them by others and, to a certain extent, who will have that information. It is widely recognized, however, that there are legitimate reasons for restricting the scope of confidentiality. It is said that the protective privilege ends where the public peril, or harm to others, begins. This includes such situations as reporting communicable disease or adhering to requirements of law. Nurses need to clarify their ethical obligations to ensure that they do not promise the patient or society more than they can deliver when protecting patient information.

Nursing Responsibilities and Strategies

Unquestionably, the most frequent users and processors of patient care information are nurses. The nursing responsibilities and strategies for safeguarding information, however, are not clearly understood. These can be addressed from the perspective of data integrity, usage integrity, and patient advocacy. With respect to data integrity, nurses are responsible for ensuring that data are accurate, reliable, valid, and complete. Here, the simplest and easiest security strategy is to control what information is collected. One should not collect more information than what is needed to compensate for not knowing what information is critical. Integrity of data can also be protected by insisting that entry of information on the computer be done as close to the source as possible. The traditional transcription of information, such as medical orders, from a written to a computerized form needs to be sacrificed for the sake of accuracy and elimination of transcription error. Each professional needs to enter his or her own data directly. This includes physicians as well as nurses.

One also needs to insist that computers allow for the correction of mistaken entries because "to err is human," and the consumer ought not to be the one who suffers from errors. Finally, "user friendly" may be interpreted to mean ease of entry as well as ease of mistake. Nurses must insist that computer systems be designed to allow the user to confirm or validate information before it is sent to the database. For example, the selection of a patient's name from a computer listing may require the user to confirm the choice so as to avoid the accidental selection of a patient with a similar name. Nurses also need to insist that software applications be tested and that they perform with close to 100% accuracy before being implemented.

With respect to maintaining usage integrity, nurses are responsible for participating in the authorization processes that control access to computer data. To guarantee security, the administration of badges, passwords, or user identifiers needs to be closely managed. The initiation, distribution, and termination processes related to these identifiers need to be clearly defined and monitored. Nurses should also be responsible for participating in the planning, organizing, directing, and evaluating of computer systems and related security measures. Internal controls need to be emphasized, with policies and penalties for abuse. This includes control over transmission of electronic communications via cellular phones, e-mail, or facsimiles. These latter technologies cannot be assumed to be secure. Risk analysis to assess threats also needs to be conducted. The responsibility and accountability for computer security and for the coordination of policies, activities, and reports through the nursing organization as well as the healthcare system also need to be clarified.

As health professionals, nurses need to insist on surveillance procedures, audit logs of computer transactions, and the monitoring of users. Computerized surveillance of systems can be implemented so that automatic sign-off for unattended terminals occurs. Educational forums on managing computer security are needed so that decisions for allocating resources, for ordering priorities, and for instituting controls can be addressed. Finally, patient advocacy is nursing's most significant responsibility. Computer strategies in this area include the following: acknowledging the right to privacy and legislative guarantees, offering explanations for the collection and uses of data, making available client access when appropriate, allowing for disclosure only on consumer's written consent, classifying the sensitivity of certain information, and clarifying the degree to which confidentiality is compromised by required disclosures to third parties.

Impact of Informatics on Nursing Roles

Informatics plays a critical role in the areas of nursing administration, clinical practice, education, and research. In the area of administration, informatics affects the role of nurse managers by facilitating communication, decision making, and resource management. For example, applications of electronic mail provide the opportunity to interact simultaneously with multiple individuals without the inconvenience of geographic barriers or the unnecessary time delays related to moving messages across space. Use of the Internet also provides ready access to information sources. Numerous software applications are available to support the decision-making process. Electronic spreadsheets and databases help the administrator convert data into meaningful information. Expert systems also provide the ability to model decision making and propose probabilities or options to pursue. In the area of resource management, information technology provides the ability to manage inventories, supplies, and manpower scheduling and utilization.

In the area of clinical practice, informatics influences data formats and structures that represent clinical care. Such structures allow for the reliability of data collection, the incorporation of standards of care into electronic databases, and the monitoring of variances of patient responses and outcomes. Clinical decision making can also be supported via access to the Internet and clinical knowledge bases. Use of such knowledge bases is becoming an expectation of clinicians. Clinical decision support systems are available to help clinicians diagnose and treat a person's health problem. The goals of these systems are to locate needed and accurate information and to make it available to the clinician in a usable form, at the point of care, in a timely manner, and without disruption to the care process. Currently, such systems are available that diagnose conditions, facilitate drug dose determination, provide preventive care reminders, and offer active diagnostic and therapeutic care advise. With the advent of telehealth and enhanced communication systems, the opportunity to communicate, assess, and treat patients via telecommunications is also becoming a reality, particularly in underserved areas.

In the area of education, patient materials can be readily accessed through the Internet. In addition, computer-assisted interactive education modules are available not only for patient education and self-assessment but also for continuing education for providers. Informatics also provides new opportunities for long-distance learning through telecommunications. The challenge to nurses is to become familiar with such technologies to integrate them as appropriate into their practice. In addition, nurses need to evaluate these technologies using appropriate criteria for learning.

In the area of research, standardization of data through the development of nursing vocabularies and taxonomies provides the infrastructure for conducting research using clinical data. Patterns and trends in populations and providers can be studied from aggregating existing electronic data in patient records without the redundant re-collection of data. Informatics also plays a critical role in facilitating the availability and accessibility of knowledge bases and library sources to allow one to assess the state-of-the-science in any particular area. Priorities for informatics research have been defined by the National Center for Nursing Research (1993) and include using data, information, and knowledge; defining and describing data; acquiring and delivering knowledge; investigating new technologies; patient–nurse–machine interactions; integrating systems for care; and evaluating effects of systems.

Summary

In summary, this chapter presented the definition of nursing informatics as a specialty with standards and certification. The role of informatics in nursing as well as issues of information management were also addressed. As we look to the role of nursing in the next millennium, we anticipate an environment that envelops us with explosions of technology. Given this, our most important challenge is to "informate," not to digress in our pursuit to automate. The roads of the information highway are being paved through the efforts of informatics nursing. The focus is on the question, "What information represents the practice of nursing, and how can we manage that information for better healthcare outcomes?" These are the challenges for both practice and education. Nursing needs to respond to the consumer demand for caring and meaningful interaction and for services that bring understanding to the human condition of suffering. Although "human" touch will be the "new" technology of the next century, informatics will allow us to harness our information and knowledge and to use it so that we meet the demands of society.

REFERENCES

American Nurses Association. (1994). *Scope of practice for nursing informatics* (NP-90, 7.5M, 5/94). Washington, DC: Author.

American Nurses Association. (1995a). *Nursing data system: The emerging framework* (NP-94, 7.5M, 5/95). Washington, DC: Author.

American Nurses Association. (1995b). *Standard of practice for nursing informatics* (NP-100, 7.5, 3/95). Washington, DC: Author.

American Nurses Credentialing Center. (1998a). *Informatics nurse certification catalog.* Washington, DC: Author.

American Nurses Credentialing Center. (1998b). *Policies and procedures for developing nurse certification offerings.* Washington, DC: Author.

Capron, H. L. (1998). *Computers: Tools for an informatics age* (5th ed.). Menlo Park, CA: Addision Wesley.

Computer-Based Patient Record Institute. (1995). *Guidelines for information security education programs* (Publication No. G595). Schaumburg, IL: Author.

Duff, L., & Casey, A. (1998). Implementing clinical guidelines: How can informatics help? *Journal of the American Medical Informatics Association* 5(3), 225–226.

Graves, J. R., & Corcoran, S. (1989). The study of nursing informatics. *Image 21*(4), 227–231.

Hays, B., Norris, I., & Androwick, I. (1994). Informatics issues for nursing's future. *Advances in Nursing Science 16*(4), 71–81.

Mills, M., Romano, C., & Heller, B. (1996). *Information management in nursing and health care.* Springhouse, PA: Springhouse Publications.

National Center of Nursing Research. (1993). *Nursing informatics: Enhancing patient care* (NIH Publication No. 93–2419). Washington, DC: US Department of Health and Human Services.

Turley, J. P. (1996). Toward a model for nursing informatics. *Image 28*(4), 309–313.

CHAPTER 11

Angeline Bushy

Diversity: A Call for Culturally Competent Practitioners

Demographers report that the largest population increase in the United States is among racial and ethnic minorities. Some demographers have even forecast that white Anglo-Americans will be in the minority before the middle of the next century. The changing complexion of American society has serious implications for healthcare providers in general, and advanced practice nurses (APNs) in particular, for planning, delivering, and evaluating services for target consumers, which are clients, patients, communities, and populations. People of color are an integral part of our national fabric, yet little is known about these and other underrepresented groups living in the United States (Ahmann, 1994; Coates, 1994; Morganthaue, 1997; National Rural Health Association [NRHA], 1994, 1997, 1998; U.S. Department of Commerce, 1996).

Health-related literature is replete with citations describing diverse minority and vulnerable populations and the concepts of multiculturalism, cultural awareness, cultural sensitivity, and cultural competency. Despite the national emphasis, the lifestyle and health beliefs of minorities within a community often remain foreign to caregivers, who most often are of Anglo-American origin (Leininger, 1969, 1978, 1984, 1985b). The predominant minorities in the United States—Africans, Hispanics, Asians, Pacific Islanders, and Native and Eskimo Americans—differ greatly in their social, political, and economic histories. Moreover, they have significant differences in their cultural beliefs, their behavior norms, and the extent of their acculturation into mainstream American culture (i.e., white, middle class, and of Anglo-European descent). Differences also exist among other underrepresented subgroups who live, work, and seek healthcare from practitioners in communities across the nation. In addition, Anglo-American consumers sometimes have beliefs and lifestyles that seem unusual to practitioners of Anglo-American origin (Andrews & Boyle, 1997; Brink, 1993; Grossman & Taylor, 1995; Leininger, 1994).

This chapter discusses the role of ethnocultural factors in an individual's perceptions of health, illness, and healthcare behaviors. The terms *multiculturalism, cultural awareness, cultural sensitivity,* and *cultural competency* are explored in relation to planning, delivering, and evaluating appropriate and acceptable healthcare to minority (i.e., underrepresented) groups. Included is historical content on self-care, folk remedies, and alternative healers. Strategies are presented that incorporate cultural factors to help APNs develop meaningful and appropriate treatment plans for culturally diverse clients.

Underserved and Vulnerable Communities

To provide care that is culturally appropriate and acceptable to a subgroup requires that practitioners make an effort to define the community or population of interest. Some subgroups are easy to identify because of geographic isolation, biologic or racial features, lifestyle, attire, religion, political views, language, leisure activity, or occupation. For example, generally it is not difficult to identify an Amish or Mennonite community in a midwestern state or the Hispanic and Asian sections of a large city. However, other groups are not obviously regionally bound or do not have an obvious distinct lifestyle, such as Laotians, Vietnamese, Italians, Poles, Irish, Jehovah's Witnesses, Orthodox Jews, Latter-Day Saints, Seventh-Day Adventist, smaller Native American tribes, or Latinos of Cuban versus Filipino versus Mexican origin. Nonetheless, the perspectives of less noticeable groups are critical to providing appropriate and acceptable services for those consumers (Barbee, 1993; Krieger, 1996; National Center for Health Statistics, 1996; Rosella, Regan-Kubinski, & Albrecht, 1994; U.S. Department of Health and Human Services [USDHHS], 1998).

Problems associated with cultural insensitivity in the healthcare system are exacerbated because a small percentage of individuals of minority origins enter the health professions, specifically as APNs. In addition to planning and delivering care, the cultural perspective also is not considered when measuring consumer satisfaction and acceptability of healthcare services for continuous quality improvement programs. This information deficit only serves to perpetuate a less than effective healthcare system because the services that are provided are neither appropriate nor acceptable to target consumers (Bushy, 1998).

Appropriate and Acceptable Care

Available and accessible services do not equate with appropriate and acceptable care. More specifically, the terms *available* and *accessible* refer to services existing within a community, with an adequate number of professional healthcare providers to deliver those services at a reasonable cost to the consumer. The terms *acceptable* and *appropriate* infer that a particular service is offered in a manner that is congruent with the ethnocultural values of a target population. This means that the care is desirable and familiar to the person receiving it, and this preference often is based on ethnic and cultural factors.

Census data reveal health professional shortage areas in the United States are most often found in the inner city and in rural counties (NRHA, 1998; USDHHS, 1996a, 1996b, 1998). Underserved areas usually include a higher proportion of racial, ethnic, religious, and cultural minority populations. Vulnerable groups in general experience high levels of poverty, limited educational opportunities, poorer overall health status, and restricted access to professionals of similar cultural and racial backgrounds. It is laudable for APNs to establish a practice in an underserved area or with a minority population. However, that in and of itself may not be sufficient to ensure that underserved populations have access to healthcare.

Cultural preferences vis-à-vis cultural barriers is not a new concept to practitioners or a novel component associated with the healthcare reform movement. Instead, the effects of cultural preferences have come to the forefront, with recent epidemiologic reports indicating that the health status of minority groups is less than desirable. Inequities are especially evident when the health status of minorities is compared with that of middle class Anglo-Americans. These epidemiologic findings are reinforced by the mandates put forth in *Healthy People 2000: National Health Promotion and Disease Prevention Objectives* (USDHHS, 1991, 1996b) specifically target the special needs of vulnerable minority populations across the United States.

Cultural factors that evoke consumer satisfaction go beyond appropriateness of dietary services, access to one's preferred pastoral care provider, or not offering an analgesic based on the belief that stoicism and suffering in silence are associated with the characteristic of machismo. Culture has been identified as a determinant in deciding the appropriate time to seek healthcare services and the manner in which a person interacts with a professional provider. Cultural values also influence a person's definition of health versus illness, choice of self-care behaviors, and perception of effective and ineffective caring behaviors. The following situations are other examples of cultural factors that may hamper acceptability of services:

- Traditions of handling personal problems (e.g., self-care practices and coping behaviors such as using over-the-counter medications, exercising, ingesting alcohol, resting, and praying);
- Beliefs about the cause of a disorder and the appropriate healer for it (e.g., doctor, nurse practitioner, neighborhood nurse acquaintance, chiropractor, herbalist, community lay healer, medicine man, voodoo priestess, homeopathy, reikke [therapeutic touch], curandero, or shaman);
- Lack of knowledge about a physical or emotional disorder and the place of formal services for preventing and treating the condition (e.g., being stoic and suffering in silence instead of seeking supportive care; paying for emergency care instead of spending money on health promotion or primary prevention; or expecting to receive a prescription, specifically an antibiotic or an analgesic, when paying to see the doctor or nurse practitioner);
- Language barriers (e.g., English as a second language, functional illiteracy [reading below the 5th-grade level—most healthcare literature is written at the 10th-grade level or higher], and nonverbal [cultural] nuances associated with terminology that is used to educate about healthcare);
- Difficulty in maintaining confidentiality and anonymity in a setting where many residents are acquainted; and
- Cultural insensitivity by health professionals, particularly APNs; this insensitivity, coupled with the usual stress experienced by consumers when seeking care, especially publicly funded care, can further exacerbate mistrust of the healthcare system.

All of these examples reinforce the notion that even if a service is available and accessible, it may not be appropriate for individuals in a target population. Moreover, consumer evaluations of services rendered usually are rated as "satisfactory," "unsatisfactory," "acceptable," or "unacceptable." This type of response does not elicit in-depth information about the client's experiences. Subsequently, this quantitative approach becomes a factor in whether the client adheres with a prescribed treatment or even uses a service that is readily available and accessible. Individual preferences ultimately can affect the overall health status of the consumer, his or her family, and the community as a whole. Ethnocultural data can provide information about the target consumer's perceptions, attitudes, values, and expectations. The need for ethnocultural data is reinforced by healthcare initiatives that promote more efficient use of existing resources, coupled with the increasing diversity in and consumers' mandate for caregivers who are culturally competent.

Culturally Competent Care

Like other skills in the APN's repertoire, cultural competency must be developed and refined. Before practitioners can become sensitive to and accommodate another's beliefs and values, however, they must first understand something about their own background. Practitioners must be aware of how their own cultural origins affect personal beliefs, behaviors, and ways of interacting with people on a professional and personal level. Of the many ways to reflect on one's circle of culture, completing a self-assessment probably is the most popular. Questions in these self-appraisals tend to be similar to the following items (Geissler, 1994; Grossman & Taylor, 1995; Yawn et al., 1994):

- How do you identify yourself in terms of race, ethnicity, religious or political beliefs, and socioeconomic class?
- What has it meant to be part of that group?
- Describe the customs or traditions in your family of origin that expressed your heritage. What special foods, gifts, songs, and ceremonies were related to events such as birth, puberty, starting school, graduation, marriage, divorce, illness, hospitalization, and death?
- How were feelings such as love and affection expressed in your family of origin?
- How were feelings such as anger and sadness expressed?
- What were the most valued and respected personal traits?
- What has been the role of women and men in your family and culture?
- How were decisions made? Who had the final say in those decisions?
- What role was fate believed to play in a person's life?
- How were time, work, leisure, health, and illness defined and valued?
- What was your first experience with feeling different?

Reflecting on these questions, first for oneself and subsequently as they apply to a client, is critical to a practitioner's developing awareness and sensitivity of the meaning of culture in everyday situations. Self-appraisal can help APNs understand personal expectations when they are ill and then compare those expectations with clients for whom they provide care. As with other problems that practitioners encounter, an initial step in resolving cultural barriers to care is to recognize factors that prevent clients from seeking care and adhering to treatment plans.

How can APNs acquire ethnocultural knowledge about groups in a particular practice setting? It is difficult to learn about people who are not part of the mainstream unless practitioners seek out subgroups within a community. Consequently, one approach is for practitioners to become highly involved and subsumed in a community's social and political activities. Even with intense involvement, it is unlikely that an outsider will learn all the important cultural facts about a minority before making at least a few blunders. Instead, over time, one learns gradually by working with clients in a particular community. Eventually, with a desire to learn, less obvious values and expectations become more obvious to the practitioner. For example, one becomes aware of and sensitive to consumers' manner of interacting with a health professional when seeking care and their preferred self-care behaviors, folk remedies, and use of alternative healers (see Exemplar 18A).

Cultural awareness and sensitivity preempts the development of cultural competence. This statement infers that practitioners have the ability to provide care that is appropriate and acceptable to a consumer even though it is not part of their own belief system. Becoming competent involves progressing from awareness and sensitivity to a more sophisticated understanding of the cultural belief systems and linguistic nuances of a minority group. The process requires a dedicated effort to learn about a group's beliefs and lifestyle preferences by interacting with individuals in their environment and by consulting outside resources that provide additional information about their lifeways and belief systems.

Ethnocultural Information Resources

The discipline of anthropology can be especially useful to practitioners desiring to glean information about a particular cultural or ethnic group. Not only is anthropologic information useful in the delivery of appropriate care but also for program planning and for measuring quality and satisfaction with care. APNs can learn a great deal by studying the language, music, and customs of a defined group. In completing a holistic group assessment, practitioners should consider social structures, including those related to religion, politics, economics, judicial systems, kinship, education, and beliefs regarding use or rejection of technology (Leininger, 1985a, 1997; Milburn, Gary, Booth, & Brown, 1992; Spradley, 1979, 1980).

Of particular interest are a minority community's geographic setting, historical roots, natural resources, economic base, food preferences, art forms, folktales, myths, symbols, and rituals. For example, practitioners might read biographies and fiction or attend plays and movies presented from a specific group's point of view. These leisure activities can provide contextual information about a minority group to an interested outsider. Individuals of a minority group vary in the extent to which they exhibit or demonstrate political, religious, ethnic, racial, or cultural traits. For instance, with immigrants and refugees, the length of time they have been in the United States often makes a difference. Language barriers in both spoken and written communication can hinder an individual's assimilation into the major culture. Generational differences, too, influence the rate of assimilation. Generally, younger persons assimilate into the American mainstream more readily than do older members of the community. Economic status also is a factor, with poor people consistently displaying more ethnocentric behaviors.

It is important to keep in mind that the healthcare system, too, has a culture of its own. Culture, in this case, influences interactions among professionals, as evidenced by the hierarchy of physicians, nurses, and technicians, and the relationship between professionals and their clients. Individuals at the top of the hierarchy function in a belief system that is defined by power and authority. Power, perceived or attributed, makes it difficult for individuals lower in the hierarchy to ask questions unless specifically given permission to do so. Hence, clients may not ask for clarification on a pertinent issue related to the care they are receiving from a practitioner they perceive as more powerful. This value is perpetuated by practitioners who inaccurately estimate what clients already know or understand, as well as the clarity and appropriateness of their own explanations.

APNs interested in reviewing or implementing research findings that focus on the culture of an underrepresented or vulnerable group are reminded that somewhat different approaches may be used for those kinds of studies. More familiar quantitative methods usually are associated with statistical analysis of surveys; experimental, quasi-experimental, or correlation studies; and epidemiologic reports. Studies using anthropologic methods, eliciting qualitative ethnocultural data, often obtain data by way of personal interviews with key informants (i.e., subjects), community focus groups, ethnographies, oral histories, case studies, and information that is disseminated by the community's media sources.

That is not to say that qualitative designs are better than quantitative designs, or vice versa. Instead, the two approaches yield complementary information. Both are important to assess cultural beliefs accurately and to measure the appropriateness of services from the consumer's perspective. For various reasons that are beyond the scope of this chapter, qualitative methods are less likely to be in the APN's repertoire. For more detailed information, the reader is encouraged to review citations included in the reference listing for this chapter.

As with any topic one wishes to learn more about, the literature review is an important step to determine what has or has not been written about a minority group. Not all information must be obtained from the professional literature, however. The popular media, including magazines such as *National Geographic* and *Newsweek,* theater productions, and television programs, can be valuable resources for APNs regarding a particular cultural group. These sources also provide perspectives about innovative programs that have been implemented to meet the group's special needs. For example, a tertiary care medical center plans to contract with the Indian Health Service to implement an alcohol treatment program for Native Americans, specifically the Cherokees. The innovative program will integrate traditional healing practices (e.g., participation of a tribal healer in the program, a sweat lodge, and other traditional rituals) with contemporary interventions (e.g., consumer-oriented education, psychotherapy, and group process). In this case, citations of probable interest to the practitioner include descriptions of similar programs for tribes in other geographic areas and general evaluation reports of other chemical dependency rehabilitation programs (Bell, 1994; Krieger, 1996; Levin, 1995; Miller, 1994; Stanhope & Knollmueller, 1997).

The lay media often includes feature articles describing innovative, cross-cultural programs that integrate traditional with contemporary healing practices. In brief, a review of the literature helps practitioners in two ways: (1) to build on the experiences of others and avoid some similar pitfalls and (2) to provide background information on the ethnocultural perspective for measuring consumer satisfaction to determine if a program is appropriate and acceptable.

Planning and Evaluation Models

Health planning and evaluation models that strictly lend themselves to the dominant (Anglo-European) culture are no longer acceptable. If consumers are expected to assume a greater role in their healthcare, planning and evaluation models must incorporate processes that consider consumers' ethnocultural heritage. To this end, anthropology, grounded theory, phenomenology, and other qualitative methods can be useful. Gradually, multidimensional data emerge that enlighten the interested outsider such as the APN. Sometimes cultural competence may not be mandatory to providing a program, but it can influence the quality of the program by providing a dimension in planning and evaluating services that targeted consumers find appropriate and acceptable. At other times, the lack of cultural competence may doom a program to failure (NRHA, 1997; 1998; Sternbert, 1997; Strickland & Strickland 1996).

For example, a group of primary care providers is deciding whether to add two outreach family planning clinics to their services. One of the proposed practice sites is located in a predominately Mexican-American community with a high percentage of migrant workers. The other proposed site is the student health center of a large university with more than 50,000 full-time students. If implemented, how can the healthcare provider be sure that these services are appropriate and acceptable to each community?

The following questions should be asked to elicit the population profile for each proposed clinic:

- What is the meaning of pregnancy to the group?
- What are the community's predominant religious denominations and community members' theologic positions regarding birth control, family planning, and pregnancy?
- What are their beliefs, values, and perceptions about public support for family planning clinics?
- What is the local fertility rate? Maternal–infant mortality rate? Adolescent pregnancy rate?
- How is an unplanned pregnancy viewed by the "typical" family? A burden? A blessing? A fulfillment of assigned gender roles?

- How are male and female gender roles defined?
- What, if any, reproductive health concepts are included in the health curricula of local schools? Who is responsible for teaching the courses? What is the instructor's background?
- What are prospective clients' preferred patterns for accessing services, particularly obstetric providers?
- What are their perceived barriers to accessing existing family planning services, including the public health clinic, physicians (e.g., family practice physician vs. obstetrician), and alternative care providers (e.g., midwife, nurse practitioner, physician assistant, or endogenous healer)?

By comparison, program planners will probably find different responses to those questions because of different demographic and cultural preferences in each of the targeted communities. The findings subsequently have implications in planning, delivering, and evaluating family planning services at each site. Once implemented, practitioners' increased cultural awareness and sensitivity will help explain puzzling or annoying differences among individuals within the context of a particular health-related behavior. In turn, meaningful ethnocultural data will enable practitioners to plan, develop, and evaluate treatment plans that articulate with client preferences. Hopefully, this will lead to more optimal outcomes in the recipients of those services, too.

Self-care, Folk Remedies, and Alternative Healers

In addition to seeking healthcare from professional practitioners, people who develop a health problem can obtain relief in several ways, including using self-care, with its folk remedies and obtaining advice from alternative healers. The resources and the rationale for those behaviors may differ depending on cultural, socioeconomic, environmental, geographic, and religious or spiritual factors. Self-care, folk medicine, and alternative healers have a strong historical basis that is common across cultures. Knowledge about this phenomenon can provide useful insights about modern self-care practices. In addition, historical perspectives can offer a frame of reference to an APN about a minority group's health beliefs. This information is a critical element of providing holistic and culturally competent care (Bushy, Grassy, Kost, & Ramsdell, 1989; NRHA, 1994, 1997, 1998).

Historical documentation generally indicates that humans have always found life to be hard and filled with numerous stressors. The essence of those stressors may change from one generation to another, but, for the most part, the outcome on health is consistent. Illness, too, was a common occurrence for our ancestors. But, unlike we contemporaries, they did not have educated health professionals to treat the sick. In cases of illness, self-care practices that integrated ritualistic behaviors with naturally occurring substances in their environment were relied on for ultimate healing. Self-care practices varied by geographic region, and many of the rituals and folk remedies had religious overtones (Thompson, 1989). Myths often had a role in directing the ritualistic use of naturally occurring substances such as animals or their body parts, plants, herbs, or personal belongings. Rituals, believed to enhance a remedy's effectiveness, usually involved repetitious behaviors, such as dancing, chanting, massaging with ointments, or ingesting the product in a carefully prescribed manner. Generally, the more complicated and severe the disease, the more complex and ritualistic was the remedy to treat it. This was especially true of treatments for communicable diseases for which no effective cure was known, such as smallpox, venereal disease, tuberculosis, whooping cough, plague, cholera, cancer, and rabies. Over time, the substance may have changed, but essentially the rituals have remained the same for generations (see Chapter 12).

INDIGENOUS COMMUNITY HEALERS

To develop cultural competence, APNs should learn about a community's traditional healers. Again, history can provide some insights regarding this topic in modern society. For example, caring for the sick was usually a task assigned to women, and some became very proficient with healing skills. Even the smallest tribes and communities had a well-known healer and experienced midwives. Terms for *healer,* such as *brauchfrua, shaman,* and *curandara,* are based on the language and cultural healing preferences of a group. Before the advent of specialized social functions, care of the sick was an individual and family responsibility. In socially and geographically isolated communities, folk medicine and good neighbors were the traditional means of treating the ill. Today this societal network is referred to as a person's "social support system."

Traditionally, most families have had a healing authority; usually this was a grandmother, aunt, or uncle with acknowledged healing skills. With the increase in the size of communities, the task of healing was eventually assigned or relinquished to specialized resources, hence the evolution of witch doctors, healers, medicine men and women, priests, shamans, physicians, APNs, and hospitals. Community members never doubted that the community healer had the power to restore health to their sick. Like the contemporary practitioner, a healer's reputation was at stake when providing services to clients. If healing did not progress in an expected manner, the healer was likely to be declared a "witch" by the community at large. Likewise, prudent contemporary health professionals also acknowledge that a satisfied customer's word-of-mouth reports probably are the most effective marketing strategy to recruit other clients.

RELIGION AND HEALING

Historically, religion and healing have long been interrelated (Thompson, 1989, Whorton, 1987; Williams, 1994). Likewise, good health and healing have often been associated with being in God's grace, ridding the body of bad spirits, or suffering in this world for one's wrongdoings. This belief system probably evolved from European priests well versed in demonology, who provided treatment for the sick. Through the centuries, religious leaders played an important role in perpetuating the belief that headaches, mental illness, epilepsy, and birth defects are the result of God's wrath or demonic possession. Modern-day faith healers are just as accessible, if not more so, through the public media, that is, radio, television, and even the Internet. Moreover, many people contribute financially to those faith healers with the belief that it can help to maintain or restore good health for themselves or family members. Common-folk always have had great respect for healers, often believing them to be God's representatives. Thus, when a family hired a healer to treat a family member, it was done to cast out evil spirits, make amends with God, and rid the person of the condition. Over time, and with repeated observations of sick people, healers gained knowledge about the patterns and symptoms of an illness as well as effective and ineffective interventions.

INTERGENERATIONAL TRANSMISSION OF HEALING PRACTICES

For posterity, healers transmitted through the oral and written word remedies that they believed were effective (Bushy, Grassy, Kost, & Ramsdell, 1989; NRHA, 1994). Thus, the healer entrusted healing secrets to subsequent generations. With the advent of the printing press, books of popular and not so well-known remedies were published and made available for public use. The *Doctor Book* was a comprehensive source of information for the prevention, treatment, and curing of ailments. A more expensive *Doctor Book* included two additional chapters, one focusing on reproductive health conditions in women and another on remedies for veterinary purposes.

For the most part, previous generations were resourceful when it came to their healthcare. For instance, because a *Doctor Book* was expensive and money was scarce, several neighbors shared in the cost of purchasing the book. Then, when someone in the family became sick, a family member was dispatched to obtain the book from the neighbor who had most recently consulted it. Interestingly, the neighbors generally knew who had that particular book at any given time. To avoid traveling in an emergency or in inclement weather, someone in the family who could read and write (again, often a female in the extended family) would copy those remedies that were believed to be most useful into the family's bible or cookbook so that the information would be available for future access.

In recent years, as part of local celebrations, groups typically comprising women (e.g., church circles, homemaker's clubs, and women's clubs) have compiled community cookbooks. It is not unusual to find several pages of "time-tested" family remedies at the end of these books. Practitioners might want to consult such books, which are yet another source of background information about a minority community.

Contemporaries are beginning to understand that emotions play an important role in healing and the body's ability to restore and maintain health. Now, as in the past, the mind–body connection probably contributes to a healer's success. Yet, folk remedies and self-care originated and have remained popular for the following reasons:

- A lack of available, accessible, affordable, and acceptable healthcare;
- Limited knowledge about body function and the disease process; and
- The reported effectiveness of a specific treatment by the highly regarded family healer.

Self-care: Where Does It Fit in the Healthcare System

Self-care is as old as humankind; therefore, it should be viewed as a healthcare resource. More than ever, as evidenced in cost-driven healthcare initiatives, society is relying on the individual and family to assume a significant role in managing their own care. APNs must, therefore, assume that most people, including health professionals, use self-care (and folk medicine) at some time in their lives. Most use more self-care treatments when they perceive themselves to be unhealthy or sick. APNs should be aware that it is not unusual for clients to use veterinary supplies for self-care, particularly antibiotics and ointments for skin and muscle conditions. Traditionally, domestic animals were of great financial value and a source of livelihood for many families. Because a remedy was safe for humans, the treatment also was deemed appropriate for animals having similar conditions. However, modern science and the U.S. Food and Drug Administration (FDA) have reversed the priority of the two. That is to say, for the most part, now a drug is first tested for safety on animals before the pharmaceutical product is approved for human use.

Although self-care and folk medicine may seem inconsistent with scientific knowledge, without such practices any system of healthcare would be swamped. For many people, the major distinction between care provided by healthcare professionals and self-care is the remuneration factor. APNs may find self-care practices ridiculous, yet well-educated consumers continue to engage in those practices (Coates, 1994; Hamburg, 1994; Miller, 1994; Whealan, 1994). Accurate data are not available, but it is estimated that Americans spend between $20 and more than $30 billion dollars on health-related products annually. Moreover, in 1997 about 40 million people tried one or more over-the-counter products. The FDA speculates that at least one in eight Americans suffers side effects from self-care treatments. The most profitable self-care products and services are arthritis remedies, spurious cancer clinics, cures for acquired immunodeficiency syndrome, weight-loss schemes, sexual stimulants, baldness remedies, nutritional cure-alls, muscle stimulators (legitimate in many cases but they do not get rid of wrinkles), treatment for "women's problems" such as premenstrual syndrome (PMS), treatment for hypoglycemia, treatment for generalized yeast infections, and feminine hygiene products. In essence, self-care and alternative providers must be considered by practitioners as integral to professional treatment plans even if these self-care interventions are not formally acknowledged by the consumer.

Categories of Self-care Practices

Self-care should be viewed from two levels: personal health behavior skills and sociopolitical skills (Bushy, Grassy, Kost, & Ramsdell, 1989). Both levels contribute to individual and family well-being. Personal self-care skills are those used to maintain or restore an individual's health. Sociopolitical skills are inherent in the self-care used by a community or a family to treat unusual conditions that occur in its members, particularly physical and emotional consequences associated with social and developmental transitions. Health promotion focuses on wellness "approach" behaviors; primary prevention involves illness "avoidance" behaviors to prevent or ward off an ailment; and illness treatments usually focus on symptom management or curing of the condition. Essentially, self-care continues to be used for health promotion, disease prevention, illness detection, and treatment of symptoms. These practices encompass a continuum of activities to retain and restore health.

Three major categories of folk remedies described in the literature are used across all cultures: folk remedies that are used to prevent or treat short-term conditions, those for chronic incurable conditions, and self-care treatments for psychosomatic conditions. Interestingly, even well-informed contemporaries continue to use variations of these remedies. This finding is evidenced by the continued popularity of self-care literature that is readily accessible in most supermarkets, bookstores, and even convenience stores.

Self-care practices in the first category are used to prevent or treat undesired physical symptoms or short-term or self-limiting conditions. Remedies in this group include (1) vitamins, minerals, and food supplements for body or muscle building; (2) remedies for warts, cold sores, minor menstrual problems, muscle aches, constipation, diarrhea, indigestion, hay fever, child growing pains, sore throats, ingrown toenails, colds, influenza, nosebleeds, insect bites, impetigo, hiccups, bumps, bruises, pimples, rashes, colic, dandruff, enuresis, ringworm, "jock itch," and athlete's foot; and (3) childrearing advice and first aid for common emergencies. These common health conditions are the focus of numerous advertisements in the popular media for an ever-increasing array of over-the-counter products used by the public to self-medicate.

Self-care practices in the second category are used to prevent or treat chronic and incurable conditions, including arthritis, hypertension, allergies, weight gain, weight loss, baldness, asthma, ulcers, gallbladder problems, impotence, infertility, sinusitis, and chronic pain, especially of the back. These chronic health conditions vary in severity depending on weather, stress, diet, and physical activity. It is not unusual, however, for a consumer to attribute improvement of the condition to a certain product used during that particular interval.

Self-care behaviors in the third category are used to prevent or treat complex conditions that often are emotional, psychosomatic, or nervous in origin, including persistent skin conditions (e.g., psoriasis, eczema, or hives), stomach ulcers, severe persistent menstrual cramps, endometriosis, migraine headaches, seizures, insomnia, neurosis, and psychosis. "Nervous" conditions have been more difficult to treat and usually are long term. Interventions for those conditions historically have been directed "at" the victim and have included praying over the afflicted person as well as physical abuse and torture through chaining, imprisonment, and shunning him or her. Often the treatment is extended to members of the client's family. The stigma associated with mental illness is an ongoing consequence of those interventions. Examples of other conditions that APNs may encounter related to this category include behavior problems in children, chronic depression, and anxiety disorders.

 Universal Healing Practices

A few self-care practices are common to several cultures. Three of the more common themes center on unusual-occurring natural phenomena, certain human behaviors, and touch. Each of these will be examined in greater detail in the next few paragraphs.

NATURAL PHENOMENA

Unusual occurrences in nature include an eclipse (or a particular position of the moon in relation to the earth or other planets), prolonged weather patterns, severe storms, dramatic changes in atmospheric pressure, and circumstantial events in daily life. At some time, most of these also have been given spiritual connotations. In some cultures, dramatic natural events are believed to affect health and healing. More significant natural phenomena are viewed as an omen or a message from God, one's spiritual guides, or angels (Thompson, 1989). Recent natural phenomena that have been attributed these qualities include the appearance of the Hale-Bopp comet, prolonged El Nino weather patterns, and several major eclipses.

Circumstantial natural events sometimes serve as a guide for childrearing or have a role in life decisions such as determining the appropriate time to marry, procreate, bury a loved one, or plant a crop. For example, an old, partially intact family bible included the following handwritten notation: "Proper weaning is done when the moon is in a zodiac sign that does not rule a vital organ—Aquarius, Pisces, Sagittarius, and Capricorn." Note the similarities between this advice and the astrologic guide published in a daily newspaper. The *Old Farmer's Almanac,* an annual publication that is available almost everywhere that popular media is sold, continues to provide similar information to modern consumers, and some precisely follow the advice provided therein. Contemporary practitioners may encounter individuals who adhere to those practices, as well as clients from other minority groups who practice voodoo, witchcraft, or have religious preferences that integrate natural phenomena into health and healing beliefs.

SELECT BEHAVIORS BY OTHERS

Another universal cultural belief relates to the concept of placing a curse or hex on another, described by some as the "evil eye." This phenomenon is believed to occur when a "spell maker" stares at another person or someone pats a child on the head. In turn, parents come to believe that the recipient of that behavior is cursed by the spell maker. It becomes a grave problem when the spell is cast on a child because the family believes that misfortune will follow this youngster.

The antidote to this imposed fate varies but often involves a ritual of anointing the cursed individual with a variety of substances, such as the saliva (spit) of the spell maker. Other rituals that people believe will improve health or ward off misfortune and illness include wearing an amulet, semiprecious stones, or colored crystals; carrying a rabbit's foot or lucky charm; wearing a select piece of clothing or a religious article of significance (e.g., crucifixes, medals of religious figures, or scapulars and some other type of garment); or hanging a bouquet of garlic in the room or near the person who is deemed to be vulnerable or ill.

TOUCH

Touch is another universal self-care behavior and healing ritual that is common across cultures. Touching rituals can involve various body parts of the healer as well as the person being healed. Touch also has symbolic or metaphoric connotations, hence the rationale for an old practice that involves touching the possession of an ill person or a blessed person. A common theme in folk healing is that certain people have a magical, God-given healing touch. For example, people of royal birth, those exhibiting unusual (bizarre) behaviors, and those having a distinguishing physical characteristic such as a birthmark or physical anomaly often are believed to have a magical or healing touch. Consequently, individuals having the "blessed touch" are sought by a community or family to treat sick members. Modern-day examples of the healing touch phenomenon have been attributed to the late Princess Diana, Mother Theresa, and popular television evangelists.

Historically, another often-cited ritual that is associated with touching was for a healer to suck on an afflicted body part to draw out evil. Bloodletting is a variation of this theme, as are several treatments for the common cold, such as placing an onion pack on the feet to draw out a cold or putting a mustard plaster on the chest to draw out germs and irritants that cause a person to cough. These remedies may seem antiquated to APNs. However, do not be surprised if some clients still espouse the curative powers of liniment, goose grease, onion packs, mustard plasters, and over-the-counter (medicated) petroleum-based salves. Some people, for instance, adhere to the practice of rubbing a mentholated ointment on the chest and feet of a person with a cold. Some think the treatment is more effective when the sick person also ingests a small dab of the ointment. Still others think that putting a small amount of the salve into a hot steamer will help purify the air, which can help the sick person breath easier.

Touch continues to be an important part of healing by contemporary health professionals. A resurgence also has occurred in research on the relationship between touch, caring, and curing. A proposed explanation is that touch promotes the generation of chemicals in the body's immune system, thereby promoting healing. Examples of therapeutic touch in which APNs may engage are the "rituals" of a routine physical examination: taking vital signs, checking the height of a fundus, providing comfort measures in the form of a back rub administered to an elderly person or premature infant, administering a therapeutic massage to relieve stress, hugging a child after administering an injection, touching the hand of a grieving person to demonstrate empathy or support, or initiating pet therapy for a lonely client.

Box 11-1 includes some commonly used self-care interventions that remain popular among Americans. Most practitioners will at some time or another encounter these self-care practices. Despite their extensive use, researchers cannot explain how and why most folk remedies work. In recent years, scientists have found several long-standing remedies to be effective. Practitioners are using a few to treat certain conditions. Even so, the treatments were used centuries before people could explain how the body responded to an intervention. For example, the remedy of placing a spider web on a wound to enhance the clotting process and help stop bleeding was used centuries before physiologists identified the clotting mechanisms of the blood. People ate rose hips for generations to help them stay healthy long before biochemists recognized the importance of vitamin C in the diet.

Many other popular remedies still do not have physiologic explanations, including wearing a copper bracelet or magnets to reduce arthritic pain, ingesting garlic to reduce high blood pressure and prevent upper respiratory tract infections, and drinking aloe vera or applying it to affected body areas for healing effects. Still, people who use these treatments typically are convinced of their effectiveness. For this reason, practitioners need to be aware that disapproval of those practices will do little to deter the client from continuing to engage in them. In fact, displaying a judgmental attitude in many cases will only serve to deter the

Box 11-1	*Common Self-care Remedies*

FOR BURNS

Scald milk and moisten a piece of bread in it. Squeeze out the excess moisture and place bread on the burned area.
Place sliced raw potato on the burned area.
Place the affected area in cold water.
Apply a leaf of the aloe vera plant to the area.

FOR BOILS

Cover the boil with axle grease three or four times a day.
Cover the boil with a piece of adhesive tape for 24 hours, then remove the tape. The core will stick to the tape.
Make a poultice with chamomile tea and apply three to four times a day to the lesion until it comes to a head and drains.

FOR DIGESTIVE/ALIMENTARY PROBLEMS

For an upset stomach and nausea, drink a tea made from ginger root or peppermint leaves.
For treating and preventing ulcers, eat fresh cabbage.
For hemorrhoids, apply witch hazel packs.

FOR BABIES WITH COLIC

Administer fennel or peppermint tea.
Massage the child's feet (based on principles of reflexology).

TO STIMULATE A BABY'S APPETITE FOR BREAST MILK

Eat fresh garlic 1 hour before breastfeeding.
Drink a can of beer while nursing.

FOR FEMININE ITCHING

Bathe with vinegar, ginger, salt, or baking soda.

FOR THE PREVENTION OF CHILDHOOD COLDS

With breakfast, give your children two cherry-flavored vitamin C tablets every day. Take an extra tablet in winter.
Daily, dissolve one or two zinc lozenges in your mouth to neutralize the cold virus.
Eat raw onions and hot peppers several times a week.

FOR THE TREATMENT OF MENSTRUAL PROBLEMS (PMS)

Take at least one tablet of each of the following daily: dolomite, multiple vitamins with iron, vitamin B_6, vitamin E, magnesium, and evening primrose oil.

FOR THE REGULATION OF BLOOD PRESSURE

Take two or three garlic tablets every day and reduce salt intake.

client from sharing this kind of information with professional caregivers. In turn, by not incorporating self-care into the treatment plan, adverse events can occur because of the interaction effects of the self-care practices with conventional medical interventions.

Trends and Implications for Advanced Practice Nurses

Despite the increased availability of healthcare services and professionals in the 20th century, self-care continues to be popular, partly because of the high cost of healthcare and the inherent skills of human survival and partly because consumers lack faith in the effectiveness of the healthcare system. The consumer movement has created a receptive audience for the distribution of a wide range of self-care literature, at-home diagnostic devices, and the ever-increasing number of over-the-counter medications.

Several contemporary self-care publications were first printed around the turn of the 20th century and probably evolved from the practice of updating early *Doctor Books*. These popular magazines still are available at many newsstands, and based on their widespread distribution, one can assume that modern consumers still are interested in the content. In perusing the content in these self-care publications, APNs will find articles on nutrition, products for illness diagnosis, and a range of treatments for common—and not so common—health problems as well as over-the-counter medications for symptom management. Consumer-focused self-care publications prescribe the most effective way to use a variety of naturally occurring substances, such as herbs, fruits, and vegetables. In each issue, one also finds an array of advertisements that inform readers how to purchase the products discussed within the edition. Some of the products are proven "fad-scams." Most, however, have never been validated as either effective or ineffective, despite the prolonged popularity of the product. Being knowledgeable about some of these fads can help APNs better understand the benefits and dangers of more popular self-care behaviors that a client may be using. In light of the widespread use of self-care and folk remedies, practitioners must be sensitive to clients' alternative conceptions of causation and remediation of illness. Then, try to work with the client to modify those behaviors so they are compatible with the conventional treatment plan.

Health professionals must accept that self-care, in many instances, may be an effective therapy. Because of ethnic diversity, many Americans use a wide range of therapeutic systems as alternatives to conventional medicine. In addition to those described in this chapter, some of the more popular remedies are psychic healing, Rolfing, chiropractic care, faith healing, therapeutic massage, osteopathy, meditation, and visualization. Perhaps a user's belief in nontraditional modalities contributes to their effectiveness.

Although practitioners of conventional Western medicine may not formally acknowledge self-care and, in many instances, deny its effectiveness, we must recognize that self-care is a significant component of healthcare. Self-care interventions, however, can interfere with and sometimes actually be detrimental to the individual. For this reason, practitioners must become informed of the fine line between folk medicine and scientifically based healthcare; but differentiating the two can become problematic in some cases.

To elicit information about a client's use of self-care and folk treatments, practitioners must learn to tactfully ask pertinent questions during the assessment phase. Practitioners should then include the information in the client's database and care plan for effective, appropriate, and acceptable education (Bushy, 1998; Geissler, 1994; Stanhope & Knollmueller, 1997). Questioning by caregivers must always be nonjudgmental and address the following themes:

■ Does the client rely on self-care or traditional folk practices? If so, what are they?
■ Which remedies does the client use for health promotion? Disease prevention? Illness intervention?

- Is the client currently being treated by a cultural healer? If so, is the person willing to share information about the nontraditional interventions?
- Does the client prefer having a cultural healer as a part of the traditional healthcare plan? If so, who is this healer and how can this individual be contacted?
- Does the client wish to have certain individuals or relatives present during treatment? What role are they to take during the healing process?

Should a client's belief system include folk remedies such as drinking herb tea, eating certain foods, using natural products, or using over-the-counter drugs or nutritional supplements, APNs should respect these beliefs and preferences. Respect, however, does not require negating the use of scientifically based treatments. Instead, it means assessing the benefits and risks of a remedy. Then, if appropriate, incorporate the self-care practice as an adjunct to prescribed scientific interventions. Or, in other instances, modify conventional treatment protocols to prevent deleterious outcomes.

APNs must be sensitive to the fact that when they present scientific knowledge that seems incompatible with a client's traditional beliefs, the client probably will accept the traditional way and reject the best health information. APNs likely can anticipate nonadherance behaviors on the part of these clients. Taking time to have the client explain, in his or her own words, the treatment plan and how to take any prescribed medicines can go a long way toward improving practitioner–client communication. Such explanation can also alert the practitioner to cultural beliefs and values that could promote or hinder client compliance with prescribed regimens. Practitioners demonstrate an even greater measure of cultural competency by asking a client for his or her point of view. This approach supports collaborating with the person rather than imposing a treatment plan, although it initially can be time consuming. A collaborative approach can prevent many follow-up phone calls or office visits because of misunderstood treatment protocols.

APNs can learn a great deal about effective client teaching from consumer-oriented self-care publications, as described in other sections of this chapter. Congruency between traditional beliefs and an emphasis on measures to promote health and prevent illness partially account for the success of self-care publications. Health information disseminated in the popular media typically is written in a clear, concise manner, making sense to the readers. Although the logic may lack scientific accuracy or at times be convoluted, the content usually has elements of truth to it. Essentially, the new information expands on what most consumers already know about a particular topic. This marketing approach is highly effective for promoting a particular product or remedy.

Efforts on the part of practitioners to collaborate and integrate self-care with scientifically based interventions is another strategy that often encourages compliance behaviors, especially if the remedy is not detrimental and will not compromise the client's therapeutic regimen. Instead of negating culturally based folk care and implementing a totally unfamiliar regimen, practitioners should consider the highly effective strategy used by popular self-care magazines. Allow the client something that is culturally familiar, such as folk remedies and self-care behaviors. As a result, the client is apt to adhere more closely to the scientifically based therapeutic regimen and to perceive that care as appropriate and acceptable to them.

Overall, cultural competency is one of the most important elements of providing holistic nursing care to clients in our culturally diverse nation. With that in mind, APNs must always be aware of, and sensitive to, the role of ethnocultural factors in an individual's perceptions of health, illness, and healthcare behaviors. Cultural competency is reflected by the coordination of a meaningful and appropriate treatment plan for a particular client and his or her family system. Cultural competency is also an important factor in planning, delivering, and evaluating appropriate and acceptable services for clients, especially those of minority origins.

REFERENCES

Ahmann, E. (1994). Chunky stew: Appreciating cultural diversity while providing health care to children. *Pediatric Nursing 20*(3), 320–324.

Andrews, M., & Boyle, J. (1997). Competence in transcultural nursing care. *American Journal of Nursing 97*(8), 16AAA–16DDD.

Barbee, E. (1993). Racism in U.S. nursing. *Medical Anthropology Quarterly 7*(4), 346–362.

Bell, R. (1994). Prominence of women in Navajo healing beliefs and values. *Nursing and Health Care 15*(5), 232–240.

Brink, P. (1993). Cultural diversity in nursing: How much can we tolerate. In J. McClosky & H. Grace (Eds.), *Current issues in nursing* (pp. 521–528). St. Louis, MO: Mosby.

Bushy, A. (1998). Social and cultural issues affecting practice. In J. Lancaster & W. Lancaster (Eds.). *Advanced nursing practice: The nurse as a change agent.* St;. Louis, MO: Mosby.

Bushy, A., Grassy, B., Kost, S., & Ramsdell, K. (1989). *Folk medicine on the prairie.* Bismarck, ND: Medcenter One.

Coates, J. (1994). The highly probable future: 83 assumptions by the year 2025. *The Futurist 28*(4), 29–38.

Geissler, E. (1994). *Pocket guide: Cultural assessment.* St. Louis, MO: Mosby.

Grossman, D., & Taylor, R. (1995). Cultural diversity on the unit. *American Journal of Nursing 95*(2), 64–67.

Hamburg, J. (1994). Can home remedies work? *Parade Magazine, July 31,* 4–5.

Krieger, N. (1996). Inequality, diversity and health: Thoughts on race/ethnicity, and gender. *Journal of American Medical Womens Association 51*(4), 133–136.

Leininger, M. (1969). Ethnoscience: A new and promising research approach for the health sciences. *Image 3*(1), 2–8.

Leininger, M. (1978). *Transcultural nursing: Concepts, theories, and practices.* New York: John Wiley & Sons.

Leininger, M. (1984). *Ethnohealth, ethnocaring and ethnonursing of six cultures.* Detroit, MI: Wayne State University Press.

Leininger, M. (Ed.). (1985a). *Qualitative research methods in nursing.* New York: Grune & Stratton.

Leininger, M. (1985b). *Transcultural care diversity and universality: A theory of nursing.* Thorofare, NJ: Charles B. Slack.

Leininger, M. (1994). Transcultural nursing education: A worldwide imperative. *Nursing & Health Care 15*(5), 254–261.

Leininger, M. (1997). Transcultural nursing research to transform nursing education and practice: 40 years. *Image: Journal of Nursing Scholarship 29*(4), 341–347.

Levin, L. (1995). The lay person as the primary health care practitioner. *Public Health Reports 91*(3), 206–210.

Milburn, N., Gary, L., Booth, J., & Brown, D. (1992). Conducting epidemiological research in a minority community: Methodological considerations. *Journal of Community Psychology 19*(1), 3–12.

Miller, L. (1994). Non-traditional medical options: U.S. spends $13 million on studies. *USA Today, August 1,* D1.

Morganthau, T. (1997). America 2000: The face of the future. *Newsweek January 27,* 58–61.

National Center for Health Statistics. (1996). *Health United States: 1996.* Washington, DC: US Government Printing Office.

National Rural Health Association (NRHA). (1994). *Conference proceedings on minority health: A shared vision, building bridges for rural heal access.* Kansas City, MO: Author.

National Rural Health Association (NRHA). (1997). *Bringing resources to bear on the changing health care system: Birmingham, Alabama conference proceedings.* Kansas City, MO: Author.

National Rural Health Association (NRHA). (1998). *Status of rural minorities health: Conference proceedings.* Kansas City, MO: Author.

Rosella, J., Regan-Kubinski, M., & Albrecht, S. (1994). The need for multicultural diversity among health professionals. *Nursing and Health Care 15*(5), 242–246.

Spradley, J. (1979). *The ethnographic interview.* New York: Holt, Rinehart & Winston.

Spradley, J. (1980). *Participant observation.* New York: Holt, Rinehart & Winston.

Stanhope, M., & Knollmueller, R. (1997). *Public health and community health nurse consultant: A health promotion guide* (pp. 211–242). St. Louis, MO: Mosby.

Sternbert, S. (1997). Study shows yawning gaps in U.S. health care: Longevity affected by environment. *USA Today December 4,* 11-A.

Strickland, J., & Strickland, D. (1996). Barriers to preventive health services for minority households in the south. *The Journal of Rural Health 12*(3), 206–217.

Thompson, C. (1989). *Magic and healing.* New York: Bell Publisher.

US Department of Commerce. (1996). *Statistical abstract of the United States.* Washington, DC: Bureau of the Census.

US Department of Health and Human Services (USDHHS). (1991). *Healthy people 2000: National health promotion and disease prevention objectives* (DHHS Publication No. PHS 91–50213). Washington, DC: US Government Printing Office.

US Department of Health and Human Services (USDHHS). (1996a). *Health United States: 1995* (DHHS Publication No. PHS 96–1242). Hyattsville, MD: Author.

US Department of Health and Human Services (USD-HHS). (1996b). *Healthy people 2000: Mid-course review.* Hyattsville, MD: Author.

US Department of Health and Human Services (USD-HHS). (1998). *Selected statistics on health professional shortage areas as of September 30, 1997.* Washington, DC: Author.

Whealan, E. (1994). *The nutritional, purely organic, cholesterol free, megavitamin, low carbohydrate, nutrition hoax.* New York: Atheneum.

Whorton, J. (1987). Traditions of folk medicine in America. *Journal of the American Medical Association 257*(12), 1632–1635.

Williams, G. (1994). The healing power of prayer. *American Legion 137*(2), 19–22.

Yawn, B., Bushy, A., Dubbels, K., et al. (1994). Making your practice palatable for your patients: Cultural competency. In B. Yawn, A. Bushy, & R. Yawn (Eds.), *Exploring rural medicine* (pp. 253–271). Newbury Park, CA: Sage Publications.

CHAPTER 12

Alternative and Complementary Therapies

Joan Engebretson

Alternative, complementary, and unconventional medicine have been used interchangeably to describe an evolving category of health resources. The terminology is confusing because the terms are not synonymous. *Alternative medicine* implies "outside of biomedicine" and is widely used to describe many of the popular activities to enhance health, including nutrition, chiropractic, massage, and use of vitamins. This term is misleading because most of these therapies are used as a complement to biomedical treatment or for health promotion. A more appropriate use would be to reserve the term *alternative* for therapies used instead of biomedical treatment. Because many of these complementary therapies meet client needs for comfort, pain, and symptom relief; facilitate coping; and focus on the holistic care of the whole patient, instead of the more narrow focus on the disease, this contemporary consumer movement has large implications for the nursing profession. Nurses are natural providers of many of these services that have previously been described as independent nursing interventions (Snyder & Lindquist, 1998).

Alternative or Complementary Therapies

It is important for nurses to distinguish between treatments used in place of biomedical care and those therapies used to complement biomedical treatment or to promote health and well-being. The definitions shown in Box 12-1 will be used for this chapter; however, the other terms may be used when citing the literature. Cassileth (1998) differentiates between alternative treatments that are seen as unproved or lacking proof of efficacy and are used in lieu of biomedical treatment and the noninvasive, gentle, pleasant, often natural and stress-reducing complementary therapies that are helpful and applicable during sickness and in health. Several biologic treatments for serious diseases, such as cancer, acquired immunodeficiency syndrome (AIDS), and heart disease, would best fall into the alternative category. These treatments often consist of use of active chemical agents or drugs that may have inherent harmful effects. Others treatments may be less toxic, such as use of a re-

Box 12-1 | *Definitions*

Alternative therapies: Therapies used instead of conventional biomedicine.
Complementary therapies: Therapies used in addition or as a complement to biomedicine or for the promotion of health.
Integrated medicine: Provision of healthcare services combining both biomedical and complementary medicine.
Disease: A specific constellation of signs and symptoms used by a provider to diagnose a disorder, explain it, and suggest a treatment.
Cure: Restoration of signs and symptoms to a normal state.
Illness: The individual's and family's experience of health and disease.
Healing: To make whole; incorporates physical, psychological, social, spiritual, and environmental health and may or may not include cure.

TABLE 12-1 *Examples of Alternative Biologic Treatments*

Apitherapy: Bee and other insect venom immunotherapy.

Used for: Chronic pain, arthritis, multiple sclerosis, migraines, premenstrual syndrome, and bladder control.

Hypothesized explanation: It stimulates an inflammatory process and activates the immune system.

How used: In products such as royal jelly, propolis, bee pollen, and raw honey.

Distribution: Through stores, mail, and the Internet.

Potential dangers: Allergic responses can be severe in certain people.

Cell Therapy: Injections of live or freeze-dried cells from animals or embryos to promote healing and youthfulness.

Used for: Overall health promotion and to repair damaged cells and organs. Often used to increase vitality and sexual function and as antidotes to aging and various diseases, such as cancer and AIDS.

Hypothesized explanation: Immune system enhancement through ribonucleic acid from healthy injected cells.

How used: 6 treatments; for restoration of youth, 6 months to 2 years.

Distribution: Not legal in the United States but available in Europe, Mexico, and the Bahamas.

Potential dangers: Immune rejection reaction (some have animal antibodies that reduce this effect).

Chelation Therapy Ethylenediaminetetraacetic Acid (EDTA): Chemicals are introduced into the bloodstream that bind to iron and are later excreted from the system. This treatment has proven effective for lead and heavy metal toxicity.

Used for: Removal of plaque from arteries and to treat thyroid disorders, multiple sclerosis, muscular dystrophy, high cholesterol, psoriasis, hypercalcemia, and cancer.

Hypothesized explanation: EDTA offers protective effects against detrimental action of free radients.

How used: May be three to four clinic visits of 3-hour duration and is offered as an alternative to angioplasty or bypass surgery.

Potential dangers: May produce toxic effects such as kidney and bone marrow damage, irregular heart rhythm, and venous inflammation.

Research: This is one of the areas targeted for further research from the National Center for Complementary and Alternative Medicine (CAM).

Colon Detoxification Therapies: Colonic irrigation using water, coffee, or herbal solutions to cleanse out built-up waste in the intestines.

Used for: As a detoxification modality it is used as a primary form of treatment, as a preventive, and as a general hygienic routine.

Hypothesized explanation: High-meat and high-fat diets that are not balanced with high fiber cause a sticky mucoid substance to remain in the colon, producing autointoxication of toxins that are carried in the bloodstream and cause various types of illnesses.

TABLE 12-1 *Examples of Alternative Biologic Treatments* (Continued)

How used: Colon therapists or colon hygienists are licensed in some states and may be members of the American Colon Therapy Association. High enemas using either gravity or machines. These treatments may be available in spas, specialty clinics, or other settings.

Potential dangers: Several cases of illness and death have been reported because of poor technique and unsanitary conditions. The American Colon Therapy Association is attempting to regulate these concerns. This therapy may also disturb normal bowel flora and be contraindicated in many medical conditions.

Research: The AMA Council on Scientific Affairs has debunked the notion of autointoxication.

Enzyme Therapy: Use of digestive enzyme supplements to aid digestion and fight illness.

Used for: Digestive aids and treatment for sore throats, hay fever, ulcers, virus, and cancer.

Hypothesized explanation: Increasing the amount of enzymes beyond that normally produced will help the body absorb more nutrients that restore health.

How used: Sold in health food stores as a food supplement to be taken between meals.

Potential dangers: Enzymes are broken down by the body and are absorbed; physiologic harm is not known.

Research: FDA investigation revealed no support for the claims and issued an injunction banning promotional material with unproved claims.

Oxygen Therapy: Use of ozone or hydrogen peroxide to treat disease.

Used for: Treatment for asthma, emphysema, AIDS, cancer, Alzheimer's disease, and a number of serious diseases.

Hypothesized explanation: Ozone and peroxide break down in the body to oxygen and provide an oxygen-rich environment that kills disease-causing microorganisms that, as lower-evolved forms of life, require a low-oxygen environment. This is based on the work of Dr. Warbug, who observed that cancer cells have lower respiratory rates than healthy cells.

How used: Intravenous infusion or injection or infusion into the rectum or vagina over a period of 1 to several weeks.

Potential dangers: Hydrogen peroxide is toxic if injected. It is not medically recommended.

Research: Clinical trials are being conducted for use in human immunodeficiency virus (HIV) based on some preliminary laboratory studies.

Shark and Bovine Cartilage: Use of exogenous cartilage.

Used for: Treatment of cancer, osteoporosis, and other bone and joint disorders.

Hypothesized explanation: A protein in cartilage inhibits angiogenesis in test tube laboratory research, thus decreasing blood supply to the tumor. The active ingredient in shark cartilage is too large to be absorbed in the bloodstream. Bovine cartilage may inhibit tumors by boosting the immune system.

How used: By mouth or by enema (shark cartilage tastes bad and is used in large doses (60–90 g/d).

Distribution: Sold in health food stores and through mail order as a food supplement.

Potential dangers: Dangerous if replaces conventional treatment; if used adjunctively, treatment interactions need to be considered.

Research: Some studies demonstrate efficacy, but more research is needed.

Biologic Cancer Treatments: Some of the more popular treatments are antineoplastins, cancell, diamethyl sulfoxide (DMSO), Essiac, Hydrazine sulfate, Livingston-Wheeler regimen, and Revici's guided chemotherapy.

Antineoplastins: Peptides are isolated from human urine and are hypothesized to convert cancer cells to normal cells. The treatment is given only by Dr. Burzynski in his clinic in Houston, TX. Although the FDA has given him permission to conduct clinical trials, the treatment has been embroiled in controversy. There are many anecdotal claims of cure.

Cancell: A treatment developed by a chemist that is popular in the Midwest and parts of Florida, with little evidence of effectiveness.

DMSO: An industrial solvent similar to turpentine. Used to relieve pain and heal injuries. It has been used by veterinarians and is currently under study for injuries and scleroderma. It has been proposed as a cancer treatment.

Essiac: An herbal preparation developed by a Canadian nurse based on a Native American mixture. Several competing products are on the market. Some of the ingredients have antitumor properties in the test tube, but studies of humans taking it demonstrate no effectiveness.

Information in this table is extracted from Cassileth (1998).

ligious ritual, but if used alternatively may delay effective medical treatment. Some of these treatments may be effective in certain circumstances, which gives added allure and promise to the user. Table 12-1 describes some common biologic treatments, with a hypothesized explanation of action and information related to use and procurement as well as potential dangers. These therapies often are invasive or include use of active chemical components and thus have the potential for harm as well as benefit. These are primarily therapies that have not undergone rigorous clinical trials for safety and efficacy; however, in many cases research is currently under way. Professional nurses must exercise caution and follow the literature in using or endorsing these treatments.

The focus of this chapter is on complementary therapies. These are generally gentle, natural, noninvasive, holistic treatments that are used as supplements to biomedical treatment or to enhance health and well-being. Many of these treatments are used to reduce stress, enhance coping, and engage the natural healing of the body. Their use parallels the public interest in self-help, human potential movements, and consumer interest in enhancing health and wellness. Although some clients may abandon biomedical treatment to pursue these treatments, most use these therapies in conjunction with biomedicine or to enhance their health and well-being.

Differentiating among the terms *disease, cure, illness,* and *healing* is necessary to better understand the relationship of these activities to biomedical and nursing care. *Disease* refers to a specific constellation of symptoms and signs that are used by a medical provider to diagnose a disorder or dysfunction, explain it, and suggest a treatment. *Curing* is the restoration of these signs and symptoms to a normal state. *Illness* refers to the individual's and family's experience of health and/or disease. *Healing* means to "make hale or whole" and implies a broader domain that may or may not include cure.

In general, biomedicine focuses on diagnosing, treating, and curing disease. This reflects the scientific base and explanatory model that underlies biomedicine. This scientific base has generated a sophisticated technology focused on increasingly precise diagnosis and treatment. Healers focus on caring for the individual through the illness experience, which is a holistic, personalized approach that is similar to the theoretical domain of nursing. Although the World Health Organization, Geneva, Switzerland, defined health beyond the absence of disease, biomedicine, in praxis, generally operates from the concept of restoration to a normal state, meaning absence of disease. In contrast, healers conceptualize health as whenever the individual is in his or her own state of health and healing as the dynamic process in which the mind, body, and spirit become whole, which may or may not include cure of disease.

Complementary and Alternative Therapies and Contemporary Healthcare

Use of alternative and complementary healing methods has been growing in popularity and now constitutes a large growth industry in healthcare. Two frequently cited studies conducted in 1990 (Eisenberg et al., 1993; Eisenberg et al., 1998) indicated an increase in the use of alternative forms of healing from 33.8% (1993) to 42.1% (1998). The greatest increases were in herbal medicine, massage, megavitamins, self-help groups, energy healing, and homeopathy. Of those users, more than 60% reported that they had not shared this information with their physician. The out-of-pocket money spent on alternative healthcare was comparable to expenditures from all U.S. physician services. Another survey of 1500 adults in the United States showed that 42% had used alternative therapies within the past year, and 67% indicated that the availability of an alternative healthcare component was important in choosing a healthcare plan (Landmark, 1998; Villaire, 1998b). A Canadian survey revealed 42% use, reflecting a doubling during the past 5 years (Villaire, 1998). In another survey of more than 1000 adults, use of alternative medicine was associated with higher education and a more holistic orientation to health, a chronic health problem, or other recent illness and having had a transformational experience that changed their world view (Astin, 1998). This group expressed a set of values and beliefs and a philosophical orientation that included commitment to environmentalism and feminism, interest in spirituality, and personal growth. Several studies described these users as generally well-educated and affluent members of the middle class (Astin, 1998; Eisenberg et al., 1993; Engebretson, 1996; McGuire, 1988).

Many healthcare plans are including options for alternative therapies, and an increasing number of hospitals are offering complementary therapies (Moore, 1997; Villaire, 1998a). In a survey of the nation's largest health maintenance organizations, 86% covered some type of alternative therapy (Goodwin, 1997). Many of these providers are able to directly bill the health plan provider without a physician's order.

This expanding interest has not been limited to the lay public. Both medicine and nursing have professional organizations that encourage incorporating select modalities into integrated practice: the American Holistic Medical Association and the American Holistic Nursing Association. A survey on American medical education indicated that 75 (60%) of the 125 medical schools are now offering courses on alternative and complementary therapies (Wetzel, Eisenberg, & Kaptchuk,1998). The Robert Wood Johnson Foundation (Marston & Jones, 1992) and the PEW Charitable Trust (PEW, 1995) established commissions to study health professions and made recommendations regarding the changing needs of healthcare delivery. These reports call for cost containment, focusing on health, using innovative and diverse provisions for healthcare, and engaging the patient as an active agent in health. The Hastings Center for Bioethics, New York, NY, in establishing priorities for the goals of medicine, called for more research on alternative therapies (Callahan, 1996). The Institute for Alternative Futures (1998) anticipates that by 2010 two-thirds of the population will use some form of complementary approaches that are well matched to the emphasis on health promotion and wellness-oriented lifestyles.

The National Institutes of Health (NIH), Bethesda, MD, in response to a mandate from Congress, established an Office for Alternative Medicine (OAM) in 1994, which was later renamed the Office for Complementary and Alternative Medicine. The OAM was established to study nonconventional therapies for potential efficacy and to disseminate information to providers and the public. In accordance with the congressional mandate, the purpose of the OAM is to identify and evaluate the effectiveness, safety, and cost of complementary and alternative healthcare therapies and modalities. The office has recently been upgraded to the National Center for Complementary and Alternative Medicine.

Ten centers have been established through the OAM to study various aspects of alternative and complementary healing (see Table 12-2). A center to study chiropractic medicine was recently added. Several peer-reviewed journals are available, and many national professional organizations—such as the American Public Health Association—have established special sections devoted to alternative therapies. In addition, many national conferences are organized around providing integrated medicine.

The OAM sponsored a working group conference to discuss the state of alternative therapy use in the United States and to make recommendations for research and practice (NIH, 1992). This group published a report, known as the Chantilly Report, that categorized and discussed complementary and alternative medicine practices into seven broad categories and made recommendations for research. The seven categories were mind–body interventions, bioelectromagnetic applications in medicine, alternative systems of medical practice, manual healing methods, pharmacologic and biologic treatments, herbal medicine, and diet and nutrition in prevention and treatment of chronic disease (see Table 12-3).

An NIH consensus panel, cosponsored by the OAM and the Office of Medical Applications of Research, evaluated scientific and medical data on the uses, risks, and

TABLE 12-2 *NIH-funded Complementary and Alternative Medicine Research Centers*

Center	Focus	Principle investigator
University of Arizona Health Science Center Tucson, AZ	Pediatric conditions	Feyez Ghishan, MD Andrew Weil, MD
Bastyr University Seattle, WA	HIV and AIDS	Leanna Standish, ND, PhD
Columbia University College of Physicians and Surgeons New York, NY	Women's health	Fredi Kronenberg, PhD
Consortial Center for Chiropractic Research[a] at Palmer College of Chiropractic Davenport, IA	Chiropractic	William Meeker, DC, MPH
Harvard Medical School Beth Israel Hospital Boston, MA	Chronic medical conditions	David Eisenberg, MD
Kessler Medical Rehabilitation University of Medicine and Dentistry Newark, NJ	Stroke and neurorehabilitation	Samuel Shiflett, PhD
Minneapolis Center for Addiction and Alternative Medicine Research Hennepin County Medical Center Minneapolis, MN	Addictions	Thomas Kiresuk, PhD
Stanford University Center for Research in Disease Prevention Palo Alto, CA	Aging	William Haskell, PhD
University of California–Davis Davis, CA	Allergies and asthma	M. Eric Gershwin MD Judith Stern, ScD
University of Maryland School of Medicine (CAMPRE) Baltimore, MD	Pain	Brian Berman, MD
University of Michigan Ann Arbor	Cardiovascular Diseases	Steven Bolling, MD
University of Texas Health Health Science Center Houston, TX	Cancer prevention and treatment	Guy Parcel, PhD
University of Virginia School of Nursing Charlottesville, VA	Pain—acute and chronic	Ann Gill, RN, EdD

[a]Added center in 1998.

TABLE 12-3 *Examples of Complementary and Alternative Medical Practices as Classified in the Chantilly Report*

Alternative systems of medical care: Acupuncture, homeopathic medicine
Bioelectromagnetic applications: Electromagnetic fields electrostimulation
Diet, nutrition, lifestyle changes: Macrobiotics, nutritional supplements
Herbal medicine: Echinacea, ginseng root
Manual healing: Chiropractic, therapeutic touch
Mind/body control: Art therapy, meditation, music therapy
Pharmacologic and biologic treatments: Antioxidizing agents, chelation therapy

benefits of acupuncture procedures for a variety of conditions. The recommendations were that acupuncture is an effective treatment for nausea caused by chemotherapy drugs, surgical anesthesia, and pregnancy and for pain resulting from surgery and a variety of musculoskeletal conditions (CAM Newsletter, 1998). Another NIH panel endorsed integrating behavioral and relaxation therapies such as meditation, hypnosis, and biofeedback into the medical management of chronic pain and insomnia (Chilton, 1996).

Historical and Cross-Cultural Approaches to Healing

All societies across cultures and historical periods have developed multiple approaches to healing. The rise of scientifically oriented biomedicine contrasted with many of the earlier fundamental explanatory models of health and illness that were oriented toward healing. These controversies are summarized in Table 12-4. The concept of the person is seen as dualistic in biomedicine, in contrast to the holistic perspective of the healing systems. Until the Age of Enlightenment, most healing systems understood health as a holistic dynamic that was subject to disorder from both the internal and the external environment. After the 17th century, the dominant academic philosophy of western Europe was epitomized by René Descartes, who attempted to resolve an ancient Greek view of reality as having two distinctly different aspects: the material, which is perceived through the senses, and the nonmaterial or pure knowledge. Descartes promoted mind–body dualism in which the

TABLE 12-4 *Fundamental Controversies in Explanatory Styles of Healing Systems*

	Biomedical Systems	Healing Systems
Concept of person	Dualistic	Holistic
World view	Reductionistic/categorical	Unified/relational
Intent	Naturalistic	Personalistic
Locus of causation	External	Internal
Organization	Professional	Community-based

body was subject to the physical mechanistic laws but the mind/spirit was subject to a different set of laws (Lovallo, 1997). Dualism subjected the body to the rigors of physical science and separated thought, emotion, and spirit from the domain of medicine. This world view also is associated with the ideas of categorical thinking and reductionism whereby one understands complex things by first studying the simpler parts. This approach of knowing more about less is contrasted with the more holistic relational or unified approaches that strive to understand complexity by looking at the larger context and the various influences on the system.

Ideas of intention and causation are also contrasted. Lacking the scientific understanding of the mechanisms of the function of the body in health and disease, a personalistic explanatory style was often used in healing systems. The personalistic model ascribes the cause of sickness to some form of intention, such as attracting the wrong energies or as a response to one's own behaviors or misperception. Thus, causation was often seen as internal. Scientific medicine used a naturalistic approach in which the causes of sickness are found in the natural world, such as germs, accidents, and other natural causes that lack specific intention (Cassidy, 1996). Biomedicine has also favored a locus of disease causation as an attack by an external agency. This is reflected in the prevalence of military metaphors used in the fighting of disease. Internal causation or degenerative disorders have not fit this framework and have presented a challenge to the biomedical model because the interventions are less prescriptive and lean toward education, prevention, and lifestyle management (Cassidy, 1996).

Finally, professional approaches that serve large, heterogeneous patient populations and are influenced by mass marketing, efficiency, and standardization contrasted with healing approaches that are more community based. The standardized professional approach is often seen in evidence-based practice, protocols for specific diseases, and other strategies used by managed care to provide efficient treatment for specific populations. The local, community-based systems are more reflective of folk medicine used by healers who have a specific treatment for multiple disorders, which is individualized to each patient.

Biomedicine, although not exclusively adhering to one side of the controversies, has been inclined toward the dualistic, reductionist, naturalistic world views with an external locus of causation. Biomedicine has also followed the professional standardized approach to treatment instead of a more local community or individualistic approach to patient care. A shift in cultural values has been evident not only in the cognitive models of the healers (Engebretson, 1996) but also in the value systems of the users (Astin, 1998). According to a large survey, nearly one-quarter of the population, labeled the "cultural creatives," held a holistic philosophy of health; valued ecology, spirituality, relationships, and self-actualization; and expressed interest in other cultures and new ideas (Ray, 1998). They tended to be highly educated and idealistic, with a higher representation of women. This shift in values corresponds well to the holistic focus espoused by many of the complementary treatment practitioners. As healthcare changes toward a more community-oriented, individualized model with a focus on prevention and health promotion, it can be anticipated that these modalities will become widely used. Many healthcare delivery models currently integrate these modalities to address the public need for more individualized health-oriented approaches that attend to the quality of life and the health–illness experience as well as diagnosis and treatment of the disease.

Multiparadigm Model of Healing

The Multiparadigm Model of Healing, illustrated in Figure 12–1, is one way of looking at the types of healing alternatives that are emerging and of understanding their relationship and similarities to each other. Not only does this model facilitate the understanding of al-

Positivist ← → Metaphysical

Material ←——————→ Nonmaterial

Modalities	Mechanical	Purification	Balance	Supranormal
Physical manipulation	Biomedical surgery	Colonics Cupping	Magnetic healing Polarity	Drumming Dancing
Applied and ingested substances	Pharmacology	Chelation	Humoral medicine	Flower remedies Hallucinogenic plants
Energy	Laser Radiation	Bioenergetics	Tai chi Chi gong Acupuncture Accupressure	Healing touch Laying on of hands
Psychological	Mind–body	Self-help (confessional type)	Mindfulness	Imagery
Spiritual	Attendance at organized religious functions	Forgiveness Penance	Meditation Chakra Balancing	Primal religious Experience Prayer

FIGURE 12-1 Explanatory Paradigms. Reprinted with permission from: *Advances in Nursing Science 20*(1), 26, 1997.

ternative healing modalities, it can also be used to better understand cultural explanatory models about health and medicine. Biomedicine is incorporated into the model, thus enabling an inclusive approach that is relevant to nursing instead of comparing alternative or biomedical views as adversarial (Engebretson, 1997). The model is organized across the horizontal axis according to explanatory paradigms that are arranged from the most materialist perspective associated with logical positivism to the most metaphysical view of knowledge based on intuition and subjectivity. The vertical axis describes the type of activity, progressing from the most concrete—physical manipulation—on top, to the most abstract—spiritual—on the bottom.

PARADIGMS

Four paradigmatic views of healing are used: mechanical, purification, balance, and supranormal. These paradigms describe an underlying belief and understanding about health, disease, and the human experience. Paradigms provide the explanatory models for cause of illness and the understanding of how and why the modality should be used. Proper understanding of these explanatory models is necessary to evaluate for appropriate use, or to research a particular modality. In the model, examples of specific modalities are used for illustration. No attempt has been made to be inclusive of all modalities that are available. Other modalities may be inserted based on an understanding of the paradigm and the type of activity.

Mechanical

The mechanical model is most closely associated with the biomedical model and is based on a fundamental approach that health and illness can be understood from an exploration of the mechanisms of the body's functions. Disease is seen as a breakdown in function and treatment serves to repair the dysfunctional part or eradicate the causative factors.

Purification

The purification paradigm views disease as caused by impurities that invade the person or toxins that build up in the body. Avoidance of pollution is the underlying rationale for many health practices cross-culturally and was a common paradigm in Western medicine until the early 20th century. This philosophy is the foundation for bloodletting and other cathartic practices and inspired the name of the prestigious British journal, the *Lancet*.

Balance

The third paradigm, balance, was the basis for Hippocratic medicine and the systems that followed, such as the Mexican belief in hot and cold balancing. It is also the paradigm that is epitomized by many Eastern systems of healing. Health is viewed as a balance of opposite forces, and treatment is based on restoring the balance. Oriental medicine is founded in the philosophy of paired opposites, yin and yang, that are always present simultaneously and give tangible expression to the otherwise uncontemplatable Dao or way. Yin and yang exist in dependence on each other, and health is correlated with the proper understanding and balance of these forces.

Supranormal

The fourth paradigm, the supranormal, is the most distant from the mechanical. This paradigm includes magical and religious healing in which illness is related to breach of a taboo, lack of integrity with higher powers, or part of a higher plan that is beyond the individual's ability to understand. Healing is based on a sacred reality that may not be understood from any of the other paradigms. Healing phenomena such as paradoxical healing, healing by distance, prayer, and so on are included under this paradigm.

ACTIVITIES

The vertical axis positions modalities along a continuum according to the type of activity involved and progresses from the most concrete—physical manipulation—on the top to the most abstract—spiritual—on the bottom. The types of activities progress from physical manipulation, applied and ingested substances, uses of energy, psychological, and spiritual actions.

Physical Manipulation

Physical manipulation is best exemplified in surgery, in which it is obvious that the healing activity is a manipulation of the physical body. Other types of physical therapy would also be included because they are best understood in a mechanical model. Physical manipulations based on a purification model would include colonic irrigation, which is a physical method of detoxification to heal a wide variety of disorders. Other types of alternative purification therapies include cupping, in which heated glass cups are placed on the skin to create suction that acts to remove impurities from the body. This practice is used in Mexico and in some European folk medicine. Many forms of body work are oriented around the idea of proper balance or alignment to prevent disease and discomfort. Physical manipulation in the supranormal paradigm could include types of drumming and dancing in which the individual, through movement, enters an altered state of consciousness in which healing may take place. Dance therapies are understood through a unity of body, mind, and spirit, which has salutogenic benefits.

Applied and Ingested Substances

Foods and pharmaceuticals are familiar applied and ingested substances to everyone in biomedicine. Mechanism of action, to understand these substances, is the bedrock of the mechanical paradigm. Many substances are also ingested or applied to purify or detoxify the body. One alternative therapy being investigated is chelation, in which chemical substances are injected into the body to form a chemical bond with unwanted elements that are then excreted, for example, plaque buildup in blood vessels. Humeral medicine, with its roots in early Greece, was based on keeping a balance in the humors for health and healing. Many nutritional practices and plant therapies are based on the concept of restoring balance, for example, balancing a hot disorder with a cold food or herb. Some substances are also used for their supranormal effects. For example, the Bach flower essences are used for their ability to modulate mental, emotional, and sometimes physical and spiritual discomforts. Hallucinogenic plants have been used in many cultures to achieve an altered state of consciousness often associated with healing.

Uses of Energy

The concept of energy is best understood from the Oriental healing systems, where it is called *Chi, Ki,* or *Qi*. According to Kaptchuk (1983), Chi is best translated as the point at which matter converts to energy or energy to matter. Ayurvedic medicine, popular in India, is based on the concept of prana, a type of vital energy. In the West, a similar concept of vitalism has historically been associated with the healing arts. This concept has not been well developed in the mechanical model. Two examples of energy use in the mechanical model are lasers and radiation. However they are largely understood for their mechanical ability, and their use is generally conceptualized as surgical or pharmaceutical. Bioenergetic modalities are based on the belief that repressed emotions are stored in the body and a combination of psychotherapy and body work can release these energies, thus purging the body of this toxic energy and restoring health. Energy is best developed in the paradigm of balance. Chi is also described as the "finest matter influences" or as "vapors arising from food." These descriptions capture the nonmaterial, but still with material attributes. The unimpeded flow of Chi through a network of meridians is associated with health, and disease is a disturbance in the Chi. Strategies such as acupuncture and acupressure are used to balance and restore the flow of Chi. Needles or massage are used to adjust the Chi along specific points on these meridians.

Energy is a concept that is also used to explain forms of healing touch, therapeutic touch, Reiki, and laying on of hands. These treatments may involve actual touching or placing the hands several inches from the body and working with the "energy field." The theoretical basis for this modality is often based on electromagnetic fields and theoretical or quantum physics. This modality has gained popularity in the nursing profession with two groups: Therapeutic Touch, founded by Dolores Krieger, and Healing Touch International, founded by Janet Metzgen. Both groups provide education and training for nurses interested in practicing this modality. Although anecdotal reports of salutatory effects abound, relatively few research studies have been published. These few study results demonstrate a lowering of anxiety and increased relaxation, and results on wound healing are equivocal. Some recent studies demonstrate that touch therapies have increased humoral immunity (Wardell & Engebretson, 1998; Olsen et al., 1997). This modality is of particular interest to the profession of nursing and warrants further study and theoretical development. Its location on the model at the juncture of the energy activity and supranormal paradigm, the two axes most alien to biomedical thinking, may explain the difficulty in understanding this modality and identifying appropriate research designs to capture effectiveness.

Psychological

Psychological actions are related to those that involve cognition or the function of the brain. Mind–body medicine is a relatively new classification of therapeutics that is a good example of techniques that primarily induce relaxation. The recent understanding of the mechanisms of psychophysiology has provided a firm base for many of these strategies to be incorporated into the mechanical model. Many forms of cognitive repatterning, biofeedback, and relaxation strategies are used for their ability to lower blood pressure and alter brain chemistry. Purification beliefs are expressed in some of the more cathartic therapies and are the foundation for some 12-step programs that incorporate a confessional format. Mindfulness is a Buddhist philosophy that provides a psychological base for being awake and living in balance. It has been popularized and applied to many therapeutic settings, such as stress reduction and cardiac rehabilitation programs. Mental imagery is a therapeutic process in which imagination and memory are used to mentally taste, smell, see, and hear the images that suggest a state of health. Several methods are used for guided imagery. Individuals may use therapists who will lead them in the practice or use commercial books and audiotapes.

Spiritual

The mechanical model often does not differentiate between spirituality and religion, which is often operationally defined as belonging to specific religious organizations or attendance at religious events. These parameters alone recently demonstrated positive health benefits (Levin, 1994). Penance and forgiveness have historically been means of spiritual purification. Forgiveness, long practiced in spiritual traditions, is emerging as a powerful healing strategy, and the Templeton Foundation recently funded research to systematically study its efficacy in healing. Forms of meditation and chakra-balancing have been practiced in many religions. These strategies use meditation as a way to quiet the mind and bring the individual into a powerfully relaxed state. Some contemporary literature describes meditation as a relaxation technique, but historically and cross-culturally it has been a spiritual practice. From either perspective, the beneficial effects on health have led to its incorporation into health practices. Prayer and primal religious experiences are spiritual actions in the supranormal paradigm. Several laboratory studies on plants and clinical studies have demonstrated effects of prayer (Dossey, 1993). Cox (1995) describes a primal religious experience that is holistic and involves physical, emotional, mental/spiritual, and social dimensions. Many Pentecostal churches use rituals of healing that engage all aspects of the individual in such a holistic experience. These types of healing activities are not well understood from a mechanical model; however, numerous anecdotal reports are available, and many people engage in these activities. Unexplained healing may baffle biomedical understanding but is indeed real to the person experiencing it.

SYSTEMS OF HEALING

The model described previously illustrates how modalities or single therapies fit into an overall framework. Systems of healing are broader and may incorporate several healing activities and modalities and may even incorporate more than one explanatory paradigm. Healing systems reflect a developed theory of the body–person as an explanatory model for understanding health–illness. This explanatory model includes the cause and suggests treatment approaches. These systems also provide for the education and preparation of practitioners and the delivery of the practice to the public. Biomedicine is the dominant medical system in Europe and North America; however, other healing systems are emerging in popularity and use. Four systems of healing will be discussed for illustration: homeopathy, Oriental medicine, Ayurvedic medicine, and shamanic healing systems (see Chapter 11).

Homeopathy

Homeopathy is a method of healing that was developed by Samuel Hahnemann (1755–1843), a German physician and chemist, based on the body's natural ability to self-heal. The word *homeopathy* is derived from the Greek prefix meaning similar. This connoted the practice of treating a disorder with medications that produced a similar symptom in a healthy person, which contrasts with the standard practice of allopathy or using medicines to counteract the symptoms, or that are unrelated to symptoms. At the time that Hahnemann practiced, principles of treatment of allopathic physicians were bloodletting, purging, or blistering of the skin. Hahnemann developed a systematic philosophy of medicine based on the Law of Similars: "Let likes be cured by likes." He also developed a method of proving, which was an innovative and rigorous system of experimentation, and established a materia medica, which now has more than 2000 remedies (Micozzi, 1996). He adhered to a belief in holism in which the totality of symptoms are interrelated and all remedies need to be individualized to the unique experience of the patient. With this in mind, he developed a tracking system regarding the course of illness and healing, with the patterns of appearance of symptoms and the movement of symptoms during recovery from head to feet, inside to outside, and more vital to less vital organs and in the reverse order of their appearance in the life history of the patient. Hahnemann adhered to a tradition of vitalism, believing that spirit was more powerful than matter; therefore, the essence (spirit) of the medicine was more important than the substance. The process of preparing the medications was to increase the dilutions of the medicine and agitate the mixture to release the essence or the active ingredient. Thus, the more powerful medication had progressively less of the substance in the solution. These preparations, some diluted beyond Avogadro's number of 10–24, are so dilute that not even a molecule of the substance can be found in the solution (Micozzi, 1996). This law of infinitesimals has remained one of the most controversial aspects of homeopathy to biomedicine, which is anchored in the allopathic tradition. Many basic science studies have been conducted with these dilutions in the areas of immunology and pharmacology. In clinical trials, however, results are equivocal. Adherents claim that in the trials, standardized treatments are given based on a biomedical diagnosis instead of the individualized treatments that are typical of clinical practice. Homeopathy is practiced widely in Europe, India, Mexico, and other parts of the world and flourished in the United States until the early 20th century. A combination of political and economic factors along with the Flexner Report in 1914, which standardized medical education and led to the American Medical Association's (AMA) ban on homeopathic medicine, phased out homeopathy in the United States. Practitioners of homeopathic medicine are currently adding homeopathic practice to an existing legal practice, which grants them a license to treat patients such as an MD or Doctor of Chiropractic.

Oriental Medicine

Oriental medicine is an energy-based system predicated on an understanding of the balance of opposites and the interrelatedness of the whole person and nature. The philosophical world views of Taoism, Confucianism, and Buddhism underlie these ancient healing arts (OAM, 1992; Kaptchuk, 1983; Micozzi, 1996). Chi, or vital energy, is understood to flow through various energy channels called *meridians* that have been mapped out over centuries of Oriental medical practice. Points along these meridians correspond to various organs or aspects of the body. Diagnosing disturbances in the Chi involves a process of observing, listening, questioning, and palpating. Emphasis is placed on palpating subtle differences in the pulse and inspecting the tongue. Treatment modalities to restore balance and unimpeded flow of Chi include acupuncture, acupressure, moxibustion, massage, touch, cupping, chigong, and herbal medicine. Acupuncture, in which fine needles are inserted at specific energy points and rotated, manipulates the energy flow along the meridians to restore balance. Acupressure involves physical pressure on these energy points, and moxibustion is the application of heat and/or herbs to energy points. Various forms of massage and touch, both contact and noncontact, are also used to manipulate and balance energy. Chigong involves using breath, movement, and meditation to cleanse, strengthen, and circulate the vital life energy and blood. A materia medica, which describes the complex practices of preparing and administering herbs, is well developed in the Orient. The most common Oriental practices currently used in the West are acupuncture, acupressure, and forms of chigong, including Tai Chi. Several states have enacted legislation that regulates and licenses acupuncturists.

Ayurvedic Medicine

Ayurvedic medicine means knowledge of life or science of longevity. Its origins are ancient, and its teachings have been passed on through the vedas, a body of ancient Sanskrit literature. Modern Ayurvedic medicine has been revived by Maharishi Mahesh Yogi and is known as Maharishi Ayurveda (Micozzi, 1996). It is holistic and is based on the concepts of balance and a vital life force. Health is based on well-being, prevention of disease, and alignment of lifestyles with one's individual constitution and personal medical history. Harmony with the environment is sought through understanding and balancing circadian rhythms, seasons, behavior, emotions, and other sensory experiences. Diet, herbs, yoga, meditation, and internal cleansing preparations are all addressed in the configuration of health. Three doshas or metabolic types exist—kapha, pitta, and vata—with one generally predominant. All doshas need to be in balance; however, the predominant dosha determines types of foods and other lifestyle practices one should incorporate. This ancient and complex system, with its focus on prevention and holistic integration, is of interest as Western biomedicine focuses more on prevention. Transcendental meditation, used in Ayurvedic medicine, has been used by many Westerners.

Shamanic Healing Systems

Shamanic healing systems refer to many of the traditional cultural healing systems. Many of these systems have multiple components, such as bone setters, herbalists, seers, massagers, and spiritual healers. These systems incorporate community in their healing practices because when one person is ill, it endangers the community and an individual's relationship to others, and the community is an important aspect of health. These systems actively fuse medicine and religion. Often the healer is called a *shaman,* whose healing powers are related to the ability to journey to nonordinary reality to receive spiritual direction for healing. The shaman enters a controlled trance through the use of drumming, repetitive sounds, meditation, or plant extractions. Healing may involve the use of physical manipulation, ingestion or application of natural substances, or supranormal actions. The shaman may be identified at or before birth, after demonstrating unusual capabilities such as forecasting the future or healing touch, or after surviving a serious illness. The shaman is often an apprentice of an elder shaman, and the calling is a lifelong commitment to the healing of the community (Micozzi, 1996; NIH, 1992). Shamanic systems most familiar to American nurses are Native American healing systems, Curanderisimo, Espiritisimo, Santeria, and African folk healing systems such as hoodoo, voodoo, and rootwork (Gordon, Nienstedt, & Gesler, 1998). Many popular healers follow shamanic practices.

Regulatory Issues

Regulation of health practices has been a controversial issue, ranging from the Jacksonian period of little regulation of medical doctors to the hegemony of medicine following the Flexner Report (Gordon, Nienstedt, & Gesler, 1998). Motives of protecting the public from harmful or ineffective treatments often coexist with those of limiting competitive practices. Osteopathic medicine used the co-optation model by adapting the prevailing biomedicine educational standards, and osteopathic practitioners are licensed and have the same legal status in all 50 states as MDs. Chiropractors, conversely, retained their professional uniqueness but have been in a legal and ideologic battle with the AMA for years. Chiropractors are now legally licensed in all 50 states.

Several federal regulatory agencies are involved in protecting the public from unsafe and ineffective treatment, including the Food and Drug Administration (FDA), the Federal Trade Commission (FTC), the U.S. Postal Service (USPS), and the Department of Justice (DOJ). The FDA plays a role in the use of all ingested or applied substances, the FTC regulates information and advertising, and the USPS regulates products and services sold through the mail that could be fraudulent. The DOJ has combined with several groups to curtail unorthodox treatment, especially for cancer (Gordon, Nienstedt, & Gesler, 1998). Issues of regulation need to balance motives of protecting the public from harmful or ineffective practice against those of limiting competetive practices.

State regulations vary and are important in both regulating and legitimizing alternative and complementary therapies and limiting practice. State provider practice acts generally regulate chiropractic practice (legal in 50 states), acupuncture (states vary regarding legality of practice and preparation of the provider), homeopathy (only a few states have homeopathy licensing, and most practitioners practice under another license such as MD or DC), massage (since 1991, several states have practice acts, but the scope of practice varies), and naturopathy (a few states license naturopaths, whereas in others the practice is illegal). Other modalities are not generally licensed, although several are working with state legislation to legitimize and regulate their practice (Gordon, Nienstedt, & Gesler, 1998). Broadly speaking, most modalities have legal sanction only if provided by a licensed health provider or clergy member (can be lay clergy). Some states do not regulate if the provider does not charge for services or the client has given consent. With the rise in numbers of modalities and providers, this issue will continue to be controversial. Healthcare providers need to be familiar with specific state laws.

REGULATORY ISSUES AND HERBAL REMEDIES

Plant-derived remedies or phytotherapies are found in all healing systems. The lay term for these basic plant-based substances is *herbal medicine*. The World Health Organization estimates that more than 80% of the world's population uses herbal medicine for some aspect of primary care (NIH, 1992). The European Economic Community, recognizing a need to standardize approval of herbal medicines, developed guidelines for quality, quantity, production, and labeling of herbal preparations. The German Federal Health Office compiled monographs from scientific literature and identified herbal products approved for use in the *Commission E,* which was recently translated into English and is available in the United States (Blumenthal et al., 1998).

Many biomedical pharmaceuticals are originally derived from plants used in folk medicine. These have been developed by isolating the active ingredient(s) and chemically synthesizing it in a lab, which allows for the control of purity and standardization. Many herbal preparations involve complex mixtures of several plants or several parts of a plant. One of the beliefs of herbalists is that use of whole plants, instead of extracted or synthesized ingredients, provides a more balanced physiologic action because other substances that modify side effects and potentiate therapeutic action are contained in the natural plant and are lost in the purification extraction process. This controversy remains unresolved for both researchers and practitioners.

Currently, most herbal products in the United States are considered food supplements by the FDA and therefore are not regulated according to the standards of clinical efficacy and safety that exist for drugs. Much controversy exists regarding the regulation issue among healers and the public as well. When stricter guidelines were proposed, a huge public protest ensued. The 1994 Dietary Supplement Health and Education Act allows manufacturers to advertise benefits of the products as long as they do not claim that the products cure or prevent specific illness. Some argue that if full drug regulations were used, individuals could be required to get a prescription for garlic. Also, herbal companies cannot afford the lengthy and expensive research and development that pharmaceutical companies invest in a drug and can regain by holding a patent.

Consumer problems occur in the absence of standardization or regulation. This poses the safety issues of presence of contamination, unstandardized dosage, and lack of guidelines regarding use, such as safety or dangers when combined with other herbs or medications. Several groups are working on a better solution to the regulation issue. The advanced practice nurse needs to be informed about phytomedicines because many patients are using them and many may be helpful. The prudent practitioner needs knowledge about these herbs to advise clients about their use and the possible contraindications and synergistic effects with medications. The FDA proposed a limit on the amount of ephedra that can be present in supplements and issued warnings on potentially dangerous herbs, including chaparral, comfrey, yohimbe, lobelia, germander, willow bark, Jin Bu Huan, and magnolia (Harvard Health Letter, 1997).

Nursing Implications for Advanced Practice

The public embrace of alternative and complementary therapies is increasing. This has implications for practice, education, and research. Nurses in advanced practice roles must first recognize the popularity of use of these therapies and elicit information from clients in their assessments. One can assume that many clients are using one or more modalities. Nurses in advanced practice need to know about various types of therapies or know where they can get more information.

It is important for nurses to assess safety issues. For example, a client with throm-

TABLE 12-5 *Sources of Information*

Books

Alternative Medicine: Expanding Medical Horizons (1992). Chantilly Report.

Blumenthal, M. (1998). The Complete German Commission E Monographs.

The Burton Goldberg Group. (1994). Alternative Medicine: The Definitive Guide.

Cassileth, B. R. (1998). The Alternative Medicine Handbook.

Collinge W. (1996). The American Holistic Health Association Complete Guide to Alternative Therapies.

Dossey, B. (Ed.). (1997). Holistic Nursing Core Curriculum.

Dossey, B., Keegan, L., Guzzetta, C., & Kolkheimer, L. (1995). Holistic Nursing: A Handbook for Practice.

Gordon, R. J., Nienstedt, B. C., & Gesler, W. M. (1998). Alternative Therapies: Expanding Options in Health Care.

Kaptchuk, T. (1983). The Web That Has No Weaver.

Micozzi, M. S. (1996). Fundamentals of Complementary Medicine.

Snyder, M. & Lindquist, R. (1998) Complementary and Alternative Therapies in Nursing.

Journals

Advances: The Journal of Mind–Body Health

Alternative Therapies in Health and Medicine

Herbalgram

Holistic Nursing Practice

Journal of Alternative and Complementary Medicine

Journal of Holistic Nursing

Websites

Acupuncture	http://www.acupuncture.com
Alternative Health News Online	http://www.altmedicine.com
American Botanical Council	http://www.herbalgram.org
American Holistic Health Association	http://www.healthy.net/ahha
American Holistic Nurses Association	http://www.ahna.org
Healing Touch International	http://www.healingtouch.net
National Center for Homeopathy	http://www.homeopathic.org
NIH Consensus Reports	http://www.nih.gov.consensus
Office of Complementary and Alternative Medicine at NIH	http://altmed.od.nih.gov/oam

bophlebitis should be cautious regarding use of massage or types of body work, and a client with hypertension should avoid herbal ecstasy, which contains ephedrine. Nurses also need to assess whether the treatment is used as an alternative to or a delay in getting scientifically proven efficacious treatment.

If the modality is not contraindicated, the nurse should be familiar with some of the low-risk modalities that are noninvasive and can be sources of comfort and healing. It would be unfortunate to advise a client against using a modality that does no harm but could be healing. Some nurses choose to develop expertise in a particular modality, such as touch therapies, and incorporate it into their practice. Others develop networks of practitioners to whom they feel comfortable referring clients. One of the best ways to gain this information is through organizations such as the American Holistic Nurses Association and nurse practitioner organizations. Several new books, journals, and websites are available to keep abreast of information (see Table 12-5). Nurses need to be familiar with state regulations in the state in which they practice that may define their role in practicing various modalities and the licensing of other modalities such as acupuncture or massage.

Little research has been conducted on many of these modalities, but because of the interest from the NIH, new research is entering journals specifically reporting on alternative and complementary therapies, as well as in mainstream journals. As alluded to previously, research on many of these modalities is difficult because the research model assumes that the variable of the diagnosed disease is uniform so that efficacy of the treatment is based on a fit between treatment and the diagnosis, whereas the healers often see the fit between the individual and the treatment. Therefore, clinical trials on clients with diabetes may not be appropriate because of the variation among the individuals and the adaptability of the intervention to the individual, not the disease. A second related concern is the difficulty of standardizing the intervention because many of these modalities adapt to individual needs of the client and use multiple combined approaches. Randomized controlled trials are often difficult because the presence of a healer may have an effect even if no action is taken and some of the activities do not lend themselves to blinded studies, the hallmark of pharmaceutical studies. Other research problems relate to the lack of developed theoretical models to explain and describe complex systems such as the immune, energetic, and spiritual/mental systems. Despite these concerns, many nurses are engaged in research, developing creative approaches based on an understanding of the modality and the explanatory paradigm from which it is framed.

Nurses, especially, should be engaged in this exciting turn in healthcare. Many of these modalities have been used by nurses through the years as part of autonomous nursing care. This is a time of opportunity for nurses to take the lead in research, education, and integration of these practices into patient care in a safe and responsible manner.

REFERENCES

Astin, J. A. (1998). Why patients use alternative medicine. *Journal of the American Medical Association* *279*(19), 1548–1553.

Blumenthal, M. Busse, W. R., Goldberg, A, et al. (Eds.). (1998). *The Complete German Commission E Monographs: Therapeutic guide to herbal medicines.* Austin, TX: American Botanical Council.

Callahan, D. (1996). The goals of medicine. *Hastings Center Report Special Supplement,* Nov-Dec, S1–26.

CAM Newsletter. (January 1998). http://odp.od.nih.gov/consensus/statements/cdc. Accessed August 5, 1998.

Cassidy, C. M. (1996). Cultural context of complementary and alternative medicine systems. In M. S. Micozzi (Ed.). *Fundamentals of Complementary and Alternative Medicine* (pp. 9–34). New York: Churchill Livingstone.

Cassileth, B. R. (1998). *The alternative medicine handbook: The complete guide to alternative and complementary therapies.* New York: W. W. Norton.

Chilton, M. (1996). Panel recommends integrating behavioral and relaxation approaches into medical treatment of chronic pain, insomnia. *Alternative Therapies in Health and Medicine 2*(1), 18–28.

Cox, H. (1995). *Fire from heaven.* Boston: Addison-Wesley.

Dossey, L. (1993). *Healing words: The power of prayer and the practice of medicine.* San Francisco: Harper.

Eisenberg, D. M., Davis, R. B., Ettner, S. L., et al. (1998). Trends in alternative medicine use in the United States, 1990–1992. *JAMA 280*(18), 1569–1575.

Eisenberg, D. M., Kessler, R. C., Foster, C., et al. (1993). Unconventional medicine in the United States: Prevalence, costs and patterns of use. *The New England Journal of Medicine 328*(4), 252–256.

Engebretson, J. (1996). Comparison of nurses and alternative healers. *Image: Journal of Nursing Scholarship. 28*(2), 95–99.

Engebretson, J. (1997). A multiparadigm approach to nursing. *ANS 20*(1), 22–34.

Goodwin, M. (1997). A health insurance revolution. *New Age Journal 1997–1998 Special Edition,* 66–69.

Gordon, R. J., Nienstedt, B. C., & Gesler, W. M. (1998). *Alternative therapies: Expanding options in health care.* New York: Springer.

Harvard Health Letter. (1997). Alternative medicine: Time for a second opinion. *Harvard Health Letter 23*(1), 1–3.

Institute for Alternative Futures (1998). The future of complementary and alternative approaches in US Health Care. Alexandria, VA. NCMIC Insurance Co. Snyder, M. & Lindquist R. (1998) *Complementary alternative therapies in nursing.* 3ed Ed. New York Springs.

Kaptchuk, T. J. (1983). *The web that has no weaver: Understanding Chinese medicine.* New York: Congdon and Weed.

Landmark Report on Public Perceptions of Alternative Care. (1998). Available at: http://landmarkhealthcare.com. Accessed 8/5/98.

Levin, J. S. (1994) Religion and health: Is there an association, is it valid and is it causal? *Social Science and Medicine 29,* 589–600.

Lovallo, W. R. (1997). *Stress and health: Biological and psychological interactions.* Thousand Oaks, CA: Sage Publications.

Marston, R. Q., & Jones, R. M. (Eds.). (1992). *Medical education in transition.* Princeton, NJ: The Robert Wood Johnson Foundation.

McGuire, M. B. (1998). *Ritual healing in suburban America.* New Brunswick, NJ: Rutgers University Press.

Micozzi, M. S. (Ed.). (1996). *Fundamentals of complementary and alternative medicine.* New York: Churchill Livingstone.

Moore, N. G. (1997) The Columbia-Presbyterian complementary care center: Comprehensive care of the mind, body and spirit. *Alternative Therapies in Health and Medicine 3*(100), 30–32.

National Institutes of Health. (1992). *Alternative medicine: Expanding medical horizons: A report to the National Institutes of Health on alternative medical systems and practices in the United States* (Publication No. 017-040-00537-7). Washington, DC: US Government Printing Office.

Olsen, M., Sneed, N., LaVia, M., et al. (1997). Stress-induced immunosuppression and therapeutic touch. *Alternative Therapies in Health and Medicine 3*(2), 68–74.

PEW Health Professions Commission. (1995). *Critical challenges: Revitalizing the health profession for the twenty-first century.* San Francisco: Author.

Ray, P. H. (1997).The emerging culture. American Demographics. Available at: http://www.demographics.com. Accessed June 1998.

Snyder, M. & Lindquist, R. (1998). *Complementary (alternative therapies in nursing.* 3rd Ed. New York: Springs.

Villaire, M. (1998a). More health plans add alternative medicine coverage. *Alternative Therapies in Health and Medicine 4*(3), 27.

Villaire, M. (1998b). Popularity of alternative medicine still growing in US, Canada, polls find. *Alternative Therapies in Health and Medicine 4*(7), 29.

Wardell, D., & Engebretson, J. (1999, in review). Reiki touch healing: An exploration of biological correlates.

Wetzel, M. S., Eisenberg, D. M., & Kaptchuk, T. D. (1998). Courses involving complementary and alternative medicine at US medical schools. *Journal of the American Medical Association 280*(9), 784–787.

Practice and Economic Imperatives in Advanced Practice Nursing

CHAPTER 13

Accountability: *The Covenant Between Patient and Advanced Practice Nurse*

Neville E. Strumpf

Meg Bourbonniere

Kristie Asimos

Accountability, the covenant between nurse and patient, is the yardstick by which we measure ourselves professionally. Subsumed within accountability are the expectations of patients, other colleagues, and society. Most important, accountability is a deeply held value intimately related to personal expectations about professional worth, responsibility for care, and meaning in one's work. As nursing evolves, and particularly as healthcare services undergo enormous transformation, accountability for practice continues to deserve both attention and vigilance.

Accountability can simply be defined as "responsibility" or "answerability" (Fry, 1991, p. 152). This definition fails, however, to capture the essence or full scope of professional practice. Responsibility and answerability alone address neither the essentialness of accountability as an integral part of nursing nor the importance of the mutual nature of a relationship between nurse and patient. Patients seek and expect accountability from providers. In today's healthcare environment, this is usually understood in terms of high-quality, cost-effective care tailored to individual needs (Sidani & Braden, 1998). Although definitions of accountability must include the broad roles of providers in diverse settings, as well as any possible regulatory or legal limits to authority or practice, the necessity to challenge or break rules responsibly is increasingly apparent (Hunt, 1997).

A finite definition of accountability is unlikely given the complexities and changes in patient–provider relationships; legal and regulatory issues; and subtle interplays created by culture, education, training, collaboration with other professionals, and work settings. In their own ways, these factors influence the nature of accountability and its articulation to patients, colleagues, and self. In this chapter, we explore various meanings and interpretations of accountability. Like the nursing profession itself, accountability also evolves to fit with the circumstances of increasingly complex care needs and systems for delivering care, especially in an era of managed care.

The themes of relationship and caring are pervasive in the historical, educational, and clinical literature and are integral to the concept of accountability in nursing. To understand accountability, one must first consider its historical roots as an early foundation for

professional nursing practice. In addition, external and self-regulatory influences on definitions of nursing and accountability have emerged in recent years.

This chapter provides a brief history of emerging ideas about accountability in nursing
and the effect of external and self-regulatory measures on perceived accountability. Existing research, barriers to accountable practice, and current understanding of accountability
are noted. The most fundamental aspect of accountability, *caring,* is also examined using
available literature on the subject and material collected during interviews with advanced
practice nurses (APNs).

Historical Evolution of the Concept of Accountability

Early discussions of accountability in nursing emphasize moral and ethical standards and
the relationship between nurse and patient. These have remained as core concepts in the
educational preparation and professional practice of nurses. Especially in the early years of
nursing's development, devotion, veracity, confidentiality, and loyalty permeated the literature and influenced education and practice.

Florence Nightingale (1859/1992), in *Notes on Nursing: What It Is and What It Is Not,*
published in 1859, understood moral and ethical principles as inherent to nursing. Nightingale's emphasis on accountability and preventive care assumed advocacy, veracity, dignity,
empathy, and confidentiality. According to Nightingale, nursing was more than "administration of medicines and the application of poultices" (p. 6). Nursing must "put the patient
in the best condition for nature to act upon him" (p. 75). Nursing ought "to signify proper
use of fresh air, light, warmth, cleanliness, quiet, and the proper selection and administration
of diet" (p. 6). Nightingale specifically mentions important moral concepts such as truthful-
ness (p. 22), trust (p. 55), confidentiality (p. 70), duty (p. 59), and responsibility (p. 24).

In describing the notion of respect for and duty to the patient, Isabel Hampton Robb
wrote in 1901 that the "nurse should always make it her rule to think of every patient as
an individual (sick) human-being, whose wishes, fancies, and peculiarities call for all the
consideration possible at her hands" (Robb, 1901). Robb added that "confidences should
always be held sacred and inviolable" and

> [the] whole conduct of the nurse should be such as to assure the patient that a mo-
> ment of weakness will never be blazoned abroad. None of the privacies of personal or
> domestic life, no infirmity of disposition or little flaw of character, observed while car-
> ing for a patient, should ever be divulged by the nurse . . . (Robb, 1901).

Similarly, Pope and Young (1934) echoed these moral and ethical aspects of accountability in a 1934 text noting that the responsibility of the nurse was to maintain "high
ethical and professional standards" (p. 3). Duty of the professional nurse to practice with
"conscientiousness" (p. 3) and with respect for patient dignity and privacy was also
emphasized.

The moral and ethical themes identified by Nightingale, Robb, and Pope were given
more immediate application in Bertha Harmer's (1925) *Text-book of the Principles and
Practice of Nursing.* Harmer noted that moral and ethical values such as reliability and
trustworthiness inspired confidence in relationships with patients and contributed to the
healing process. She viewed prevention as a crucial aspect of nursing and understood the
work of nursing as holistic in nature.

> Nursing is rooted in the needs of humanity and is founded on the ideal of service. Its
> object is not only to cure the sick and heal the wounded but to bring health and ease,
> rest and comfort to mind and body, to shelter, nourish and to protect and to minister
> to all those who are helpless or handicapped, young, aged, or immature. Its object is
> to prevent disease and to preserve health (p. 3).

Virginia Henderson attributed her ethically based humanistic approach to nursing to her teacher, Annie W. Goodrich, Dean of the Army School of Nursing at Walter Reed Hospital. Henderson (1966) described visits by Goodrich to the unit as moments when sights were lifted "above techniques and routines. . . . She never failed to infect us with the ethical significance of nursing" (p. 7). Henderson's now classic description of the nature of nursing considers holistic care of the patient as an explicit outcome of the relationship between patient and nurse. The nurse is seen as a

> substitute for what the patient lacks to make him complete, whole, or independent . . . in mind and body. . . . She is temporarily the consciousness of the unconscious, the love of life for the suicidal, the leg of the amputee, the eyes of the newly blind, a means of locomotion for the infant, knowledge and confidence for the young mother, the "mouthpiece" for those too weak or withdrawn to speak (Henderson, 1966).

Accountability is implied in complete obligation to the patient and in the relationship between nurse and patient. Contemporaneous with Henderson, Gertrude Ujhely (1968) described general agreement in the nursing literature that the "main concern of nursing is, or should be . . . care of the whole patient" (p. 86). Regardless of setting and diversity of role, or of sophistication in technology, Doris Schwartz (1988), a leader in public health and an advocate of advanced practice nursing in geriatrics, urged that the humanistic, moral, and ethical values inherent in comprehensive patient care never be relinquished.

In contrast to these more philosophical explications, accountability was also defined in a program review report under provisions established by the U.S. Public Health Service in the federal Nurse Training Act of 1964. In this report, it was "for the care of patients that nursing is accountable to society" (U.S. Department of Health, Education, and Welfare [USDHEW], 1967, p. 15). The report sought to determine the "nature of nursing practice . . . what it is today and what it will be tomorrow" (p.15). Reflecting a continuum of greater complexity in nursing and in the healthcare environment, this statement concerning professional accountability extended beyond traditional moral or ethical and medical models. It emphasized the concept, first alluded to by Florence Nightingale, that professional practice in nursing is theory-oriented more than technique-oriented and is founded on a body of knowledge derived from scientific investigation. The role of the nurse was described as "doing for the patient what temporarily cannot be done alone" and helping "to develop and use physical and emotional resources effectively to move toward being well" (p. 16). These statements echo and expand on the sentiments of early nurse educators that nursing accountability involves a holistic sense of caring.

Today, schools of nursing uniformly emphasize caring and empathy as foundational aspects of professional practice at all levels. Separate courses and integration of content related to nursing ethics and values are required components of the curriculum, and students are evaluated clinically on provision of care that demonstrates accountability to patients, peers, and self. This accountability refers to the "sense of overriding concern for the whole process of nursing care," including concepts of duty, autonomy, service, competence, authority, and commitment (Claus & Bailey cited in Omerod, 1993, p. 730).

Definitions of nursing have traditionally recognized patients' physical and emotional needs and have viewed both as essential to quality care. Despite the growth and evolution of more technical and scientifically based practice, meeting the basic physical and emotional needs of patients remains paramount in nursing.

Scope and Standards of Practice

Although ethical and moral values, technical skill, and holistic approaches to care were addressed as components of professional nursing by early nurse educators, tremendous variability nevertheless existed in the early years of nursing in training, education, and skill. Persons with varied backgrounds who cared for the sick were referred to as "nurses" regardless of the quality of the programs from which they had graduated. In time, the need for greater consistency in education and skill became apparent.

SELF-REGULATION

With the formation of permanent American schools of nursing in the 1870s, nursing was legitimized as a vocation, and the movement toward regulation began. Regulatory efforts were clearly a response to extreme needs for trained nurses with standardized skills who could minister to the sick, as well as for better conditions in late 19th and early 20th century hospitals, where "nurses" could still be relatively unsupervised workers waiting on patients (Goodnow, 1943).

As nursing care of hospitalized patients improved, hospitals proliferated, along with the schools of nursing frequently associated with them. Nurses increasingly wished to define the mission of a growing profession and to organize and communicate with one another.

The first national meeting of nurses in the United States was held at the Chicago World's Fair in 1893. It resulted in formation of the American Society of Superintendents of Training Schools, a name that was later changed to the National League of Nursing Education. At about the same time, in 1896, with Isabel Hampton Robb as its first president, a general society of graduate nurses was formed: the Nurses' Associated Alumnae of the United States and Canada. The name was changed in 1912 to the American Nurses Association (ANA) (Goodnow, 1943). The Association, in 1897, stated its purpose as follows: "(1) to establish and maintain a code of ethics, (2) to elevate the standards of nursing education, and (3) to promote the usefulness and honor, the financial and other interests of the nursing profession" (Deloughery, 1977, p. 114).

By 1920, every state had an association of nursing that, in addition to setting standards and identifying scopes of practice in association with the ANA, was given responsibility to secure registration laws. Over time, the functions of registration and regulation of practice increasingly shifted toward external regulation by the states.

Today, the profession still establishes standards and scopes of practice for its members. Standards, which are continually revised and evaluated, commonly exceed minimum guidelines set by the state. In addition to the profession's code of ethics for nurses, more than 20 other publications of the ANA describe nursing standards and scopes of practice in various practice settings and are a gold standard by which educators, clinicians, and consumers can measure accountability in practice.

In addition to setting standards and scopes of practice, to which all nurses hold themselves accountable, specific criteria for certification in advanced practice in a specialty are also set by the profession. Almost all certification for advanced practice by the various credentialing bodies prescribes specific educational criteria, usually a master's degree in nursing from an accredited college or university. One such certifying body, the American Nurses Credentialing Center (1998), offers certification examinations in three generalist, six clinical specialist, one nursing administration, and six nurse practitioner specialties. An increasingly common requirement to employment in an advanced practice role is certification based on a credentialing process (usually an examination) by a professional association.

EXTERNAL REGULATION

Along with optimal standards set through self-regulation by the profession, as described above, legislative and regulatory bodies have increasingly played a role in establishing at least minimal standards for professional practice. The trend toward external regulation began around 1920, when requirements for registration as a professional nurse were set forth in state law. In 1944, a few states administered the first uniform multistate nursing board examination; this was followed by development of state board pool tests, which have been used in all states since 1950 (Deloughery, 1977). Now known as NCLEXs (National Council Licensure Examinations), these examinations provide consistent and uniform testing of knowledge essential to performance as an entry-level professional nurse.

Health professions, including nursing, are regulated by means of state rules for licensure and practice. Licensure controls admittance into the profession, and practice acts define scope of practice for those who are licensed. This protection issues from the legislature, which speaks for the state, with authority often delegated to a state board of nursing. Functions of the board include determination of eligibility requirements for initial licensure of professional and practical nurses, approval and supervision of educational institutions of nursing, development of rules and regulations concerning practice, and enforcement of restrictions (Deloughery, 1977). In determining licensure and practice, these regulatory boards have contributed to current understanding of accountability.

Although each state has fairly consistent legislation regarding entry-level practice, regulation for advanced practice nursing varies from state to state (Pan, Straub, & Geller, 1997), in sharp contrast to the professional guidelines for standards and scope of practice. The latter are consistent for each specialty and clearly transcend the discrepancies in role or authority that may be prescribed at the state level. Among many possible criteria for advanced practice, a state board of nursing may accept professional certification as sufficient to meet advanced practice regulations, may determine which schools have acceptable curricula for advanced practice, or may have additional requirements, for example, specific continuing education programs and various tests of competency. In addition, the parameters of practice on a state-by-state basis can also vary widely, especially regarding prescriptive privileges and practice protocols (Pearson, 1998; Pan, Straub, & Geller, 1997). Although opponents of broadened practice guidelines charge that the public's health would be jeopardized if APNs were allowed to prescribe drugs, studies show that APNs make appropriate decisions when prescribing medications (Hamric, Worley, Lindebak, & Jaubert, 1998; Mahoney, 1994).

BALANCING INTERNAL/EXTERNAL REGULATION

The current trend toward advanced practice nursing is clearly a response to profound changes in needs for healthcare and systems for delivering services. Consistency between the profession's standards and scope of practice and state regulations is essential if the skills of APNs are to be used.

Accountability in advanced practice nursing is measured against established professional standards for education and expertise. Thus, the educational base for advanced practice, assuming it is uniform throughout the profession for a particular specialty, should mean that any APN is accountable to provide similar care regardless of the state in which he or she practices (Pearson, 1998).

Depending on state regulations, barriers to practice contribute greatly to the uncertainty of consumers and other professionals concerning expanded roles for nursing. Restrictive practice environments that attempt to control professional autonomy interfere with accountability in advanced practice (Brown, 1998; Brush & Capezuti, 1997; Hunt, 1997; McDermott, 1995; Pan, Straub, & Geller, 1997). Guidelines developed by the ANA or other professional organizations need to be more fully used by legislative and regulatory bodies charged with redefining the legal parameters of advanced practice, including accountability and authority. Similarly, as state legislatures respond to societal healthcare needs and remove barriers to fully accountable advanced practice, care must be taken to ensure that arbitrary practice restrictions are not imposed by local agencies (Mahoney, 1995).

Truly accountable practice requires and incorporates both internally and externally imposed standards and regulations, but it also must extend beyond them. Katims (1993) describes nursing as holding two primary values: caring and excellence. These values shape nursing actions in significant ways. Although caring is foundational to the nurse–patient relationship, excellence addresses particular skills, moral and ethical obligations, and professional standards (Katims, 1993). Understandably, the profession of nursing adheres to standards that exceed the requirements imposed by state regulation. As the skills of advanced practice and practice "privileges" come under greater legal scrutiny, the profession must strengthen its commitment to the caring relationship as integral to all accountable practice.

The Nurse–Patient Relationship

Much of the nursing literature and nursing research focuses on the nurse–patient relationship.

> Each time a nurse encounters a patient, something happens. The meeting is never a neutral event. It is the power of the nurse–patient relationship that makes nursing exciting and . . . not a series of automatic performances. . . . The . . . nurse must understand that every patient encounter is meaningful, that it always has impact, that it always affects both the patient and the nurse. The effect may be dramatic or it may be subtle, but something—either positive or negative—always occurs (Kenner, Guzzetta, & Dussey, 1985, p. 9).

Indeed, one bond uniting nurses, regardless of diversity in backgrounds, experiences, and roles, is attention to the nurse–patient relationship. This relationship is central to the provision of nursing care (Peplau, 1997). It is through this that nurses intervene to assist patients as they move through transitions that affect health and well-being. "The essence of nursing is the caring connection that transcends time and culture" (Rawnsley, 1994, p. 189).

Growing concerns about dehumanization in the healthcare encounter (Carper, 1979) have led to greater interest in caring. Compassion, the genuine capacity to feel and to "share in the pain and anguish . . . understanding . . . what sickness means . . . together with a readiness to help and to see the situation as the patient does" (Pellegrino, 1974, p. 1289), is necessary to an authentic sense of caring. Such authenticity by healthcare professionals is frequently perceived by patients as an important factor in the quality of healthcare (Carper, 1979). As technology and specialization contribute to a greater sense of depersonalization, caring behaviors—patience, trust, honesty, humility, hope, compassion, courage, knowledge, and flexibility—are increasingly desired by consumers. Relationship and continuity between provider and patient may actually be lost in the trade-off between more personalized versus more specialized care.

The importance of relationship is increasingly evident in the current healthcare environment, in which emphasis is shifting to greater collaboration between patients and providers, with both working jointly to determine goals and weigh alternative courses of action and approaches to healthcare (Kasch, 1986; Mackenzie, Strumpf, Johnson, & Sands, 1998). Consumers seem to value in their healthcare providers the fusion of curing and caring and the inclusion of clinical excellence as well as healing art. Patients are no longer content to be passive recipients of healthcare. These changing perceptions of patients must be considered in any definition of holistic and accountable practice.

Managed care will no doubt intensify concerns about patient–provider relationships (Thomasma, 1996). Choice, communication, competence, compassion, and continuity will be essential (Emanuel, Mezey, & Dubler, 1993). Compassionate delivery of competent and effective primary healthcare is fundamental to accountable practice of the whole patient. With accountability comes a sense of responsibility for providing continuity that exceeds a set time or a set problem.

In this emerging healthcare market, as APNs seek and reclaim autonomy, credentialing is viewed as a means to ensure accountable practice (Rustia & Bartek, 1997). In managed care organizations, the scrutiny afforded by credentialing will assure consumers of cost-effective, high-quality care. Rustia and Bartek argue that, through this type of accountable practice, APNs will "complete the transformation to a responsive and accountable health system" (p. 103).

However, the tensions brought to bear on the nurse–patient relationship in managed care can alter the traditional covenant. Accountable practice exists at the core of this tension. As healthcare has rapidly transformed, patients seek and expect accountability from providers in the form of high-quality, cost-effective care that is also tailored to meet individual patients' needs (Sidani & Braden, 1998). In managed care, the relationship moves from covenantal to contractual (Raines, 1997). Care previously provided without regard to compensation or reciprocity is today based on an exchange of goods for services. The provider no longer determines the quantity of care; instead, the amount of care is predetermined. The ensuing struggle then becomes one of balancing responsibility to the system with traditional responsibility to the patient. Maintaining quality relationships with individual patients, as well as advocating for larger groups of patients, especially those most vulnerable, remains preeminent (Varon, 1996; Ware et al., 1996).

Ethical Base for Accountability

The conceptual framework and moral dimensions of accountability for nursing practice are based on certain ethical principles and are integral to education and practice. The traditional principles of nonmaleficence, beneficence, autonomy, justice, and veracity can be expanded to include concepts such as advocacy, loyalty, care and caring, compassion, and human dignity (Creasia & Parker, 1991; Strumpf & Paier, 1992). These concepts are frequently discussed in the nursing literature as intrinsically connected to nursing's work. Although critical to the concept of accountability, such "caring" concepts are difficult to measure and quantify.

The covenant between patient and nurse is largely unspoken and based on traditional nursing values and ethics, for example, caring and empathy. Much of what is viewed as responsibility and accountability to and for patients is intimately associated with a caring relationship. Although elements of the relationship and the accompanying ethical values are felt by patient and nurse, they are not easily defined; instead, they are understood. Patients consistently describe this relationship as essential to responsive practice and care by a nurse, although "caring, the essence of nursing, defies measurement" (Baer, 1993, p. 109).

With continued emphasis in all health systems on resource allocation, nurses are challenged to maintain a philosophy of care that includes ethical and moral principles as well as caring behaviors. As Raines (1997) suggests, ethical conflict will arise as more nurses become employed by managed care organizations and duty to the system collides with duty to the patient. Withholding care or assigning blame are consequences of cost containment and resource allocation. In a recent study examining the effects of patient responsibility on the nurse–patient relationship, Olsen (1997) found that nurses tempered their relationships, and thus their caring and concern for patients. Mitigating and conferring fault for the clinical situation were the influential factors. Whatever form it takes, accountability in practice requires maintenance of a provider–patient relationship.

Research Related to the Nurse–Patient Relationship

In available studies of patient outcomes, findings to date point to the importance of relationship and indirectly to accountability in practice. Much more investigation, however, is needed to tease out the impact of the nurse–patient relationship on outcomes of care.

This type of research is hampered by numerous methodologic problems, among them defining specific nursing interventions and using measures that truly capture outcomes of care.

In the narratives of nurses in 88 caring situations, Astrom, Norberg, Hallberg, and Jansson (1993) sought to interpret the meaning and impact of caring actions on patients, from both the patients' and the nurses' points of view. Consistently, patients and nurses agreed on which caring actions made a difference. Typically, these situations involved a well-developed nurse–patient relationship characterized by empathy from the nurse, along with knowledge of the patient's personality and preferences.

Ongoing research concerning comprehensive discharge planning for hospitalized elderly patients has shown the positive effect of APNs on patient outcomes after discharge. In one randomized clinical trial conducted at a large medical center, 276 patients and 125 caregivers were assigned to intervention and control groups (Naylor et al., 1994). Patients in the control group received the hospital's routine discharge plan, and those assigned to the intervention group received, in addition to the hospital's routine plan, a comprehensive, individualized discharge plan designed specifically for elderly patients and implemented by gerontologic nurse specialists. Patients in the intervention group were seen by the nurse specialist within 24 to 48 hours of admission and every 48 hours thereafter to revise and implement the discharge plan. The last hospital visit was made within 24 hours of discharge. After discharge, the nurse specialist made home visits and was available by telephone for 2 weeks. From the initial hospitalization until 6 weeks after discharge, patients in the intervention group had fewer readmissions, fewer total days rehospitalized, lower readmission charges, and lower charges for healthcare services after discharge. The results of this study suggest the importance of a relationship with the nurse, of continuity and trust, and of individualization of care.

In another study of 87 persons infected with human immunodeficiency virus, patients' perceptions of clinic care by APNs, compared with physicians, were explored. Patients were assigned to either APNs or physicians for their periodic visits. Patients followed by the APNs experienced greater satisfaction with their healthcare, as evidenced by significantly fewer reports of problems with their care providers. Although patients in both groups experienced symptoms between visits, patients were more likely to report these symptoms to the APNs (Aiken et al., 1993). These findings suggest the importance of a trusting provider–patient relationship in acquiring information and achieving optimal healthcare.

A pilot study representing a collaborative effort between an advanced practice psychiatric–mental health nurse and primary care providers identified depressive symptoms in a group of 33 young women seeking attention for physical complaints. Interventions were then based on interpersonal nursing theory and used the nurse–patient relationship to decrease depression scores and to increase self-esteem in the young women (Beeber & Charlie, 1998). Although limited by sample size and design, the study nevertheless suggests that collaboration between providers and extending to patients limits specialist referral and protects continuity of care.

Other studies demonstrate effective advanced practice nursing interventions with return to work, smoking cessation, and reduced stress and dependency after myocardial infarction (Burgess et al., 1987; Pozen et al., 1977); lower symptom distress, increased independence, and fewer hospital readmissions in patients diagnosed as having progressive lung cancer (McCorkle et al., 1989); discharge planning with hospitalized older adults (Naylor, 1990; Naylor et al., 1994; Neidlinger, Scroggins, & Kennedy, 1987); reduction in weight and blood pressure in hypertensive adults (Ramsay, McKenzie, & Fish, 1982); and reduced physical restraint use in nursing homes (Evans et al., 1997). Although limited in number, studies linking nurse interventions and relationships to patient outcomes of care are a first step in quantifying the significance of a caring relationship.

Barriers to Accountable Practice

BARRIERS TO CARING

Caring, which should serve as a unifying concept for healthcare providers, is unfortunately an undervalued commodity. Reasons for this devaluation are complex. Certainly the explosion of science and technology are contributing factors, but perhaps more important, the changes wrought by these advances have had a significant and probably detrimental impact on caring relationships.

The historical progression of "nursing care," as described by Susan Reverby (1987) in *Ordered to Care: The Dilemma of American Nursing, 1850–1945,* illustrates the myriad factors contributing to the undervaluation of caring. Reverby suggests that a crucial dilemma exists in contemporary American nursing: "the order to care in a society that has refused to value caring" (p. 1). Nursing developed within a set of cultural expectations about caring as part of women's duties to family and community. When training for nursing was introduced in the late 19th century, it was based on this understanding of women's duty but not of women's rights (Reverby, 1987).

Unquestioning subservience and acceptance of orders under the watchful control of hospitals and physicians became increasingly unacceptable as trained nurses gained knowledge and a sense of advocacy and independent accountability to patients. Conflict soon developed among physicians, nurses, and others regarding the appropriate role of the nurse (Reverby, 1987). Despite desires for increasing autonomy and accountability, nurses often had little of either as the economic and cultural power of hospitals and physicians increased throughout much of the 20th century. Nursing's "educational philosophy, ideological underpinnings, and structural position made it difficult to create the circumstances from which to gain a recognized claim of rights" based on caring (Reverby, 1987, p. 203).

More recently, social, political, and economic conditions have permitted greater autonomy in decisions regarding practice. Increased technical expertise has given nurses more "ability to integrate and synthesize volumes of differentiated knowledge in order to translate that knowledge into coordinated, safe patient care" (Reverby, 1987, p. 204). The increasing acceptance of women's rights has enhanced respect for the role of women in society and in the professional world. What still remains, however, are potent barriers to the valuing of much of women's work, especially that related to nurturance and care. As already discussed, these are essential elements of accountable practice that challenge nursing professionals who struggle to deliver both technically proficient and humane care.

CONSTRAINTS IN HEALTHCARE SYSTEMS

In addition to the undervaluation of caring, or perhaps associated with it, the healthcare system itself can impede accountable practice. Such system constraints as time, access, reimbursement, and models of care are often complicating factors. All can negatively affect fundamental elements of the ideal provider–patient relationship and, hence, patient satisfaction and optimal healthcare.

Both managed care and reimbursement issues potentially threaten choice in healthcare. In managed care plans, decisions may be and often are determined to a great extent by insurers or case managers. Limits on reimbursement for specific diagnostic and treatment alternatives can affect choices in providers, facilities, and options for care. Although much is to be applauded in reforming healthcare to include more integration of services and providers, greater continuity, and curtailment of unnecessary costs, these changes represent remarkable departures from the ways in which healthcare has been delivered for nearly a century. Such changes will inevitably and dramatically affect the practices and decisions of all providers, including physicians and APNs.

Potential risks associated with the outcomes of inadequate care (e.g., complications associated with delayed treatment) worry many providers about accountability and malpractice. Given the access and care issues inherent in the existing healthcare delivery system, one is reluctant to dismiss the changes now taking place; however, many questions are raised for providers about practice in accountable and caring ways in these highly cost-driven systems. Regardless of changes already here, or yet to come, one hopes that financial considerations will not eliminate compassion in clinical decision making.

BARRIERS TO COLLABORATION

Historically, nurses were viewed as "helpers and agents of physicians; not co-workers or colleagues" (Reverby, 1987, p. 131). Thus, collaboration, even with APNs, remains difficult for many physicians to embrace (Kassirer, 1994). In providing care for the "whole" person, nursing has accepted accountability for aspects of care that overlap with the accountability and authority of other professions (Ujhely, 1968), especially physicians. Overlaps in professional accountability frequently cause confusion regarding authority and responsibility, feelings of competition, and inhibition of the collaborative effort necessary in accountable healthcare (Brush & Capezuti, 1997; Fagin, 1992; Mundinger, 1994).

It is not surprising that issues stemming from historical antecedents in nurse–physician relationships have also contributed to inconsistency from state to state regarding practice roles and privileging. These political and competitive pressures, often driven by the medical and nursing associations, contribute to feelings of resentment and reluctance to collaborate and have been difficult to overcome.

In their book *Nurse–Physician Collaboration: Care of Adults and the Elderly,* Eugenia Siegler and Fay Whitney (1994) refer to their frustrations in promoting and maintaining collaborative practice in settings that are often indifferent and occasionally hostile. Physicians and nurses receive different educations and thus think differently. But both disciplines must cope with "expanding knowledge bases, rapid technological changes, increasing complexity of patient care inside and outside of the hospital, and difficult fiscal-management and policy issues" (p. 19). Paradoxically, the need to collaborate "grows exponentially" as the system becomes more complex, but the priority to teach principles of collaboration "falls in the wake of the pressure to disseminate new knowledge" (p. 19). Thus, those professionals who do practice collaboratively must overcome many barriers at professional, institutional, and legislative levels (Siegler, Hyer, Fulmer, & Mezey, 1998). Collaborative practice, although largely misunderstood, rarely valued by academic institutions, and currently not compensated by third-party payers, is a necessary ingredient in accountable advanced practice nursing and in the solution to America's continuing healthcare crisis.

*C*ASE VIGNETTES

The following three vignettes, describing APNs in home care, a community-based family health center, and an emergency department, respectively, are based on interviews and illustrate many of the themes discussed in this review of accountability.

Vignette 1
J. Konick-McMahon, MSN, RN, Gerontological APN in Discharge Planning, School of Nursing, University of Pennsylvania

Konick-McMahon is part of the staff for a research project, "Home Follow-up of Elderly Patients With Heart Failure." The setting for her work is a large, tertiary care medical center and the surrounding urban community. The focus is acutely ill elderly patients with heart failure who are at "high risk" because of multiple chronic conditions, age (>65 years), and frequent or recent hospitalizations.

A major goal of the comprehensive discharge planning protocol is maintenance of function during and after hospitalization. This is accomplished by careful monitoring and evaluation throughout hospitalization and follow-up at home as often as necessary for 3 months after discharge. During home visits, APNs manage acute problems as they arise, assess and resolve a wide range of concerns about function, and respond to caregiver concerns. Referrals are made as necessary, and a close relationship is maintained with several home care agencies to which patients have been assigned.

Key to the success of the intervention is development of a trusting relationship with clear communications, one which permits understanding of personal preferences, assessment of needs, and determination of realistic outcomes mutually agreeable to patients and their families. Each case requires individualized care planning and creativity. Among the varied problems that can arise are the need to follow specific drug regimens, to overcome environmental barriers, or to cope with acuity associated with rapid discharge from the hospital (the average length of stay is 3.7 days for acute heart failure).

In this unusual role, the barriers to practice faced by Konick-McMahon often center on explaining to colleagues from all disciplines the nature of her role, gaining trust, and obtaining cooperation in implementing necessary interventions. Bridging the gaps from hospital to home and maintaining continuity of care can be exceedingly challenging. Konick-McMahon believes that one of the most urgent changes needed in healthcare is greater accountability by hospital staff for discharge planning and greater responsibility for outcomes after hospitalization. Collaboration with physicians, many of whom do not know the APNs or are unfamiliar with the skills of APNs or the project, can be difficult. For APNs who so clearly see the needs of patients and experience so intimately the barriers created by the system of care, frustration can be intense.

Nevertheless, this role provides an opportunity for the APN to establish a plan of care with the patient and caregiver and to bring it to fruition. Each encounter reinforces the need for a model of services based on transitional care, and findings from the study increasingly document that such services performed by an APN produce positive, cost-effective outcomes (Naylor et al., 1994). In addition, the need for reimbursement or managed care arrangements for these services are clearly evident.

Accountability to the patient is 24 hours a day, 7 days a week. It requires collaboration with other providers and commitment to improved function, reduction in complications, and avoidance of rehospitalization. Konick-McMahon describes the extraordinary sense of responsibility that accompanies management aimed at achieving these goals with frail elderly patients in the community, as the following example attests.

Mrs. R, 76 years old, was hospitalized for heart failure. Six months previously she suffered a myocardial infarction (MI) that further complicated her recovery from a left-sided stroke. Her two daughters assumed responsibility for cooking, cleaning, and transportation so that she could remain in her first-floor apartment. Throughout intensive rehabilitation for the stroke, her subsequent hospitalization for an MI, and the episode of heart failure, Mrs. R's chief goal was to be able to walk outside and to care for her garden.

As Konick-McMahon assumed care, she became accountable for actions undertaken to prevent complications and rehospitalization. A time period of 3 months for intervention by the APN meant that a trusting relationship had to be quickly established to (1) coordinate medications prescribed by the cardiologist and the primary physician, (2) foster communication between providers and patients and family members regarding management, (3) coach the patient and family to assume an empowered role in managing symptoms of heart failure, and (4) assist the patient to reframe perceived barriers to goal attainment. A philosophy of accountability in advanced practice is essential throughout these processes and emphasizes collaboration, communication, and follow-up. Although Mrs. R was unable to meet her personal goal—to return to gardening—she and her daughters were able to meet other health goals, resulting in no need for rehospitalization.

Vignette 2
Melinda Jenkins, PhD, RN, Family Nurse Practitioner

A nurse-managed center located in a public housing complex provides family healthcare to residents in one of Philadelphia's poorest neighborhoods. APNs see patients of all ages, including prenatal, pediatric, adult, and elder care. Jenkins characterizes accountability for care at the center, and responsibility of the APNs, as congruent with the ANA's Social Policy Statement: "The profession of nursing serves the public and in so doing contributes to the good of society" (ANA, 1995). Relationships between a committed tenant counsel and staff of the center are strong, and a sense of shared accountability exists for services rendered and received.

Recently, APNs at the center found themselves in a complex struggle over interpretation of rules governing Medicaid contracts to health maintenance organizations in Pennsylvania. Although the APNs had been following patients covered by two managed care contracts for several years and had been re-imbursed, stringent interpretation of the state regulations could have prevented APNs from continuing to serve as primary providers to Medicaid patients as the state moved to mandatory Medicaid managed care. In the balance of this decision were more than 800 nursing center patients having trusting relation-ships with their APNs, a coherent service successfully meeting community needs, and survival of the center itself. APNs at this nursing center and in other community nursing centers were successful in their efforts to have APNs recognized as primary care providers in a technical advisory from the Depart-ment of Health and later in health maintenance organization legislation. Jenkins believes that a central role of primary care APNs is one of contributing to the development of regulations that allow direct pa-tient access to APNs.

Currently, the focus of attention concerning advanced practice in Pennsylvania is on prescriptive au-thority, as regulated jointly by Pennsylvania's Boards of Nursing and Medicine. Jenkins and her col-leagues at the center remain frustrated by restrictive prescriptive ability that limits the care provided and even thwarts the process of care once assessment and diagnosis are complete. Accountability in pre-scribing remains cloudy because APNs are required to use prescriptions that feature the name of the col-laborating physician, who is paid an hourly rate for consultation but has little first-hand knowledge of patients and no direct responsibility for the plan of care.

Such circumstances, no doubt being repeated elsewhere, illustrate continuing and as yet unresolved barriers to accountable advanced practice. What happens when providers must tell patients that their in-surance plan no longer covers the care they have been receiving or that they must change plans or providers to receive care? The irony, of course, is that APNs, especially in managed care arrangements serving similar populations, are best able to respond to changing incentives for delivering services, namely, health promotion and disease prevention aimed at reducing expensive hospital care.

An example is the case of a young woman followed by Jenkins for prenatal care. After delivering a healthy baby, Ms. B came in for routine well-woman and pediatric care only. One day, just as the center was about to close, Ms. B called Jenkins in great alarm over the extreme fatigue and sudden 30-lb weight loss of her fiancé. The fiancé was reluctant to seek care, but because Ms. B trusted the APNs at the center, he agreed to see Jenkins, who also felt it was an emergency. A quick history and examina-tion revealed 4+ glucose in the urine and a random blood glucose of 400. Hospitalization for a diabetic crisis was averted. Jenkins is convinced that this successful outcome depended greatly on accountability for care and the relationship with patient and community.

Vignette 3

Michael Clark, MSN, RN, Nurse Practitioner in Emergency Services, Hospital of the University of Penn-sylvania

As part of emergency services provided by the Hospital of the University of Pennsylvania, a walk-in clinic staffed by APNs in collaboration with physicians has been established for persons requiring less emergency care. Protocols help delineate practice parameters, but it is experience gained over time and the ability and confidence "to think on one's feet" that most defines what the practitioners do. In this setting, the dialog between APNs and physicians concerning decision making is an ongoing one.

First and foremost, APNs view their primary obligation and accountability to patients. Frequently, this takes the form of advocacy, especially with a patient population that has problems accessing more appropriate primary care services. Most clinic patients have Medicaid coverage or its equivalent; helping them overcome barriers experienced in obtaining care is often the focus of interventions by APNs. Thus, Clark queries all patients about the reasons they are in the emergency department and not somewhere else. Often it is "last straw" phenomena—long-standing dissatisfaction with providers, enormity of healthcare problems, exhaustion and frustration, or declining resources (personal and financial)—that precipitate visits to the emergency department.

Although patients struggle with barriers related to access, APNs work against numerous time and volume constraints to maximize what is likely to be a single patient encounter. For practice to be truly responsive to the public, Clark believes that patients coming to the walk-in clinic must be empowered with information to care for themselves. Although these patients can benefit from services and expertise unique to an academic medical center, it is translation of that knowledge, quickly and in pragmatic terms, that is essential. Many factors must be considered as to which interventions will be useful, feasible, and cost-effective.

Clark related the story of an older couple who arrived in the triage area. The wife was immaculately groomed and refined in her manner; the husband was extremely agitated and demanded that his wife "be tested for drugs." Immediately, the nurse practitioner made a decision to separate the couple for purposes of assessment and possible admission to the hospital. In eliciting a history from the wife, he learned that her husband had been physically assaultive for the past few weeks. Psychiatric consultation was arranged for the couple, which ultimately led to resolution of some family stresses and problems. This story represents the kind of situation that could easily be dismissed in an emergency department as bizarre and a waste of time. In this case, however, commitment to look beyond superficial behavior and appearance, and to gather additional data, made a difference in quality of life for the couple and potentially prevented serious injury.

Each of these examples of advanced clinical practice is shaped by setting, characteristics of and constraints on particular practices, and perceptions of accountability and responsibility. Whether care is acute and episodic or continuous over time, a consistent theme emerges: The focus of the APNs is holistic and devoted to principles of primary care. Accountability is understood in terms of ethical commitments to honor and respect individuals and their needs, to remain nonjudgmental, to empower through information sharing and advocacy, and to be true to community and societal expectations and trust.

Summary and Conclusions

The covenant between APN and patient is rooted in the profession's moral and ethical foundations and its abiding commitment to persons in need. As healthcare changes and as nursing advances its knowledge base, the boundaries of practice continuously expand. Practice is influenced by professional standards and external regulations designed to protect the public. These forces both facilitate and constrain practice and are constantly evolving.

In its statement of graduate outcomes for primary care APNs, the National Organization of Nurse Practitioner Faculties (NONPF) (1993) identifies as critical competencies caring, advocacy, support, relationships, therapeutic communication, interpersonal skills, and ethics. In addition, as discussed here, the NONPF considers as part of accountable practice professional and legal standards, collaboration and consultation with others, and maintenance of certification.

Embedded within accountable practice is responsibility for excellent care, a caring relationship, and commitment to positive outcomes for individuals and for society. APNs are challenged daily by both the complexities of patient care and certain barriers to practice, but the rewards include the satisfaction associated with truly accountable care. The essence of that accountability, so beautifully illustrated in the case vignettes, is eloquently captured in a single, simple sentence from Doris Schwartz's (1995) personal story of 50 years in nursing: "Caring *about* a patient can be as important as providing care *for* the patient" (pp. 213–214).

REFERENCES

Aiken, L. H., Lake, E. T., Semaan, S., et al. (1993). Nurse practitioner managed care for persons with HIV infection. *Image: Journal of Nursing Scholarship 25,* 172–177.

American Nurses Association. (1995). *Nursing's social policy statement.* Washington, DC: Author.

American Nurses Credentialing Center. (1998). Certification catalog. Available at: http://www.ana.org/ancc/index.html.

Astrom, G., Norberg, A., Hallberg, I. R., & Jansson, L. (1993). Experienced and skilled nurses' narratives of situations where caring action made a difference to the patient. *Scholarly Inquiry for Nursing Practice: An International Journal 7,* 183–193.

Baer, E. D. (1993). Philosophical and historical bases of primary care nursing. In M. D. Mezey & D. O. McGivern (Eds.). *Nurses, APNs: Evolution to advanced practice* (pp. 102–118). New York: Springer.

Beeber, L. S., & Charlie, M. L. (1998). Depressive symptom reversal for women in a primary care setting: A pilot study. *Archives of Psychiatric Nursing 12,* 247–254.

Brown, S. J. (1998). A framework for advanced practice nursing. *Journal of Professional Nursing 14,* 157–164.

Brush, B. L., & Capezuti, E. A. (1997). Professional autonomy: Essential for nurse practitioner survival in the 21st century. *Journal of the American Academy of APNs 9,* 265–270.

Burgess, A. W., Lerner, D. J., D'Agostino, R. B., et al. (1987). A randomized control trial of cardiac rehabilitation. *Social Science Medicine 24,* 359–370.

Carper, B. A. (1979). The ethics of caring. *Advances in Nursing Science 1*(3), 11–19.

Creasia, J. L., & Parker, B. (Eds.). (1991). *Conceptual foundations of professional nursing practice.* Philadelphia: Mosby.

Deloughery, G. L. (1977). *History and trends of professional nursing* (8th ed.). St. Louis, MO: Mosby.

Emanuel, E. J., Mezey, M. D., & Dubler, N. N. (1993). *The provider–patient relationship under the new health care system.* Unpublished manuscript.

Evans, L. K., Strumpf, N. E., Allen-Taylor, L., et al. (1997). A clinical trial to reduce restraints in nursing homes. *Journal of the American Geriatrics Society 45,* 675–681.

Fagin, C. M. (1992). Collaboration between nurses and physicians: No longer a choice. *Academic Medicine 67,* 295–303.

Fry, S. T. (1991). Measurement of moral answerability in nursing practice. In C. F. Waltz and O. L. Strickland (Eds.). *Measurement of clinical and educational nursing outcomes: Vol. 4.* New York: Springer.

Goodnow, M. (1943). *Nursing history in brief* (rev. ed.). Philadelphia: Saunders.

Hamric, A. B., Worley, D., Lindebak, S., & Jaubert, S.

(1998). Outcomes associated with advanced nursing practice prescriptive authority. *Journal of the American Academy of APNs 10,* 113–118.

Harmer, B. (1925). *Text-book of the principles and practice of nursing.* New York: Macmillan.

Henderson, V. (1966). *The nature of nursing: A definition and its implications for practice, research, and education.* New York: Macmillan.

Hunt, G. (1997). The human condition of the professional: Discretion and accountability. *Nursing Ethics 4,* 519–526.

Jurchak, M. (1990). Competence and the nurse–patient relationship. *Critical Care Nursing Clinics of North America 2,* 453–459.

Kasch, C. R. (1986). Establishing a collaborative nurse–patient relationship: A distinct focus of nursing action in primary care. *Image: Journal of Nursing Scholarship 18*(2), 44–47.

Kassirer, J. P. (1994). What role for APNs in primary care? *New England Journal of Medicine 330,* 204–205.

Katims, I. (1993). Nursing as aesthetic experience and the notion of practice. *Scholarly Inquiry for Nursing Practice: An International Journal 7,* 269–278.

Kenner, C. V., Guzzetta, C. E., & Dussey, B. M. (1985). *Critical care nursing: Body-mind-spirit* (2nd ed.). Boston: Little-Brown.

Mackenzie, E. R., Strumpf, N. E., Johnson, J. E., & Sands, R. (1998). Selecting and preparing team training educators. In E. L. Siegler, K. Hyer, T. Fulmer, & M. Mezey (Eds.). *Geriatric interdisciplinary team training* (pp. 51–62). New York: Springer.

Mahoney, D. F. (1994). Appropriateness of geriatric prescribing decisions made by APNs and physicians. *Image: Journal of Nursing Scholarship 26*(1), 41–46.

Mahoney, D. F. (1995). Employer resistance to state authorized prescriptive authority for NPs (results of a pilot study). *Nurse Practitioner: The American Journal of Primary Care 20,* 58–61.

McCorkle, R., Benoliel, J., Dondalson, G., et al. (1989). A randomized clinical trial of home nursing care for lung cancer patients. *Cancer 64,* 1375–1382.

McDermott, K. C. (1995). Prescriptive authority for advanced practice nurses: Current and future perspectives. *Oncology Nursing Forum 22* (8 Suppl), 25–30.

Mundinger, M. O. (1994). Advanced practice nursing: Good medicine for physicians? *New England Journal of Medicine 330,* 211–214.

National Organization of Nurse Practitioner Faculties. (November 1993). *Primary care nurse practitioner graduate outcomes.* Washington, DC: NONPF Education Committee.

Naylor, M. D. (1990). Comprehensive discharge planning for hospitalized elderly: A pilot study. *Nursing Research 39,* 156–161.

Naylor, M., Brooten, D., Jones, R., et al. (1994). Comprehensive discharge planning for the hospitalized elderly: A randomized clinical trial. *Annals of Internal Medicine 120*(12), 999–1006.

Neidlinger, L., Scroggins, K., & Kennedy, L. (1987). Cost evaluation of discharge planning for hospitalized elderly. *Nursing Economics 5*, 225–230.

Nightingale, F. (1859/1992). *Notes on nursing: What it is and what it is not* (commemorative edition). Philadelphia: J. B. Lippincott.

Olsen, D. P. (1997). When the patient causes the problem: The effect of patient responsibility on the nurse–patient relationship. *Journal of Advanced Nursing 26*, 515–522.

Omerod, J. A. (1993). Accountability in nurse education. *British Journal of Nursing 2*, 730–733.

Pan, S., Straub, L. A., & Geller, J. M. (1997). Restrictive practice environment and APNs' prescriptive authority. *Journal of the American Academy of APNs 9*, 9–15.

Pearson, L. J. (1998). Annual update of how each state stands on legislative issues affecting advanced nursing practice. *Nurse Practitioner, 23*(1), 14–16, 19–20, 25–26.

Pellegrino, E. D. (1974). Educating the humanist physician. *Journal of the American Medical Association 227*, 1288–1294.

Peplau, H. E. (1997). Peplau's theory of interpersonal relations. *Nursing Science Quarterly 10*, 162–167.

Pope, A. E., & Young, V. M. (1934). *The art and principles of nursing*. New York: G. P. Putnam's Sons.

Pozen, M. N., Stechmiller, J. A., Harris, W. A., et al. (1977). A nurse rehabilitator's impact on patients with myocardial infarction. *Medical Care 15*, 830–837.

Raines, D. A. (1997). From covenant to contract: How managed care is changing provider/patient relationships. *Lifelines, August*, 41–45.

Ramsay, J., McKenzie, J., & Fish, D. (1982). Physicians and APNs: Do they provide equivalent health care? *American Journal of Public Health 72*(1), 55–56.

Rawnsley, M. M. (1994). Response to "The nurse–patient relationship reconsidered: An expanded research agenda." *Scholarly Inquiry for Nursing Practice: An International Journal 8*(2), 185–190.

Reverby, S. M. (1987). *Ordered to care: The dilemma of American nursing, 1850–1945*. Cambridge, MA: Cambridge University Press.

Robb, I. H. (1901). *Nursing ethics: For hospital and private use*. Cleveland, OH: J. B. Savage.

Rustia, J. G., & Bartek, J. K. (1997). Managed care credentialing of advanced practice nurses. *Nurse Practitioner 22*(9), 90, 92, 99–100, 102–103.

Schwartz, D. R. (1988). In T. M. Schorr & A. Zimmerman (Eds.). *Making choices, taking chances: Nurse leaders tell their stories* (pp. 311–320). Washington, DC: Mosby.

Schwartz, D. (1995). *Give us to go blithely: My fifty years of nursing*. New York: Springer.

Sidani, S., & Braden, C. J. (1998). *Evaluating nursing interventions: A theory-driven approach*. Thousand Oaks, CA: Sage Publications.

Siegler, E. L., Hyer, K., Fulmer, T., & Mezey, M. (1998). *Geriatric interdisciplinary team training*. New York: Springer.

Siegler, E. L., & Whitney, F. W. (1994). *Nurse-physician collaboration: Care of adults and the elderly*. New York: Springer.

Strumpf, N. E., & Paier, G. (1992). Ethical issues. In T. Fulmer & M. Walker (Eds.). *Critical care nursing of the elderly* (pp. 296–305). New York: Springer.

Thomasma, D. C. (1996). The ethics of managed care: Challenges to the principles of relationship-centered care. *Journal of Allied Health 25*, 233–246.

Ujhely, G. B. (1968). *Determinants of the nurse–patient relationship*. New York: Springer.

United States Department of Health, Education, and Welfare. (1967). *Nurse Training Act of 1964: Program review report* (USDHEW Public Health Service, no. 1740. pp. 15–18). Washington, DC: Author.

Varon, J. (1996). Managed care for real people: Consequences of political and financial government decisions. *Journal of Long-Term Home Health Care 15*(2), 24–32.

Ware, J. E., Bayliss, M. S., Rogers, W. H., et al. (1996). Differences in 4-year health outcomes for elderly and poor chronically ill patients treated in HMO and fee-for-service systems: Results from the Medical Outcomes Study. *Journal of the American Medical Association 276*, 1039–1047.

CHAPTER 14

JoAnne Kirk Henry

Political Activism: Moving the Profession Forward

The political environment today is one of increasing cynicism that discourages many from increasing their involvement in the political process. Any discussion of politics conjures up visions of power brokers, primarily men, in private rooms trading favors and negotiating influence. Politics is more than this. Opening the political process to new leaders is essential to the changes that nurses desire. Politics is not an individual activity: politicians are team players. Nurses have the skills needed to be team players in the political arena. Nurses have to learn about the environment of politics and then apply their nursing skills.

This is a period of rapid change in government as well as healthcare. Over the centuries, Americans have shown an amazing capacity to reinvent the political system (Sabato & Simpson, 1996). Today is no exception. New influences can become the power for the future. Nurses have unique contributions to make to this evolving system.

"Nursing has two notable strengths in the political arena: the large number of RNs and their tremendously positive image. Numbers translate into political strength" (Harrington & Estes, 1997, p.171). Nurses are regarded positively by the public and political leaders. They are not seen as self-interested but as interested in the public good. This is a critical time for advanced practice nurses (APNs) to assume leadership roles.

Increasing Nursing's Political Power

The public is confused about nursing. Advanced practice nursing is not well understood, and the descriptions of various groups of APNs—nurse practitioners (NPs), clinical nurse specialists (CNSs), certified nurse–midwives, and certified nurse–anesthetists—often increase rather than decrease this confusion. To increase the public's understanding of nursing, the focus must be on the common elements of nursing. Then, brief and clear statements about the differences among nurses can be added. Focusing on agreed-on common elements and goals will maximize nursing's power. Nurses lose political power when they argue among themselves.

Political Power

A continuum of political involvement is presented in this chapter. It can be used to increase nursing power throughout the policymaking process. The focus of this chapter is on government and politics, but the principles can be used in the community as well. APN reimbursement, a key policy issue, is used to describe the actions of nursing along the continuum of political involvement. The model of political involvement is presented, and the political action strategies for nurses are outlined.

Political power is the ability to influence or persuade the individuals who have the power to work toward the goal that nurses' desire. Nurses use political power in the work place and successfully persuade others to support the goals of nursing. Transferring these skills to professional organizations and the community will enhance nursing power.

Governmental leaders have positive regard for nursing, and this provides a base of good will that can be built on by skilled, committed APNs. The political process provides the vehicle for nurses to work for change in government and health policy. The political process is not necessarily a fair or objective process. It is dynamic and changeable. Policy is formed by compromise, and the language of policy may be intentionally vague to allow for differing interpretations. "Policy is not written in stone. It is dynamic, a potpourri of laws (often vague), of regulations (often late), government officials' interpretations (often conflicting, sometimes wrong), court decisions (sometimes bizarre) and, in the final analysis, the level of compliance" (Weissert & Weissert, 1996). These are the determining factors in the impact of policy with the law. It is easy to see how unintended consequences are a frequent outcome. Therefore, policy evolves and changes. Nurses work for legislation and celebrate its passage but frequently ignore the regulatory process that determines the specific impact of the policy. Regulations remove the ambiguity of policy and are vital to policymaking.

Political Activism

Political power is increased through political activism. Political decisions influence many aspects of our lives and have a significant influence on healthcare and on advanced practice nursing. When nurses fail to participate in the political process, they allow decisions to be made by people who are seeking control for their own reasons, and nurses' interests are unrecognized (Harrington & Estes, 1997). These influential people frequently have different goals than nurses.

Policy is formed by compromise. Policies may be left deliberately vague and the specifics added within the agencies that are responsible for implementation (Weissert & Weissert, 1996). This is an advantage to APNs who have numerous places to influence nursing and health policy. In government, the legislature is often the first place that nurses try to change policy. It is not always the appropriate place to effect change. The executive branch of government, through its agencies, defines policy through regulation. Influencing the boards of health and health professions, the insurance commission, and the Medicaid and social services divisions may be the more appropriate places to create change. To do this, APNs must be knowledgeable about these agencies and how they function.

Activism exists along a continuum, and most nurses are politically inactive. One measure of activism is membership in professional organizations. The American Nurses Association (ANA) reports that only 200,000 of the 2.5 million registered nurses belong to the ANA (DeVries & Vanderbilt, 1996). Of these nurses, only a small number are actively involved in the organization. The active involvement of all 2.5 million nurses is not required to achieve political power, but the current level of involvement is too low. A greater percentage of APNs are thought to be active than the percentage of registered nurses without advanced practice preparation. APNs are professional leaders. Their graduate preparation has provided skills that are essential in the political arena—knowledge of the issues, research and writing skills, and skills in presenting their ideas clearly and succinctly. Educational preparation, leadership skills, and practice knowledge prepare APNs to increase their political involvement. APNs have not necessarily mastered other skills essential in the political arena; they must work to be knowledgeable, sophisticated participants in the political process.

Nursing's Influence

APNs are the leaders in nursing. Their individual power is much less than their collective power. The model, A Continuum for Political Involvement (Table 14-1), can be used to determine the APN's current level of political activism. Goals can be set for increasing involvement and the model used to determine the appropriate steps for increasing activism. Moving to higher levels on the continuum expands nursing's collective power as nurses move from individual to collective action.

Most nurses are at levels 0—unaware—and 1—aware. Moving from level 0 to 1 should be a commitment that every nurse makes. It is a commitment for life and not just for today. Registering to vote and voting thoughtfully demand little time and make a significant difference. Joining a professional organization demands little but increases the power of nursing. Professional organizations are only as strong as their budgets allow. Increasing the number of members increases the ability of the organization to lobby for nursing and to influence healthcare. This support for a professional organization ensures a voice for nursing in healthcare policy changes.

TABLE 14-1 *Continuum of Political Involvement*

Levels of Activity

0 Unaware	1 Aware	2 Involved	3 Participant	4 Leader
Not registered to vote	Registered to vote			
Does not know names of elected officials	Knows names of elected officials	Contacts legislators Offer assistance on issues	Known to elected officials	Active in a political party
Not a member of professional organizations	Belongs to professional organizations	Active in organizations	Leader in professional/ community/political organizations	Appointed government committee or board
	Follows selected political issues	Works in organizations to influence the outcome of selected political issues	Works in political arena to influence leaders for outcome of issues	Contributes to or works on campaigns
		Joins coalitions	Presents testimony on issues	Elected to public office

Movement to level 2—involved—is the beginning of leadership in the political arena. Nurses work at this level to understand the issues and the differing points of view, writing or talking to elected officials about the issues, becoming leaders in professional organizations, and working for change. Level 2 is the place where most active nurses remain. Few nurses move to levels 3—participant—and 4—leader. At levels 3 and 4, nurses are leaders in the political arena. Are nurses reticent to take risks that keep them from moving into more visible leadership roles?

Level 3—participant—is the level where influence is achieved. It demands higher visibility and greater commitment. Chalich and Smith (1992) describe the process as moving up the rungs of a ladder. They describe the need for building confidence and credibility by beginning with civic involvement through local groups like the Parent-Teacher Organizations or neighborhood groups. Nurses most frequently work through local nursing groups to achieve the same skills. After skill and confidence are built in these groups, APNs can move to leadership roles in advocacy. Participation in broader community groups is the next step and increases nursing's influence. The satisfaction of knowing that a change has occurred as a result of your work moves many to the next level on the continuum. Networking and leading groups are more advanced but still short of the ultimate goal, which is to achieve long-term influence.

Level 4—leader—is the most advanced level of participation. Active participation through campaigning for oneself or others and agenda setting for local or state government are the characteristics of nurses who achieve this level. Involvement at this level requires participation in partisan politics. Not all nurses will wish to be involved in partisan politics, but greater involvement of a few nurses has an enormous payoff for all nurses. Supporting colleagues who are candidates for election is a means of being vicariously active.

APNs are active simultaneously on several levels in the continuum. For nursing to achieve greater influence, more nurses must be active in all areas of levels 3 and 4. Most APNs who have moved to higher levels of the model have been influenced by colleagues who are active at higher levels on the continuum. One strategy to increase the involvement of nurses is to invite colleagues to work with you in an organization or on a project.

Issues in Advanced Practice Nurse Reimbursement by Medicare

Reimbursement for APN care is presented as the example of success in the political arena. It is an important issue for nursing. Reimbursement is important not only for the reimbursement dollars but because reimbursement records are frequently used by researchers to study quality and effectiveness of care. If APN care cannot be identified separately from physician's care, then the care that they provide remains invisible and the quality of that care cannot be studied.

In the evolving healthcare system, reimbursement for healthcare services has become increasingly important to employers of APNs as well. In the mid-1990s, attempts to eliminate healthcare billing fraud and abuse have made it clear that the actual provider of care must be the one to bill for services. Physicians bill for services provided by other healthcare providers under the "incident to" rule. These billings have been questioned by healthcare insurers unless the physician actually cared for the patient.

The Health Care Financing Administration (HCFA) defines *incident to* as "any service furnished as an integral, although incident, part of the physician's personal professional services in the course of diagnostic or treatment of an injury or illness" (HCFA, 1998). Under this rule, APN care was billed by the physician using the physician's provider number. To ensure that the billing provider is, in fact, the provider of care, a physician review of all APN care has been implemented in many practice settings. This has been done not to ensure quality of care but to ensure that care could be reimbursed.

APNs practice independently or with collaborative agreements for the care that they provide. Physicians do not care for or need to care for most of the patients who receive care from APNs. The requirements for physicians to see patients cared for by APNs increased the barriers and access to care. A change was needed.

WORKING TOWARD ADVANCED PRACTICE NURSE REIMBURSEMENT

After 8 years of work by a coalition of the ANA and specialty nursing organizations, the Balanced Budget Act of 1997 (P.L.105–33) included the provision for reimbursement of physician's assistants, NPs, and CNSs. They will be reimbursed for services of the type that have been considered physician services under federal definition and are within the APNs' scope of practice (Minarik, 1998). Medicare beneficiaries can have access to the services of APNs no matter where they live. This process of achieving third-party reimbursement was filled with frustrations and barriers, but the tenacity of nursing's leaders achieved a successful outcome.

Individual nurses working for reimbursement policy change worked primarily at levels 1 and 2 of the Continuum of Political Involvement (Table 14-1). They were aware of the issue and belonged to professional organizations. Their dues supported the nursing organizations that lobbied for APN reimbursement. At level 2, the APN contacted legislators and worked within the organization or coalitions to influence legislators to support reimbursement for APNs. Few nurses have been active at levels 3 and 4. If they had been lobbying legislators, associations would have been more effective and nurses would have had greater influence in the political system. Nursing organizations had the major responsibility to develop networks of members who would work at levels 1 and 2, and organization staff worked to ensure that communication was coordinated in lobbying.

The focus for third-party reimbursement has been at the federal level because states and private insurers use the federal requirements as models for their own insurance regulations. If federal regulation did not include the requirement to reimburse APNs for the care that they provide, then it is much more difficult to achieve reimbursement at the local level.

REGULATIONS FOR ADVANCED PRACTICE NURSE REIMBURSEMENT BY MEDICARE

Effective January 1998, provisions of the Balanced Budget Act of 1997 (P.L. 105–33) removed the restrictions on types of areas and settings in which the NP and CNS services could be reimbursed by Medicare Part B. Payments are allowed for services furnished by these nonphysician providers in all settings and areas permitted under the applicable state licensure laws. This provision expanded the reimbursement to NPs and CNSs by authorizing them to bill the program directly for their services. The provision maintains the current policy that no separate payment may be made to nonphysician providers when a facility or other provider charge is also made for the services and the "incident to" rules are unchanged (HCFA, April 1998). Some care provided by APNs remains billable under the "incident to" regulation.

Reimbursement is set at 80% of the actual charge or at the level of 85% of the physician reimbursement rate, whichever is smaller. In March 1998, the HCFA released the memorandum notifying all local Medicare carriers and intermediaries of the change and provided instructions on its implementation. NPs and CNSs must apply for their own provider numbers from their local Medicare carriers.

The process of providing for reimbursement of APN care has brought the issue of the definition of collaboration into question because it includes supervision by a physician as a component of the definition of collaboration. Many state regulatory boards and health insurers use this language to restrict the practice of APNs.

Collaboration is a process in which the NP or CNS works with a physician to deliver healthcare services within the scope of the practitioner's professional expertise, with medical direction and appropriate supervision as provided for in the jointly developed guidelines or other mechanisms as defined by the law of the state in which the services are performed. CNSs are not required to practice with the supervision of a physician. Before the 1998 change in HCFA regulations, each state's definition of scope of practice was the determining factor in whether a service was appropriate for the NP or CNS to provide independently or with supervision. It is important to work at the state level to ensure that no further practice restrictions are put in place. Changing the federal definition of collaboration is the next task to be achieved.

Medicare provides reimbursement through contracts with private healthcare insurers who each have their own requirements. Although they are required to comply with the federal regulations, some insurers create barriers that delay or obfuscate the intent of the federal intent. Nurses must continue to work to ensure that the regulations being written in HCFA, part of the executive branch of government, will support the legislative intent. The HCFA, through its advisory board, will be influential in the process of change in the definition of collaboration. It is important to know about this board and its members. Do they have vested interest in maintaining the status quo? Are they nurses? How can nurses change the composition of this advisory board? The appointment of nurses within government is key to ensuring that progress continues and that nursing's voice is stronger. Who are the nurses who are ready for appointment to a national board?

Medicaid Reimbursement—Interwoven Barriers

Medicaid is a joint federal–state program that provides healthcare services to people with low incomes. The federal government allows states to determine the services that can be reimbursed, and it allows states to broaden the categories of providers who can receive reimbursement for services. Ensuring that APNs receive Medicaid reimbursement required a shift in focus for nursing's lobbying effort from the federal to the state level. APNs can no longer rely on their national organizations to work for them. The action is at the state level.

To ensure that APNs can be reimbursed for the care that they provide to individuals who have Medicaid insurance, coalitions of nurses must work in each state. This is the level at which APNs can be active and influential. Finding out how the system works in your state is essential to change. How does your state regulate APN practice? Is it through the board of nursing, medicine, or joint boards? What are the roles of Medicaid, the health department, and the insurance commission in determining which healthcare providers can receive reimbursement for services? Does the definition of primary care provider determine who can receive reimbursement? Can APNs be primary care providers in your state?

How does nursing lobby for change in your state or local area? Is it through the state nurses association? Is there a coalition or alliance of nursing organizations? Do APNs work through the state nurses association? Are there paid lobbyists for nursing? Who speaks for nursing? APNs can find out the answers to these questions through their state nursing associations.

Learning About the Political Process

Increasing political involvement necessitates learning more about the systems. One way to do this is through the local or state nursing organizations. There are also numerous books that describe the political process and the points of influence in the process. These books are published by professional organizations, by groups like the League of Women Voters, and by state and local government. APNs can contact local resources to get these materials. Joining a group that has a public policy action agenda and participating in the educational sessions is helpful. It may provide an opportunity to meet government representatives as well because local officials are often presenters. Work in community organizations is another way to learn and to build support for nursing.

A resource for political knowledge is the Internet. Most professional nursing organizations have websites that provide information about legislative and health policy issues. Local and state government websites may also provide helpful information about elected and appointed officials and a way to contact them directly by e-mail. Many websites for government agencies include agendas and dates for meetings, legislation that is in process or has been passed, and regulations. This evolving resource is changing rapidly and is an excellent means for education and communication. Caution is needed in using e-mail for communication with government officials. The same rules of formal address and communication style should be applied to electronic communication as apply to written communication that is delivered by mail.

Progress of Involvement—Nurses Make a Difference

The following example is compiled from the experiences of several nursing groups and does not represent an individual nurse. People become active when issues are important to them. For nurses, issues of decreased access to care or increased cost of care frequently move them to act. Political rules (see Box 14-1) provide a guide for action.

Changes to healthcare that increase the bureaucracy and result in increasing use of emergency care frustrate nurses. Nurses frequently see people who do not understand how to use their managed care system and inappropriately use emergency department services. Changes in the rules for managed care were needed. Nurses work to change the system; at times they work ineffectively. Working as individuals, they call legislators without clearly understanding the issue or what can be achieved through legislation. The result is frustration for all.

A more effective way to influence policy is to choose an issue that is important to you. Learn not only about the issue but also about the policy process. Do not work alone. Find out who else in your community is concerned about this issue. Be sure to let people know that you are a nurse. Increasing nursing's visibility is important to its collective power (see Exemplar 17D).

Changes in the healthcare system confused patients and led them to increase their emergency department use. Several emergency department nurses became concerned about this inappropriate emergency department use. They started by talking to each other. They contacted the Emergency Nurses' Association for information about how to change care. They talked to others in their community. They discovered that physicians, hospitals, rescue squads, and managed care organizations shared the same concern about emergency department use. Nurses joined other community members in meetings to determine a strategy and to increase their influence. They learned from others. They found that not all of the groups who shared their initial concern saw the same solutions. Groups had different ideas. This made the work more difficult because the different groups proposed different solutions. Nurses found that other nurses shared their ideas, and they worked with other nurses. In the end, the outcome was not specific to emergency department use at all. The coalition of concerned people worked for a policy change that required managed care organizations to educate their members about how to use healthcare services appropriately. An additional requirement was that the educational materials be written at a level that all could read. This was a transitory coalition that focused on a particular issue. The coalition disbanded after the policy change was implemented.

| Box 14-1 | *Political Rules to Live By* |

DETERMINE THE IMPRESSION THAT YOU WANT TO MAKE:

Determine how should you dress

Decide if you will you have a fact sheet

Rehearse the way you will present your ideas

DO THE OBVIOUS:

Show up

Do your homework

Know the system

Plan your strategy

Be honest and admit if you do not know

DO NOT ASSUME THAT ANYONE SHARES YOUR POINT OF VIEW

Ask questions

BE DEPENDABLE

NETWORKS ARE IMPORTANT:

Process is as important as content

Never surprise your friends

Work indirectly

Negotiate

Take public credit but do not take too much

PERCEPTIONS ARE REALITY BUT THEY CAN BE CHANGED

Nurses Act Together—The Coalition of Virginia Nurses

The Coalition of Virginia Nurses is an example of the effectiveness that can be achieved when nurses work together. Virginia nursing organizations have worked for more than 20 years building connections between the multiple state and local nursing organizations. This work has taken various forms. At times the relationships between the organizations have been positive and effective, and at other times they have been contentious and divisive. There are more than 20 nursing organizations that have local officers in Virginia. The Virginia Nurses' Association is the only organization in the state that has full-time staff, and as a result, it has provided leadership.

Virginia has developed two coalitions. The Alliance of Nursing Organizations, formed in the mid-1980s, focuses on nursing issues and problems that require collective action, but it does not lobby for legislation. In the late 1990s, it became clear that changes in the health-care system required active involvement of Virginia's nurses in political action. Leaders from the Alliance held organizational meetings. The result was the formation of the Coalition of Virginia Nurses. Critical to the initial formation of the Coalition was the high level of trust among leaders that had been established by their participation in the Alliance.

The Coalition has as its purpose the creation and implementation of a legislative action agenda. Two additional goals are to educate nurses about legislative issues and to promote the appointment of nurses to state policymaking boards and commissions. The Coalition has organizational and individual members and a clear voting mechanism. The linkages within nursing groups are strong. The linkages to other health-related coalitions are less clear. At meetings, Coalition members report not only on the political issues for their nursing organization but also on the actions of other coalitions. The Nursing Coalition has supported the actions of these other groups, which has broadened the influence of the Nursing Coalition. To date, no issues have been addressed that would divide nursing groups. Issues have drawn nurses together.

More than 20 nursing organizations have dues-paying members, and representatives of most of these organizations attend meetings. Individuals may join and are full participants. Communication is primarily through e-mail and fax because that communication is prompt and inexpensive. The Coalition has elected officers, decided on modest dues, and invited members of the Board of Nursing, the Virginia Nurses' Association Political Action Committee, and lobbyists for nursing organizations to participate in its meetings and deliberations.

APNs are active participants in the Coalition and have proposed numerous issues for action. In fact, the primary legislative agenda has addressed issues that most directly affect APNs. There are clear differences in priorities for legislative action among the APN groups. The Coalition has served as a forum for discussion of the issues and differing perspectives. An example is that certified nurse–midwives within the state set a goal of changes in the definition of physician supervision as an immediate priority. The NPs raised concerns that addressing this issue in the same year that the sunset for the ratios of physicians and NPs in prescriptive authority was to be voted on could result in a loss of prescriptive authority for all APNs. The result of the discussion was that a 2-year plan was developed to focus initially on prescriptive authority and then to build a strategy for proposing legislation to change the definition of supervision within the Nurse Practice Act.

The coalition work has made it obvious that nursing does not have clear, effective communication links to legislators. As a part of the long-term strategy, the Coalition sponsored an invitational political action summit for nurses who wanted to be more active. The goal was to move more nurses to levels 3 and 4 of the Continuum of Political Involvement. Individual nurses were recommended by their organizations and invited to attend. Nurses who attended agreed to work with a legislator and develop a key contact relationship and serve as a resource to the legislator on health and nursing issues. The focus was to apply the political rules (see Box 14-1) and to establish a network of nurses who are known resources to legislators and seen as key contacts. This summit was the first action by the Coalition to develop the key contact network of nurses for legislators. Follow-up action included small-group sessions to discuss experiences and successes and to enlarge the network. The long-term goal was to achieve a network of nurses who are committed to working for healthcare change through legislative action, political involvement, and membership on governmental boards and commissions. The ultimate goal was to identify and support nurses who run for elected office.

BUILDING AN EFFECTIVE COALITION

Coalition building is widely discussed and is seen as an effective mechanism for achieving influence in the political arena. Coalition formation and action are means to achieve power through connections and collective action. In the 1980s healthcare providers had to learn to compete, and this made these providers aware that they had to collaborate and compete at the same time if their goals were to be achieved. It also changed the alliances among healthcare groups. Narrowly focused coalitions for specific purposes emerged as a result.

"Coalition formation and utilization is all about responding to change and complexity through connections" (Sullivan, 1998, p. 253). Coalitions bring key individuals or organizations together in a formal structure to pursue agreed-on goals and outcomes that could not be achieved by one member acting alone. Coalitions have formal structures to determine the areas of agreement, power sharing, and communication strategies. They are widely used in the healthcare setting. These dynamic structures may be formed as short-term structures around specific issues or may have long-term goals that result in stable organizations. Coalitions must address their reasons for forming, issue of goals, membership, structure, approaches to problem solving, power sharing, levels of interagency collaboration, functions and tasks to be performed, and outcomes to be achieved. Coalitions are not necessarily linear in their development. These are noisy organizations where mixed signals abound. Given the conflicting demands of the like-minded and diverse-minded members gaining trust, making decisions and taking action is not easy. The goals are greater than the capacity of one organization to achieve, and members have to subjugate their interests toward the common goal (Sullivan, 1998, p. 255).

Most of the literature about coalitions describes their formation and is anecdotal. Reports of coalitions show the widely varying forms that they take. The literature provides little or no evidence of successful outcomes of coalition activity and few evaluation models. One critical factor gleaned from the literature is that successful coalitions are developed voluntarily by the members and are not required by an external body (Sullivan, 1998, p. 259–261).

APNs who wish to form coalitions can find guidance in the literature (DeVries & Vanderbilt, 1992; Mason & Talbott, 1985; Sullivan, 1998). At the local level, the state nurses association is a good place to begin building membership in a nursing coalition. Coalitions of interested people form around specific issues, for example, mental health, children's health, breast cancer, and access to care. These groups often have individual and organization members. They are good places for nurses to gain experience in the political process. Coalitions formed around specific issues may be transitory. They form, address the issue, and disband.

Coalitions may also be formed to develop policy rather than to respond to policy problems. Nurses need to build constituents who support nursing and issues of importance to nursing from outside of nursing. This is a more advanced stage of coalition formation and participation (Cohen et al., 1996). Success in working with a coalition increases the member's skills and power and prepares the members to assume leadership roles in the future.

Advanced Practice Nurses—Take the Next Step

Nurses must use their power more effectively if the perspective that they bring to healthcare and governmental reform is to be included in policy. This chapter presents a model and strategies for change. It is not exhaustive. Nursing and public literature provide numerous resources for APNs who wish to move forward as leaders for political change.

What will you do? How will you work with organizations? Review the continuum and determine where you are now. Where do you want to be? Decide on a plan to achieve your goal.

Are you the leader who will seek appointed or elected office to ensure that the values of nurses are heard in political debate and implemented in policy? Or do you prefer to work behind the scenes?

There are more experienced colleagues who will help. Do not limit your activity to nursing organizations. The contributions that APNs make to the broader community help not only the community but also the public perception of nurses. This chapter focuses on professional organizational development, but the principles can be used in any setting.

REFERENCES

Chalich, T., & Smith, L. (1992). Nursing at the grassroots. *Nursing & Health Care 13*(5), 242–244.

Cohen, S. S., Mason, D. J., Kovner, C., et al. (1996). Stages of nursing's political development: where we've been and where we ought to go. *Nursing Outlook 44*(6), 259–266.

DeVries, C., & Vanderbilt, M. (1992). *The grassroots lobbying handbook*. Washington, DC: American Nurses Association.

Harrington, C., & Estes, C. (1997). *Health policy and nursing*. Sudbury, MA: Jones and Bartlett Publishers.

HCFA, DHHS. (April, 1998) Program Memorandum Transmittal No. AB-98-15 Change Request #202. http://www. hcfa.gov/pubforms/transmit/AB981560.html.

Mason, D. J., Cohen, S. S., O'Donnell, J. P., et al. (1997). Managed care organizations' arrangements with nurse practitioners. *Nursing Economics 15*(6), 306–314.

Mason, D. J., & Talbott, S. W. (Eds.). (1985). *Political action handbook for nurses*. Menlo Park, CA: Addison-Wesley Publishing Co.

Minarik, P. A. (1998). Medicare and Medicaid Reimbursement: New Law and New Legislation. *Clinical Nurse Specialist 12*(2), 83–84.

Sabato, L., & Simpson, G. (1996). *Dirty little secrets*. New York, NY: Times Books.

Sullivan, T. (1998). *Collaboration: A health care imperative*. New York, NY: McGraw-Hill.

Thomas, P., & Shelton, C. (1994). Teaching students to become active in public policy. *Public Health Nursing 11*(2), 75–79.

Weissert, C., & Weissert, W. (1996). *Governing health*. Baltimore, MD: The Johns Hopkins University Press.

What is ANA-PAC? Information sheet. Washington, DC: American Nurses Association Political Action Committee.

CHAPTER 15

The Research Basis for Practice:
The Foundation of
Evidence-based Practice

Vicki L. Kraus

Descriptions of advanced practice nursing have traditionally included research as a professional-role activity. The dilemma for the advanced practice nurse (APN) has been how to incorporate research activities into what have become increasingly complex and intense practice responsibilities. In recent years, the research-role component for APNs has been more commonly described as one consisting of the transfer of research into practice, that is, research utilization. The conduct of research is done collaboratively as a member of a team composed of other nurses and professionals from other disciplines. APNs with advanced research knowledge and skills may conduct research independently or serve as the principle investigator for an independent or collaborative research project.

This chapter discusses the role of the APN in the conduct and utilization of research. Models for research utilization are presented as a foundation for the promotion of evidence-based practice. Collaborative research examples are described to demonstrate opportunities for APN participation in the conduct of research.

Research Role of the APN

SCOPE AND STANDARDS OF ADVANCED PRACTICE NURSING

The scope and standards of advanced practice registered nursing, developed by the American Nurses Association (ANA) (1996), describe the research responsibilities of APNs. The integration of research and practice is evident in the standards of care, and research is identified as a professional-role activity in the standards of professional performance. The standard of professional performance for research focuses on the utilization of research "to discover, examine, and evaluate knowledge, theories, and creative approaches to health care practice" (ANA, 1996, p. 19). Indicators of competent research practice are described as including the critical evaluation of existing practice using current research findings; the identification of research questions in practice; and the dissemination of research findings through practice, education, or consultation. Research utilization has been integrated into other standards of professional performance, including use of research findings in the evaluation of the quality and effectiveness of care and in developing and maintaining current knowledge and skills in specialty practice areas. The conduct of research has been included as an interdisciplinary activity of the APN (ANA, 1996).

RESEARCH UTILIZATION AND THE APN

Cronenwett (1986) and Hickey (1990) affirmed the research utilization role of APNs. Being a clinical expert makes it appropriate for the APN to have a major role in the research utilization process, including identifying clinical problems and developing and implementing research-based protocols to alleviate problems or minimize their effects. In addition, the APN participates in establishing standards and maintaining or improving the quality of care for a patient population. These accountabilities depend on and are enhanced by using research findings to validate or change practice (Hickey, 1990). Cronenwett (1986) recommended that the APN work with nursing administration to set appropriate and attainable expectations for research-related activities. Expectations should be based on an assessment of the organization's readiness and commitment and the competence and commitment of the APN to the conduct of nursing research (Cronenwett, 1986). Assessment of these same topics related to the utilization of research would be essential for specifying expectations for APN research-role performance.

RESEARCH COMPETENCIES OF ADVANCED PRACTICE NURSES

McGuire and Harwood (1996) described three areas of research competence: interpreting and using research, evaluating practice, and conducting research. They propose that these competencies will be "exceedingly important in defining, implementing, refining, validating, and evaluating advanced nursing practice" (McGuire & Harwood, 1996, p. 189). These authors emphasize that these competencies are not levels of expectation or performance and differentiate between a basic and an advanced level of performance for each competency. Basic-level activities for interpreting and using research means incorporating relevant research findings appropriately into the APN's own practice and assisting others to incorporate research into individual or unit practice. An advanced-level activity for this competency means developing a departmental research-utilization process. Basic-level activities for evaluating practice are using existing data to evaluate nursing practice for individual patients or a patient population and collaborating in the conduct of evaluation studies. An advanced-level activity for this competency means identifying or developing a practice-specific package of outcome criteria. A basic-level activity for conducting research means participating in collaborative research. An advanced-level activity for this competency means conducting independent research. The APN would be expected to perform basic activities in all three competencies on completion of graduate school. The advanced level of activity for each competency would be developed later through academic study, mentoring, and self-study (McGuire & Harwood, 1996).

Three levels of research utilization competencies are included in the Stetler–Grady model: beginner, competent, and proficient. The proficient user of research is likely to be the APN because the knowledge and skills required include in-depth knowledge of a specialty area, knowledge of theories of planned change, and advanced-level course work on the conduct and utilization of research as well as statistics (as cited in McGuire & Harwood, 1996). Stetler (1997) described five domains of behavior in the Stetler–Grady model: (1) inquiry (focused reviews of practice- and research-based literature), (2) exploration (critique of the literature), (3) application (translation of research findings into usable form), (4) evaluation (use of research as a process and assessment of the effectiveness of targeted use of research findings), and (5) diffusion (dissemination of findings and extension of validated use of research findings). For each of these domains, the knowledge, skills, and behaviors are defined for each level of user (Stetler, 1997).

A descriptive study of current research utilization behavior among clinical nurse specialists was conducted by Stetler and DiMaggio (1991). The question asked in this research was what is the extent and nature of utilization of research-based information by clinical nurse specialists in terms of level and related frequency of use, types of use, sources of information, and criteria for utilization. A descriptive field survey design was used for the research. Twenty-four CNSs completed a semistructured interview designed to measure the level and nature of self-reported utilization behavior relative to specific cases. Seventy-five percent of the sample reported that they used research to improve their understanding or influence their way of thinking on a clinical issue. Twenty-one percent reported that they usually applied specific parts of studies directly to their practice, usually after making some modification so as to adapt the findings to the clinical situation. One CNS reported not routinely considering research-based information in her practice. The types of research use included application in direct patient care situations via either consultation or direct involvement, development or revision of a program or exploration of new activities for a generic problem or a patient population, and development or provision of a rationale for departmental documents, for example, policies. The CNSs used a variety of research-based and non–research-based information for application in practice. Slightly more than half of these CNSs (58%) said they used a set of criteria for determining applicability of research findings to practice. These criteria included those related to the soundness of the research, assessing the applicability of research results to practice, and the presence of substantiating evidence, that is, replicated research (Stetler & DiMaggio, 1991). These findings pointed to an opportunity for improvement of research utilization competencies of clinical nurse specialists.

In an effort to enhance research utilization by clinical nurse specialists, Stetler, Bautista, Vernale-Hannon, and Foster (1995) established and evaluated research utilization forums in two settings. These forums were designed to accomplish the following objectives: (1) to enhance research utilization knowledge and skills and (2) to explore strategies for systematic integration of the research utilization into the role of the clinical nurse specialist. The primary emphasis of the forum was the use of the practitioner-oriented Stetler–Marram Model for Application of Research Findings (Stetler & Marram, 1976). The forums were effective in accomplishing the objectives and had a positive impact on the self-perceived research utilization competencies of the participants. The forums also resulted in a refinement and expansion of the Stetler–Marram model (Stetler, Bautista, Vernale-Hannon, & Foster, 1995), which is described later in this chapter.

Research Utilization

The conduct and utilization of research are interdependent processes (Horsley, Crane, Crabtree, & Wood, 1983). Research utilization is the transfer of specific research-based knowledge into clinical practice, whereas the conduct of research is the production of knowledge that is generalizable beyond the population directly studied (Haller, Reynolds, & Horsley, 1979). Research utilization is problem-focused and institution-focused, and the conduct of research is knowledge-focused and theory-focused (Stetler, 1992). Research utilization uses research processes to transfer research products into clinical practice (Stetler, 1985). Ultimately, both the conduct of research and research utilization are directed toward improvement in the quality and effectiveness of the care provided to patients and families.

The nature of research utilization in clinical practice varies (Stetler, 1994; Stetler & Marram, 1976; Tanner, 1987). Stetler (1994) describes three levels of utilization of research findings: instrumental, conceptual, and symbolic. *Instrumental* research utilization is the concrete or direct application of research-based knowledge and may take the form of assessment criteria, an intervention, or institutional standards. *Conceptual* research utilization means changing the level of understanding or the way a nurse thinks about a situation. This is a less specific way of using research in practice but over time leads to gradually accumulating more in-depth knowledge of a topic. *Symbolic* or political research utilization is using information derived from research to legitimize a policy or a currently held position (Stetler, 1994). Tanner (1987) described a continuum of research-based knowledge utilization, with conceptual use of knowledge on one end and instrumental use on the other end. Conceptual use of research-based knowledge results in improved understanding of clinical problems or of the dynamics of an intervention and exerts an influence on thinking. Instrumental use of research-based knowledge results in actually changing practice, that is, use in clinical decision making for a specific patient (Tanner, 1987).

The scope of research utilization activities varies widely. Research utilization can occur at the individual or the organizational level (Cronenwett, 1987). The individual nurse can apply research findings in the care of a specific patient, or an organization can make a research-based practice change that will affect the care of multiple patients (Cronenwett, 1987; Tanner, 1987). Research utilization models reflect this variable scope and describe the complex set of activities that are required to transfer research-based knowledge into clinical practice.

MODELS FOR THE UTILIZATION OF RESEARCH

Models of research utilization in nursing provide APNs with frameworks for the integration of research and practice. Three of these models are described: (1) the model from the Conduct and Utilization of Research in Nursing (CURN) Project (Haller, Reynolds, & Horsley, 1979; Horsley, Crane, & Bingle, 1978; Horsley, Crane, Crabtree, & Wood, 1983), (2) the Stetler Model of Research Utilization (Stetler, 1983, 1985, 1994; Stetler & Marram, 1976), and (3) the Iowa Model for Research in Practice (Titler et al., 1994).

The Conduct and Utilization of Research: A Nursing Model

The CURN Project was designed to develop and test a model for using research-based knowledge in clinical practice settings. In the CURN model, research utilization is viewed as an organizational instead of an individual process, that is, making research-based practice changes is the responsibility of the department of nursing and not of individual nurses. Planned change processes are integrated throughout the research utilization process and are considered essential to establishing research-based practice (Horsley, Crane, Crabtree, & Wood, 1983).

Research utilization is described as a systematic series of activities, including (1) identification and synthesis of multiple research studies in a common conceptual area (research base), (2) transformation of the knowledge derived from this research base into a solution or a clinical protocol, (3) transformation of the clinical protocol into specific nursing actions (innovations), and (4) clinical evaluation of the new practice to see if it produced the expected outcome. A protocol is a document that transforms all of the studies in the research base into a synthesized whole, translates the research language into clinical language, and addresses the realities of using the new knowledge in practice (Horsley, Crane, Crabtree, & Wood, 1983).

The research utilization process consists of the following seven steps: (1) systematically identifying patient care problems; (2) identifying and assessing research-based knowledge to solve the identified patient care problems; (3) using the research base to design a nursing practice innovation; (4) conducting a clinical trial and evaluating the effectiveness of the innovation; (5) deciding whether to adopt, alter, or reject the innovation; (6) developing a means to diffuse the practice innovation to beyond the trial unit; and (7) developing mechanisms to maintain the innovation over time (Horsley, Crane, Crabtree, & Wood, 1983).

The evaluation of research studies is described in detail in the CURN model, and the importance of this process in preventing the misutilization of research is emphasized. A research base is defined as "a synthesis of knowledge resulting from several studies whose findings corroborate, extend, or delineate the concept(s) investigated in the studies" (Horsley, Crane, Crabtree, & Wood, 1983, p. 35). Three sets of criteria are used to evaluate research bases for clinical utilization: (1) determination of the validity or generalizability of the knowledge, (2) determination of the practice relevance of the research base, and (3) determination of whether the research base includes the measurement instruments that can be used to evaluate the practice change. Criteria for determining validity and generalizability included replication, scientific merit, and potential risks to patients. Criteria for determining practice relevance included clinical merit, clinical control, feasibility, and cost-benefit. Criteria for determining whether the research base includes the necessary measurement instruments included availability, clinical control, and scientific merit (Horsley, Crane, Crabtree, & Wood, 1983).

Stetler Model of Research Utilization

The Stetler Model of Research Utilization (Stetler, 1994) is a refinement and expansion of the Stetler–Marram Model for Application of Research Findings (Stetler, 1976; Stetler & Marram, 1976). The primary focus of the model is the application of research findings at the individual practitioner level. The model has six phases: (1) preparation, (2) validation, (3) comparative evaluation, (4) decision making, (5) translation and application, and (6) evaluation (see Fig. 15-1). Critical thinking and decision making at the practitioner level is emphasized during each phase (Stetler, 1994). An excellent guide to help proceed through the phases of the Stetler model and facilitate education about research utilization is available (Stetler, Bautista, Vernale-Hannon, & Foster, 1995).

The preparation phase consists of specifying the purpose and context of the research review. The research review may be initiated for a variety of reasons, including the need to solve a clinical or managerial problem, to update knowledge, to validate or revise a practice standard, or to prepare an educational program. Specifying the purpose or focus of the research review enables the identification of measurable outcomes (Stetler, 1994).

The validation phase includes conducting a utilization research critique. The end points of this critique are to accept or reject. Once a study is accepted, that is, has scientific merit and is usable for current needs, a statement that summarizes applicable findings is developed. This statement should reflect how likely the findings of the study are applicable in the current situation and how relationships or variables could be used in daily practice. The variables are defined in operational terms and related to relevant details of practice (Stetler, 1994).

Comparative evaluation involves the use of four criteria to determine whether it is desirable or feasible to apply the validated research findings in practice. The fit of the setting criterion examines the similarity of the study sample and environment to the patient population and the clinical setting. The feasibility criterion considers the 3 Rs: risks, resources, and readiness. The current practice criterion looks at whether the knowledge from the research does or can provide a relevant basis for practice and whether the level of effectiveness of current practice calls for a change. The substantiating evidence criterion incorporates both research- and non–research-based knowledge in the comparative evaluation. Multiple research studies with congruent findings provide the strongest evidence for application of research in practice, and other sources are used to supplement the research base, including expert opinion and standards and guidelines from professional organizations (Stetler, 1994).

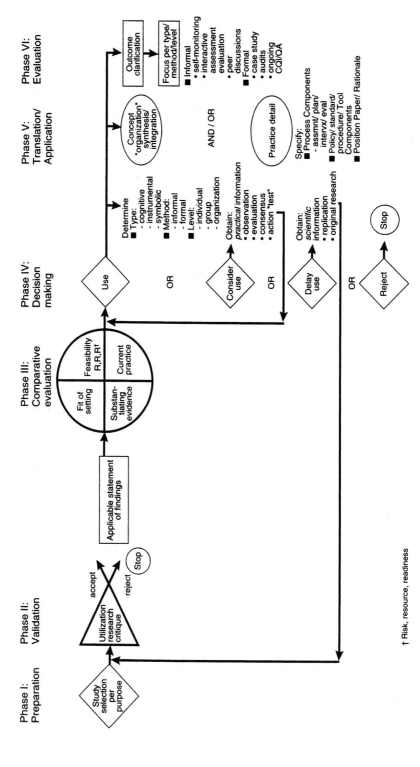

FIGURE 15-1 The Stetler Model for Research Utilization. From: Stetler, C.B. (1994). Refinement of the Stetler–Marram model for application of research findings to practice. *Nursing Outlook 42*(1), 15–25.

Decision making consists of making a decision based on the integration of the original purpose of the review and the results of the comparative evaluation. The four potential decisions are (1) to use, (2) to consider use, (3) to delay use, or (4) to reject or not use. When the decision made is to use the research knowledge, the type, method, and level of use is determined. The type of use may be instrumental, cognitive, or symbolic, and the method may be formal or informal. The level of use may be the individual, a group, or the organization. If the research findings look like they are applicable but uncertainty still exists about use, additional practical information should be sought, including conducting trials with individual patients and accumulating information about effectiveness, consulting with experts, or getting a consensus of opinion from key stakeholders. If too little research exists, the results are conflicting, or too much risk is involved if applied in clinical practice at this time, use of the research would be delayed contingent on research replication with congruent results. Finally, a decision to reject or not use the research is made if too many risks or costs were involved, if consistent and strong findings were lacking, or if current practice was strong (Stetler, 1994).

The translation and application phase consists of taking the findings and other relevant information from the research and transforming it into action terms. The first step of this phase is the conceptualization of the common threads or factors that are evident across all of the research. There is an "integration or synthesis of interrelated findings and relationships into a generalization" (Stetler, 1994, p. 23). The next part of this phase involves the identification of the way the research will be used in practice. The research-based generalization may affect an entire department, a group of patients, or an individual practitioner's practice. The use of the research-based generalization may be instrumental, cognitive, or symbolic. It may provide ideas or suggestions for a specific aspect of practice, management, or education. It may be used to focus assessments, enhance care planning, provide components of an algorithm for decision making, or provide direction for the selection of interventions. It may be used to provide a background for future decisions or a rationale for a position taken on a practice issue (Stetler, 1994).

The evaluation phase consists of clarification of expected outcomes and differentiation of formal and informal application. The outcomes are derived from the purpose defined in the preparation phase, and define the evaluation process. How the evaluation is conducted depends on whether the application was informal or formal. Evaluation of the informal application of research findings by an individual nurse may include routine monitoring of practice or discussions with peers. Evaluation of the formal application of research findings on a unit may include case study analyses and ongoing quality improvement activities (Stetler, 1994).

Iowa Model of Research in Practice

The Iowa Model of Research in Practice is a heuristic model used for infusing research into practice to improve the quality of care (Titler et al., 1994). It is an outgrowth of the Quality Assurance Model Using Research (QAMUR) (Watson, Bulechek, & McCloskey, 1987). In this model, research utilization is an organizational process, and planned change principles are used to integrate research and practice (see Fig. 15-2). The model is currently being revised to incorporate concepts related to evidence-based healthcare provided by a multidisciplinary team (Kleiber & Titler, 1998).

The Iowa Model of Research in Practice identifies knowledge- or problem-focused triggers as the forces that provide the impetus for research-based practice changes. Problem-focused triggers include risk management and quality improvement data, total quality management programs, and identification of a clinical problem. Knowledge-focused triggers are activated by new information, including standards and practice guidelines from national agencies or organizations, philosophies of care, recent research publications or meta-analyses, or expert opinions. Once a problem- or knowledge-focused trigger is identified,

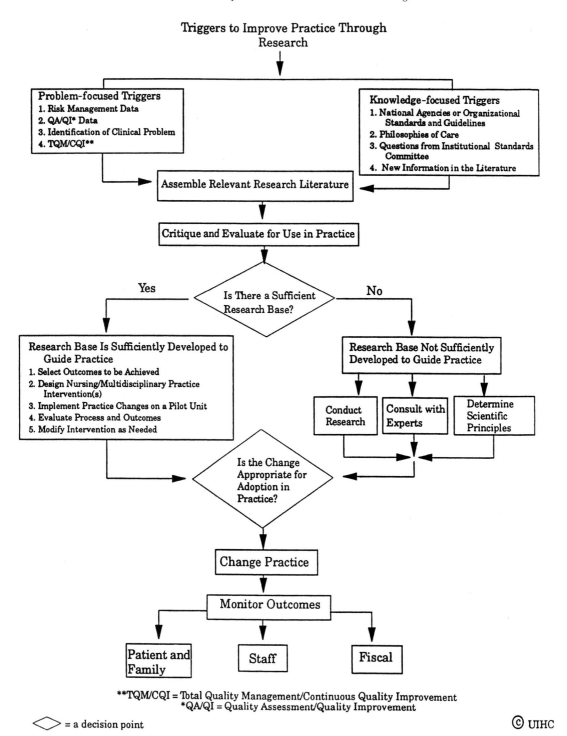

FIGURE 15-2 The Iowa Model: Research-based Practice to Promote Quality Care.
Adapted from: Titler, M.G., Kleiber C., Steelman, V., et al. (1994). Infusing research into practice to promote quality care. *Nursing Research 43*(5), 307–313.

relevant research and related literature is assembled, critiqued, and evaluated for applicability to the practice setting (Titler et al., 1994).

The first decision point in the model is whether a sufficient and appropriate research base exists to change practice. If the answer is yes, the steps needed to transfer the research findings into practice are implemented: (1) clarify the expected outcomes and document the baseline or current status of these outcomes, (2) design nursing and multidisciplinary practice innovations, (3) implement the research-based practice changes on a pilot unit, (4) evaluate practice change from a process and outcome perspective, and (5) modify practice intervention and implementation methods as needed for implementation on other units. If the answer is no, that is, the research base is not sufficiently developed to guide practice, the conduct of research is indicated. Practice changes must then be based on other types of knowledge i.e., expert opinion or scientific principles. The model recommends consultation with experts currently investigating the problem and application of scientific principles (Titler et al., 1994).

The second and final decision point in the model is whether the change is appropriate for adoption in practice throughout the organization. This decision is based on the consideration of many factors: costs and cost savings, impact on quality of care, risks to the patient, competency of staff to carry out research-based practice, and administrative support. If the decision is to adopt the practice change, the process of planned change is used to implement the research-based practice innovation, and continuous monitoring of process and outcome data takes place. This continuous monitoring facilitates providing feedback to staff and promotes the maintenance of the practice change (Titler et al., 1994).

EVALUATION OF RESEARCH-BASED PRACTICE

Evaluation is identified as a component of each of the research utilization models (Horsley, Crane, Crabtree, & Wood, 1983; Stetler, 1994; Titler et al., 1994). The purpose of evaluation is to determine the effectiveness of the research-based practice change in the natural clinical setting. This evaluation has two components: (1) the determination of whether the intervention was implemented as intended and identification of barriers that prevented its implementation and (2) the determination of whether the intervention resulted in the expected outcomes. Process and outcome data are collected and analyzed and used to decide whether to accept, reject, or modify the research-based intervention (Goode, 1995).

Goode (1995) outlined the steps for the evaluation of a research-based practice change: (1) specify the variables to be measured (process and outcome); (2) determine data collection methods, design data collection forms or questionnaires, and establish content validity; (3) determine frequency and method of data collection, identify and train data collectors, and establish interrater reliability; (4) determine sample size needed for data collection before and after implementation; (5) provide encouragement and support during the evaluation process; and (6) report the results of the evaluation and decide whether to accept, reject, or modify the intervention (Goode, 1995).

The evaluation of a research-based practice change is described in detail in the CURN model (Haller, Reynolds, & Horsley, 1979; Horsley, Crane, Crabtree, & Wood, 1983) and is expanded by Goode (1995). The evaluation of patient outcomes is done before and after implementation of the research-based practice change. The dependent variables from the research base are measured as outcomes. Other outcome variables of importance in the evaluation of the effectiveness of a practice change are usually added, for example, patient satisfaction and cost. The evaluation of the process component is done during the implementation of the research-based practice change. The independent variables from the research base determine the process indicators that will be used to determine whether the practice change has been implemented accurately and consistently and to identify the barriers, if any, that stood in the way of the implementation (Goode, 1995; Haller, Reynolds,

& Horsley, 1979; Horsely, Crane, Crabtree, & Wood, 1983). Measurement of process and outcomes is repeated until we are assured that the intervention is being carried out as intended and is effective in producing the expected outcomes. This monitoring is included in the continuous quality improvement or quality management activities of the organization and is used to provide feedback to appropriate groups (administration and staff) about the cost-effectiveness of the practice change (Goode, 1995; Horsely, Crane, Crabtree, & Wood, 1983; Stetler, 1994; Titler et al., 1994).

Evidence-based Practice

The culture of healthcare is shifting to decision making on the basis of evidence. No longer is it acceptable to base decisions on opinion, past practice, and precedent. Instead, in an effort to improve effectiveness and reduce costs, science, research, and the best available evidence is being used to guide clinical decision making (Kleiber & Titler, 1998). Research utilization is the transfer of research findings into practice. Evidence-based practice promotion goes beyond research utilization and uses other sources of evidence as a basis for decision making in healthcare. Research utilization is, however, the foundation of evidence-based practice.

Definitions of evidence-based practice come from medicine. Sackett et al. (1996) defined evidence-based medicine as the "conscientious, explicit and judicious use of current best evidence in making decisions about the care of individual patients" (p. 71). The best available evidence is used to answer a specific clinical question (DiCenso, Cullum, & Ciliska, 1998). Evidence that may be used in clinical decision making is comprised of research, clinical expertise, patient preferences, and other available sources of economic and scientific evidence (DiCenso, Cullum, & Ciliska, 1998; Mulhall, 1998; Sackett, 1997; Sackett et al., 1996). Research utilization models are being expanded to include nonresearch sources of evidence to validate or change current practice (Goode & Piedalue, 1999; Kleiber & Titler, 1998; Stetler et al., 1998). Research results include research syntheses: integrated research reviews and meta-analyses (Goode, 1995; Stetler et al., 1998) as well as the results of individual studies (Stetler et al., 1998). Methods for evaluating the strength of the evidence are available (Guyatt et al., 1995; Stetler et al., 1998). Nonresearch sources of evidence include performance data, for example, benchmarking data, risk management data, quality improvement data, report cards, peer review reports, program evaluations, focus group and questionnaire results, consensus recommendations of local and national experts (Goode, 1995; Stetler et al., 1998), clinical expertise, pathophysiologic data, and cost-effectiveness analyses (Goode & Piedalue, 1999). Stetler and colleagues (1998) also include affirmed experience as a source of evidence. This is the sharing of accumulated experiences "for purposes of reflection, verification, evaluation, and growth" (Stetler et al., 1998, p. 48). Although research utilization remains the foundation for evidence-based practice, other sources are given deliberate consideration in the clinical decision-making process.

Conduct of Research

The clinical expertise of the APN creates opportunities for participation in collaborative research. Often this collaboration takes the form of research team membership. APN research team membership has benefits for the team as well as for the APN. The APN serves as an essential clinical resource for the research team and contributes to every step of the research process: identifying and defining the research problem, reviewing the literature, developing a conceptual framework, selecting a design and developing the methodology, collecting and analyzing the data, and interpreting and communicating the results. As a member of a research team, the APN gains valuable research knowledge and skills by participating with nurses and other professionals with research expertise. Ultimately, this mentorship, along with advanced course work in research and statistics, prepares the APN for a more independent role in the conduct of research.

APNs at the University of Iowa Hospitals and Clinics, Iowa City, IA, have had the opportunity to participate as members of research teams in the College of Nursing at the University of Iowa, Iowa City, Iowa. Two of these teams will be used as examples: Nursing Interventions Classification (NIC) and Nursing Outcomes Classification (NOC). This APN has participated on both of these teams as a research assistant (NIC), a doctoral student member (NIC and NOC), a clinician member (NIC and NOC), and a focus group member (NOC).

In 1987, Drs. Joanne McCloskey and Gloria Bulechek formed a research team at the University of Iowa to define and categorize nursing interventions. The work of this team is ongoing. The research team has received internal funding from the University of Iowa, Iowa City, Iowa, as well as two grants from the National Institute of Nursing Research, National Institutes of Health, Bethesda, MD. The first 3-year grant (1990–1993) was for the development of the nursing interventions classification and the construction of the taxonomy. A 4-year continuation grant (1993–1997) was awarded to refine, validate, and code the taxonomy and to field-test implementation of the standardized language. Members of the NIC team represent a wide range of research, education, administration, informatics, and clinical knowledge and experience. Many APNs, representing a variety of specialties, have participated actively on the NIC team since its beginning and have contributed to completion of its work, which has included developing and refining the initial list of interventions; developing intervention labels, definitions, and defining activities based on literature review and clinical experience; conducting expert surveys and interpreting the results; participating in focus group work to develop, review, and revise interventions; classifying the interventions and developing the structure for the taxonomy; identifying linkages between nursing diagnoses and interventions; and facilitating implementation of NIC language in clinical practice. The results of this work have been disseminated in two books and numerous presentations and journal articles. To date, 433 interventions, a taxonomy, and linkages between nursing diagnoses and interventions have been published (McCloskey & Bulechek, 1992, 1996). A third edition of the Nursing Interventions Classification is in press and will include 486 interventions (McCloskey & Bulechek, in press).

The NOC research team was formed by Marion Johnson and Meridean Maas in 1991 to conceptualize, label, and classify nursing-sensitive patient outcomes. The work of this team is also ongoing. Grants from Sigma Theta Tau International, Indianapolis, IN, and the Office of Nursing Research, University of Iowa, Iowa City, IA, funded pilot work and the beginning development of the NOC. The research team has received two grants from the National Institute of Nursing Research, National Institutes of Health. The first 4-year grant (1993–1997) was awarded to develop the classification, construct the taxonomy, and field-test the outcomes (Johnson & Maas, 1997). A second 4-year grant has recently been awarded to evaluate the sensitivity, reliability, and construct validity of the outcome measures and for continued development of individual patient outcome measures as well as family-level outcome measures and for initial development of risk factors for selected outcomes (Johnson & Maas, 1997). Membership on the NOC team is also diverse. The investigators have all of the areas of expertise represented on the NIC team as well as the benefit of the experience to date at the College of Nursing in developing standardized language. The more than 20 master's-prepared APNs from hospitals, nursing, and community health agencies are assisting with the development and refinement of the outcomes and indicators through focus group participation. Each of eight focus groups was assigned a category of outcomes that had been extracted from literature review and clinical information systems: social and role status; physical functional status; safety; perceived well-being; physiologic status; psychological and cognitive status; health attitudes, knowledge, and behavior; and family caregiver status. Each focus group took all of its assigned outcomes and used a modified concept analysis to refine the outcome labels and develop the definition and indicators for the label. APNs were recruited as working members of every focus group to ensure input of expert clinicians. Focus group responsibilities included the following: (1) reviewing literature and measurement tools related to the outcome category; (2) reviewing the outcome labels in the category and collapsing similar labels or adding new labels as needed; (3) developing a label, proposing a definition, and creating a list of indicators for each outcome; and, (4) presenting the outcome label, definition, and indicators to the principal investigators and the entire research team for approval. This focus group work resulted in the development of 190 nursing-sensitive patient outcomes (Johnson & Maas, 1997). The results of this work have been disseminated in a book (Johnson & Maas, 1997) and numerous presentations and journal articles. A second edition of the Nursing Outcomes Classification is in press and will include 260 nursing-sensitive patient outcomes (Johnson, Maas, & Moorhead, in press).

An interdisciplinary research team at the University of Iowa Hospitals and Clinics has been awarded internal funding to conduct a pilot study of an intervention to improve the effectiveness of symptom management in persons with chronic disease. Initial work on the research proposal was done by the Nursing Research Committee, which is composed of the Director of Research, Quality, and Outcomes Management, a PhD-prepared nurse scientist; a College of Nursing faculty member, a PhD-prepared academician and researcher; and six APNs, two who are PhD-prepared and four who are in various stages of PhD preparation. This committee has identified building a program of research on symptom management as a means of aligning the Department of Nursing's conduct of research with the strategic plan of the organization: improving patient care while also reducing costs and assuming a leadership role in providing preventive health services and initiating health enhancement activities. Ultimately, an intervention to enhance the effectiveness of symptom management will maximize the health of persons with chronic disease. The pilot study results will be used to write a grant proposal for multiple patient populations. In this example, APNs are afforded the opportunity to collaborate with nurse scientists, other APNs, and other disciplines to enhance the quality of care for selected patient populations.

Summary

The research role of the APN includes research utilization and the conduct of research. The APN participates in or provides leadership for research utilization at the organizational level. Clinical expertise, along with research competencies and leadership skills, positions the APN for an essential role in the organizational change process inherent in this level of research utilization. The APN also continuously integrates research into clinical practice on an individual level while both providing direct patient care and educating and consulting with staff members. The conduct of research is done collaboratively as a member of a research team as well as independently as a principal investigator for independent or collaborative research.

REFERENCES

American Nurses Association. (1996). *Scope and standards of advanced practice registered nursing*. Washington, DC: Author.

Cronenwett, L.R. (1986). The research role of the clinical nurse specialist. *Journal of Nursing Administration 16*(4), 10–11.

Cronenwett, L. R. (1987). Research utilization in the practice setting. *Journal of Nursing Administration 17*(7,8), 9–10.

DiCenso, A., Cullum, N., & Ciliska, D. (1998). Implementing evidence-based nursing: Some misconceptions. *Evidence-Based Nursing 1*(2), 38–40.

Goode, C. J. (1995). Evaluation of research-based nursing practice. *Nursing Clinics of North America 30*(3), 421–428.

Goode, C. J., & Piedalue, F. (1999). Evidence-based clinical practice. *Journal of Nursing Administration 29*(6), 1–7.

Guyatt, G. H., Sackett, D. L., Sinclair, J. C., Hayward, R., Cook, D. J., & Cook, R. J. (1995). Users' guides to the medical literature: IX. A method for grading health care recommendations. *Journal of the American Medical Association 274*(22), 1800–1804.

Haller, K. B., Reynolds, M. A., & Horsley, J. A. (1979). Developing research-based innovation protocols: Process, criteria and issues. *Research in Nursing and Health 2*, 45–51.

Hickey, M. (1990). The role of the clinical nurse specialist in the research utilization process. *Clinical Nurse Specialist 4*(2), 93–96.

Horsley, J. A., Crane, J., & Bingle, J. D. (1978). Research utilization as an organizational process. *Journal of Nursing Administration, July,* 4–6.

Horsley, J. A., Crane, J., Crabtree, M. K., & Wood, D. J. (1983). *Using research to improve practice.* Orlando, FL: Grune & Stratton.

Johnson, M., & Maas, M. (Eds.) (1997). *Nursing outcomes classification (NOC).* St. Louis, MO: Mosby-Year Book.

Johnson, M., Maas, M., & Moorhead, S. (Eds.) (in press). *Nursing Outcomes Classification (NOC)* (2nd ed.). St. Louis, MO: Mosby-Year Book.

Kleiber, C., & Titler, M. G. (1998). Evidence based practice and the revised Iowa Model. *Fifth national research utilization conference* (April 23–24). Iowa City, IA: University of Iowa Hospitals and Clinics.

McCloskey, J. C., & Bulechek, G. M. (Eds.). (1992). *Nursing interventions classification (NIC).* St. Louis, MO: Mosby-Year Book.

McCloskey, J. C., & Bulechek, G. M. (Eds.). (1996). *Nursing interventions classification (NIC)* (2nd ed.). St. Louis, MO: Mosby-Year Book.

McCloskey, J. C., & Bulechek, G. M. (Eds.). (in press). *Nursing interventions classification (NIC)* (3rd ed.) St. Louis, MO: Mosby-Year Book.

McGuire, D. B., & Harwood, K. V. (1996). Research interpretation, utilization, and conduct. In A. B. Hamric, J. A. Spross, & C. M. Hanson (Eds.). *Advanced nursing practice. An integrative approach* (pp. 184–211). Philadelphia: W. B. Saunders.

Mulhall, A. (1998). Nursing, research, and the evidence. *Evidence-Based Nursing 1*(1), 4–6.

Sackett, D. L. (1997). Evidence-based medicine. *Seminars in Perinatology 21*(1), 3–5.

Sackett, D. L., Rosenberg, W. M. C, Gray, J. A. M., Haynes, R. B., & Richardson, W. S. (1996). Evidence-based medicine: What it is and what it isn't. *British Medical Journal 312,* 71–72.

Stetler, C. (1997). Evidence-based nursing practice, research utilization, and related competencies. *Fourth national research utilization conference,* (April 27). Iowa City, IA: University of Iowa Hospitals and Clinics.

Stetler, C. B. (1983): Nurses and research responsibility and involvement. *National Intravenous Therapy Association, Inc. 6* (May/June), 207–212.

Stetler, C. B. (1985). Research utilization: Defining the concept. *Image: The Journal of Nursing Scholarship XVII*(2), 40–44.

Stetler, C. B. (1992). Nursing research and quality care. In M. Johnson (Ed.). *The delivery of quality health care: Series on nursing administration, volume 3* (pp. 191–207). St. Louis, MO: Mosby-Year Book.

Stetler, C. B. (1994). Refinement of the Stetler/Marram model for application of research findings to practice. *Nursing Outlook, January/February,* 15–25.

Stetler, C. B., Bautista, C., Vernale-Hannon, C., & Foster, J. (1995). Enhancing research utilization by clinical nurse specialists. *Nursing Clinics of North America 30*(3), 457–468.

Stetler, C. B., Brunell, M., Giuliano, K. K., Morsi, D., Prince, L., & Newell-Stokes, V. (1998). Evidence-based practice and the role of nursing leadership. *Journal of Nursing Administration 28*(7/8), 45–53.

Stetler, C. B., & DiMaggio, G. (1991). Research utilization among clinical nurse specialists. *Clinical Nurse Specialist 5*(3), 151–155.

Stetler, C. B., & Marram, G. (1976). Evaluating research findings for applicability in practice. *Nursing Outlook 24*(9), 559–563.

Tanner, C. A. (1987). Evaluating research for use in practice: Guidelines for the clinician. *Heart and Lung 16*(4), 424–430.

Titler, M. G., Kleiber, C., Steelman, V., Goode, C., Rakel, B., Barry-Walker, J., Small, S., & Buckwalter, K. (1994). Infusing research into practice to promote quality care. *Nursing Research 43*(5), 307–313.

Watson, C. A., Bulechek, G. M., & McCloskey, J. C. (1987). QAMUR: A quality assurance model using nursing research. *Journal of Nursing Quality Assurance 2*(1), 21–27.

CHAPTER 16

Economics and Healthcare Financing

Peter I. Buerhaus

Beginning in the late 1980s and accelerating throughout the 1990s, government cost-containment initiatives and private sector pressures stimulated the development of price competition among healthcare providers in many parts of the country. Before this period, the health insurance and delivery systems were dominated by fee-for-service plans and providers who did not compete on the price of their premiums and services. Consequently, providers faced few incentives to act in a financially accountable manner or to minimize the costs of producing their services. In the 1990s, however, a variety of managed care plans developed; not only did they begin to charge deductibles and copayments and limit the use of high-cost procedures by plan members, but they also stimulated a powerful surge in price competition. For employers, the development of competition among managed care plans allowed them to search aggressively for lower premiums and richer benefit packages to offer employees. The resultant effect on healthcare spending was profound: From 1993 through 1997, the rate of increase in national healthcare spending decelerated each year, and total spending on healthcare stabilized at approximately 13.5% of the gross domestic product. This was the longest period in which the health sector grew no faster than the rest of the country during the past three decades (Levit, 1998).

Thus far, the ability of market competition to slow the rate of increase in healthcare spending has dampened the interest of Congress to develop legislation creating a national health system or to implement much else in the way of health reform. This is not to suggest that Congress has or will ignore healthcare in the future; instead, the recent containment of steep yearly increases on healthcare spending has enabled legislators to focus on addressing the financial problems facing the Medicare program, which accounts for nearly 12% of each year's federal budget. In 1997, Congress passed the Balanced Budget Act (BBA) (P.L. 10533), which contains the most sweeping set of changes in the Medicare program since 1983, when Medicare implemented its prospective payment system that began paying acute care hospitals according to diagnosis-related groups (DRGs). Under the BBA, Medicare will develop a program called Medicare+Choice, which will expand the range of healthcare plans for beneficiaries and significantly change how Medicare pays both managed care and traditional plans. The BBA also directed the Department of Health and

Human Services to implement prospective payment systems for skilled nursing facilities, hospital outpatient departments, long-term care hospitals, home health agencies, and rehabilitation facilities. In addition, the BBA provides for direct Medicare payment to nurse practitioners and clinical nurse specialists (at 80% of the level paid to physicians), regardless of geographic setting. Taken together, these changes in Medicare are expected to slow the program's spending by $115 billion during the 5-year period from 1998 through 2002 (Medicare Payment Advisory Commission, 1998).

Looking ahead, advanced practice nurses (APNs) can anticipate that market competition will be the dominant force guiding the production, delivery, and consumption of healthcare services. The federal government will probably confine its role to passing legislation in the area of consumer protection, ensuring quality of care, and making subsidies available to providers to help ensure access to care for vulnerable populations. The evolution of price competition and the growth of managed care will transform the way society receives healthcare services, define new roles for providers and health professionals, reshape the attitudes of leaders of healthcare organizations, and change policymakers' notions about the delivery of healthcare in contemporary American society.

If APNs are to succeed in a competitive healthcare environment, then they must understand the forces that led to its emergence, anticipate the expected consequences of price competition, and implement strategies to take advantage of the many opportunities that it is likely to create. Thus, this chapter begins by discussing the development of economic competition in healthcare and the economic concepts and relationships underpinning price competition. Next is a discussion of the sources of costs that APNs in independent group practice need to consider when making decisions on the price to charge for their services. This is followed by an analysis showing how the pricing decisions made by APNs can positively affect their incomes and capacity to stay in business. The chapter concludes with a discussion of the likely effects of APNs' pricing decisions on physicians and consumers.

Development of Economic Competition in Healthcare

At the beginning of the 1980s, several private and public sector initiatives sprang forth and acted both independently and together to stimulate the beginning of economic competition among providers of personal healthcare. The first of these initiatives occurred as a result of American businesses facing double-digit inflation during the Carter administration, followed by a sharp economic recession during the first Reagan administration. During both of these jolts, the volume of lower-priced imported goods rose substantially, as did competition from Japan and other countries. For the first time, many American businesses became aware of and concerned about steadily rising healthcare premiums' effect on increasing the costs of labor. More employers started to fear that, if left unchecked, then rising healthcare costs could thwart the ability to price their products competitively in a marketplace that was becoming increasingly global.

To combat the rise in health insurance premiums, some companies began to form business coalitions, to collect data on health plans and providers, and to reduce costly inpatient hospital stays by beginning programs that mandated prehospital testing and screening, utilization review, requiring second opinions for surgical procedures, and pressuring insurance companies to cover the provision of less costly outpatient settings—even before Medicare implemented DRGs, these private sector actions were causing a decline in hospital occupancy rates and admissions (Feldstein, 1993).

A second precursor of competition in healthcare was the increasing realization that various federal and state regulatory programs, developed in the 1970s to constrain healthcare expenditures, had failed. Among theses were state certificate-of-need programs, voluntary and state health systems planning agencies, professional standards peer review organizations, hospital rate setting, and other initiatives that were part of numerous health systems planning laws. Because of their overall failure, many policymakers and academicians began to seriously question the reliance on a predominantly regulatory-driven approach to constrain healthcare costs. Not surprisingly, health planning legislation was significantly scaled back during the 1980s under the Reagan administrations.

A third precursor involved several state and Supreme Court rulings that decided that antitrust laws were applicable to healthcare, thereby removing real and perceived legal barriers to economic competition. A fourth precursor to the development of competition was the substantial amount of excess hospital capacity (i.e., too many unfilled beds—which regulations had failed to remove) and the rising supply of physicians. And finally, the Medicare program became a more prudent buyer of hospital care when it replaced its inflationary, cost-based reimbursement system with a prospective payment system based on DRGs. Over time, these developments fueled the growth of health maintenance organizations (HMOs) and what later became known as the managed care revolution. By the late 1980s, many healthcare providers were beginning to talk about the spread of competition in healthcare.

Emergence of Price Competition in the 1990s

Although the development of economic competition in healthcare and implications to nurses and APNs are discussed elsewhere (Buerhaus, 1992, 1994a, 1994b, 1994c), it is important to clarify the meaning of competition in an economic sense. This can best be explained by contrasting price competition with nonprice competition. Nonprice competition refers to activities such as hospitals' attempting to attract physicians to join their medical staff for the purpose of expanding the hospital's access to patients and keeping its beds occupied. To attract and compete for physicians, hospitals have paid off physician loans, provided rent-free office buildings, built new facilities, added services, and acquired the latest technology, although in many cases it was duplicative, expensive, marginally effective, and frequently underused. But these forms of nonprice competition are not what is meant by competition in the sense that economists use the term.

To an economist, economic competition is based on the price and quality of the products and services that are sold in the marketplace. By competing on the basis of price, firms (suppliers) have strong incentives to produce goods and services using the least costly combination of labor and capital (buildings and equipment). By keeping production costs low, the firm can price its products below or roughly equal to the price of similar products offered by rival firms. This allows the firm to sell more of its products and earn higher profits. However, if the firm fails to keep its production costs low, then it will be unable to price its products competitively, resulting in fewer sales and smaller profits. To stay in business, the firm must adjust its production processes to lower costs or switch to producing a different product. Because firms in competitive industries face the prospect of going out of business if they fail to minimize their costs, economists argue that this helps ensure that society's resources are, for the most part, used in their most productive manner: If firms use methods of production that are too costly and wasteful, then their price will be too high and the firm, unable to sell enough of its products, will go out of business and thereby free up resources that can be used more efficiently by other producers.

Because purchasers (demanders) consider the price and quality of the products and services they buy, firms must keep a sharp focus on both production costs and the quality of their products. If the product is lacking in quality in the eyes of consumers, then the firm will be unable to sell its products and services and, unless it makes changes, will ultimately go out of business. Thus, firms invest considerably in marketing activities to discover the needs of potential purchasers and their evaluation of the quality of its products. In addition, advertisement and promotional activities are aimed at pointing out the various qualitative attributes of its products, especially those that distinguish them from competitors. Successful firms combine such information with improvements and innovations in production processes so that they minimize their cost structure, keep quality high, and therefore increase their chances of remaining price competitive in an environment characterized by rapid development of cost-reducing technologies and constantly changing consumer tastes and preferences.

When thinking about these economic incentives in relation to the production and consumption of personal healthcare services, it is apparent that, up until recently, little economic competition existed among providers on the basis of price. For reasons described elsewhere (Buerhaus, 1994a), most hospitals and physicians resisted the development of price competition, large employers and labor unions knowingly and in some cases unwittingly took actions that retarded its development, and certain government regulations (demanded by those threatened by economic competition) erected barriers to competition. However, the cumulative effects of government cost containment and private sector forces that were strengthening during the 1980s, discussed earlier, were able to overcome this resistance. Moreover, in the early 1990s, the managed competition approach to reforming the healthcare system espoused by Enthoven (Enthoven, 1993; Enthoven & Kronick, 1989a, 1989b, 1991) raised the intellectual level of the debate over the virtues and drawbacks of price competition, focused policymakers' and employers' attention on the barriers to its development and how they could be removed, and offered practical strategies for business and government to deal with the potentially negative outcomes of price competition. Consequently, many members of Congress and the Clinton administration adopted elements of managed competition in formulating proposals to reform the nation's healthcare system. Following the demise of the Clinton plan for national healthcare reform, the development of market competition accelerated rapidly, leading to the transformation of the U.S. healthcare system.

Looking ahead, market competition will continue to evolve, augmented by a number of public and private sector forces, chiefly tightening Medicare and Medicaid payments; provisions under the BBA to extend prospective payment to nonhospital providers; a $5 trillion federal budget deficit requiring large annual interest payments paid for by tax dollars; steady elimination of providers' capacity to cost-shift; eradication of costly excess capacity; influence of scientifically obtained knowledge on outcomes and the quality of healthcare; and growth in the number of people enrolled in HMOs and other managed care organizations. The healthcare system is evolving in ways that should enable society to obtain greater value (more per dollar) from the resources it allocates to healthcare. This transformation means that APNs and other nurses will face new economic and clinical opportunities as well as significant challenges and threats. To be sure, APNs will have to carefully consider how they price their services if they are to compete successfully and thrive in the years ahead. The next section addresses the economic concepts that APNs should consider when contemplating their responses to increasingly cost-conscious purchasers of healthcare who are demanding greater value for their dollar.

Pricing Services Provided by Advanced Practice Nurses

In economics, the meaning of the term *price* is probably comparable in depth and breadth to what the word *health* means to nurses: Both are so vital and fundamental to their respective disciplines, yet neither term will probably ever be adequately explained. For example, at a global conceptual level, the price system enables a society's economic system to perform four basic tasks: allocate resources among competing uses; determine how to combine and process resources to produce the desired amount of goods and services; determine how various goods and services are distributed throughout society; and determine how to ensure future economic growth (Mansfield, 1982). Entire books and theoretical and applied courses examine the workings of the price system, and even Nobel Prizes have been awarded to economists for their contributions to understanding how the price system influences firms, individuals, and governments to accomplish these four tasks. However, when considering the issues involved in determining the price of APN services, it is necessary to step down the ladder of abstraction and examine several concrete factors. Even then, the issues involved are not simple or straightforward. After reviewing the determinants of the price of services produced by APNs, the pricing decisions of APNs will be examined to see how they are likely to affect their chances of surviving and growing in a price-competitive marketplace.

PRACTICE ENVIRONMENTS THAT ADVANCED PRACTICE NURSES MUST CONSIDER IN DETERMINING THE PRICE OF SERVICES

As the economic environment of healthcare becomes increasingly price competitive and hence more receptive to APNs because of their comparative cost advantage over physicians, some APNs are likely to decide to practice independently. Others may form group practice arrangements that may or may not collaborate with physicians or other health professionals. APNs in independent practice might establish contracts with large employers, HMOs, or insurance companies to provide a defined set of health services. Alternatively, other APNs may become employees of managed care firms, but because these entities receive prepaid capitated payments, the APN will not have to make pricing-related decisions. This does not mean that APNs will be exempt from certain competitive risks—quite the opposite. However, these threats will be considered later as the discussion that follows next is confined to the sources of costs that APNs must consider in setting their prices.

COSTS OF PRODUCING SERVICES

APNs need to understand and calculate the costs associated with overhead (rent, maintenance, utilities, office equipment, and insurance [for fire, theft, and accidents]), malpractice insurance, personal health insurance, the number of employees required and their wages, employee benefits, special equipment and supplies, individual and practice licenses and other fees, payment of principal and interest on loans, and other expenses or financial obligations. APNs must also decide the amount to reserve for contingency or emergency expenditures and whether any bonus or incentive pay will be provided. For the APN firm to be profitable, the total costs of the practice must be exceeded by the revenues that are generated by providing services.

UNIT OF SERVICE

APNs will need to decide if they are going to price each service separately or bundle services together and price them as a package (obviously, a payer's policies will influence this decision). If an APN firm anticipates providing care to consumers who mostly pay out of pocket, then it will have to determine the costs of administration and bookkeeping that are involved in billing and collection for individual versus bundled services and compare these costs to the revenues that realistically can be received by either method.

MARKET DEMAND CHARACTERISTICS

APNs must understand the characteristics of the market, particularly the kind of services needed, by whom, and by how many people. APNs should analyze the geographic area where they intend to practice and determine the number of potential consumers, their healthcare needs, age and income distribution, and other community- and individual-level health deficits that they can address. The objective of such an assessment is to determine whether enough people have the type of health problems, incomes, and health insurance that can pay for the volume and kind of APN services the firm can produce.

STRUCTURAL BARRIERS

APNs must ascertain whether any structural barriers to their practice exist. These could take the form of state practice acts that restrict APNs from performing certain activities that would be critical to the economic and clinical vitality of the practice or regulations and city codes that directly or indirectly raise the costs of the practice. Other barriers might include the absence of physicians who will collaborate with APNs and the existence of any social or culturally rooted customs or beliefs that might cause people to be unwilling to purchase healthcare from APNs, regardless of economic circumstances. If barriers exist, then APNs must decide if they can be removed and how much this will cost in terms of time, effort, and dollars.

PRESENCE OF COMPETITORS

It is essential that APNs understand who their competitors are, how many exist, where they are located, what services they offer, how much they charge, how they are paid, and how profitable they are. This information tells the APNs a great deal about what other providers are doing and what seems to work (or not work), which can spare the APN practice from making time-consuming and costly mistakes. Knowing as much as possible about the competition will also make it possible for APNs to determine whether any gaps in service exist that they can fill, how to take advantage of market niches, and how they might do things differently and for less cost, all of which can increase their chances of economic survival.

PAYMENT AMOUNTS

APNs need to know who will pay for their services. If most of the likely consumers have private individual or employer-provided insurance plans, it is essential to know whether insurers will pay for services provided by APNs. If they do, then APNs must understand the payment rate and how soon after submitting bills they can expect to receive payment. However, if many people in the practice area are enrolled in HMOs, then APNs can expect that most will be unwilling to become clients because of the out-of-plan charges plan members must pay. In that case, it would be wise for the APN firm to negotiate with the HMO to see if APNs can contract for certain services.

If the practice is locating in an underserved or low-income area, then APNs need to understand the means by which providers are customarily paid for their services. Payments could involve accepting Medicaid fees that are less than the costs of providing services, small amounts of out-of-pocket cash, or in-kind services (e.g., snow shoveling, lawn care, maintenance, and so on). An APN firm must decide the amount of uncompensated care it can provide (charity care and services for which they do not expect to be paid by people able to do so), determine whether cost-shifting opportunities are available, and ascertain the level of in-kind payments it can accept without imposing financial harm. APNs should investigate grants and donations offered by state, county, city, or private philanthropic organizations to help pay for care provided in underserved areas.

ADVERTISING

For APNs to break into the market and attract new clients, particularly when provider–client relationships already exist, advertising will be essential to inform potential consumers that APN services are available, where the office is located, and how much services cost. Information on the qualifications of members of the practice, together with descriptions of the unique services, philosophy on health, and other attributes that can distinguish the firm from its competitors, should be part of initial promotion efforts.

OTHER SOURCES OF COSTS

Undoubtedly, other sources of costs need to be considered beyond those already identified. However, APNs must realize that the importance of many of these costs will change over time and will vary with an APN's practice pattern or location of the group or solo practice (rural, metropolitan, or inner city), and so on. Some of the costs could exert a great bearing at certain times. For example, if the price of malpractice insurance increases, an APN firm might have to consider raising prices, especially if it believes that clients will not switch to another provider. Unfortunately, no exact or precise method exists by which to calculate the price to charge for their services; this is a complex decision that, in addition to the preceding information, involves a fair amount of guesswork and intuition, trial and error, and a strong set of nerves. Ultimately, however, the value that consumers attach to the services provided by APNs will indicate how much they are willing to pay. If they perceive that APN services are valuable, consumers will be more willing to pay a higher price and vice versa. To add further complexity, consumer preferences are constantly changing, as is their willingness to pay for services offered by APNs.

The bottom line is that if APNs in either solo or group practice arrangements are to survive in a competitive market, they will have to be alert, seek ways to innovate and minimize costs, and be willing to make frequent adjustments in the quality of their services and how they price and market them. Although it is virtually impossible to specify the "correct" (profit maximizing) price that APNs should charge for their services, APNs would be wise to initially set their prices below the prevailing market price of services provided by physicians or their nearest competitor. Why this is so is explained next.

Economic Consequences of Advanced Practice Nurses' Pricing Decisions

This section focuses on the potential economic consequences of the pricing decision of an APN group practice, including the anticipated effects on physicians and consumers. However, to adequately explain these, it is necessary to first discuss the key economic terms and concepts that underpin the relationship between price and the firm's demand, amount of total revenues, profitability, and the economic responses by physicians of consumers.

PRICE, QUANTITY DEMANDED AND SOLD, TOTAL REVENUE, AND PRICE ELASTICITY OF DEMAND

The total revenue (amount of dollars) that is earned by the APN practice is simply the product of the quantity of services sold multiplied by the price of each service. The quantity of services could be measured by the number of visits, billable procedures, treatments, min-

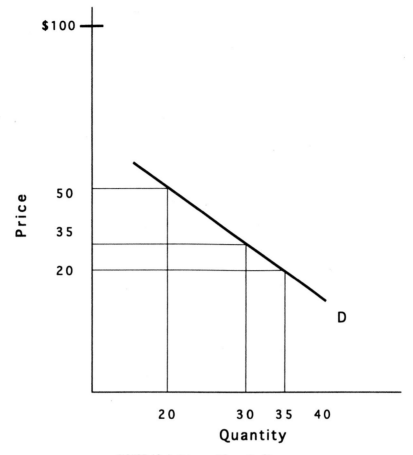

FIGURE 16-1 Price and Quantity Changes.
D, demand.

utes, or whatever unit of service the firm decides. Figure 16-1 shows the price of services on the *y* axis and the quantity of services sold on the *x* axis. Holding other things constant (e.g., incomes of consumers, prices of other goods and services, and so on), the relationship between the quantity sold and price is shown by a downward sloping line (D), which is the demand curve for the particular service provided by the APN. For example, at $50 per service, the firm could sell 20 units and generate revenue equal to $1000 ($50 × 20). Notice that as the price falls, to say $20, the practice can sell more services (35 units), and total revenue falls to $700 ($20 × 35). The firm's profitability is determined by calculating total revenues and subtracting total costs, and what remains is profit (or loss).

A critically important determinant of the amount of revenue obtained is the degree to which changes in the quantity of services sold are sensitive to changes in their price. Economists use the term *price elasticity of demand* to refer to the sensitivity or responsiveness in the relationship between quantity sold and price changes. For some goods or services, a small change in price results in a large change in the quantity sold, whereas for other goods or services, a small change in price results in hardly any or no change in quantity sold.

The underlying relationship between quantity sold and price changes and the resultant impact on total revenues are illustrated graphically in Figure 16-2. Once again, the price of the APN service is shown on the *y* axis and the quantity sold is depicted along the *x* axis. In Figure 16-2a, notice that when the price is $35, the number of units sold is 30, and the

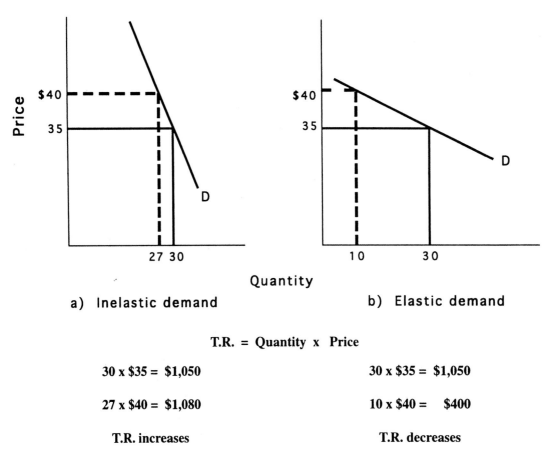

FIGURE 16-2 Total Revenue When Demand Is a) Inelastic and b) Elastic.
D, demand.

corresponding revenue equals $1050. However, when the price increases to $40, the quantity sold decreases to 27, but note that revenue increases to $1080. Now consider Figure 16-2b, which also shows that when the price is $35, 30 units are sold and total revenue is $1050. However, when the price is increased to $40 the amount sold decreases considerably, to only 10 units, and total revenue falls to $400. It should be clear that the same $5 increase in price, from $35 to $40 in Figure 16-2a and 16-2b, results in vastly different decreases in the quantities sold and hence in the total revenue obtained ($1080 compared with $400).

These results should make it clear that the sensitivity of the relationship between quantity sold and price—the price elasticity of demand—is a monumentally important determinant of the amount of the firm's total revenue and hence profitability. Graphically, when the relationship between quantity sold and price is like that depicted in the steeply sloped demand curve of Figure 16-2a, the demand for the product or service is referred to as *inelastic*, which means that the relationship is not very sensitive. The less steeply sloped demand curve shown in Figure 16-2b shows a much more responsive relationship between quantity and changes in price and is referred to as an *elastic* demand curve. Because the degree of sensitivity of the relationship between quantity and price is such an important determinant of total revenue, and hence the firm's profitability, it is important to consider what influences whether the underlying relationship is sensitive or not very sensitive (or in economic terms, whether demand is elastic or inelastic).

DETERMINANTS OF THE PRICE ELASTICITY OF DEMAND

The sensitivity of the relationship between price and quantity sold depends on three factors. First, and foremost, is the *number* and *closeness* of substitutes. The greater the number of close substitutes that are available for a particular good or service, the more its demand (quantity sold) is likely to be sensitive to changes in price. For example, if the price of a certain brand of television were to increase substantially, an individual would have an economic incentive to purchase a television produced by a different manufacturer. In this case, the demand for a particular television is likely to be sensitive to changes in price, as would be depicted by the relatively elastic demand curve in Figure 16-2b. However, if few substitutes are available for a particular good or if the substitutes are not close, a producer can raise the price of the good and, although this will normally lead to a decrease in quantity sold, total revenues will not decrease—see the inelastic demand curve in Figure 16-2a. In healthcare, few close substitutes to physicians exist; consequently, their inelastic demand curve is an important reason that physicians have been able to raise prices without experiencing a large decrease in total revenues or net incomes.

Second, the price elasticity of demand also depends on the importance of the commodity in a consumer's budget. To illustrate, the demand for commodities such as thumbtacks, salt, and pepper is likely to be quite inelastic (i.e., not very sensitive). Thus, if the price of salt goes up, then the consumption of salt is unlikely to fall much, if at all. But if an individual is buying a major appliance or an automobile, which would have a much greater impact on the person's budget, then the selection and purchase of the automobile are more likely to be sensitive to price.

The third determinant of the sensitivity of the relationship between quantity sold and price changes is the length of time over which the commodity is demanded by consumers. The longer the period, the easier it becomes for consumers or firms to substitute one good for another. Over a long period (versus a shorter period), few commodities do not have substitutes, and the longer the commodity is being produced and sold, the easier it becomes for firms to find ways to produce new substitute goods, and people to learn how to make substitutions by themselves. For example, in healthcare, consider how magnetic resonance imaging has substituted for computerized axial tomography, which has substituted for radiographs. Likewise, consider that cardiac catheterization can be a substitute for certain types of cardiac surgery or that lithotripsy can substitute for surgery to remove kidney stones and gallstones.

EFFECT OF ADVANCED PRACTICE NURSES' PRICING DECISIONS ON PHYSICIANS AND CONSUMERS

To understand how price, quantity sold, total revenue, and price elasticity of demand will ultimately determine APNs' ability to successfully compete in a competitive environment, suppose that several APNs develop a formal group practice and, after considering all of the determinants of price discussed earlier, conclude that it is economically feasible to charge a lower price than that charged by physicians in the market for the same or similar services. Charging a lower price would be an economically rational decision because the relationship between the price charged and the quantity of APN services sold is likely to be quite sensitive, or elastic (in the eyes of consumers, physicians are close and available substitutes to APNs). Given an elastic demand, consumers need an economic incentive to purchase care from APNs, which would be provided by APNs who are charging a lower price than physicians. Moreover, charging a lower price will have important economic effects on APNs, physicians, and consumers. Consider Figure 16-3, which shows the two providers, APNs and a medical group, in a market competing for patients.

Assume that P_1 in Figures 16-3a and 16-3b is the existing market price for physician ser-

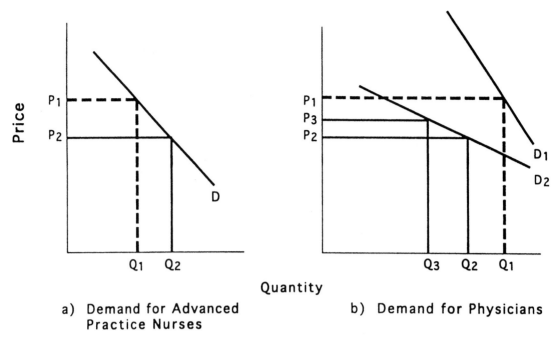

a) Demand for Advanced Practice Nurses

b) Demand for Physicians

FIGURE 16-3 Effects of Price Change on Demand for Physicians.
D, demand; P, price; Q, quantity.

vices. APNs can provide identical or nearly equivalent services (any differences are not significant to patients) but decide to charge a lower price, P_2 in Figure 16-3a. Notice that the demand curve for APNs is relatively elastic, which reflects the influence of primary care physicians as available, close, and well-known substitutes. Consequently, the relationship between quantity sold and price of APN services is quite sensitive. However, the physicians' demand curve (D_1) in Figure 16-3b is less elastic (more steeply sloped), which reflects the assumption that most people in the market are less familiar with APNs and may not view them as close substitutes.

The fact that APNs offer their services at lower prices (P_2) than their medical competitors (P_1) will result in stimulating some initial demand for their services. Provided that APNs attract additional consumers at this price and obtain a favorable reputation and that knowledge of their availability spreads through word of mouth and by advertising, more services will be sold (Q_2) and APN revenues will expand to $P_2 \times Q_2$. If, however, APNs did not offer their services at a lower price, then they would not provide increasingly cost-conscious consumers and insurers an economic incentive to direct their subscribers to APNs, let alone give HMOs or large employers an incentive to contract for a defined set of health services for their enrollees. Without consumers buying and payers purchasing APN services, the APN group will go out of business.

Assuming again that APNs initially charge a lower price (P_2) for the same or similar services that are offered by their competitors, this will create negative economic effects on physicians who are practicing in the same market. As more patients respond to the lower prices charged by APNs, the demand for physicians will fall (in microeconomics, this relationship between the change in price of one product and change in demand for another is referred to as a *positive cross-price elasticity of demand*). The reduction in demand for physician services is shown by the demand curve shifting inward and to the left (D_2). Notice that this decline in total demand is different from a change in quantity demanded, which results solely from a *price* change, in which case the movement in quantity sold would be along the stationary demand curve. The reduction in total demand to D_2 will exert two significant economic effects on physicians: (1) along the new demand curve, D_2, physicians will always sell less (see Q_2 or Q_3 in Fig. 16-3[b]), even if they lower their prices, compared with what they could have sold when demand was previously reflected by D_1, and (2) the reduction in quantity of services sold means that physicians' total revenues will be less, as will be net income.[1]

The presence of APNs in the market, and their use by consumers in response to lower prices, will exert an additional and important effect on the economic interests of physicians. Notice that not only does the demand curve shift inward and to the left to D_2, but the elasticity of the new demand curve increases, which means that the relationship between quantity demanded and price changes has greater sensitivity than what existed previously along D_1. As explained earlier with reference to Figure 16-2(a), physicians' relatively inelastic demand curve has long enabled them to increase the price of most services without diminishing total revenues (incidentally, to maximize total revenues, physicians in private practice have favored policies that would limit the supply of physicians or other competitors, thereby ensuring an excess demand for their services). But as APNs become available and act as close substitutes for many of the services provided by physicians, physicians' comparatively inelastic demand curve will become more elastic. As demand becomes more elastic, physicians will find that if they increase their price to compensate for the loss in revenue, then they are likely to experience a substantial decrease in the quantity of services sold, and total revenues will decline even further. The lost revenues, however, will be gained by APNs as their lower prices attract patients who formally purchased services from physicians.

From the perspective of physicians, the presence of close substitutes (APNs) in the market creates negative changes in their economic position: demand is likely to decrease, as will total revenues and net income. In addition, the relationship between future quantity changes and price increases will have greater sensitivity (i.e., physicians' demand curve would become more elastic). The expected economic response of physicians would be to lower their prices, increase advertising, and perhaps even improve the qualitative aspects of their medical practice. It is also conceivable that physicians might try predatory pricing by dropping their prices so low that APNs could not match the lower price and still remain in business. But because these changes would impose new costs to the medical practice, physicians would probably try less costly and more permanent solutions by trying to remove their competition by attempting to have the practice of APNs declared illegal; obtaining regulations that restrict the number or type of procedures and activities; blocking APNs from obtaining hospital admitting privileges (or removing them if they have them); boycotting insurance companies, HMOs, or other physicians who recognize or collaborate with APNs; or trying to influence payer policies toward APNs. Thus, as more APNs start group practice arrangements and the healthcare delivery system becomes more price competitive, APNs must anticipate these responses. Addressing these responses will take time and impose additional costs. For these and other reasons, it is essential that APNs are familiar with antitrust provisions and their application in healthcare.

EFFECT ON CONSUMERS

With APNs successfully competing in the market, consumers benefit in at least three ways. First, the presence of APNs gives consumers new choices, and some are likely to find that they derive more satisfaction with the purchase of healthcare from APNs (e.g., consumers might find that APNs spend more time during visits, communicate better than physicians, and offer a different perspective about health). Second, consumers would be paying less for

[1]When demand is strong, the practice is well established, and APNs are working close to full capacity, it would then be appropriate to consider increasing the price of their services.

healthcare and hence have more of their income left to save, invest, or use to purchase other items that increase their total satisfaction derived from using their money resources. Third, as the success (i.e., profitability) of more APNs provides an incentive for others to start independent practice arrangements, more price competition will develop, which would help to dampen future healthcare cost increases than what would otherwise be the case.

The price of healthcare is likely to rise at a slower rate (even for patients seen by physicians) because if any one provider raises prices too much in a competitive market, then consumers, who can be expected to become more price-sensitive as they steadily pay more out-of-pocket healthcare costs, are more likely to shop around and switch to a lower-priced provider (assuming provider quality differences are not large). Such behavior would send a powerful and unmistakable message to all providers to keep their prices as low as possible. When summed over many providers and over time, the cumulative effect of price competition can be substantial, and the future rate of price increases is likely to be constrained.

Advanced Practice Nurses in Prepaid Capitated Firms

As much of the content of this chapter has attempted to convey, the forces that evolved in the 1980s and early 1990s and culminated in the development of price competition largely came about because it has become in the economic interest of increasingly cost-conscious purchasers to obtain greater value for each dollar spent on healthcare. In the years ahead, APNs can expect that more of the clinical and economic forces that shape their practice and determine their personal income will be driven by impersonal and unambiguous incentives that govern price-competitive industries: providers and health professionals will be rewarded only to the extent that they keep their prices low and quality high.

The manifestation of a more competitive environment in healthcare is expected to take the form of increasing enrollment in prepaid capitated healthcare firms, such as HMOs, and the formation of larger integrated systems. Their growth will be aided by continuing regulatory and market-based adjustments designed to make sure that providers compete fairly and on the basis of price and quality. The evolution of the managed care industry is a significant and generally positive development for APNs, whether they are employed by managed care firms or decide to compete independently as solo providers or in group practice arrangements. From the economic perspective of APNs, the major difference between practicing as an employee of an HMO or practicing independently is that, as an employee, the APN functions as an economic complement, whereas APNs in independent practice function largely as economic substitutes to an HMO or medical group practice. This section focuses on APNs as economic complements and briefly identifies some of the opportunities and challenges that many are likely to face as price competition develops among healthcare providers.

APNs are an economic complement if providing their services increases the productivity of the managed care firm and the profits of its owners. The complementary role is not unlike that of hospital-employed nurses whose nursing practice functions to increase the productivity of physicians by allowing them to both treat inpatients and maintain an office-based practice, thereby increasing physicians' revenues and net income. Because an HMO operates according to a prepaid capitated budget, it has an economic incentive to keep the total costs of providing healthcare as low as possible. In this way, any amount of unspent dollars can be retained as profit. Thus, HMOs have an economic interest to provide its enrollees with more preventive care and health education so that it can reduce future consumption of HMO resources to treat preventable acute and chronic illness. In addition, HMOs try to reduce admissions to costly hospitals, negotiate discounts on the purchase of pharmaceuticals and medical devices, and pursue other methods to minimize its costs (including enrolling younger and more healthy people who are less likely to consume resources and thereby help lower total costs).

A feature unique to HMOs is the use of primary care health professionals as gate-keepers. The economic objective of the gatekeeper is to ensure that the HMO uses its re-sources efficiently. At the same time, gatekeepers must ensure that plan members receive the appropriate kind and amount of healthcare, because if they do not, then HMO costs are likely to increase as treatable conditions and ailments worsen and eventually require ad-ditional resources. However, the gatekeeper, like other physicians and health professionals employed by the HMO, incurs costs that are associated with salary, benefits, and year-end bonus or incentive pay. Because it has a strong economic incentive to keep its labor costs as low as possible, the HMO will want to find the cheapest and most effective way to fill gatekeeping roles and provide appropriate healthcare services.

Many of the clinical services that APNs provide can closely substitute for those pro-vided by generalist and some specialty physicians. Because APNs are less costly to an HMO in terms of salary and benefits requirements, they are economical alternatives to physicians in gatekeeping and other provider roles. As employers pressure HMOs to lower and con-strain the growth of premiums charged per member, price competition among HMOs will intensify. Thus, HMOs will face even more pressure to minimize their costs, which should increase the demand for APNs even further. However, this does not mean that APNs will totally replace physicians because physicians provide certain medical services that APNs cannot provide. The point is that the spread of price competition should materially increase HMOs' demand for APNs in the future. Moreover, because managed care firms must keep premiums competitively priced, it can be anticipated that they will develop new roles for APNs and experiment with delivery models that will be tailored extensively around APNs to find new ways to lower costs and at the same time increase enrollees' satisfaction and at-tainment of desired clinical outcomes.

For at least two economic reasons, however, APNs must anticipate that primary care physicians and physician assistants will resist the increasing employment of APNs. First, as more APNs become available, the total supply of primary care health professionals will in-crease relative to the number of available managed care positions. Consequently, this will place downward pressure on the salaries that managed care firms are able to offer and still hire all the providers they want. As the supply of generalist physicians increases, specialty physicians become trained as primary care providers, and practicing medicine in managed care firms becomes increasingly acceptable to more members of the medical profession, ad-ditional physicians will be seeking employment in managed care firms and, therefore, com-peting for available positions with APNs, who have a comparative cost advantage. A sec-ond reason to expect physicians to resist the expansion of APNs in managed care is that many firms might adopt policies directing that APNs' caseloads comprise mostly the "less difficult cases." But by having to take care of the "difficult cases," primary care physicians may be unable to obtain appropriate outcomes or levels of patient satisfaction to qualify for year-end bonus or incentive payments. Thus, APNs must understand that although they present economic benefits to the owners of HMOs, they represent an increasingly vis-ible economic threat to primary care and specialist physicians. For these reasons, it will not be surprising if organized medicine takes actions aimed at decreasing the supply of APNs in the same way, as discussed earlier, that physicians may attempt to eliminate APNs in group practice from the marketplace to prevent price competition.

Conclusion

In contemplating the likelihood that the opportunities for APNs that have been described in this chapter will actually materialize, it is important to reflect on the number and inten-sity of economic forces that have been discussed. These include the effects of federal bud-get deficits; the expansion of the Medicare prospective payment system to nonhospital providers; new and increasingly restrictive physician payment policies; the adoption of government regulatory efforts and other cost-containment innovations by the private sector; the growth of resistance to cost shifting; effective use of purchasing power by more employers to stimulate price competition among managed care firms; and an invigorated federal health services research agenda.

These forces are compelling the development of true price competition in healthcare, serious and pervasive cost-control initiatives, and the beginning of competition over quality and patient outcomes. As these forces grow, so too will the power and economic will to sweep away barriers that have existed in healthcare since the mid-1960s and that have served all too well to protect the economic interests of traditional providers. The future will be vastly different and will offer many opportunities for APNs and the entire nursing profession to elevate its role and visibility as providers of healthcare services.

REFERENCES

Buerhaus, P. I. (1992). Nursing, competition and quality. *Nursing Economic$ 10*(1), 21–29.

Buerhaus, P. I. (1994a). Economics of managed competition and consequences to nurses: Part I. *Nursing Economic$ 12*(1), 10–17.

Buerhaus, P. I. (1994b). Economics of managed competition and consequences to nurses: Part II. *Nursing Economic$ 12*(2), 75–80, 106.

Buerhaus, P. I. (1994c). Health care reform, managed competition, and critical issues facing nurses. *Nursing & Health Care 15*(1), 22–26.

Enthoven, A. C. (1993). The history and principles of managed competition. *Health Affairs 12*, (Suppl on Managed Competition: Health Reform American Style?), 24–48.

Enthoven, A. C., & Kronick, R. (1989a). A consumer choice health plan for the 1990s: Universal health insurance in a system designed to promote quality and economy. *New England Journal of Medicine 320*(1), 29–37.

Enthoven, A. C., & Kronick, R. (1989b). A consumer choice health plan for the 1990s: Universal health insurance in a system designed to promote quality and economy. *New England Journal of Medicine 320*(2), 94–101.

Enthoven, A. C., & Kronick, R. (1991). Universal health insurance through incentives reform. *Journal of the American Medical Association 265*(19), 2532–2536.

Feldstein, P. J. (1993). *Health care economics* (4th ed.). Albany, NY: Delmar Publishers Inc.

Levit, K. (January/February 1998). National health spending trends in 1996. *Health Affairs 17*(1), 35–51.

Mansfield, E. (1982). *Theory and applications* (4th ed.). New York: W. W. Norton.

Medicare Payment Advisory Commission (MedPAC) (March 1998). *Report to the Congress: Medicare payment policy. Volume I: Recommendations.* Washington, DC: Author.

The Advanced Practice Nurse: Roles and Innovative Models for Caring

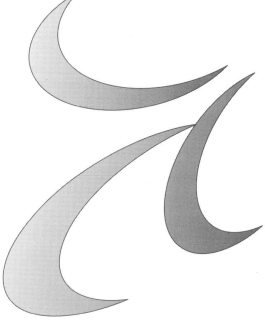

CHAPTER 17

Primary Care: Improving Health Promotion and Disease Prevention

Exemplars

17A *Occupational Health Nursing Strategies for Health Promotion*

17B *An Entrepreneurial Faculty Practice Plan*

17C *Advanced Practice Nursing in the Department of Veterans Affairs: A Model for the Future*

17D *Monitoring Clinical Outcomes and Satisfaction in Patients of Psychiatric Clinical Nurse Specialists in Private Practice*

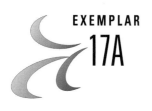

Occupational Health Nursing Strategies for Health Promotion

Bonnie Rogers
Elizabeth Lawhorn

Occupational health nursing practice has been in existence since the late 1800s. During this period, industrial nurses, as they were called then, provided care to ill and injured workers. In fact, Ada Mayo Stuart, touted as the first industrial nurse hired by a company, the Vermont Marble Company, not only provided on-site healthcare services to workers but made home visits, provided care to families of workers, and provided school healthcare services throughout the factory town (Rogers, 1994).

More than 100 years have elapsed since the beginnings of the specialty of occupational health nursing, and the practice has evolved and expanded enormously. Professional nurses are constantly being called on to change and enlarge their roles increasing their knowledge to meet the demands of the client and the profession. Occupational health nursing practice is autonomous; nurses practice mostly independently, collaborating with physicians, industrial hygienists, safety specialists, and others as needed to ensure a safe and healthful work environment and quality healthcare to meet worker needs. Occupational health nursing is a profession that recognizes and prevents work-related disease. Those individuals who practice occupational healthcare are principally concerned with the effects of work on health and supporting a work environment that supports a health concept.

The scope of occupational health nursing practice is broad, and elements and their descriptions are shown in Box 17A-1 (Rogers, 1994). During the 1970s, not only were occupational health nurses involved with determining the health and ability of employees to safely perform the job, but increased emphasis was placed on a health environment as an integral part of occupational health. Our current healthcare system concentrates on the diagnosis and treatment of medical problems after they occur. Many companies cannot afford illness and have realized that a well-designed health promotion program is a powerful cost-containment tool. The best long-term solution to controlling healthcare costs and improving health is fostering healthy lifestyle choices.

Most of the 110 million people who make up the American workforce spend the major portion of their day at the worksite. Occupational health nurses have made significant

| BOX 17A-1 | *Scope of Practice in Occupational Health Nursing* |

WORKER/WORKPLACE ASSESSMENT AND SURVEILLANCE

Placement of workers into jobs that match their skill; monitoring the worker for adverse work-related health effects, and the workplace for health hazards.

HEALTH PROMOTION–DISEASE PREVENTION

Use of health promotion, health protection, and control strategies to prevent illness and injury.

PRIMARY CARE

Provision of healthcare, both occupational and nonoccupational, including treatment, first aid, and referral as necessary.

CASE MANAGEMENT

Provision of comprehensive, cost-effective, care to the worker from the beginning of illness or injury to optimal return to work.

COUNSELING

Provision of individual and group counseling for anticipatory guidance, preventive care, and crisis management.

INJURY/ILLNESS INVESTIGATION

Determination of trends in illness and injuries for worker and workforce health management.

MANAGEMENT/ADMINISTRATION

Policy development, strategic planning, and operational oversight for occupational health services.

COMMUNITY ORIENTATION

Utilization of community resources consistent with the mission, programs, and services of the occupational health unit.

LEGAL/ETHICAL

Knowledgeable about the laws governing occupational health and nursing practice; uses an ethical framework for practice.

RESEARCH

Integrates new knowledge into practice and participates in research as appropriate.

progress in the past 20 years in educating the workforce about health risks and using the worksite to promote healthy behavior. The primary health promotion goal, beyond awareness, is a positive change in the individual's behavior (Pellitier, 1993). This exemplar outlines the strategies for worksite health promotion, the occupational health nurse's role and strategy implementation, and ways to improve employees' health through education and nursing interventions.

Health promotion and disease prevention have major emphasis in this specialty practice, particularly because the worksite venue provides a great opportunity to discuss lifestyle, demographic, and environmental determinants that impact health. For example, Table 17A-1 identifies specific lifestyle behaviors and related health risks. The occupational health nurse, who usually manages the occupational health center, is the key healthcare provider at the worksite, who not only develops and implements targeted health promotion programs, but also implements nursing interventions designed to assist the employee to achieve specified health outcomes (Childre, 1997). It is vitally important that goals and outcomes be delineated so that both the employee and the employer know what to expect in terms of reduced health risk, reduced healthcare costs, and improved employee and employer satisfaction with both healthcare delivery and health status (AWHD, 1994; Wachs, 1997).

Many companies provide a wide range of risk assessment and screening programs, with services ranging from a simple health risk appraisal (HRA) to on-site health testing, which may incorporate health screening at the worksite. Within the context of health promotion and risk reduction, the use of HRAs has been beneficial and satisfying in health improvement (Donnelly, 1993).

HRAs were formally introduced in the 1970s and have been used for many years in health education and health promotion programs, especially at the worksite. The HRA is a tool administered in the form of a questionnaire that asks questions about health history and health behaviors. Figure 17A-1 presents examples of questions for the category of motor vehicles (Staywell, 1996). The tool identifies the likelihood of developing preventable disease within a specific period of time based on several personal and health-related lifestyle behaviors. Several biometric measurements can be taken, such as total blood cholesterol level, height, weight, blood pressure, or body fat content, depending on which tool is used. The results are then calculated and printed to provide to employees, in booklet form, their "risk age" and their achievable risk age, based on aggregate risk data. The occupational health nurse can use the group aggregate data to determine appropriate established specific goals for risk factor modification and for use with supportive educational materials.

TABLE 17A-1 *Diseases and Their Consequences*

Lifestyle Behaviors	Risk
Alcohol, drugs	Motor vehicle accidents
Elevated cholesterol, blood pressure	Heart disease, arteriosclerosis
Alcohol abuse	Cirrhosis of the liver
No seatbelt use, speeding	Motor vehicle accidents
Lack of exercise	Heart disease, high blood pressure, obesity
Stress	Ulcers, neck and back problems, heart disease, asthma
Cigarette smoking	Emphysema, lung cancer, coronary heart disease, asthma

Motor Vehicles –
Mark the best response to each question:
48. How would you best describe the vehicle you drive or ride in the most often?
 a. Motorcycle...
 b. Compact or subcompact car...
 c. Midsize or full car..
 d. None of the above..

49. About how many miles per year do you drive or ride as a passenger?

MILES PER WEEK	=	MILES PER YEAR
a. more than 500	=	more than 30,000
b. 401 to 500	=	20,001 to 30,000
c. 301 to 400	=	15,001 to 20,000
d. 201 to 300	=	10,001 to 15,000 (average person's mileage)
e. 101 to 200	=	5,001 to 10,000
f. 40 to 100	=	2,001 to 5,000
g. less than 40	=	2,000 or less

50. How often do you exceed the posted speed limits, either driving or riding as a passenger?
 a. Most of the time...
 b. Sometimes...
 c. Rarely or never...

51. How many traffic tickets (moving violations) have you had within the last 2 years?
 a. Four or more...
 b. Three..
 c. Two...
 d. One...
 e. None..

52. What percentage of time do you wear a seatbelt when riding or driving a motor vehicle?
 a. 75% or more of the time...
 b. 50% to 74% of the time..
 c. 25% to 49% of the time..
 d. Less than 25% of the time..

53. Do you request that all passengers in your motor vehicle wear seatbelts?
 a. Yes...
 b. No...

54. Where do you drive or ride as a passenger most of the time?
 a. On highways...
 b. On city streets..
 c. Both equally...

55. How often do you drink and drive, or ride with a driver who may have had too much to drink?
 a. Frequently..
 b. Sometimes...
 c. Rarely...
 d. Never..

FIGURE 17A-1 Example of HRA Questions for Motor Vehicles.

The HRA provides individuals with recommendations for reducing risk related to lifestyle behavior and for promoting desirable changes in health behavior. Corporate benefits can range from improved health, reduced absenteeism, lower healthcare costs, decreased disability, decreased mortality, and improved morale among workers. Two examples of employees with their HRA-generated information and occupational health nursing interventions at the worksite follow.

John Preston, a 54-year-old employee, participated in an HRA program at a large manufacturing facility and learned how important it is to follow recommended lifestyle changes to reduce his risk of developing serious cardiovascular disease. After John completed the process, the HRA-processed and individualized report was generated based on his self-reported responses to the questions and clinical data. The occupational health nurse at the site discussed general results of the HRA report in a group interpretation session. Those at high risk and with multiple risk factors were asked to schedule an individual counseling session with the occupational health nurse to formulate a plan to address strategies for risk reduction. Goal-setting and follow-up meetings were scheduled. John found out from his HRA that his age risk was accelerated and that his excessive weight of 50 lbs was putting him at greater risk for a heart attack, heart disease, arthritis, back disorders, and joint pain. Nursing recommendations included evaluating John's motivation for weight reduction and determining appropriate strategies for weight loss.

The Clinical Guidelines on the Identification, Evaluation, and Treatment of Overweight and Obesity in Adults (National Heart, Lung, and Blood Institute, 1997) provided valuable information to help John. The first step was to explore with John realistic goals for weight loss; reasons for previous unsuccessful attempts at weight reduction; social and family supports; understanding of the causes of obesity and its health impact; and attitude toward and willingness to engage in physical activity. John believed he needed to reduce his weight because of health consequences and that his family was supportive and concerned. In consultation with John's primary care physician, the plan of care focused on diet and exercise, with a goal to achieve 50% weight reduction in 6 months, or 25 lb (1 lb per week). John's wife was involved in the diet counseling sessions because she did the cooking. Counseling focused on calorie reduction of 300 to 500 kcal/d including reductions in saturated fat with total fats not exceeding 30% of total calories. In addition, a reduction in carbohydrates and an increase in fruits and vegetables was discussed. An individualized diet plan was developed with the input and approval of John and his wife.

An increase in physical activity is an essential component of a weight-loss program. Although most weight loss occurs because of decreased caloric intake, regular exercise helps prevent weight gain and reduces cardiovascular and diabetes risks. Given that John had no exercise program, the occupational health nurse recommended a gradual increase in physical activity over time, beginning with walking 30 minutes 3 days per week and increasing to 5 days per week after 3 weeks or alternating with swimming, which John had enjoyed previously. He had access to a swimming pool daily. In addition, using stairs instead of elevators, particularly for shorter distances, was encouraged.

The role of the occupational health nurse was to help motivate John to make small changes at first, understanding adequate information about his health status and ways to learn how to make appropriate changes. Eliciting information to improve the nurse–patient relationship is important; however, at the worksite many occupational health nurses know individuals on a personal basis so a rapport is already established. John was encouraged to learn positive substitutes for the behaviors that had created his long-term health risks. Knowledge about his views and behaviors was used to design a more effective plan. Particular emphasis was placed on his social network and support system, given that his wife prepared the meals. Because counseling is often complex and compliance is essential, the occupational health nurse scheduled four weekly appointments to discuss the rationale for reducing risk behaviors and reinforcing positive behaviors. In this situation, employees have the advantage of being on-site, with time and resources for follow-up for wellness activities.

The discussions of detailed dietary instruction and physical activity took place during several visits. Emphasis was placed on maintaining healthy diet and nutrition behavior to keep the weight in check. Careful attention to his weight was performed at follow-up visits, and progress toward achieving his goals was monitored through scheduled visits and telephone calls. At 3 months, John's weight was reduced by 28%, at 6 months by 55%.

Another major health issue that affects all people is cancer. One specific health problem facing many women is breast cancer. About 54% of women in the United States older than 18 years work outside the home, making the workplace an excellent setting for health promotion programs for women (Caplan & Coughlin, 1998). In 1997, it was estimated that 180,200 women were diagnosed with invasive breast cancer, with nearly 44,000 dying of the disease, making breast cancer the second most common malignancy for women and the second leading cause of death in the United States (Parker, Tong, Bolden, & Wingo, 1997). Through early detection, breast cancer screening reduces mortality in women, with mammography screening accounting for 20% to 39% of mortality reduction in women aged 50 to 74 years (Kerlikowske et al., 1995). Still, many women are not screened for breast cancer, citing lack of knowledge about mammography benefits; no physician recommendation; and travel, distance, cost, and time as barriers (Colditz, Hoaglin, & Berkey, 1997). Using the workplace as a venue for breast cancer screening is ideal because of the potential to reach large numbers of women, including those who might not otherwise practice preventive health behaviors or have access to screening venues (Reimer, 1997).

With this information in mind, the occupational health nurse had implemented a breast cancer screening program at the worksite. One employee, Mary Lister, a 50-year-old African-American working in a manufacturing facility, knew she should have a mammogram. Her family had been encouraging her to have one performed. The occupational health nurse provided breast examination clinical services at the worksite for employees interested in this service. The occupational health nurse also provided instruction on breast self-examination to be performed once monthly and about 1 week after menses, with emphasis on making breast self-examinations a lifetime habit. Pamphlets explaining the procedure were also available at the company. Mary had felt a lump in her breast while taking a shower and had come to see the occupational health nurse on the day the nurse was implementing a workplace mammography screening program. The nurse examined her, validated the lump, and advised her to have a mammogram. When the van appeared at the workplace, Mary was ready for the mammogram, which was performed in the mobile van. The nurse counseled her about the risks and benefits and possible outcomes. After several days her report was sent directly to the worksite to the occupational health services department in a confidential envelope. The mammogram was suspicious, with a proliferate lesion identified and reported. The occupational health nurse discussed the findings of the report, provided reassurance and a listening atmosphere, and advised and assisted with referrals. The need to inform, explain, and advise is essential primary care, and the occupational health nurse provided intervention strategies to help employees cope with sensitive situations. The occupational health nurse contacted Mary and discussed her personal and family history and her understanding of the risk and the meaning of the risk. The nurse discussed the report and explored Mary's feelings about fear, frustration, and lack of control over the situation and her supportive family.

The occupational health nurse advised Mary that a breast biopsy may need to be performed and counseled her on the importance of early treatment. Mary was referred to a specialist, and a fine-needle aspiration was performed. Abnormal cells were found, and a lumpectomy was performed. The occupational health nurse visited Mary at the hospital and in her home to assess her status and reassure her about her job. Community services were available to her, but her family was available to provide care. Mary was placed on 6 weeks of disability after the surgery and progressed well without complications. The occupational health nurse has the responsibility to be knowledgeable about all jobs and their demands, to determine fitness for work, and to determine the type of accommodations necessary for the employee. Before returning to work, the nurse visited Mary and cleared her to return full-time with several accommodations. Mary was placed on 8 hours a day, no lifting with the right arm of more than 5 lbs, and no excessive lifting overhead for 6 weeks. Mary visited the occupational health unit and discussed her progress with the occupational health nurse in terms of recovery and optimal return to work. Gradually, over several months, Mary was able to return to her job without restriction. The occupational health nurse played a vital role in providing information, collaborating with the physician, counseling Mary, and providing follow-up and return-to-work services at the workplace.

Various on-site occupational health nursing programs may differ in methods, but they offer an opportunity to increase the employee's knowledge and adherence to preventive care. The occupational health nurse activities within the worksite provide for earlier detection of health-related conditions that otherwise may not be detected and, more importantly, may help reduce morbidity and premature mortality. Healthcare costs are estimated to decrease with on-site occupational health nursing programs.

Summary

Preventive and primary care services are widely provided by occupational health nurse clinicians and practitioners. Within the context of the business environment, workers are exposed to a variety of work-related hazards and also bring with them lifestyle health issues that may, alone or in interaction, increase their risk of adverse health effects. Health promotion and health protection interventions are important strategies to reduce health risks and improve health status. The occupational health nurse practices within a prevention framework and as such uses primary, secondary, and tertiary prevention approaches to manage a variety of employee health risks. The worksite is an ideal setting to develop and implement these interventions to improve worker health. The occupational health nurse has a splendid opportunity to make a change to foster positive behaviors.

REFERENCES

Association for Worksite Health Promotion. (1994). *Guidelines for employee health promotion programs* (p. 2). Champaign, IL: Human Kinetics.

Caplan, L. S., & Coughlin, S. (1998). Worksite breast cancer screening programs. *AAOHN Journal 46*(9), 443–453.

Childre, F. (1997). Nurse managed occupational health services: A primary care model in practice. *AAOHN Journal 45*(10), 484–490.

Colditz, G. A., Hoaglin, D. C., & Berkey, C. S. (1997). Cancer incidence and mortality: The priority of screening frequency and population coverage. *The Milbank Quarterly 75*, 147–173.

Donnelly, W. J. (1993). Health risk appraisals can reduce health care costs. *Journal of Compensation and Benefits September–October*, 22–26.

Kerlikowske, K., Grady, D., Rubin, S. M., et al. (1995). Efficacy of screening mammography: A meta-analysis. *Journal of the American Medical Association 273*, 149–154.

National Heart, Lung, and Blood Institute. (1997). *Clinical guidelines on the identification, evaluation, and treatment of overweight and obesity in adults.* Washington, DC: US Government Printing Office.

Parker, S. L., Tong, T., Bolden, S., & Wingo, P. A., (1997). Cancer statistics 1997. *CA: A Cancer Journal for Clinicians 47*, 5–27.

Pelletier, L. R. (1993). A review and analysis of the health and cost-effective outcome studies of comprehensive health promotion and disease prevention programs at the work-site: 1991–1993 update. *American Journal of Health Promotion 8*(1), 50–62.

Reimer, B. K., Barrett, E., & Rosen, J. (1997). *Weighing the evidence about mammography for women in their forties and fifties.* Durham, NC: Blue Cross/Blue Shield.

Rogers, B. (1994). *Occupational health nursing: Concepts and practice.* Philadelphia: W. B. Saunders.

Stay Well. (1996). *Health path management survey.* St. Paul, MN: Author.

Understandings of Health: How individual perceptions of health affect health promotion needs in organizations. *AAOHN Journal 45*(7), 330–336.

Wachs, J. E. (1997). Nurse-managed occupational health centers: An overview. *AADHN Journal 45* (10), 477–483.

Woods, M. (1996). Health promotion program strategies responsive to workplace change: Successful program. *AAOHN Journal 44*(9), 447–453.

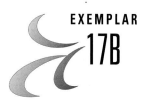

17B

An Entrepreneurial Faculty Practice Plan

Ginette A. Pepper
Maureen R. Keefe
Amy Barton
Patricia Hinton Walker

This exemplar describes the evolution of Health Care Partners (HCP), the faculty practice plan at the University of Colorado Health Sciences Center School of Nursing (SON) in Denver. HCP comprises multiple diverse practices that provide advanced practice nursing care. Following an overview of the literature on faculty practice that explains the context in which the program at the University of Colorado evolved, the development and evolution of HCP is delineated. Using table format, populations served, services provided, collaborative relationships, reimbursement mechanisms, and student involvement are summarized. The emphasis of this exemplar is on issues unique to multicomponent academic nursing faculty practice plans. The exemplar concludes with a profile of the transformation of the faculty practice plan to address changes in education and healthcare in the 21st century.

Faculty Practice

Faculty in approximately 64% of schools of nursing engage in practice activities (American Association of Colleges of Nursing [AACN], 1993; Barger, Nugent, & Bridges, 1993). Although the term *faculty practice* has only been used in the nursing literature for about 20 years, a considerable volume of articles, chapters, proceedings, and books has emerged. Chicadonz and associates (1981), Walker (1995), and Broussard, Delahoussaye, and Poirier (1996) have critically reviewed existing research on faculty practice and academic nursing centers. This section overviews the definition and history of faculty practice; summarizes existing opinion and research on the benefits, barriers, and facilitators to development of faculty practice; and outlines models of faculty practice.

DEFINITION AND PURPOSE OF FACULTY PRACTICE

Definitions of faculty practice in the nursing literature reflect diverse assumptions about its purpose. Just, Adams, and DeYoung (1989) identified two opposing positions on the focus of faculty practice: (1) clinical competence of faculty to support student learning or (2) benefit of the recipients through the advance of nursing care. More recently, authors define faculty practice as a source of revenue to enhance education and research rather than merely funding the individuals who provide the nursing services (Barger, 1995; Littlefield, Keenan, & Skillman, 1988; Rudy, 1995; Walker, 1994).

Many authors maintain that faculty practice requires direct patient care (Algase, 1986; Anderson & Pierson, 1983; Collison & Parsons, 1980; Kent, 1980; Mauksch, 1980; Rudy et al., 1995). Other definitions subsume indirect as well as direct nursing care as long as the focus is on activities that improve patient care or occur in a service setting (Barger & Bridges, 1987; Ford & Kitzman, 1983; Joel, 1983; Millonig, 1986). Student supervision in the clinical setting is considered faculty practice by some definitions (Durand, 1985; Just, Adams, & DeYoung, 1989; Potash & Taylor, 1993), but not by others (Algase, 1986; Barger, Nugent, & Bridges, 1993; Bennett, 1990). Similarly, practice conducted as an employee of an organization other than the educational institution ("moonlighting" and temporary summer employment) is included in some definitions (Anderson & Pierson, 1983; Just, Adams, & DeYoung, 1989; Potash & Taylor, 1993; Turner & Pearson, 1989) and excluded in others (Barger, Nugent, & Bridges, 1993; Batey, 1983; Durand,1985; Rudy et al., 1995). Some authors consider scholarship in the form of publication and research as the defining characteristic of faculty practice, differentiating it from practice by nurses who happen to be faculty or are practicing only to maintain clinical skills (Algase, 1986; Ford & Kitzman, 1983; Joel, 1983; Millonig, 1986; Sherwen, 1998). Although faculty practice usually involves faculty functioning in advanced practice roles, few definitions limit faculty practice to advanced practice nursing (Munroe, Sullivan, Lee, & Sarter, 1987; Stainton, Rankin, & Calkin, 1989). Clinical research, research utilization, consultation, in-service training, and continuing education of nursing staff are also identified in various descriptions of faculty practice (Burke, 1997; Keefe, 1993; Kirkpatrick, 1992; Miller, 1997; Potash & Taylor, 1993; Walker & Walker, 1995). Taylor (1996) differentiated faculty practice—the delivery of nursing services as part of the faculty role—from the faculty practice plan, which is the business strategy and organizational structure through which faculty implement the practice mission and allocate revenues to faculty, departments, and schools.

APPRAISING FACULTY PRACTICE

Much of the literature on faculty practice appraises the benefits and obstacles to faculty practice and suggests strategies to overcome the obstacles. Few of the hypothesized benefits, barriers, and strategies are supported by research, although numerous anecdotal reports in the literature suggest that many schools of nursing have had common experiences in establishing faculty practice.

Benefits of Faculty Practice

Table 17B-1 lists benefits of faculty practice reported in the nursing literature, categorized according to beneficiary: (1) clients, including patients and agency partners; (2) students; and (3) schools of nursing and faculty. Numerous investigators have reported high patient satisfaction with care in academic nursing centers and other sites of faculty practice (Adams & Partee, 1998; Gale, 1998; Gersten-Rothenberg, 1998; Lang, Evans, Jenkins, & Matthews, 1996; Neil, 1995; Schroeder & Neil, 1992). A few studies have documented quality and cost-effective patient outcomes, although research designs lacked randomization and control groups (Adams & Partee, 1998; Gale, 1998; Lang, Evans, Jenkins, & Matthews, 1996; Schroeder, 1993).

Although few studies have been done on the benefits of faculty practice to students, it is the most compelling research on faculty practice. Pugh (1988) established that students prefer faculty who are clinical role models. Kramer, Polifroni, and Organek (1986) documented higher professional craftsmanship among baccalaureate students taught by faculty

TABLE 17B-1 *Benefits of Faculty Practice*

Clients and Partners	Students	Faculty and School of Nursing
Agency Partners	Increased relevance of classroom instruction	Bridge the gap between service and academia
Access to scarce expertise		
Intellectual stimulation of staff	Socialization on business of advanced practice	Enhance credibility of faculty with clinical colleagues
Increased research activity	Practice in nursing theory-based environment	Enhance credibility of faculty with students
Theory-based practice		
Evidence-based practice	Increased student satisfaction	Fulfill community service mission
Improved communication with educators	Enhanced professionalism	
Contribute to education of new graduates	Clinically current content in classroom	Maintain faculty's clinical competence
	Experience evidence-based practice	Improved communication with clinical colleagues
	Participate in nursing research utilization	Generate topics for research and scholarship
Patients	Increased access to clinical training sites	Maintain clinically relevant curriculum
Improved access to care		Revenue enhancement for institution and individuals
Holistic, client-centered services		Faculty collaboration with physicians and other healthcare providers
Health promotion focus		
Improved outcomes		Recruit graduate students
Improved quality of care		Increased faculty satisfaction
Improved patient satisfaction		Develop and evaluate models of care
Access to alternative and complementary modalities		Implement theory-based practice

Sources: Bennett, 1990; Budden, 1994; Gersten-Rothenberg, 1998; Joachim, 1988; Kirkpatrick, 1992; Lambert & Lambert, 1988a; Littlefield, Keenan, & Skillman, 1988; Maurin, 1986; Miller, 1997; Millonig, 1986; Mundinger, 1996; Potash & Taylor, 1993; Ryan, 1997; Walker, Starck, & McNeil, 1994.

who practice. Areas in which these students surpassed students taught by faculty not currently involved in practice were self-rated professional characteristics, self-concept and self-esteem, internal locus of control, professional and bicultural behavior, and autonomy.

Research findings on the benefits of practice to faculty are contradictory. Most have shown higher satisfaction among practicing faculty (Just, Adams, & DeYoung, 1989; Maurin, 1986; Nugent, Barger, & Bridges, 1993; Steele, 1991), but one study found no differences (Acorn, 1991). Ryan and Barger-Lux (1985) found greater scholarly productivity among faculty who practiced compared with nonpracticing faculty, but other researchers (Acorn, 1991; Barger & Bridges, 1987) found no differences. Various studies comparing role strain of practicing and nonpracticing faculty have reported greater strain in practicing faculty (Higgs, 1988), less strain in practicing faculty (Steele, 1991), and no difference between the two groups (Acorn, 1991; Lambert & Lambert, 1993).

Obstacles to Faculty Practice

Barriers to faculty practice cited in the nursing literature, as well as strategies to overcome these obstacles, are summarized in Table 17B-2. Survey research studies consistently evidence lack of support structures for faculty practice (Anderson & Pierson, 1983; Barger, 1986; Barger & Bridges, 1987; Barger, Nugent, & Bridges, 1992; Higgs, 1988; Nugent, Barger, & Bridges, 1993; Potash & Taylor, 1993. Only 10% of schools had a written faculty practice plan. Cross-sequential surveys showed no improvement in the structural support for faculty practice during a 5-year period (Barger & Bridges, 1987; Barger, Nugent, & Bridges, 1992).

HISTORY OF FACULTY PRACTICE

Under the Nightingale model that dominated nursing education in many countries well into the 1960s, teachers practiced and clinicians taught (Henry, 1995). Faculty practice was proposed in the United States to correct the schism between education and service that developed when nursing education moved from the hospital into the university beginning in the 1940s (Christy, 1980; Just, Adams, & DeYoung, 1989; Mauksch, 1980). The relocation of nursing education to academic institutions resulted in a similar gap between education and service in other industrialized countries, such as Canada and Britain (Baillie, 1994; Fairbrother & Ford, 1998; Joachim, 1988). The faculty practice movement gained impetus in the United States when 13 prominent leaders in nursing issued the Statement of Belief Regarding Faculty Practice (1979), which triggered nursing organizations to conduct national meetings and issue position papers supporting faculty practice. Several analyses of the history of faculty practice and its impact on the unification of nursing service and nursing education have been published (Christy, 1980; Lambert & Lambert, 1988a; Millonig, 1986).

MODELS OF FACULTY PRACTICE

Four models of nursing faculty practice have been identified (Bennett, 1990; Millonig, 1986; Potash & Taylor, 1993; Stainton, Rankin, & Calkin, 1989). Although moonlighting is sometimes labeled a faculty practice model, it is not considered here because the faculty member practices outside the assigned faculty duties and no direct impact on the school of nursing is experienced.

Unification Model

The unification model involves consolidating the administration, budgets, and governance of the clinical agency and the school of nursing. Members of the faculty have appointments both as clinicians and teachers. Two successful unification structures implemented in 1972 at Rush-Presbyterian University in Chicago, IL by Luther Christman (1979) and the University of Rochester in Rocheser, NY by Loretta Ford (1980) remain unique examples of this model.

Collaboration Model

In the collaboration model, the administration of the school of nursing and clinical agency are separate, but some of the teachers and clinicians have joint appointments with responsibilities both in service and academia. Examples of this model include the School of Nursing at Case Western Reserve University in Cleveland, OH (Schlotfeldt & MacPhail, 1969), the primary affiliation partnerships at the University of Southern California in Los Angeles, CA (Munroe, Sillivan, Lee, & Sarter, 1987), joint appointments at the University of Calgary in Alberta, Canada (Stainton, Rankin, & Calkin, 1989), and the University of Iowa Iowa City, IA Collaboration Model (Kelly et al., 1990).

TABLE 17B-2 *Barriers to Faculty Practice and Strategies to Overcome Barriers*

Barriers to Faculty Practice*	Strategies to Overcome Barriers
Financial Vulnerability of School	
Lack of business expertise of faculty	Develop business plan using consultants as needed (Barger, 1995; Walker, 1994)
University policies preclude assuming financial risk	Cultivate community involvement (Barger, 1995; Phillips & Steel, 1994; Walker, 1994)
Lack of access to third-party payment	Seek grants from private foundations and government (Elsberry & Nelson, 1993; Phillips & Steele, 1994)
Decreased revenues from tuition, state, and university to underwrite faculty practice and nursing centers	Develop a marketing plan (Barger, 1995; Walker, 1994)
	Set adequate fees (Elsberry & Nelson, 1993)
	Diversify services (Finkler, Knickman, & Hanson, 1994; Walker, 1994; Walker, Starck, & McNeil, 1994)
	Develop partnerships to share risk (Elsberry & Nelson, 1993; Mackey & McNeil, 1996)
	Merge with an established medical faculty practice plan to access payers (Lambert & Lambert, 1988b; Parsons, Felton, & Chassie, 1996)
	Ensure adequate information management systems for business, clinical, and research needs and document cost and quality outcomes (Walker & Walker, 1995)
Faculty Work Load Issues	
No release from usual responsibilities to practice	Financial plan includes coverage for weekends, evenings, vacations, and substitute classroom teachers (McNeil & Mackey, 1995)
Conflict between needs of students and needs of patients if concurrent teacher and practitioner roles	
Requirement to work evenings, weekends, holidays, and school breaks	Integrate research and education into clinical activity (Potash & Taylor, 1993; Ryan, 1997)
Role strain and burnout	Adjust work load to accommodate faculty practice responsibilities (Barnes, Duldt, & Green, 1994)
Decreased quality of family life	
Competition with activities required to attain tenure	Computerized information systems to facilitate teaching and research roles as well as patient care (Lundeen, 1995; Walker & Walker, 1995, 1996)
Lack of appropriate clinical sites; instability of nursing centers	
	Develop broad definition of practice to capitalize on faculty expertise (Bennett, 1990, Lambert & Lambert, 1988b)
	Flexible scheduling by agency or clinical site (Nugent, Barger, & Bridges, 1993)
	Use practice revenues for expenses to support activities of other missions, e.g., computers, teaching assistants, research assistants, and replacement faculty (McNeil & Mackey, 1995)

TABLE 17B-2 *Barriers to Faculty Practice and Strategies to Overcome Barriers*

Barriers to Faculty Practice*	Strategies to Overcome Barriers
Lack of Incentives and Rewards	
Perceived lack of administrative support	Develop criteria for scholarly practice and develop structures for evaluating practice activity (Sherwen, 1998)
No financial incentive	
Not rewarded in tenure and promotion criteria	Allow sabbaticals to involve clinical practice activity (Lassan, 1994)
Peer resentment	Develop practice plans for revenue sharing with practicing faculty (AACN, 1993; McNeil & Mackey, 1995; Williamson, McDonough, & Boettcher, 1990)
Faculty may need to retool for advanced practice roles	
Difficult to keep up with advances with part time practice	Revise promotion and tenure criteria to value scholarship of application or develop dual (clinical and tenure) tracks (Walker, Starck, & McNeil, 1994)
	Develop broad definition of practice to capitalize on faculty expertise (Bennett, 1990; Walker, 1994)
-	Promote research on barriers and model reward systems (Barger, Nugent, & Bridges, 1993)
Opposition from the Medical Profession	
Fear of competition	Multisite, rigorous cost and outcome studies (Barger, Nugent, & Bridges, 1993; Gersten-Rothenberg, 1998; Riesch, 1992)
Concerns about quality of care	Establish mechanisms for communication and collaboration with the medical community (Mundinger, 1996; Phillips & Steel, 1994; Potash & Taylor, 1993)

*Sources: AACN, 1993; Barger, 1993; Barger & Crumpton, 1991; Barnes, Duldt, & Green, 1994; Broussard, Delahoussye, & Poirrier, 1996; Budden, 1994; Gersten-Rothenberg, 1998; Kirkpatrick, 1992; Lambert & Lambert, 1993; Nugent, Barger, & Bridges, 1993; Rodgers & Peake-Godin, 1988; Rudy et al., 1995

Integrated Model and Academic Nursing Centers

In the integrated model, faculty and students share responsibility for patient care in an academic nursing center that is an integral part of the school of nursing. Nursing centers, also called *nurse-managed centers, community nursing organizations,* or *nurse-run clinics,* are defined by the following characteristics: (1) nurse control of practice; (2) direct access by the patient or client to nursing care; and (3) holistic, client-centered, reimbursed services (Barger & Bridges, 1990; Riesch, 1992).

Of the approximately 250 nursing centers in the United States, it has been estimated that 40 to 80 are affiliated with schools of nursing (Barger, Nugent, & Bridges, 1993; Lockhart, 1995; Phillips & Steele, 1994). Nearly all academic nursing centers involve practice by faculty who are advanced practice nurses (AACN, 1993; Phillips & Steele, 1994). The variety of services provided in academic nursing centers, predominantly to underserved populations, include health promotion and disease prevention, developmental assessment and counseling, treatment of acute minor and major illnesses, initial evaluation and follow-up of chronic health problems, case management and care coordination, prenatal and post-partum care, mental health counseling, behavioral interventions, family planning and pre-scription services, student and employee health services, prison healthcare, nontraditional alternative and complementary therapies, and home care (AACN, 1993; Aydelotte et al., 1987; Adams-Davis & Fitzpatrick, 1995; Barger, 1993; Coggiola & Walker, 1995; Gilti-

TABLE 17B-3 Summary of Faculty Practice Sites, University of Colorado Health Sciences Center School of Nursing

Practice Name	Population	Students/wk	H/wk	No. of Exam Rooms	Annual No. of Visits	Year Initiated	Medical Collaboration	Payer Mix	Partners
Carin Clinic	0–18 y	8	12	4	1100	1993	MDPN	Uninsured 90%, self-pay 5%, Medicaid 5%	Hospital, school district, city government
Jefferson Hills	Adolescent, high risk, 12–18 y	4	8	2	1000	1994	Private practice MD	Medicaid 90%, private 10%	Private facility
Sheridan School Based Clinic	10–20 y	10	40	2	1379	1994	MDPN	Medicaid 7%, self-pay 2%, uninsured 89%	Hospital, city government, grants
Adams County School District #50	3–11 y from district	2	40	2	2500	1998	Private physician practice	Medicaid 10%, CHP Plus 2%, uninsured 88%	School district, 4 hospitals, county health department, county mental health department, grant from foundation
Gilliam	Incarcerated youth 12–18 y	10	40	2	4680	1995	Private practice MD	Data unavailable	Colorado Division of Youth Services
Family Tree/Golden	0–21 y	3	8	2		1996	MDPN	Data unavailable	Hospital, family resource center
Jeffco Action Center	Homeless children & adults	3	8	2	672	1995	MDPN	Medicaid 20%, uninsured 80%	Hospital, Jefferson Action Center
Women in Crisis (battered women's shelter)	Women & children	3	8	2	472	1995	MDPN	Medicaid 30%, uninsured 40%, insured, self-pay 30%	Hospital, HMO
CNM's University Hospital	Employees, students, OB/GYN	1–2	Clinic: 16, hospital: 168	2	700	1973	Medical School Department of OB/GYN	Medicaid 77%, insurance 11%, self-pay 2%, discount 9%	University Hospital & Department of OB/GYN
CNM's Fitzsimons	OB/GYN Military	1	Clinic: 8, hospital: 168	2	250–300	1997	Medical School Department of OB/GYN	Military 90%, Medicaid 10%	University Hospital & Department of OB/GYN

Program	Population				Volume	Year	Medical director	Funding	Affiliation
CNM's Aurora	GYN annual exams	1	8	1–2	250–300	1998	Medical School Department of OB/GYN	Military 60%, other insurance 40%	University Hospital & Department of OB/GYN
CNM's Littleton	GYN annual exams & OB visits	0	8	1–2	100	1998	Medical School Department of OB/GYN	Military 90%, other insurance 10%	University Hospital & Department of OB/GYN
Boulder Internal Medicine	Adult, geriatrics	1	8	5	750	1998	MD	Medicare, Medicaid, private insurance	None
Littleton Health & Wellness	Family, obstetrics, pediatrics	2	40	3	1350	1993	University-affiliated family medicine practice	Self-pay 90%, Medicaid 8%, Medicare/other 2%	Community Center, recreation district
Jefferson County Jail	Inmates	New	20	2	New	1998	Denver Health & Hospitals	N/A	Jefferson County
Partnership in Prevention (PIP)	At-risk middle school youth	2	28	N/A	Variable	1993	N/A	N/A	Colorado Alcohol & Drug Abuse Division Schools district
Brighton Senior Center	Older than 55 y	1–2	8–10	2	1000	1982	N/A	Donation	City government
Children's Hospital Pain Team	0–20 y	1/wk	168	N/A	350	1992	Interdisciplinary & anethesiologist	Private insurance, Medicaid, HMO, Medicare, etc.	Hospital (joint appointment)
Denver Women's Correctional Facility	Inmates	New	40	2	New	1998	NA	NA	Colorado Department of Corrections
Samaritan House	Homeless adults & pediatrics	5	16	2	1200	1998	Private MD	Grants	Hospital, city government, Catholic Charities

N/A indicates not available.

nan & Murray, 1992; Hale, Harper, & Dawson, 1996; Patton, Conrad, & Kriedler, 1995; Phillips & Steele, 1994; Richie et al., 1996; Smerke, 1990; Tranzillo, 1995; Walker, 1994).

Unfortunately, surveys indicated that academic nursing centers have frequently been short lived, generated less income than other forms of faculty practice, and often failed to survive the termination of grant support (Barger, Nugent, & Bridges, 1993; B. Dunn & J. K. Henry, personal communication, June 10, 1997; Gersten-Rothenberg, 1998; Higgs, 1988). Several authors analyzed this trend and recommended strategies to promote survival of academic nursing centers (Barger, 1995; Gersten-Rothenberg, 1998; Walker, 1994).

Entrepreneurial Model

Faculty determine goals and services in the entrepreneurial model and implement the services as part of the faculty role. Although the entrepreneurial model is also called the *private practice model,* types of services, client population, practice setting, and business arrangements vary widely and frequently do not resemble those of private practice. Student education and clinical research are usually integral to practices in the entrepreneurial model in academic settings. Examples of faculty practice plans in the entrepreneurial model include the University of Tennessee College of Nursing in Memphis (Potash & Taylor, 1993), the Medical College of Georgia School of Nursing in Augusta (Williamson, McDonough, & Boettcher, 1990), the College of Nursing at the University of South Carolina in Columbia (Parsons, Felton, & Chassie, 1996), the University of Utah College of Nursing in Salt Lake City (Amos, 1996), and the community coalition at Arizona State University in Tempe (Gale, 1998). A growing number of schools of nursing have mixed-model faculty practice. In addition, the distinctions between integration and entrepreneurial models are increasingly ambiguous. It is likely that distinctions among models of faculty practice will continue to blur in the future as more schools of nursing develop multifaceted practice activities.

Evolution of Health Care Partners Faculty Practice Plan

This exemplar describes three phases in the evolution of HCP: (1) initial design and development, (2) interim maintenance, and (3) transformation. Each phase approximately corresponded with the leadership of a different dean and practice administrator. HCP is most appropriately characterized as an entrepreneurial faculty practice model because it comprises multiple practice sites, each initiated by an individual faculty member or small group of faculty. Table 17B-3 summarizes the current practice sites of HCP, excluding sites that closed in the 5 years since the plan was initiated.

ENVIRONMENT

The University of Colorado Health Sciences Center SON, one of the oldest university-affiliated schools in the United States, was established in 1898 on the Boulder campus and moved to the Health Sciences campus in Denver in 1924. The SON offers Bachelor of Science in Nursing (BSN), Masters of Science (MS), Doctor of Philosophy (PhD), and Nursing Doctorate (ND) degrees, as well as post-Master's certification in advanced practice nursing and other postgraduate professional development offerings. In the mid-1960s the SON began the first nurse practitioner program in the world in partnership with the School of Medicine. The SON also shares the research-intensive campus with the School of Dentistry, School of Pharmacy, Graduate School, two hospitals, and numerous centers and institutes. The School of Medicine has a well-established faculty practice plan, and the other professional schools have developed faculty practice plans within the past 2 to 8 years. The University is governed by an elected Board of Regents. Each of the four campuses has a separate budget and administrative governance under the direction of a chancellor.

In the 1980s when Jean Watson was dean, the SON adopted a collaborative faculty practice model. Chief nursing officers of four closely affiliated clinical agencies were appointed as associate deans for clinical practice by the Board of Regents. Five nurse researchers with adjoint or joint appointments established the Denver Collaborative Research Network between the SON Center for Nursing Research and clinical agencies (Keefe, Pepper, & Stoner, 1988). Other joint appointments and clinical faculty designations have included practitioner–teachers, clinical teaching scholars, and clinical teaching associates (De Voogd & Salbenblatt, 1989; Phillips & Kaempfer, 1987). Watson's (1985, 1988, 1990) philosophy and science of human caring was the conceptual framework for the educational and practice activities of the SON.

The SON established its first nurse-managed practice in the 1970s as a nursing clinic in a senior center in Brighton, a rural town northeast of Denver. Midwifery practice was an integral part the midwifery Master's specialty option beginning in the 1980s, supported by a federal division of nursing training grant, practice revenues, and hospitals. The Denver Nursing Project in Human Caring (the "Caring Center"), a nursing center for human immunodeficiency virus (HIV) and acquired immunodeficiency syndrome (AIDS) care, was founded in 1988 as a collaboration of three hospitals and the SON (Smerke, 1990). The Caring Center subsequently received Division of Nursing Special Projects grants, foundation grants, contracts, and donations (Neil, 1995). In addition, many faculty members were practicing under a Universitywide faculty policy called "The 1/6th Rule," which allows full-time faculty to expend one-sixth of their effort in consultation or other community service and to retain remuneration with approval of their dean or department chair. The SON identified three faculty tracks (tenure, research, and clinical), with separate criteria for promotion in the 1980s. Although the mission of the campus included patient care and much practice activity took place in the SON, before 1992 faculty practice was still marginal and practice was not a primary mission of the SON.

PHASE I: DESIGN AND DEVELOPMENT

In 1992, the position of associate dean for practice was created and charged by the dean, Claire Martin, PhD, FAAN, with the development and implementation of a faculty practice program to serve the SON education and research missions. Beginning in January 1992, a faculty task force began to work with the administrators through a seven-step planning process: initial assessment and survey, definition of purpose, creation of a definition, development of membership guidelines, exploration of organizational options, development and approval of a concept paper, and formulation of bylaws. Concurrently, strategic planning for development of new practice sites was conducted.

Initial Assessment of Practice Activity

The first action of the task force was to survey faculty and inventory existing faculty practice activity. The survey identified 20 different clinical projects and faculty practice activities, which were classified into the following revenue categories: fee for service, contract, grant, and pro bono. More than half of the activity was pro bono practice that did not involve student learning or research opportunities. Other early activities of the task force included review of the literature, analysis of faculty practice plans from other professional schools on the campus and from schools of nursing nationwide, and arranging for consultants from schools with established practice plans to work with faculty in development of the plan.

Defining Purpose and Benefits

The task force identified eight priorities that formed the rationale for proceeding to develop a plan and served as the core of the concept paper. These priorities included developing and testing innovative care delivery models, improving access to care for underserved individuals, enhancing student learning experiences, ensuring continuing clinical expertise of the faculty, showcasing nursing expertise in health promotion, increasing community involvement, engaging in outcome research, and contributing additional revenue. The consensus of the task force was that the implementation of a faculty practice plan would allow the SON to carry out its mandates more effectively in the areas of nursing education, research, and service.

Faculty Practice Definition

Faculty of the SON favored a broad definition of faculty practice that included families, groups, organizations, and communities within the definition of client; recognized consultation as practice; and stipulated a nursing theory context. The following definition of faculty practice provided a guiding philosophical statement:

> Faculty practice is the art, science and application of theory and research in service to clients, families and communities. Faculty practice includes, but is not limited to, provision of direct nursing services to individuals and groups, as well as technical assistance and consultation to health care providers and community agencies to the end of advancing health in individuals, groups and communities. Faculty practice in this framework encompasses health promotion and disease prevention activities, acute and episodic care, restorative and rehabilitative services, long-term chronic disease management, and care across the life span. It may include first contact, but will emphasize continuity and coordination of care. A distinguishing characteristic of faculty practice within the School of Nursing is the focus on human caring and the delivery of health care service addressing the whole person within a human caring and healing context.

Defining Faculty Membership and Enrollment Criteria

From the outset of planning, one of the most contentious issues was enrollment criteria for HCP. Campus administrators advised emulating the School of Medicine faculty practice plan requirement that members waive the 1/6th Rule (see the "Environment" section) so that no ambiguity would exist in what activities were covered by the plan. Most SON faculty opposed requiring waiver of the 1/6th Rule, which had been a faculty right since the 1940s. In addition, faculty identified other barriers to practice, which have been described in the literature and summarized previously. As a result of these concerns, faculty supported two levels of membership. All faculty, as defined in the SON bylaws, were members of HCP, eligible to vote and serve on the governing board. Faculty who had signed the member agreement and were practicing at approved practice sites as part of their faculty assignment were accorded governmental immunity from civil liability and were covered by the University of Colorado Self-Insurance and Risk Management Trust. These members were also eligible for incentives such as professional development support; salary supplement; research assistant support; and equipment purchases such as computers, software, and publications. Faculty practicing under the 1/6th Rule were not accorded these benefits. Revenues such as royalties, episodic honoraria, grant review stipends, and expert witness fees were excluded from reportable practice plan income.

Selecting Among Legal Entity Options

The task force had to determine whether the faculty practice should be structured as an entity within the University or as a separate legal entity, a 501c.3 nonprofit corporation. The SON could either establish a new 501c.3 nonprofit corporation for its faculty practice or merge with the medical practice plan (University Physicians Incorporated) as affiliate members. A new tax-limiting referendum in Colorado had placed a limit on growth in revenues and expenditures of state governmental agencies, except within a new legal entity called an *enterprise*. Establishing the practice plan within the University structure meant either a cap on growth, which was hardly desirable for a new venture, or forming an enterprise that would still be subject to government bureaucracy and policies for hiring, purchasing, and accounting. The task force elected to form a new 501c.3 nonprofit corporation to accommodate the diversity of services and payment mechanisms anticipated, to promote the flexibility that would be required to respond to healthcare reform initiatives that were paramount in 1992, and to maintain the autonomy necessary to distinguish the unique contributions of advanced practice nursing.

Concept Paper and Approval

During the May 1993 general faculty meeting, the faculty unanimously voted to seek administrative and Regental approval to develop bylaws and create a practice entity. The resolution was forwarded to the chancellor, and then to the president and regents of the University, and included the concept paper and a set of 5-year business pro forma on all existing and proposed practice sites. The Board of Regents approved the development of a practice plan for the SON in October 1993 with the recommendation that the plan be initiated as an enterprise auxiliary of the University instead of as an independent nonprofit corporation.

Organizational Structure and Bylaws

The task force recommended the establishment of a standing committee of the faculty governance to address practice issues, just as the Research Council and Curriculum Committees addressed other missions. With faculty approval, the Practice Council was initiated and worked with administrators, campus legal council, and campus fiscal officers to write bylaws, which included the sections outlined in Box 17B-1.

Governance and Administration

The governance and administration of HCP was vested in three interlinked structures: the Practice Council, the Governing Board, and the Faculty Practice Office. Community involvement through an external advisory board was also stipulated in the concept paper and bylaws to ensure SON commitment to increasing involvement with a variety of sectors of the community. The Governing Board consisted of the five-member Practice Council representing each of the faculty teams, two faculty-elected members-at-large, the dean, and the associate dean for practice. The budget officer of the SON and the University legal counsel were ex officio members. Responsibilities of the Board included setting policies for the professional, legal, and business conduct of the practice; approving practice sites; and being accountable for the fiscal status of the practice plan. A Faculty Practice Office was established under the direction of the associate dean for practice to provide administrative, planning, budgeting, contracting, and billing support for the practice plan. Initially, staff included a special projects director, an administrative assistant, and a part-time research assistant.

Practice Site Development

The selection of sites, populations served, and services provided was based on several criteria, including unmet healthcare needs of the population, faculty expertise and interest, the degree to which the site could contribute to student learning, opportunity for research and

---

BOX 17B-1 | *Articles of Health Care Partners Bylaws*

Mission statement, including definition and purpose
Membership, including eligibility, liability, and work load agreements
Organizational structure, including legal entity and governance
Financial mechanism, including revenue sources and disbursement guidelines
Amendment process

nursing innovation, administrative and fiscal sustainability, and the extent to which the sites and services fit with the overall mission and goals of the SON. Potential practice sites were initially identified by faculty, but once the community became aware of the SON faculty practice plan, community and governmental agencies also proposed projects. Some practice ventures emerged from the Community Assessment Project, a 20-year project of SON community health faculty and graduate students involving an in-depth analysis of the health needs of a different community each semester or year (Stoner, Magilvy, & Schultz, 1992). Based on the initial needs assessment, a comprehensive proposal was developed for each proposed site, including summary of professional services, business plans and pro formas, and marketing plans. Approximately 50% to 75% of these initial proposals proceeded to the contract stage. The staff of the Faculty Practice Office also assisted the community partners and faculty in writing grant proposals to support the practice sites. The rapid growth and diverse revenue profile of the HCP practice sites reflected in Table 17B-3 represents the effectiveness of combining entrepreneurial commitment with administrative support.

Revenue Disbursement

A separate account was maintained for each practice site or contract, but overall revenues exceeded $1.2 million in the first year of the practice plan. Funds generated through the faculty practice plan were disbursed in accordance with the following priorities:

1. Costs incurred by the practice such as personnel (faculty, support staff, and consultants), operating, travel, and equipment costs. Indirect costs were identified for each project, including fees to cover site-specific services of the Practice Office.
2. Assessments, including (1) a University fee of approximately 4% on all expenditures to pay for personnel, accounting, and other services; (2) a Practice Office fee of 5% of revenues to cover general services of the Practice Office; and (3) the Academic Enrichment Fund (AEF) assessment of 5% of revenues, used at the discretion of the dean for practice, education, and research initiatives. AEF assessment could be increased by the Governing Board to a maximum of 10%.
3. Funds for salary supplements and incentives such as professional development, research or teaching assistants, and equipment such as computers.

Research and Information Systems

Based on needs analysis, information system requirements for computerized patient records, administration and billing, and research functions were specified. Practice Office staff and Practice Council members used these specifications to review clinical information software demonstrated by vendors. Because faculty members were interested in the impact of nursing systems on outcomes, it was essential that data could be output into a relational database. The system produced by MedicaLogic of Portland, OR, was most congruent with these expectations. The company agreed to supply site licenses for a nominal fee for ClinicaLogic and Logician, the Windows-based version then in development. This system included modules for the electronic patient record, pharmacology reference, laboratory interface, patient education, and appointment scheduling. In exchange, HCP contracted to provide the company with consultation on modifying the software to meet the unique needs of nursing centers. Although practicing faculty members were enthusiastic about the system, inadequate hardware and computer networking in the practice sites precluded full benefit from this partnership for either party, so the contract was terminated in 1995.

PHASE II: INTERIM MAINTENANCE

When the dean and associate dean for practice accepted leadership positions at other universities in 1995, the SON experienced an interlude with an interim dean and a temporary practice administrator. Typical of such periods in academic units, the goal was to maintain programs and avoid commitments that would limit the options of the next dean. The primary activities in HCP during this interval were managing growth, revisiting the legal entity dilemma, and performing general maintenance functions.

Managing Growth

Practice sites were opened and expanded during the interim period. One of the problems with this positive growth was a shortage of qualified nurses who had the 2 years of advanced practice clinical experience required for SON faculty appointment. This policy was meant to ensure that faculty have adequate clinical experience before they are charged with clinical supervision of students. Shortage of qualified faculty prompted proposals for modification of criteria for appointment in the clinical track or establishment of advanced practice nurse residencies within the faculty practice, which were not implemented because the shortage resolved.

More challenging was negative growth, that is, closure of sites, attributable to the changing healthcare environment. Two hospitals eliminated the position of nurse researcher when the faculty in the joint appointments took other jobs, reflecting a national trend of eliminating research and education positions in hospitals. Revolutionary changes in the care of HIV and AIDS patients caused by new drug treatments abolished the mandate for the Caring Center. The hospital hosting one of the midwifery practices closed without advanced notice. Although the midwives relocated to another hospital, patient volume and revenues fell significantly. University rules governing faculty appointments did not allow the midwifery faculty to be laid off until the next contract cycle, resulting in an $80,000 financial liability to the practice plan that had to be retired through an additional assessment on other practices. Because these revenues would have been expended on salary supplements and incentives to faculty in the successful practices, the assessment affected the morale of even the most enthusiastic supporters of the practice plan. SON administration and HCP governing revised personnel procedures to minimize future risk of similar occurrences. Closure of practice sites also required new policies for storage and retention of patient records and accumulation of vacation, which constituted a financial liability when faculty resigned and had to be paid for accumulated vacation time.

Revisiting the Legal Entity Dilemma

Based on the recommendation of the Board of Regents, HCP was organized as an enterprise within the University of Colorado. As a result, policies governing faculty appointment and termination, designed to protect academic teaching faculty who can only start a job at the beginning of a semester, applied to faculty in clinical positions. This caused untenable financial liability to the practice plan. A proposal for partnership of the HCP enterprise with the Faculty Practice Plan of the School of Medicine offered numerous advantages in contracting, financial accounting, and personnel policies but met resistance from nursing and medical faculty similar to that reported by others (Parsons, Felton, & Chassie, 1996). Administrators of the medical faculty practice plan terminated the collaboration when they learned that they were to undergo financial audit by the federal government, fearing the partnership might increase their exposure to the high fines that have been assessed on other medical school practice plans. At this point, the HCP Board of Governor's requested administrative approval to pursue 501c.3 application because formation of a nonprofit, tax-exempt corporation afforded the optimal opportunity for financial success.

Performing Practice Maintenance Functions

Barger (1995) described seven major implementation issues that schools face as they develop or expand nursing centers: funding, integration into the community, service, marketing, legal and regulatory, faculty, and research issues. Although all of these were relevant to HCP, two required the most attention during the interim phase. Legal and regulatory issues such as Clinical Laboratory Improvement Amendment (CLIA) compliance, Occupational Safety and Health Administration (OSHA) regulations on exposure to bloodborne pathogens, and prescriptive authority were managed through partnerships. For example, a nurse who worked for one of the collaborating hospitals helped SON faculty establish clinics operated in partnership with the hospital. She set up the policies and ensured compliance with CLIA and OSHA standards, standards for storage of vaccines, and other routine quality monitors. HCP contracted with the hospital for the services of the nurse to assist other sites to achieve compliance. Similarly, HCP contracted with Metropolitan Denver Provider Network (MDPN), a federally qualified community health center, for medical consultation and backup for several practice sites. MDPN physicians signed protocols before prescriptive authority for nurses in Colorado, served as collaborating physicians once faculty attained prescriptive authority, and participated in quality management committees. In return, HCP contracted to provide midwifery services to MDPN patients.

How to credit faculty work load for teaching in a faculty practice context was another challenging issue, particularly in practices operating in deficit or close to the break-even point. HCP faculty were generally expected to generate revenues to cover their salary, benefits, and practice assessments for the time spent in practice. Faculty estimated it took about 20% longer to provide care in concert with a student, depending on the level and ability of the student. Thus, the presence of students decrease the potential income in a practice site. In contrast, faculty who practiced in settings without students but visited students in external clinical practice sites received separate work load credit for each activity. Although faculty who taught students in the faculty practices sites were convinced it is optimal clinical education, many challenged the equity of applying traditional faculty work load formulas to this model of clinical teaching. Several remedies were proposed and piloted, but the issue persisted through the interim period.

PHASE III: TRANSFORMING FACULTY PRACTICE FOR A NEW CENTURY

The arrival of a new dean, Patricia Hinton Walker, PhD, FAAN, marked an opportunity for faculty to rethink strategies for integrating the missions of the school in light of anticipated changes in healthcare and education in the next century. Four practice-inquiry foci were defined to structure curriculum, research, and practice: human experience of health, illness, and healing; human–technology interface; environmental contexts of health and healthcare delivery; and quality and cost-effective outcomes. Reorganization was initiated to realign programs with the core missions of the school and to enhance resource coordination. For faculty practice, this involved creation of the International Center for Integrative Caring Practice. This "center without walls" is an umbrella structure to be organized as a 501c.3 nonprofit corporation that incorporates faculty practice, international health programs, and the former Center for Human Caring. An organizational chart for the new center is shown in Figure 17B-1.

Faculty Practice Into the 21st Century

Faculty practice at the SON will continue to emphasize community partnerships, provision of primary care, and consultative services. Consultative services are arranged based on the expertise of individual faculty members. The fastest growing area of practice is within the corrections environment. The SON currently has contracts with the state department of corrections, the state division of youth services, a county jail, and a privately operated juvenile detention facility. Most of the practices are funded through contracts with collaborating agencies. The practice also has contracts with Medicare; Medicaid; and Colorado Access, a Medicaid health maintenance organization. In addition, third-party payers are billed for services at two sites. A local billing agency submits claims and provides monthly reports at minimal cost. A standardized quality improvement plan is used to provide support to the nurse

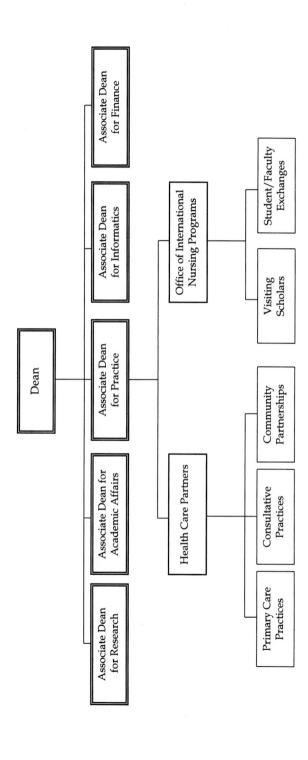

FIGURE 17B-1 Organizational Structure of the International Center for Integrative Caring Practice at the University of Colorado Health Sciences Center School of Nursing, Denver.

practitioners across primary care sites. Two to three standard indicators are selected annually, providing individual sites with the option of adding their own indicators.

International Programs

The Office of International Nursing Programs facilitates interdisciplinary activities in diverse cultures and global healthcare. In concert with the campus Office of International Health Care Programs, the SON is engaging in the enhancement of primary healthcare training. Office staff provide assistance to international scholars in structuring visits to the campus. In addition, this office organizes faculty and student exchange with international communities.

The Center for Human Caring visiting scholars program was established to bring together faculty with scholars from the humanities, arts, and social and behavioral sciences to enhance the study, research, and practice of human caring knowledge. It is a multidisciplinary focal point for generating philosophy, theory, research, advanced clinical practice, and ethics related to human caring. Inclusion of this entity within the broader international center promotes collaboration in the implementation of theory-guided research, education, and practice. Currently, research is under way to measure the outcomes of caring practice.

The International Center for Integrative Caring Practice is under the direction of Amy Barton, PhD, RN, associate dean for practice. The Center is staffed by Jean Watson, PhD, FAAN, distinguished professor, and Phyllis Updike, DNS, RN, interim coordinator of international nursing programs.

Creating an Informatics Infrastructure

Facilitating the infrastructure for primary care practices has been challenging because of the extent of collaborative relationships that are required to provide care to vulnerable populations. A major challenge faced by faculty nurse practitioners is that the patient charts are usually owned by the partner agencies and not by the SON. This requires that data be recorded on different forms for each site. As a result, faculty practitioners find themselves in a situation similar to many of their colleagues across the country: necessary data are not available to describe patient problems that nurses manage, actions that nurses take to prevent or resolve problems, or resources that nurses use to accomplish patient outcomes (Delaney & Moorhead, 1995). This also impedes research in practice settings.

The SON clinical faculty members have adopted use of the Omaha System to describe and document their practice. The Visiting Nurse Association (VNA) of Omaha developed the Omaha System. It is a community practice–based language that was developed over 20 years based on 11 years of federally funded research (Martin & Scheet, 1995). The Omaha System has three components: the Problem Classification Scheme, the Intervention Scheme, and the Problem Rating Scale for Outcomes (Martin & Scheet, 1992). Since its inception, the system has been implemented beyond the VNA environment to sites such as community-based nursing clinics (Coenen, Marek, & Lundeen, 1996), schools of nursing (Bednarz, 1998), ambulatory care centers, homeless clinics, residential centers, and correctional centers (Martin & Scheet, 1992).

The SON is in the process of standardizing minimum data collection across sites to effectively assess patient health outcomes. This will be accomplished through design of a standardized face sheet that will incorporate the Nursing Minimum Data Set (NMDS) elements (Werley & Lange, 1988; Werley, Lange, & Westlake, 1986; Werley, Ryan, & Zorn, 1995). The 16 items that comprise the NMDS are categorized as nursing care items, patient demographic items, and service items. The benefit of using the Omaha System for faculty practice is that the framework allows for the inclusion of specific assessment tools for research projects without having to modify the structure of the system. Thus, practice-based research is becoming a reality at our clinical sites, as indicated by the partial list of current projects shown in Box 17B-2.

BOX 17B-2	*Examples of Recent Research at Health Care Partners Faculty Practice Sites*

Prescriptive practices of nurse practitioners

Outcomes of otitis media treatment in nursing clinics

Cost and outcomes of a nursing center for HIV and AIDS care

Comparison of student learning in faculty practice nursing centers and physician offices and clinics

Development of a caring-based patient satisfaction instrument

HIV education for incarcerated youth

Rate of exposure of children to second-hand tobacco smoke

Group therapy for children of drug-addicted adults

Mentorship for at-risk youth

 ## Conclusions

This exemplar overviewed three phases of the evolution of a multicomponent faculty practice plan. The development of HCP illustrated concepts from the nursing literature on faculty practice, including diverse purposes of faculty practice, barriers and facilitators, and models of practice. Other themes from the literature present in this exemplar included issues of structural support for practicing faculty; the imperative for information systems to support scholarship; and the need for diversification, sound business planning, marketing, and partnerships to ensure financial stability.

Essential Points to Remember

- Major purposes of faculty practice are improving client health, enhancing student learning, promoting clinical scholarship, advancing the nursing profession, promoting scholarship and research, maintaining faculty competence, and generating revenues;
- Models of faculty practice are unification, collaboration, integration, entrepreneurial, and "moonlighting";
- Although research on faculty practice is limited, studies have shown benefit to patient outcomes and student learning. Studies show contradictory results on benefit to faculty and lack of support structure for practicing faculty;
- The term *faculty practice plan* refers to the business strategy and organizational structure through which faculty implement the practice mission and allocate revenues to faculty, departments, and schools;
- Diversification of sites, services, and revenue sources promotes success of faculty practice plans; and
- Information system development is crucial for scholarly productivity in faculty practice.

REFERENCES

Acorn, S. (1991). Relationship of role conflict and role ambiguity to selected job dimensions among joint appointees. *Journal of Professional Nursing* 7(5), 221–227.

Adams, S. M., & Partee, D. J. (1998). Integrating psychosocial rehabilitation in a community-based faculty nursing practice. *Journal of Psychosocial Nursing & Mental Health Services 36*(4), 24–28, 47–48.

Adams-Davis, K., & Fitzpatrick, J. J. (1995). The nursing health center: A model of public/private partnership for health care delivery. In B. Murphy (Ed.). *Nursing centers: The time is now* (pp. 83–96). New York: National League for Nursing Press.

Algase, D. (1986). Faculty practice: A means to advance the discipline of nursing. *Journal of Nursing Education 25,* 74–76.

American Association of Colleges of Nursing. (1993). *1992–1993 Special Report on Institutional Resources and Budgets in Baccalaureate and Graduate Programs in Nursing.* Washington, DC: American Association of Colleges of Nursing.

Amos, L. K. (1996). Education/practice models: University of Utah College of Nursing. In *The power of faculty practice: Proceedings of the American Association of Colleges of Nursing 1995 and 1996 Faculty Practice Conferences* (pp. 29–32). Washington, DC: American Association of Colleges of Nursing.

Anderson, E. R., & Pierson, P. (1983). An exploratory study of faculty practice: Views of those faculty engaged in practice who teach in NLN-accredited baccalaureate programs. *Western Journal of Nursing Research 5,* 129–140.

Aydelotte, M. K., Barger, S. E., Branstetter, E., et al. (1987). *The nursing center: Concepts and design.* Kansas City, MO: American Nurses Association.

Baillie, L. (1994). Nurse teachers' feelings about participating in clinical practice: An exploratory study. *Journal of Advanced Nursing 20*(1), 150–159.

Barger, S. E. (1986). Academic nursing centers: A demographic profile. *Journal of Professional Nursing 2,* 246–251.

Barger, S. E. (1993). The delivery of early and periodic screening, diagnosis and treatment program services by NPs in a nursing center. *Nurse Practitioner 18*(6), 65–68.

Barger, S. E. (1995). Establishing a nursing center: Learning from the literature and the experiences of others. *Journal of Professional Nursing 11*(4), 203–212.

Barger, S., & Bridges, W. (1987). Nursing faculty practice: Institutional and individual facilitators and inhibitors. *Journal of Professional Nursing 3*(6), 338–346.

Barger, S. E., & Bridges, W. C. (1990). An assessment of academic nursing centers. *Nurse Educator 15*(2), 31–36.

Barger, S. E., & Crumpton, R. B. (1991). Public health nursing partnership: Agencies and academe. *Nurse Educator 16*(4), 16–19.

Barger, S. S., Nugent, K. E., & Bridges, W. C., Jr. (1992). Nursing faculty practice: An organizational perspective. *Journal of Professional Nursing 8*(5), 263–270.

Barger, S. S., Nugent, K. E., & Bridges, W. C. Jr. (1993). Schools with nursing centers: A 5-year followup study. *Journal of Professional Nursing 9*(1), 7–13.

Barnes, N. J., Duldt, B. W., & Green, P. l. (1994). Perspectives of faculty practice and clinical competence: A trilogy of paradox. *Nurse Educator 19*(3), 13–17.

Batey, M. V. (1983). Structural consideration for social integration of nursing. In K. E. Barnard (Ed.). *Structure to outcome: Making it work* (pp. 1–11). Kansas City, MO: American Academy of Nursing.

Bednarz, P. K. (1998). The Omaha System: A model for describing school nurse case management. *Journal of School Nursing 14*(3), 24–30.

Bennett, S. J. (1990). Blending the entrepreneurial and faculty roles. *Nurse Educator 15*(4), 34–37.

Broussard, A. B., Delahoussaye, C. P., & Poirrier, G. P. (1996). The practice role in the academic nursing community. *Journal of Nursing Education 35*(2), 82–87.

Budden, L. (1994). Nursing faculty practice: Benefits vs. costs. *Journal of Advanced Nursing 19*(6), 1241–1246.

Burke, L. M. (1997). Teachers of nursing: Presenting a new model of practice. *Journal of Nursing Management 5*(5), 295–300.

Chicadonz, G. H., Bush, E. E., Korthus, K., & Utz, S. W. (1981). Mobilizing faculty toward integration of practice into faculty roles. *Nursing & Health Care 2,* 548–553.

Christman, L. (1979). On the scene: Uniting service and education at Rush-Presbyterian-St. Luke's Medical Center. *Nursing Administration Quarterly 3,* 7–40.

Christman, L., Diers, D., Fahy, E. T., et al. (1979). Statement of belief regarding faculty practice. *Nursing Outlook 27,* 158.

Christy, T. (1980). Clinical practice as a function of nursing education: A historical analysis. *Nursing Outlook 28,* 493–497.

Coenen, A., Marek, K. D., & Lundeen, S. P. (1996). Using nursing diagnoses to explain utilization in a community nursing center. *Research in Nursing & Health 19,* 441–445.

Coggiola, P., & Walker, P. H. (1995). Building an entrepreneurial multi-site autonomous practice in a rural community. In B. Murphy (Ed.). *Nursing centers: The time is now* (pp. 117–134). New York: National League for Nursing Press.

Collison, C., & Parsons, M. (1980). Is practice a viable faculty role? *Nursing Outlook 28,* 672–679.

Delaney, C., & Moorhead, S. (1995). The Nursing Minimum Data Set, standardized language, and quality. *Journal of Nursing Caring Quality 10*(1), 16–30.

De Voogd, R., & Salenblatt, C. (1989). The clinical teaching associate model: Advantages and disadvantages in practice. *Journal of Nursing Education 28*(6), 276–277.

Durand, B. A. (1985). Defining faculty practice: A look

at theory–practice relationships. In K. E. Barnard & G. R. Smith (Eds.). *Faculty practice in action* (pp. 38–43). Kansas City, MO: American Academy of Nursing.

Elsberry, N., & Nelson, F. (1993). How to plan financial support for nursing centers. *Nursing and Health Care 14*(8), 408–413.

Fairbrother, P., & Ford, S. (1998). Lecturer practitioners: A literature review. *Journal of Advanced Nursing 27*(2), 274–279.

Finkler, S. A., Knickman, J. R., Hanson, K. L. (1994). Improving the financial viability of primary care health centers. *Hospital & Health Services Administration 39*(1), 117–131.

Ford, L. (1980). Unification of nursing practice, education, and research. *International Nursing Review 27*(8), 178–183.

Ford, L., & Kitzman, H. (1983). Organizational perspectives on faculty practice: Issues and challenges. In K. E. Barnard (Ed.). *Structure to outcome: Making it work* (pp. 13–29). Kansas City, MO: American Academy of Nursing.

Gale, B. J. (1998). Faculty practice as partnership with a community coalition. *Journal of Professional Nursing 14*(5), 267–271.

Gersten-Rothenberg, K. (1998). Should schools develop nursing centers? *Clinical Nurse Specialist 12* (2), 59–63.

Giltinan, J. M., & Murray, K. T. (1992). Meeting the health care needs of rural elderly: Client satisfaction with a university-sponsored nursing center. *Journal of Rural Health 8*(4), 305–310.

Hale, J. F., Harper, D. C., & Dawson, E. M. (1996). Partnership for nurse practitioner–directed student primary care center. *Journal of Professional Nursing 12*(6), 365–372.

Henry, B. (1995). The education-service system is nursing is broken. *Image: Journal of Nursing Scholarship 27*(4), 254.

Higgs, Z. R. (1988). Academic nurse-managed center movement: A survey report. *Journal of Professional Nursing 4*, 422–429.

Joachim, G. (1988). Faculty practice: Dilemmas and solutions. *Journal of Advanced Nursing 13*, 410–415.

Joel, L. A. (1983). Stepchildren in the family: Aiming toward synergy between nursing education and service: From the faculty perspective. In K. E. Barnard (Ed.). *Structure to outcome: Making it work* (pp. 43–57). Kansas City, MO: American Academy of Nursing.

Just, G., Adams, E., & DeYoung, S. (1989). Faculty practice: Nurse educators' views and proposed models. *Journal of Nursing Education 28*(4), 161–168.

Keefe, M. (1993). An integrated approach to incorporating research findings into practice. *The American Journal of Maternal-Child Health Nursing 18*, 65–66, 68, 70.

Keefe, M. R., Pepper, G., & Stoner, M. (1988). Toward research-based nursing practice: The Denver Collaborative Research Network. *Applied Nursing Research 1*(3), 109–115.

Kelly, K., Gardner, D., Johnson, M., et al. (1990). Adjunct executive appointment for faculty: An innovation in nursing collaboration. *Journal of Nursing Administration 20*(10), 35–42.

Kent, N. A. (1980). Evaluating the practice component for faculty rank and tenure. In *Cognitive dissonance: Interpreting and implementing faculty practice roles in nursing education* (pp. 21–26). New York: National League for Nursing.

Kirkpatrick, M. K. (1992). The ABCs of maintaining clinical competence. *Nurse Educator 17*(3), 5–6.

Kramer, M., Polifroni, E. C., & Organek, N. (1986). Effects of faculty practice on student learning outcomes. *Journal of Professional Nursing 2*(5), 289–301.

Lambert, C. E., & Lambert, V. A. (1988a). Faculty practice: Unifier of nursing education and nursing service? *Journal of Professional Nursing 4*(5), 345–355.

Lambert, C. E., & Lambert, V. A. (1988b). The economic relevance of nursing faculty practice programs. *Nursing Economics 6*(6), 291–296.

Lambert, C., & Lambert, V. A. (1993). Relationships among faculty practice involvement, perception of role stress, and psychological hardiness of nurse educators. *Journal of Nursing Education 32*(4), 171–179.

Lang, N. M., Evans, L. K., Jenkins, M., & Matthews, D. (1996). Adminstrative, financial, and clinical data for an academic nursing practice: A case study of the University of Pennsylvania School of Nursing. In *The power of faculty practice: Proceedings of the American Association of Colleges of Nursing 1995 and 1996 Faculty Practice Conferences* (pp. 79–100). Washington, DC: American Association of Colleges of Nursing.

Lassan, R. (1994). Nursing faculty practice: A valid sabbatical request? *Nursing Forum 29*(2), 10–14.

Littlefield, V. N., Keenan, C., Skillman, L. (1988). Academically based practice: Seizing opportunities, enhancing outcomes. *Journal of Professional Nursing 4*(5), 329–338.

Lockhart, C. A. (1995). Community nursing centers: An analysis of status and needs. In B. Murphy (Ed.). *Nursing centers: The time is now* (pp. 1–18). New York: National League for Nursing Press.

Lundeen, S. P. (1995). Information systems for community nursing centers: Issues of clinical documentation. In B. Murphy (Ed.). *Nursing centers: The time is now* (pp. 47–55). New York: National League for Nursing Press.

Mackey, T. A., & McNeil, N. O. (1996). Negotiating private sector partnerships with academic nursing centers. In *The power of faculty practice: Proceedings of the American Association of Colleges of Nursing 1995 and 1996 Faculty Practice Conferences* (pp.

61–68). Washington, DC: American Association of Colleges of Nursing.

Martin, K. S., & Scheet, N. J. (1992). *The Omaha System: Applications for community health nursing.* Philadelphia: W. B. Saunders.

Martin, K. S., & Scheet, N. J. (1995). The Omaha System: Nursing diagnoses, interventions, and client outcomes. In *An emerging framework: Data system advances for clinical nursing practice* (pp. 105–113). Washington, DC: American Nurses Publishing.

Mauksch, I. (1980). Faculty practice: A professional imperative. *Nurse Educator 5*(3), 21–24.

Maurin, J. T. (1986). An exploratory study of schools of nursing that assume patient care responsibilities. *Journal of Professional Nursing 2*(6), 359–364.

McNeil, N. O., & Mackey, T. A. (1995). The consistency of change in the development of nursing faculty practice plans. *Journal of Professional Nursing 11*(4), 220–226.

Miller, V. G. (1997). Coproviding continuing education through faculty practice: A win-win opportunity. *Journal of Continuing Educationin Nursing 28*(1), 10–13.

Millonig, V. (1986). Faculty practice: A view of its development, current benefits, and barriers. *Journal of Professional Nursing 2*, 166–172.

Mundinger, M. O. (1996). New alliances: Nursing's bright future. *Nursing Administration Quarterly 20* (3), 50–53.

Munroe, D. J., Sullivan, T. J., Lee, E. J., & Sarter, B. (1987). Establishing an environment for faculty practice: The primary affiliation. *Journal of Nursing Education 26*(7), 297–299.

Neil, R. M. (1995). Evidence in support of basing a nursing center on nursing theory. In B. Murphy (Ed.). *Nursing centers: The time is now* (pp. 33–46). New York: National League for Nursing Press.

Nugent, K. E., Barger, S. E., & Bridges, W. C., Jr. (1993). Facilitators and inhibitors of practice: A faculty perspective: The role of faculty practice. *Journal of Nursing Education 32*(7), 293–300.

(1991). *Nursing's agenda for health care reform.* New York: National League for Nursing.

Parsons, M. A., Felton, G. M., & Chassie, M. B. (1996). Success stories: Faculty practice plan entrance strategy for nursing. *Nursing Economics 14*(6), 373–376, 382.

Patton, J. G., Conrad, M. A., Krieldler, M. C. (1995). *Nursingconnections 8*(1), 27–35.

Phillips, D. L., & Steele, J. E. (1994). Factors influencing scope of practice in nursing centers. *Journal of Professional Nursing 10*(2), 84–90.

Phillips, S. J., & Kaempfer, S. H. (1987). Clinical teaching associate model: Implementation in a community hospital setting. *Journal of Professional Nursing 3,* 165–175.

Potash, M., & Taylor, D. (April 1993). *Nursing faculty practice: Models and methods.* Washington, DC: National Organization of Nurse Practitioner Faculties.

Pugh, E. J. (1988). Soliciting student input to improve clinical teaching. *Nurse Educator 15*(5), 28–33.

Richie, M. F., Adams, S. M., Blackburn, P. E., et al. (1996). Psychiatric nursing faculty practice: Care within the community context. *N&HC:Perspectives on Community 17*(6), 317–321.

Riesch, S. K. (1992). Nursing centers: An analysis of the anecdotal literature. *Journal of Professional Nursing 8*(1), 16–25.

Rodgers, M. W., & Peake-Godin, H. (1988). Implementing faculty practice in an atmosphere of retrenchment. *Journal of Nursing Education 27*(2), 87–88.

Rudy, E. B., Anderson, N. A., Dudjak, L., et al. (1995). Faculty practice: Creating a new culture. *Journal of Professional Nursing 11*(2), 78–83.

Ryan, M. C. (1997). Integrating practice, education, and research: Killing three birds with one stone. *Clinical Excellence for Nurse Practitioners 1*(4), 244–249.

Ryan, S., & Barger-Lux, M. (1985). Faculty expertise in practice: A school succeeding. *Nursing Outlook 28,* 75–78.

Schlotfeldt, R., & MacPhail, J. (1969). An experiment in nursing: Rationale and characteristics. *American Journal of Nursing 69,* 1018–1023.

Schroeder, C. A. (1993). Nurses' response to the crisis of access, costs, and quality in health care. *Advances in Nursing Science 16*(1) 1–20.

Schroeder, C. A., & Neil, R. M. (1992). Focus groups: A humanistic means of evaluating an HIV/AIDS program based on caring theory. *Journal of Clinical Nursing 1,* 265–274.

Sherwen, L. N. (1998). When the mission is teaching: Does nursing faculty practice fit? *Journal of Professional Nursing 14*(3), 137–143.

Smerke, J. M. (1990). Healing and wholeness: A case study of a nurse-managed AIDS center: In *Perspectives in nursing: 1989–91* (pp. 67–90). New York: National League for Nursing.

Stainton, M., Rankin, J., & Calkin, J. (1989). The development of a practicing nursing faculty. *Journal of Advanced Nursing 14,* 20–26.

Steele, R. M. (1991). Attitudes about faculty practice, perceptions of role, and role strain. *Journal of Nursing Education 30*(1), 15–22.

Stoner, M. H., Magilvy, J. K., & Schultz, P. R. (1992). Community analysis in community health nursing practice: The GENESIS model. *Public Health Nursing 9*(4), 223–227.

Taylor, D. (1996). Faculty practice plan or faculty practice groups? In *The power of faculty practice: Proceedings of the American Association of Colleges of Nursing 1995 and 1996 Faculty Practice Conferences* (pp. 33–35). Washington, DC: American Association of Colleges of Nursing.

Tranzillo, M. J. (1995). A nurse managed student health center: From idea to reality. In B. Murphy (Ed.).

Nursing centers: The time is now (pp. 203–213). New York: National League for Nursing Press.

Turner, D. M., Pearson, L. M. (1989). The faculty fellowship program: Uniting service and education. *Journal of Nursing Administration 19*(10), 18–22.

Walker, P. H. (1995). Faculty practice: interest, issues, and impact. *Annual Review of Nursing Research 13*, 217–236.

Walker, G. C., Starck, P. L., McNeil. N. O. (1994). The Houston Linkage Model 1992: An update. *Nurse educator 19*(5), 40–42.

Walker, P. H. (1994). A comprehensive community nursing center model: Maximizing practice income: A challenge to educators. *Journal of Professional Nursing 10*(3), 131–139.

Walker, P. H., & Walker, J. M. (1995). Community nursing center informatics for business, practice, research, and education. In B. Murphy (Ed.). *Nursing centers: The time is now* (pp. 57–82). New York: National League for Nursing Press.

Walker, P. H., & Walker, J. M. (1996). Determining the right questions and calculations in forecasting cost and risk in managed care. In *The power of faculty practice: Proceedings of the American Association of Colleges of Nursing 1995 and 1996 Faculty Practice Con-ferences* (pp. 11–18). Washington, DC: American Association of Colleges of Nursing.

Watson, M. J. (1985). *Nursing: The philosophy and science of caring.* Boulder: Colorado Associated University Press.

Watson, M. J. (1988). *Nursing: Human science and human care.* New York: National League for Nursing.

Watson, M. J. (1990). Transperson caring: A transcendant view of the person, health, and healing. In M. W. Parker (Ed.). *Nursing theories in practice* (pp. 277–288). New York: National League for Nursing.

Werley, H. H., & Lang, N. M. (1988). *Identification of the nursing minimum data set.* New York: Springer.

Werley, H. H., Lang, N. M., & Westlake, S. K. (1986). The Nursing Minimum Data Set: Executive summary. *Journal of Professional Nursing 2*(4), 217–224.

Werley, H. H., Ryan, P., & Zorn, C. R. (1995). The Nursing Minimum Data Set (NMDS): A framework for the organization of nursing language. In *An emerging framework: Data system advances for clinical nursing practice.* (pp. 19–30). Washington, DC: American Nurses Publishing.

Williamson, N. B., McDonough, J. E., & Boettcher, J. H. (1990). Nurse faculty practice: From theory to reality. *Journal of Professional Nursing 6*(1), 11–20.

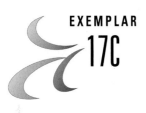

17C

Advanced Practice Nursing in the Department of Veterans Affairs: A Model for the Future

Nancy M. Valentine
Deborah Antai-Otong
Deborah B. Kupecz
Marilyn M. Lynn
Mary Chaffee

 ## Welcome to the "New" VA

The U.S. Department of Veterans Affairs (VA) operates the largest federal integrated healthcare system, and is one of the largest employers of nurses, in the world. The VA health system enrolls more than 3.8 million American veterans and provides service to 2.7 million. In addition, in the event of a national emergency or extensive wartime casualties, the VA provides back-up care for the U.S. Department of Defense.

Nearly 200,000 staff serve in the VA at approximately 1,100 sites in 171 medical centers throughout the United States, including Alaska, Hawaii, and Puerto Rico. More than 38,000 nurses provide care in the VA system, including nearly 1,500 nurse practitioners (NPs) and 900 clinical nurse specialists (CNSs) (Valentine, 1998, p. 5). Nearly 550 certified registered nurse anesthetists (CRNAs) provide anesthesia for VA patients. (CRNA practice will not be addressed in this exemplar.)

Advanced practice nurses (APNs) have practiced in the VA system since the early 1970s. However, the VA has navigated a period of significant reinvention and restructuring since 1994 that has significantly impacted APN practice. Care shifted to an outpatient-based model from the previous hospital-based delivery model. Forty-six VA medical centers were consolidated within the 22 integrated VA network systems nationwide, eliminating duplication of services and producing more than $75 million in savings. Resources were shifted to increase the number of outpatient visits for populations with growing needs, including homeless patients, mental health and substance abuse patients, and blindness rehabilitation patients. More than 23,000 acute care beds were eliminated, and admissions decreased by more than 250,000 per year. Inpatient bed-days of care were reduced by more than 50%. During the same time, ambulatory care visits have increased by more than 7 million per year. New points of service include 188 community-based clinics, with additional sites planned.

Trends Favoring Increased Demand for Advanced Practice Nurses in the VA

SHIFT TO PRIMARY CARE

A major initiative in the redesign of the VA health system is to provide every veteran with a primary care provider. With 2.7 million veteran users and 14,000 physicians, it was evident that the traditional model of physician-led team care could not be directly converted to primary care and would require greater use of nonphysician clinicians. Today, the change in philosophy is evident. Current guidelines mandate provision of primary care, specifying that every patient enrolled in primary care must have a provider who is a physician, APN, or physician assistant.

MARKET FORCES

The demand for family practice physicians has increased, and the VA has found itself competing with the private sector. APNs were well known within the system and had demonstrated that they were both quality and cost-effective providers.

QUALITY INDICATORS

Best of all, patients have expressed satisfaction with providers such as APNs, and outcomes of care are equivalent. The literature indicates that other providers' skills and abilities to achieve quality are equivalent to, if not better than, those of physicians (Lardner, 1998).

COMFORT WITH OUTPATIENT SETTINGS

As demand for care in outpatient settings increased, the APN role has expanded. APNs are often more comfortable and experienced than other healthcare providers in providing care in homes and other places in the community.

THE IMPACT OF RESTRUCTURING

The impact of health systems reengineering directly impacted all VA employees. Today, 25,000 fewer employees work in the VA than just a few years ago. Rightsizing is anticipated to continue as the VA seeks to balance achievement of the goals of quality, access, cost, customer satisfaction, and attainment of greatest functional ability for patients with identification of the types and numbers of staff required to achieve these results. The impact on the number of nursing staff is anticipated to continue as more beds close. Most decreases in nursing positions resulted from attrition related to a combination of expected turnover and financial incentives for early retirement. Nurses who are educated to provide care in primary and community-based models enjoy more employment options and will continue to handle system transition more successfully. Restructuring has been a threat to the employment of some nurses, whereas it has been a bonanza of opportunities for others, especially APNs.

The Evolution of Advanced Practice Nursing in the VA

A WAKE-UP CALL

The VA has long been an APN advocate and was one of the earliest employers of APNs. However, most APNs in the early years were recognized on a local level, and their impact was difficult to assess on a national scale. Recently, the VA Under Secretary for Health (the chief executive officer of the VA healthcare system) directed that there be a 200% increase in providers other than physicians in the VA during a 2-year period. In a system that has relied on physicians to deliver healthcare, the shift to using other healthcare providers was a systemwide wake-up call. The Under Secretary for Health's goal (a courageous act for a physician executive) stimulated a flurry of action, as well as criticism from some physician colleagues and associations. It was pivotal in creating strategies designed to organize APNs in the VA. In 1994, when the plan to increase primary care providers was outlined, VA APNs had no national organizational structure. Hiring, job responsibilities, and compensation issues were determined locally, and no national VA guidelines existed.

ADVANCED PRACTICE NURSING ISSUES IDENTIFIED

Anecdotal reports suggested that APNs had several professional concerns. These included concerns about how to obtain privileges, organizational and professional identity issues, variations in job responsibilities when working in a nursing service versus a medical service, role acceptance by physicians and other nurses, prescriptive privileges, and practice guidelines. APNs identified the need for communication, networking, consistent policies to clarify their roles, and support and formal sanctioning of advanced practice roles.

ASSESSMENT OF APN NEEDS

The VA Under Secretary for Health's directive was the impetus to analyze the status of APNs and to design their role in the future. Assessment was accomplished by coupling anecdotal reports with a national survey of existing NPs and CNSs. This survey provided data to determine the numbers, practice locations, and demographics of APNs practicing in the VA. Questions elicited feedback about perceived barriers to recruitment, retention, and practice. The responses were important in determining the number of APNs required to meet the VA Under Secretary of Health's goal to increase primary care providers by 200%.

Surveys were distributed in December 1995 to 1903 APNs in 171 VA facilities, and the response rate was 87%. The responses demonstrated that all but 5 VA facilities used APNs. Respondents identified several barriers to practice, including inadequate prescriptive authority, lack of understanding by others of the role of APNs, and lack of administrative support. Despite these perceived barriers, 93% of VA APNs surveyed reported satisfaction with their jobs. The survey results confirmed anecdotal reports, and planning became a collective effort of a constituency of nurses and other interested stakeholders. Plans were designed with measurable outcomes. Two years later, the goal of increasing the number of primary care providers was realized, with APNs providing the bulk of these new providers.

CREATION OF THE ADVANCED PRACTICE NURSING COUNCIL

An important step in the process of optimizing the role of the APN was the creation of the Advanced Practice Nursing Council. The Nursing Strategic Healthcare Group, located in Washington DC, provides national leadership in administering nursing services in the VA. The Nursing Strategic Healthcare Group's board of directors is composed of field-based leaders (individuals from VA sites around the country) representing constituents in five areas: administration, education, research, clinical practice, and informatics. A field-based leader from the clinical practice component was selected to coordinate all APN efforts through an Advanced Practice Nursing Council (APN Council). The APN Council chair was joined by a diverse group of NPs and CNSs representing sites throughout the country.

THE ADVANCED PRACTICE NURSING COUNCIL'S EARLY EFFORTS

In 1995, the first retreat of APN Council members took place in Denver, CO. In its first year, the APN Council rewrote and updated the VA guidelines for APN practice in the form of a utilization statement. It described how APNs could be used more effectively in their clinical settings to maximize care, quality, access, and cost-effectiveness. The utilization statement defined minimum APN credentials and offered suggestions on optimizing the APN role in the organization. Suggestions included individualizing scope of practice in accordance with expertise, identifying barriers to practice, establishing privileging mechanisms, and developing collaborative relationships with colleagues. The utilization statement recommended increased organizational support for APN mentorship, professional consultation, and professional development. The utilization statement was approved by the VA Under Secretary for Health in July 1997.

As the APN Council continued its work, further issues were identified. These included development of competitive pay rates for APNs, strategies for enhancing the availability of APNs, a best practice model, processes for credentialing and privileging, networking through a nationwide VA electronic mail system, and analysis of APN workload.

THE CENTER FOR ADVANCED PRACTICE NURSING

The Center for Advanced Practice Nursing (CAPN) was instituted as an information and networking center for VA APNs. The center is a "virtual organization" comprising experts from around the country. Its mission is to shape and influence the professional practice and utilization of APNs within the VA heathcare system. The CAPN is a national information resource and provides consultation relating to task force work, licensure, and scope of practice. The CAPN establishes standards and charters bylaws of the APN Council. Activities of the CAPN are directed by the APN Council.

RESTRUCTURING ACCOMPLISHMENTS

In just 4 years, VA APNs developed a national council (1994), designed a study of APNs in the VA (1995), conducted the study (1996), and analyzed and published the study results (Domine et al., 1998, p. 16) while also working on six organizational strategies. These efforts have had tremendous impact on the current role and utilization of APNs in the VA.

APN PARTICIPATION ON THE VA MULTIDISCIPLINARY PRACTICE ADVISORY BOARD

Despite the excellent work of the APN Council, it was recognized that both APNs and others were still meeting resistance in effecting change in administrative policies. To address this issue, the VA under secretary for health convened a Multidisciplinary Practice Advisory Board. This group, composed of APNs, clinical pharmacy specialists, physicians, physician assistants, and administrators, examines barriers to practice, develops strategies, makes recommendations, and oversees implementation of their task force work. Two members of the APN Council have been appointed to the Multidisciplinary Practice Advisory Board and serve as expert consultants on APN issues.

The Clinical Nurse Specialist in the VA

CNSs are a vital link in providing cost-effective, safe, and high-quality healthcare to veterans. During this time of role evolution within the VA, the CNS has emerged as a viable and important asset of the organization. In the VA healthcare system, diverse roles of the

CNS include advanced clinical practice, consultation, education, research, and administrative leadership. The CNS scope of practice varies by VA facility.

CNSs provide direct patient care to diverse populations. They perform physical examinations, obtain histories, and order and interpret laboratory and diagnostic studies and procedures. Many prescribe, administer, and evaluate pharmacotherapeutic and nonpharmacotherapeutic treatments. CNSs have implemented innovative strategies to provide education to patients, families, and other healthcare providers. CNSs are involved in carrying out continuous quality improvement activities (Forbes, Rafson, Spross, & Koziowski, 1990, p. 65). Like other APNs in the VA, CNSs work collaboratively with other healthcare professionals to maximize resources and provide quality care to veterans (see Tables 17C-1 and 17C-2).

THE UNIQUE ROLE OF THE CLINICAL NURSE SPECIALIST IN THE VA

The CNS role is highly valued in the VA system. CNSs have demonstrated their flexibility and creativity by developing new roles and practice skills. Some CNSs administer clinics in which their activities include medication management and patient and family education.

TABLE 17C-1 *Conditions Commonly Managed by VA Clinical Nurse Specialists*

Acute stress reactions
Alcohol abuse and dependence
Alcohol detoxification
Anxiety disorders
Asthma
Bereavement
Bipolar disorders
Chronic obstructive pulmonary disease
Chronic pain syndromes
Chronic renal failure
Coronary artery disease
Depression
Diabetes mellitus
Genitourinary system diseases
Hypertension
Infectious diseases
Nutritional diseases
Obesity
Personality disorders
Posttraumatic stress disorder
Schizophrenia
Schizoaffective disorders
Sexual erectile disorders
Sleep apnea
Substance abuse and dependence
Urologic disorders

TABLE 17C-2 *Specialty Areas of VA Clinical Nurse Specialist Practice*

Psychiatric mental health (acute and chronic care)

Conscious sedation recovery

Diabetes mellitus

Employee assistance program/health promotion

Geriatrics

Gastroenterology

Hematology-oncology

Hypertension

Infectious disease

Nephrology

Neurology

Nicotine dependency

Pain management

Pulmonology

Urology

Women's health

New roles continue to emerge as healthcare shifts from acute care inpatient settings to community, ambulatory, and primary care settings. Some CNSs choose to pursue NP training.

INNOVATIONS IN CLINICAL NURSE SPECIALIST PRACTICE IN THE VA

The following are examples of innovations of CNS practice within the VA system.

The Medical–Surgical Clinical Nurse Specialist: General Surgery, Oncology, and Breast Care

The CNS in this role provides health education to women and men regarding breast self-examination, annual screening, and mammography. The CNS focuses on cancer prevention, health promotion, and maintenance, as well as managing and directing the care of more than 80 veterans diagnosed with colorectal disease. The CNS provides consultation to clinicians in hematology, medical oncology, radiation oncology, and home health and community health agencies.

This role includes research and healthcare services that improve the quality of life for veterans with cancer. These efforts link veterans with necessary services that improve the quality of their lives. The CNS recognized a need to provide critical services to female veterans who had undergone mastectomy or lumpectomy and formed a local Reach for Recovery support group. The CNS guides volunteers who provide greatly needed emotional support to veterans in their homes and communities. Currently, this CNS is participating in research with hemicolectomy patients, which has been funded by outside educational grants.

The Medical–Surgical Clinical Nurse Specialist in the Urology Clinic

In a urology clinic, a CNS manages two screening clinics for initial consultations and provides therapy for bladder outlet obstruction in collaboration with other health professionals. The CNS educates veterans on incontinence, erectile dysfunction, and other urologic conditions. The CNS administers immunotherapy for bladder cancer and participates in urologic diagnostic testing. The CNS's coordination of healthcare services reduces fragmentation of care and enhances both patient and family satisfaction.

The Medical–Surgical Clinical Nurse Specialist: Conscious Sedation Recovery

A CNS serves as coordinator of conscious sedation recovery. This program provides innovative, high-quality, and cost-effective healthcare to veterans in an ambulatory care unit. Responsibilities of the CNS include performing recovery procedures and providing follow-up care to veterans who undergo conscious sedation. The CNS educates veterans and their families about procedures and provides consultation to nurses and other clinicians about conscious sedation. The CNS conducts research to measure treatment outcomes and conducts quality improvement activities. This approach to managing patients in ambulatory care units instead of in inpatient settings has saved the VA system more than $1200 per procedure.

The Psychiatric Mental Health Clinical Nurse Specialist: Program Director of the Employee Support Program

A psychiatric CNS serves as program manager of an employee support program. An ideal role for a psychiatric CNS, it affords the opportunity to develop comprehensive health promotion and prevention strategies for employees experiencing personal and job-related stress and substance abuse–related problems. This CNS-staffed program provides continuous healthcare to employees and their families. It serves more than 3000 employees and provides access to confidential primary, secondary, and prevention services. The motto of the program is "Keeping healthy employees healthy."

Primary services of the employee support program include comprehensive biopsychosocial assessment; psychoeducation; case management; crisis intervention; grief counseling; brief psychotherapy; financial assistance through community referrals; educational opportunities to employees, managers, and new employees; and new supervisors' training. Education offerings include programs on assertiveness training, the drug-free workplace, conflict resolution, time management, and anger management. The CNS provides consultation about workplace tension, enhancing interpersonal relationships, stress management, and workplace violence. A unique feature for those employees with addiction problems is a 12-month relapse prevention program that focuses on psychoeducation about addiction and managing triggers, 12-step principles, and stress reduction techniques. Ongoing research on treatment outcomes and productivity are integral parts to this innovative program. In an organization with more than 200,000 employees, programs such as these are vital.

The Psychiatric Mental Health Clinical Nurse Specialist: Substance Abuse Treatment Program

Psychiatric CNSs provide a wide range of services to veterans with substance abuse–related disorders, including psychotherapy to veterans and their families. CNSs perform physical and psychosocial assessments, prescribe medications, and manage the care of dually diagnosed veterans being admitted for inpatient and outpatient substance abuse–related disorders. CNSs are used in both the Alcohol Abuse Rehabilitation and Residential Treatment programs.

❧ *The Nurse Practitioner in the VA*

The Denver Veterans Administration Medical Center (VAMC) serves as an exemplary model of the evolution of NP roles within the VA system. Both clinical roles and administrative issues demonstrate an innovative use of advanced practice nursing.

A NURSE PRACTITIONER PROTOTYPE

In 1973, a prototype for NP practice was established by a national VA task force that unveiled a model for a more humanized approach to patient care. The nurse in this model, soon to be known as an NP, was responsible for continuity of care. The nurse would have initial patient contact and assume primary responsibility for determining the patient's health needs. Along with 11 other sites, the Denver VAMC participated in implementing the new model. A partnership between the Denver VAMC and the University of Colorado Schools of Nursing and Medicine prepared nurses to become NPs with expertise in adult and geriatric care. The functional role of these early NPs included triage for routine health problems, emergency care, evaluation of the need for specialty care, and episodic care for patients managed in an ambulatory care clinic. As care delivery shifted to outpatient settings, NPs managed chronic illness in addition to providing health maintenance. Although the initial arena for NPs was the admission–triage area, it became apparent that their skills could be used throughout the healthcare facility (Kupecz, 1994, p. 29).

The original group of NPs at the Denver VAMC numbered six, and grew to 28 by 1998. The population served by the NPs covers a wide range of ages and clinical conditions. Patients may initially present to an NP as young adults with few health problems. The NP often witnesses the progression of multiple illnesses as the patient ages. Because NPs have practiced at the Denver VAMC for the past 25 years, many veterans have had only an NP as their primary care provider (see Table 17C-3 for conditions commonly managed by VA NPs).

An innovative characteristic of the Denver setting is the total integration of NPs and the medical staff. Since the inception of primary care clinics, NPs have been assigned individual caseloads similar to their physician colleagues. Caseloads range from 300 to 600 patients. NPs and physicians are audited using identical standards of practice. Audits demonstrate similar outcomes in NP and physician practice.

TABLE 17C-3 *Conditions Commonly Managed by VA Nurse Practitioners*

Alcohol dependence

Asthma

Atrial fibrillation

Coronary artery disease

Congestive heart failure

Chronic obstructive pulmonary disease

Chronic pain syndromes

Chronic renal failure

Degenerative joint disease

Diabetes mellitus

Gastroesophageal reflux disease

Hypertension

Hyperlipidemia

Infectious diseases

Obesity

TABLE 17C-4 *Specialty Areas of Practice for VA Nurse Practitioners*

Acute care
Dermal ulcer care
Dermatology
Diabetes
Geriatrics
Hypertension
Infectious disease
Multiple sclerosis
Nephrology
Nicotine dependency
Occupational health
Oncology
Orthopedics
Pain management
Rheumatology
Urology
Women's health

NURSE PRACTITIONER CLINICAL SPECIALTY PRACTICE IN THE VA

Because of the wide acceptance of NPs as primary care providers at the Denver VAMC, many have developed expertise in specialty areas (see Table 17C-4). Diabetes care and women's health clinics are two examples of specialized NP practice. NPs not only provide specialty care but also are sought out for expert consultation by clinicians throughout the medical center.

NURSE PRACTITIONER–MANAGED DIABETES CARE

Before 1975, patients with diabetes were evaluated and treated in the VA by endocrinologists. As the demand for diabetic care increased, an NP-managed diabetes clinic was instituted. NPs provide primary care for patients with diabetes and coordinate their referrals. They provide diabetic education in both group and individual sessions and serve as consultants to physicians who refer patients with diabetic management needs. Two additional clinics were added to the original diabetes clinic. A diabetes education clinic, managed by an NP, provides ongoing education to patients and families, and the diabetic foot clinic specializes in care for patients with diabetic foot and dermal ulcers. The NP in this clinic is recognized throughout the medical center as the clinical expert for resolving diabetic foot problems.

WOMEN'S HEALTHCARE

An unusual characteristic of the VA population is the gender composition of VA patients. Approximately 95% of veterans are male, so many VA clinicians have limited experience with women's healthcare. NPs have assumed a leadership role in managing woman veterans' special needs. Each VAMC now has a women veterans coordinator who assists female patients access resources in the medical center. The coordinator, either an NP or a social worker, acts as a liaison between the VA and veterans service organizations, including the Veterans of Foreign Wars, Disabled Veterans of America, and the American Legion, to obtain maximum support for female veterans. At the Denver VAMC, an NP serves as the women veterans coordinator and is essential in providing comprehensive care for female patients. NPs assessed the needs of female patients and initiated a women's screening clinic in 1997. This NP-managed clinic provides health screening, evaluation, and treatment for uncomplicated gynecologic problems. By increasing clinic availability, the women's screening clinic increases access to care.

GERIATRIC CARE

As the numbers of geriatric veterans has increased, the demand for experienced gerontological NPs (GNPs) has increased. In the Nursing Home Care Unit at the Denver VAMC, the GNP is the primary care coordinator for all nursing home residents. GNPs assess new patients, conduct weekly rounds on stable residents, and coordinate ancillary services and referrals.

GERONTOLOGICAL NURSE PRACTITIONER—MANAGED RESPITE CARE

An extremely valuable program managed by GNPs is a respite program for caregivers of homebound patients. During a 1- to 2-week hospital admission, the GNP assumes responsibility for all patient care. This service is invaluable for caregivers, who are provided a break from the demands of home care. Patients benefit from preventive care provided during the admission.

ADMINISTRATIVE EVOLUTION OF ADVANCED PRACTICE NURSES

As the numbers of APNs at the Denver VAMC increased throughout the 1990s, it was apparent that a peer review mechanism was needed. In 1996, an APN peer review board was instituted, consisting of nine APNs representing CNSs, NPs, and nurse anesthetists. A policy was created to define the appointment, utilization, qualifications, standards, and scope of advanced practice. The peer review board ensures compliance with the peer review policies.

Since its inception, the APN peer review board has reviewed all records of VA APNs as well as the records of candidates for employment. The group has provided guidance to medical center administration about scope and standards of practice. It has made recommendations to expand or limit practice in individual cases and has become a resource for APNs seeking clinical guidance. The peer review policy has served as a nationwide prototype for other VAMCs.

INDEPENDENT PRACTICE

On recommendations of the Joint Commission on Accreditation of Healthcare Organizations, 10 NPs at the Denver VAMC sought Licensed Independent Practitioner status. The chief executive board granted these privileges for a 1-year period while an independent audit was performed to monitor standards of practice. Following the 1-year trial period, all NPs were granted full independent clinical privileges. A member of the APN peer review board was invited to become a standing member of the Medical Staff Professional Standards Board. Now when an APN requests Licensed Independent Practitioner status, the APN member of the medical board reviews the individual's application and makes a recommendation for appointment. The APN appointment to the medical board also permits APN input into the medical center bylaws. APNs can now be recognized as members of the active medical staff with voting privileges.

Although the Denver VAMC is presented as an example of innovative NP practice, many VAMCs use NPs in a similar manner. NPs participate in nearly every aspect of patient care, including inpatient and short-stay acute care. NP responsibilities commonly include admitting patients, making daily patient rounds, adjusting treatments, and discharging patients. Care has been extended into the community through satellite clinics where NPs serve as administrators while still maintaining an active clinical role.

National Perspectives

DISTANCE LEARNING OPPORTUNITIES

As the role of the APN in the VA has flourished, VA administration identified ways to support their professional growth. A distance learning project resulted from the focus on APN development. A collaborative resource-sharing arrangement was designed between the VA and the Uniformed Services University of the Health Sciences, located in Bethesda, MD. This 18-month program is targeted to CNSs who desire NP training. CNSs are able to access this program at seven VA medical centers, with future expansion on the drawing board. In 1997, 36 students were enrolled, with a projected increase in enrollment to 50 students in 1998. The first graduating class in 1999 has yielded the first group of cross-trained advanced practice nurses. The program symbolizes the VA's commitment to its nurses through innovative education. It also represents an example of collaboration between the VA and the Department of Defense in the service of American military veterans.

AN APN MODEL FOR PATIENT-CENTERED CARE

The VA APN Best Practice Model Task Force designed a model for APN practice. This innovative model resulted from the efforts of 14 APN task force members from across the country and can be incorporated into any healthcare system. It is most useful in a setting in which APNs are present throughout the system, are able to practice in primary care roles, and are highly valued by patients and staff.

Future Challenges

APNs in the VA have accomplished a great deal, but many challenges lie ahead. An ongoing challenge is to educate other healthcare professionals that APNs are not a threat to their practice. A few physicians who desire restraint of the growth of the APN role have lobbied the U.S. House of Representatives and Senate Veterans Affairs Committees to institute limits. In clinical settings, though, indications are clear that more physicians are working collaboratively with APNs, and they are forging new relationships in an effort to provide high-quality care. APNs seem to be greatly respected for their skills and expertise. Some physician executives in the VA are working to hire as many APNs as budgets will allow (Glaser, 1994, p. 44; Lowes, 1998, pp. 124, 127). Additional data that demonstrate the value of APNs and other healthcare providers will encourage enhanced professional collaboration.

The partnership between APNs and the VA is a proud one that has improved healthcare for American veterans. The combination of committed APNs with the support of organizational leadership that values the APN will encourage excellence in patient care for America's veterans for many years to come.

Acknowledgment: The authors would like to acknowledge Brian Westfield, nurse executive of the Salt Lake City, UT, VAMC, for his leadership as chair of the APN Council, and the members for their contributions: Barbara Zicafosse, Salem, VA, VAMC, and Deborah Antai-Otong, Dallas, TX, VAMC, cochairs; Loraine Domine, Portland, OR, VAMC, consultant; and members-at-large Patricia Quigley, Tampa, FL, VAMC; Marilyn Lynn, Denver VAMC; Margaret Kruckemeyer, Dayton, OH, VAMC; Jennifer, Dardy, Birmingham, AL, VAMC; and Janell Christenson, Fargo, ND, VAMC.

The authors also wish to thank the staff of the VA National Center for Cost Containment, Milwaukee, WI, for their assistance in conducting the national study of APNs in the VA.

The views expressed in this exemplar are those of the authors and do not reflect the official policy or position of the Department of Veterans Affairs, Department of the Navy, the Department of Defense, or the US government.

REFERENCES

Domine, L. M., Siegal, M., Zicafoose, B., et al. (1998). Survey of advanced practice nurses employed by the veterans health administration (VHA). *The Nurse Practitioner 23*(4), 16–23.

Forbes, K., Rafson, J., Spross, J., & Koziowski, D. (1990). The clinical nurse specialist and nurse practitioner: Core curriculum survey results. *Clinical Nurse Specialist 4,* 63–66.

Glaser V. (1994). Does your practice need a midlevel provider? *Family Practice Management September,* 43–52.

Kupecz, D. B. (1994). The nurse practitioner movement in the VA. *VA Practitioner 11*(8), 29–30, 32–33.

Lardner, J. (1998). It's a test insurers are backing: Can primary care work without doctors? *US News and World Report July 27,* 58–59.

Lowes, R. L. (1998). Making midlevel providers click with your group. *Medical Economics April 13,* 123–138.

Valentine, N. M. (1998). APNs make their mark in today's VA. *The Nursing Spectrum 5* (February 9), 11.

Monitoring Clinical Outcomes and Satisfaction in Patients of Psychiatric Clinical Nurse Specialists in Private Practice

Janet Garvey Baradell

A review of the literature revealed no research on clinical outcomes and satisfaction of patients of psychiatric clinical nurse specialists (CNSs) (Baradell, 1995). Reasons for conducting research that demonstrate clinical outcomes and patient satisfaction with the psychotherapy provided by CNSs include describing the population of patients seen by advanced practice nurses; illustrating current practice; comparing the patient population, outcomes, and satisfaction with that of other professionals; improving practice; shaping health policy; informing managed care companies; identifying educational needs; and providing data in legal proceedings.

For a comprehensive review of psychiatric nursing research, refer to Merwin and Mauck (1995). Their data indicate that psychiatric nurses have tested specific approaches to care and changes in systems for delivering care, but nurses have not addressed clinical outcomes and patient satisfaction with psychotherapy provided by psychiatric CNSs. Barrell, Merwin, and Poster (1997) provide an excellent review of tools relevant to psychiatric nursing outcomes research and detailed information on how to obtain those tools. For a comprehensive review of tools used to measure patient satisfaction with nursing care, see McDaniel and Nash (1990). That review demonstrates that satisfaction with nursing care, in general, is often confused with satisfaction with services other than those provided by nurses. In addition, no valid and reliable tools for measuring satisfaction with psychotherapy provided by CNSs were identified. For an example of evaluation of a system of care provided by psychiatric CNSs, refer to Moller and Murphy (1997). Finally, examples of single-case research designs, used to determine the clinical outcomes of psychiatric CNS care, can be found in Baradell (1990) and Saur and Ford (1995).

In 1994, six CNSs in private practice in North Carolina volunteered to participate in a study to examine the clinical outcomes and patient satisfaction with psychotherapy provided by psychiatric CNSs. Following is an illustration of one method used to monitor the quality of care provided by CNSs in private practice. Full details of the study are provided elsewhere (Baradell, 1995).

Description of the Research

Before beginning the study, a proposal was developed and reviewed by a panel of three nursing experts (one content, one theory, and one methodology expert) to ensure the ethical treatment of human subjects. Research in the private sector is not reviewed by an institutional review board, which exists to review proposed studies involving patients in institutions receiving federal funding.

INSTRUMENTS

The first task was to identify what to measure. Given that managed care was emerging, two large, managed mental health care companies were approached. Each was willing to share the tools used to monitor outcomes and satisfaction. It was clear that symptoms and patient satisfaction were the variables of interest to them. However, neither company used a valid and reliable instrument to monitor changes in clinical symptoms. Each company used similar tools to monitor patient satisfaction.

The Patient Satisfaction Survey (PSS) (Baradell, 1995) was adapted, from the client satisfaction questionnaire (Nguyen, Attkisson, & Stegner, 1983), to measure satisfaction with psychotherapy provided by a CNS. This eight-item questionnaire had two subscales—one for satisfaction with the interpersonal relationship and one for satisfaction with the psychotherapy services.

In addition, the Profile of Mood States–Short Form (POMS-SF) (McNair, Lorr, & Droppleman, 1992) was selected to measure clinical symptoms. The POMS-SF is a 30-item questionnaire that measures clinical symptoms defined as mood states: anxiety, depression, anger, vigor, fatigue, and confusion.

Also, it was decided to evaluate the impact of psychotherapy on patients' quality of life (QOL). This variable is of interest to nurses as well as other mental health providers (Lehman, 1991; Sederer, Hermann, & Dickey, 1995). The QOL questionnaire selected was an adaptation of the Quality of Life Interview (Lehman, 1991). This 15-item instrument used three subscales to measure subjective QOL in three domains: family relations, social relations, and work. Together, the POMS-SF and QOL were used to examine clinical outcomes.

As with any material that is under copyright, written permission was obtained before using each instrument for research purposes.

Each CNS was provided a cover letter to send out to patients with the research instrument. The letter explained the nature of the study, sought voluntary participation, and assured privacy. The three questionnaires—POMS-SF, QOL, and PSS—composed the research instrument that was mailed to patients. The directions on the questionnaires instructed the patient to complete the POMS-SF and QOL twice, indicating how they felt at the beginning of therapy and how they felt, in general, since the end of therapy.

Demographic data were needed to describe the patient population and treatment characteristics. These data were obtained from the CNSs using a code number for each client to protect privacy. A CNS data collection form (DCF) was used to record information and included data such as age, sex, multiaxial diagnosis, length of therapy, number of sessions by treatment modality, and type of termination (planned or unplanned).

METHODS

The study methods were the next consideration. Since no existing data were available, a retrospective mail survey was chosen for this pilot study. Data were collected only from patients who had completed psychotherapy so as not to influence treatment. Each CNS was provided a cover letter, research instruments, and DCFs. Then, the CNS mailed the cover letter and research instrument to each client who had terminated treatment in 1994. The CNS completed a DCF for each patient and returned it to the project statistician. The advantages of this design were that it was economical of CNS and patient time, was inexpensive, and ensured privacy for the CNSs and patients. CNSs voluntarily paid postage and shared the cost of data analysis. In return for their participation, each CNS received outcome and satisfaction data on her practice.

RESULTS

Demographics of Patients Seeing Clinical Nurse Specialists

There were 100 usable surveys returned of the 223 original patient sample, yielding a response rate of 45%. The sample was predominantly female (82%), and the average age was 37 years. Individual therapy was the treatment modality for 43%, group therapy for 9%, and couples therapy for 8%. More than one treatment modality was used for 40% of patients. The median number of sessions was 16. In this survey, 25% of patients had terminated by the 8th session, another 25% by the 16th session, and another 25% by the 30th session.

The primary diagnoses listed by the CNSs for patients were affective disorders (46%), adjustment disorders (34%), anxiety disorders (10%), and "other" (10%).

The CNSs indicated that 61% of patients participated in planning for their terminations.

Clinical Outcomes and Patient Satisfaction

Derived from patients' responses to questionnaires, patients reported a high level of satisfaction with the psychotherapy provided by CNSs and excellent clinical outcomes.

Percentages are used to describe the patients' level of satisfaction with the psychotherapy services of the CNS (Table 17D-1). The first four items measured the patient's satisfaction with the interpersonal relationship with the therapist. Patients' responses indicated that 98% felt the therapist was excellent, very good, or good when asked if the therapist "listened closely to you." Especially noteworthy is the finding that no patient rated the CNS as a poor listener. When asked if the therapist understood the problem and the patient's feelings, 96% responded that the therapist was excellent, very good, or good. Ninety-three percent of the patients reported an excellent, very good, or good "match between the therapist's skills/specialty and your concerns." When asked if the therapist was willing "to help you obtain other care (if needed)," 95% of patients rated the therapist as excellent, very good, or good. Nine patients either omitted this item or wrote in "not applicable."

The final four items on the satisfaction questionnaire ascertained the patient's level of satisfaction with the CNSs' services. Eighty-two percent of patients reported that therapy met almost all or most of their needs. Ninety-seven percent responded that therapy with the CNS helped a great deal or helped somewhat. No patient felt that therapy had made things worse. Ninety-five percent of patients reported that, overall, they were satisfied with the services received. Finally, when patients were asked if they would return to the CNS if they needed help again, 91% percent reported "yes, definitely" or "think so."

Each of the clinical symptoms measured on the POMS-SF—depression, anxiety, anger, fatigue, vigor, and confusion—experienced significant improvement (Table 17D-2), as did all three domains of QOL—family, social, and work (Table 17D-3).

DISCUSSION

From these data, it is possible to describe the demographics, satisfaction, and clinical outcomes of patients of CNSs and to compare these data with those of other mental health professionals. It was found that the patients of CNSs are similar to those reported in other recent, mental health samples: they are predominantly female and in their late 30s, and most

TABLE 17D-1 *Percent Responses on PSS: Interpersonal Relationship and Service Items (n=100)*

Item	Excellent	Very Good	Good	Fair	Poor
Interpersonal Relationship					
Listened	69	22	7	2	0
Understood problems & feelings	51	37	8	3	1
Therapist–client match	47	36	10	6	1
Obtain other care, if needed*	54	29	12	3	2
Service	**Almost All**	**Most**	**A Few**		**None**
Extent of needs met	34	48	16		2
	A Great Deal	Helped Somewhat	No Help		Made Worse
Helped to Deal with Problems	67	30	3		0
	Very Satisfied	Mostly Satisfied	Mild Dissatisfaction		Quite Dissatisfied
Overall Satisfaction with Service	77	18	3		2
	Yes Definite	Think So	No		Definitely Not
If needed, would see CNS again	65	26	8		1

*n=91, because of missing values.

have affective or adjustment disorders (Achievement and Guidance Centers of America, 1993; U.S. Behavioral Health, 1994, 1995). This represents a shift from studies during the past 10 years in which the most frequently reported diagnoses were depression and anxiety (Betrus & Hoffman, 1992; Knesper, Belcher, & Cross, 1989; Knesper, Pagnucco, & Wheeler, 1985; Pelletier, 1984; U.S. Department of Health and Human Services, 1988).

Compared with data provided by managed mental health care companies (Achievement and Guidance Centers of America, 1993; U.S. Behavioral Health, 1994, 1995), the patients' reports of satisfaction with the relationship and psychotherapy services provided by the CNSs exceeded the level of satisfaction reported by patients of providers on managed mental health care panels for every item.

No data were available for comparing clinical outcomes because the managed mental health care companies that provided outcome data had not used valid and reliable tools to examine clinical symptoms or QOL.

IMPLICATIONS

The results of this study suggest that the use of CNSs as mental health providers would prove less expensive, extremely effective, and highly satisfactory to patients when substituted for the more expensive mental health services of psychiatrists and psychologists.

Furthermore, the data from this study indicate that CNSs are accepted by other healthcare providers. The most frequently cited referral source was other healthcare providers (doctors, nurse practitioners, physician assistants, and other mental health providers).

TABLE 17D-2 *Results of t Tests for the Differences in Means for POMS-SF Before and After Psychotherapy With Clinical Nurse Specialists (n=100)*

Symptom	Mean			t	P
	Before	After	Difference		
Anxiety	12.25	5.19	7.06	15.27	<.0001
Depression	12.75	5.10	7.65	15.72	<.0001
Anger	10.63	5.27	5.35	10.88	<.0001
Confusion	11.32	4.80	6.53	16.79	<.0001
Fatigue	12.74	5.23	7.51	14.44	<.0001
Vigor	5.33	11.10	5.77	12.87	<.0001

The possible range of scores for the six subscales of the POMS-SF is 0–20.

Monitoring your individual practice can provide a description of the population of patients that you see. Nurses who participated in this study each received a profile of their patients' average age, percentage of patients by gender and ethnicity, a diagnostic profile, average number of sessions, and average length of treatment. Each CNS received results of the changes reported by their patients' in clinical symptoms and QOL, as well as their patients' reports of satisfaction. Many patients offered written feedback to their therapists that highlighted strengths and weaknesses for individual CNSs. These data allow individual nurses to understand and improve their practice.

This type of monitoring has additional uses. CNSs can provide data to managed care companies describing their practice, outcomes, and patient satisfaction. In addition, faculty who teach in graduate schools can use outcome and satisfaction data to design curriculum to prepare graduates for today's practice arena. These data indicate that expertise in managing depression and adjustment disorders in adult females is essential. Furthermore, expertise in individual psychotherapy is necessary, but not sufficient. Treatment of almost half of the patients in this sample required the use of more than one psychotherapeutic modality.

TABLE 17D-3 *Results of t Tests for the Differences in Means for Quality of Life Before and After Psychotherapy With Clinical Nurse Specialists (n=100)*

Domain	Mean			t	P
	Before	After	Difference		
Family	16.74	19.65	2.91	6.32	<.0001
Social	26.86	30.51	3.65	6.21	<.0001
Work*	23.19	24.43	1.20	2.47	.008

The possible range of scores for each of the QOL domains are as follows: family, 4–28; social, 6–42; and work, 5–35.
  *n=89, because of missing values.

Finally, data of this type may be useful in defending your practice in legal proceedings. As more CNSs enter private practice, the risk of being a defendant in a lawsuit increases. Data illustrating the quality of your work and your patients' responses to that work may offer a different view from that offered by a plaintiff's attorney.

THE FUTURE: RESEARCH

A second clinical outcomes and satisfaction study is nearing completion in North Carolina (Baradell & Bordeaux, 1999). Many changes were made to improve the methods and instruments.

A more representative sample was drawn by obtaining CNS volunteers from across the state. The design was changed from ex post facto to prospective. Measures of clinical symptoms were taken at the beginning of psychotherapy, at termination, and 6 months after termination. This refinement is designed to demonstrate the range and severity of symptoms and the QOL at initiation of psychotherapy, the impact of psychotherapy on symptoms and QOL, and the duration of the impact of treatment.

The POMS-SF was used again to measure clinical symptoms. However, the QOL tool was revised by adding three new domains to examine functioning in daily life, health, and school (when applicable). Revisions of the PSS were designed to facilitate ease of patient response.

The research questions were expanded to encompass the impact of psychotropic medication use on clinical outcomes, patient satisfaction, and characteristics of psychotherapy (i.e., length of treatment and number of sessions). Given that the scope of practice of CNSs includes management of medications, this study obtains a record of psychotropic medications used by patients, examines the effectiveness of medications, records side effects, and identifies education provided to patients. The impact of psychotropic medication use on psychotherapy is of great interest to nurses, third-party payers, and pharmaceutical companies.

Funding from an external source was essential to pay for a study of this magnitude. External funding was obtained from Glaxo Wellcome Inc.'s Nursing Research Program, Research Triangle Park, NC and from Sigma Theta Tau, Alpha Alpha Chapter, University of North Carolina School of Nursing, Chapel Hill, NC.

Additional research is needed to further clarify the impact of psychotherapy provided by psychiatric CNSs. A large sample of CNSs and their patients from across the country would be more representative. Also, a study that compares a "treatment" with a "no-treatment" control group is needed. This type of study would be unethical for CNSs in private practice because treatment would be delayed for the sake of research. However, because of waiting periods for treatment in the outpatient mental health section of tertiary care hospitals, mental health centers, or managed mental health care companies, this type of study may be feasible.

THE FUTURE: SHAPING LEGISLATION AND PUBLIC POLICY

CNSs in North Carolina pursued direct reimbursement through the legislature in 1985 and 1991 after discovering that many insurers refused to acknowledge their statutory scope of practice. Reimbursement was denied for services unless CNSs were employed and supervised by a psychiatrist or psychologist. Blue Cross and Blue Shield of North Carolina, for example, used the following guidelines to restrict the practice of psychiatric CNSs:

> Blue Cross and Blue Shield of North Carolina benefits are payable for psychotherapy personally rendered by an eligible doctor or by an allied mental health professional in the employ of an eligible doctor. Employment is interpreted to mean that a normal salaried employer/employee relationship exists and that services are not on a per case consultant contractual agreement or referral basis. A salaried employer/employee relationship is further defined to include payment of Social Security, federal and state taxes.
> For coverage to be paid for psychotherapy rendered by an allied mental health profes-

sional, the eligible doctor must be personally responsible for the services, and the services must be provided under the direction and supervision of the eligible doctor. Direction and supervision by the eligible doctor include initial evaluation of the patient by the doctor and regular contact between doctor and patient and employee (BSBSNC, 1991).

Efforts to educate insurers about the education, experience, national certification, and statutory scope of practice of the CNS, as well as the impact of their policies on access and cost, did not bring about change in reimbursement policies. Attempts to work with the insurance commissioner and attorney general to gain equity in reimbursement also failed. Legislative mandate became the only viable alternative. In 1993, North Carolina passed legislation mandating direct reimbursement for psychiatric CNSs, nurse practitioners, and nurse anesthetists. However, the legislation had a sunset clause that allowed mandatory direct reimbursement to expire in 5 years.

During the attempt to get legislation passed in 1991, it became apparent that data on the cost and effectiveness of psychotherapy by CNSs were needed. The first effort to secure cost data was in 1991, when a phone survey was conducted to determine the average fee for psychotherapy provided by CNSs. These data indicated that CNSs' fees were 20% to 40% lower than those of psychologists and psychiatrists in North Carolina (Baradell, 1991, 1994). These data were used to help educate policymakers about cost-effectiveness. The sunset clause was an incentive to demonstrate to legislators the quality of psychiatric CNSs care and led to the pilot study described in this exemplar and to the study recently completed (Baradell & Bordeaux, 1999). In 1997 the sunset clause was removed.

We now find ourselves in a position to educate members of the U.S. Congress and the Health Care Financing Administration (HCFA) about the statutory scope of practice as well as the clinical outcomes and satisfaction reported by patients of psychiatric CNSs. The passage of the Balanced Budget Agreement in August 1997 opened Medicare reimbursement to psychiatric CNSs regardless of geographic location or practice site.

However, the proposed rules implementing the changes in Medicare that were published by HCFA (*Federal Register*, June 5, 1998) were profoundly regressive. The proposed rules required physician supervision for the psychotherapy services that have long been provided independently by psychiatric CNSs.

Efforts to educate policymakers at HCFA resulted in revisions to the proposed rules permitting the independent practice of psychotherapy to CNSs (*Federal Register*, November 2, 1998). By redefining the term "collaboration," HCFA has acknowledged the statutory scope of practice for CNSs. This has been a long struggle and was finally won by intense lobbying by the American Psychiatric Nurses Association and Virginia Trotter Betts, Department of Health and Human Services Senior Advisor on Nursing.

It is critical that we continue to educate policymakers about our statutory scope of practice and QOL provided by psychiatric CNSs, if we are to remain viable in the mental health arena.

Summary

Monitoring clinical outcomes and patient satisfaction in your practice is feasible. Select variables that are relevant to your patient population. Defining those variables will guide tool selection and assist in interpretation of results. Working with an experienced nurse researcher to develop a proposal, especially determining methods, is essential for the beginning researcher or clinician. Submitting your proposal to an expert panel provides you with a review to ensure ethical treatment of patients as well as valuable feedback about your methods. Adaptation of a prospective design, use of tools relative to your individual practice, and collaboration with a statistician will get you started.

Participating in a research study is one level of involvement, and conducting studies is another level of involvement. Some elements to consider in implementing clinical research are building a research team; having access to literature; committing time and money; identifying funding sources; recruiting clinicians to participate; and coping with within-group conflict and out-of-group controversy.

Psychiatric CNSs have a legitimate role in providing mental health care. Monitoring the quality of our care is a new role for many of us, and the pressure to provide these data is mounting.

Essential Points to Remember

- Formal monitoring of outcomes and satisfaction is a new role;
- Select tools relevant to your patient population;
- Write definitions of variables;
- Decide on methods;
- Seek external review for ethical treatment of patients and to obtain feedback on methods;
- Work with an experienced nurse researcher;
- Consider hiring an expert to enter data and conduct statistical analyses; and
- Use data to improve your practice, market to managed care companies, shape legislation and public policy, and defend yourself in legal matters.

REFERENCES

Achievement and Guidance Centers of America (now Medco Behavioral Care System Corp). (June–August 1993). *Patient Satisfaction Survey: North Carolina/South Carolina area*. St. Louis, MO: Author.

Baradell, J. (1990). Client-centered case consultation and single-case research design: Application to case management. *Archives of Psychiatric Nursing 4*(1), 12–17.

Baradell, J. (1991). Fee survey for clinical specialists. *Pacesetter 18*(2), 4.

Baradell, J. (1994). Cost-effectiveness and quality of care provided by clinical nurse specialists. *Journal of Psychosocial Nursing and Mental Health Services 32*(3), 21–24.

Baradell, J. (1995). Clinical outcomes and satisfaction of patients of clinical nurse specialists in psychiatric–mental health nursing. *Archives of Psychiatric Nursing 9*(5), 240–250.

Baradell, J. & Bordeaux, B. (1999). Clinical outcomes and statisfaction of patients of certified specialists in psychiatric-mental health nursing. Manuscript submitted for publication.

Barrell, L., Merwin, E., & Poster, E. (1997). Patient outcomes used by advanced practice psychiatric nurses to evaluate effectiveness of practice. *Archives of Psychiatric Nursing 11*(4), 184–197.

Betrus, P. & Hoffman, A. (1992). Psychiatric–mental health nursing: Career characteristics, professional activities, and client attributes of members of the American Council of Psychiatric Nurses. *Issues in Mental Health Nursing 13*, 39–50.

Blue Cross Blue Shield of North Carolina. (1991). *Guide lines for filing claims for psychotherapy services provided by employees of physicians and clinical psychologists*. Durham, NC: Blue Cross Blue Shield of North Carolina.

Federal Register. (1998). Proposed Rules Section 410.78 Clinical Nurse Specialist Services. (June 5, Vol. 63, No. 108). Washington, DC: US Government Printing Office.

Federal Register. (1998). Medicare program: Revisions to payment policies and adjustments to the relative value units under the physician fee schedule for calendar year 1999. (November 2,: Vol 63, No. 211). Washington, DC: U. S. Government Printing Office.

Knesper, D., Belcher, B., & Cross, J. (1989). A market analysis comparing the practices of psychiatrists and psychologists. *Archives of General Psychiatry 46*, 305–314.

Knesper, D., Pagnucco, D., & Wheeler, J. (1985). Similarities and differences across mental health services and practice settings in the United States. *American Psychologist 40*(12), 1352–1369.

Lehman, A. F. (1991). *Quality of Life Interview: Core version manual*. Baltimore, MD: University of Maryland Medicine Center, Department of Psychiatry.

McDaniel, C., & Nash, J. (1990). Compendium of instruments measuring patient satisfaction with nursing care. *Quality Review Bulletin, May,* 182–188.

McNair, D., Lorr, M., & Droppleman, L. (1992). *Profile of Mood States*. San Diego, CA: Educational and Industrial Testing Service.

Merwin, E., & Mauck, A. (1995). Psychiatric nursing outcome research: The state of the science. *Archives of Psychiatric Nursing 9*(6), 311–331.

Moller, M., & Murphy, M. (1997) The three R's rehabilitation program: A prevention approach for the management of relapse symptoms associated with psychiatric diagnoses. *Psychiatric Rehabilitation Journal 20*(3), 42–48.

Nguyen, T., Attkisson, C., & Stegner, B. (1983). Assessment of patient satisfaction: Development and refinement of a service evaluation questionnaire. *Evaluation and Program Planning 6*, 299–314.

Pelletier, L. (1984). Nurse psychotherapists: Whom do they treat? *Hospital and Community Psychiatry 35*(6), 1149–1150.

Saur, C., & Ford, S. (1995). Quality, cost-effective psychiatric treatment: CNS-MD collaborative practice model. *Archives of Psychiatric Nursing 9*(6), 332–337.

Sederer, L., Hermann, R., & Dickey, B. (1995). The imperative of outcome assessment in psychiatry. *American Journal of Medical Quality 10*(3), 127–132.

US Behavioral Health. (December 1994). *Use of goal focused treatment planning expands: Network news.* Emeryville, CA: Author.

US Behavioral Health. (January 1995). *Goal focused treatment planning member survey results.* Emeryville, CA: Author.

US Department of Health and Human Services. (1988). *National health survey 1985* (Publication No. 88–1755). Hyattsville, MD: National Center for Health Statistics.

CHAPTER 18

Management of High-risk and Vulnerable Populations

Exemplars

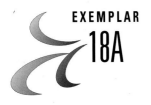

18A

Providing Inclusive
Healthcare Across Cultures

Shotsy C. Faust

It is very difficult to know people and I don't think one can ever really know any but one's own countrymen. For men and women are not only themselves; they are also the region in which they were born, the city apartment or farm in which they learned to walk, the games they played as children, the old wives tales they overheard, the food they ate, the schools they attended, the sports they followed, the poets they read, the god they believed in. It is all these things that have made them what they are, and these are the things that you cannot come to know by hearsay: you can only know them if you lived them (Maugham, 1944).

More than 50 years ago, the English writer Somerset Maugham underscored the difficulty of trying to understand people from different backgrounds and experiences. In clinical practice, nurse practitioners (NPs) encounter many kinds of patients who present with languages other than English and come from a variety of cultures. When confronted with this diversity, the NP might question how to best meet patient needs safely and with sensitivity. This exemplar outlines the following three goals: (1) to examine the process of migration and how it affects clinical care, (2) to explore ways of identifying and incorporating the patient's health belief system into the therapeutic regimen in a culturally sensitive and clinically effective manner, and (3) to evaluate the effect of the bilingual interpreter on the patient–practitioner relationship. Achievement of these goals will enhance the practitioner's ability to care for patients cross-culturally. These goals are presented in the form of the problem-oriented model geared toward the practicing clinician: the SOAP (Subjective, Objective, Assessment, Plan) process.

The traditional Western medical model teaches healthcare practitioners to identify pathophysiologic processes that cause the patient's complaint. Frequently, this disease focus fails to consider the broader context of the patient's health beliefs or practices. When working cross-culturally, it seems simpler to focus on the quantifiable, measurable processes of the body because there are so few guidelines or experiences to assess the context or culture of the patient's complaints. Unfortunately, a focus on the disease itself to the exclusion of its context can lead to frustration for both patient and practitioner. Symptoms and conditions that cannot be explained by our medical tradition and are not readily quantifiable by examination or laboratory testing are easily overlooked or dismissed.

A disease focus also reinforces the view of newcomers as victims rather than as individuals with strengths and resources as survivors (Meucke, 1992). Most practitioners attempt to understand the cultures of newcomers they see in practice. Practitioners often assume, however, that there is a degree of homogeneity among groups who share the same ethnicity or language. For example, Southeast Asians represent different countries, languages, religions, and cultural identities but are sometimes viewed as being the same. Each patient who comes to a clinic for care brings an individual worldview that is formed by education, class background, urban or rural upbringing, and exposure to Western healthcare (Nydegger, 1983). Newcomers also vary in their motivations to emigrate. Thus, although patients may share language or ethnicity, each patient brings a unique set of beliefs and expectations to the clinical setting.

Clinical Care Plan: Integrating the Migration Process Into Clinical Care

This section addresses the two essential aspects of eliciting the history or subjective information from the patient. Understanding the newcomer's migration status and the psychological stage within the migration process are critical to the provision of appropriate care.

NEWCOMER'S STATUS

It is useful to understand the difference between immigrants and refugees. Immigrants and refugees leave their homeland for different reasons and have different experiences of flight and resettlement (Westermeyer, 1990). Immigrants come to a new land seeking opportunity for a better life. They may have time to plan the emigration; choose the country in which to settle; and bring material goods, resources, and family with them. Although immigration can be overwhelming and stressful, immigrants move toward a perceived goal and future. Conversely, refugees flee persecution or death. Having little or no time to plan for their flight, they often leave everything, including family, behind. They spend considerable time, sometimes years, in a refugee or detainment camp awaiting asylum in a country not always of their choosing. Refugee patients commonly will have been imprisoned or tortured or will have lost other family members to a violent death (DeLay & Faust, 1987). Their focus is to flee from something or someone rather than to reach for a new goal. Refugee patients, therefore, are at higher risk for physical and emotional crises after arrival than are immigrant patients. It is often at this time that refugee patients first come to the clinic.

At the first visit, the NP should ascertain, without exploring details, whether the patient is a refugee or immigrant and how long he or she has resided in the United States. The practitioner's description of the patient as an immigrant versus a refugee should be based on the newcomer's motivation for migration and his or her emotional status rather than on the patient's political or legal qualifications. Many undocumented newcomers or illegal aliens fear that questions about immigration status could result in deportation or reprisal. Consequently, it is important that the NP explain that legal status is not germane to the clinic visit and will not be reported or documented. Patients should be reassured that information about the circumstances of their immigration is only used to gauge the stress or duress they have experienced.

MIGRATION HISTORY

Carlos Sluzki, a physician who has worked extensively with migrant families, developed the Migration History model of migration (Sluzki, 1979, 1992). The Migration History is a helpful tool in the collection of historical information from the patient and is a useful predictor of potential patient distress experienced during each stage in the migration process. Practitioners can also use it as a predictor of physical and emotional distress after the new-comer's arrival. However, practitioners must evaluate each patient individually. This tool is meant to provide general guidelines for assessing the stresses of migration. Practitioners should not use the Migration History to generalize about all individuals who migrate from one country to another. When applied judiciously, the Migration History can help practitioners understand the individual patient's psychology and craft a care plan that is specific to individual patient needs. Sluzki divided migration into the following five stages: (1) Planning Stage, (2) Act of Migration, (3) Period of Overcompensation, (4) Period of Decompensation, and (5) Resolution Stage or Stage of Intergenerational Support.

The Planning Stage may be a prolonged one for immigrants. During this stage, immigrants make their plans to emigrate to the country of destination. The time between recognition of the need to flee to the act of migration itself often is abbreviated to minutes, hours, or days.

The Act of Migration refers to the duration of transit from the country of origin to the country of destination for immigrants. For refugees, migration is a time of intense stress and uncertainty because their destination is unknown. Refugees may spend months to years in a refugee or detention camp waiting for permanent placement in a third or permanent country of asylum.

Soon after arrival (the Period of Overcompensation), both refugees and immigrants begin to learn the essentials of daily life in their new country. They focus on obtaining housing, using public transportation, receiving welfare assistance, enrolling children in school, and finding healthcare. Psychologically, newcomers are often relieved at "having arrived" and are hopeful about prospects in the new country. Worries or concerns about past experiences and losses are supplanted by the mastering of tasks necessary for survival in their adopted country. In addition, a newcomer's social services agency or individual sponsor may arrange for a health screening. NPs complete typical screening for tuberculosis or hepatitis as well as immunization updates; newcomers often have few health concerns or complaints.

The Period of Decompensation occurs when the newcomers have mastered basic skills, usually 6 months to 1 year after arrival, and the reality of making a life in their new country becomes more apparent. Newcomers typically speak little, if any, English and have few transferable job skills. Housing might be limited to overcrowded rooms in a low-income area. Memories of the homeland, of dead loved ones or loved ones left behind, or of the flight experience itself, may surface. Hopelessness and despair frequently ensue. It is often at this point that patients come to a clinic for care. Their complaints are commonly somatic, including headache, weakness, dizziness, fatigue, or exacerbations of preexisting conditions (Westermeyer, Bouafuely, Neider, & Calleis, 1989).

The Stage of Intergenerational Support is related to resolution of migration crises. Families are able to come together to provide strength and support to members, and the process of adjustment or acculturation continues. Practitioners do not often witness the Resolution Stage or Stage of Intergenerational Support because their patients frequently are not in crisis. Patients may reexperience the psychological crises of migration in various stages if other life stresses intensify.

First Clinic Visit

The following discussion addresses how practitioners use the Migration History model during the first three clinic visits. The patient may come to the first clinic visit (Table 18A-1), unless it is a screening visit that was not arranged to address a complaint, because he or she has been experiencing symptoms of crisis, which may present as multiple somatic complaints, vegetative symptoms of depression, or symptoms of posttraumatic stress disorder.

In addition to the symptom-focused medical history, the practitioner elicits information about migration in the reverse order of occurrence, starting with the present living sit-

TABLE 18A-1 *Format for Three Sample Clinic Visits*

Visit No.	Subjective	Objective	Assessment	Plan
1	Obtain medical history Obtain migration history Apply the explanatory model	Provide a complete or focused examination Look for signs of folk treatment	Perform a differential diagnosis Relabel diagnosis using patient's terminology	Include family in treatment Provide treatment (including symptomatic or over-the-counter) Explain test, lab results Advise on diet Discuss appropriate nontraditional therapies Schedule follow-up visit
2	Follow up complaints Add immediate past of migration history (arrival to USA) Obtain more extensive psychosocial history	Assess blood pressure, pulse, other vital signs Check lab tests results	Hone differential diagnosis Begin to consider psychiatric diagnosis, if appropriate	Adjust medications or treatments; consider other therapies Refer, if needed, to support groups and so forth Schedule follow-up visit
3	Evaluate symptoms Probe migration history/Premigration flight	Assess vital signs	Continue to assess problems Evaluate healthcare maintenance needs	Adjust medications or treatments Refer, if needed, to specialist (e.g., cardiologist) Teach healthcare maintenance Schedule follow-up visit

uation only, unless the patient volunteers more. Illustrative questions are, Where are you living? Do you live alone or with family or friends? Do you have any means of income or assistance? The patient may view questions about the past or about earlier stages of migration as intrusive and personal because the patient has yet to form a relationship with the practitioner. Furthermore, inquiring about the reasons for fleeing and evaluating torture or abuse may trigger or intensify symptoms.

The patient has come specifically for treatment of particular physical complaints; it is paramount that the practitioner focus on the symptoms at hand because the patient may perceive questions about emotional issues as suggesting mental or emotional disorder. Western culture is unique in its separation of psyche and soma. In other healing traditions, it is uncommon for practitioners to ask probing or psychological questions that seem unrelated to the problem at hand (Westermeyer, Bouafuely, Neider, & Calleis, 1989). Patients and healers in most other cultures do not distinguish so clearly between emotional and physical events, and they do not attribute psychological causes to experience in the Western manner. Patients do not complain of "depression" or "sadness" but rather of headache, abdominal pain, or other somatic ailments (Chung & Kagawa-Singer, 1993; DeLay & Faust, 1987). Many cultures equate expression of psychological distress with mental illness or "craziness." A psychiatric diagnosis can reflect and have social consequences not only on that individual but on the family as a group.

Explanatory Model

Western health practitioners often do not understand the value patients place on certain symptoms or treatments; however, patient responses to questions about their health beliefs can be revealing (Patcher, 1994). Practitioners at times may find the patient's description of a symptom (e.g., "hotness in the body") unfamiliar or meaningless. Rather than pursue a fruitless medical evaluation of a misunderstood entity, it is better that they explore the patient's beliefs about the symptom.

Arthur Kleinman, an anthropologist and cross-cultural psychiatrist at Harvard University, developed a series of questions for eliciting the explanatory model that underlies the patient's health beliefs. Practitioners will find it useful to ask these questions (especially 1, 2, and 8) during the first clinic visit when they take the medical history. They should note the patient's phrases or words for describing the symptom (e.g., "hotness") to be used later when the practitioner's health beliefs are joined with those of the patient to formulate a shared assessment and plan. It is helpful to use the questions with patients from Western culture as well because everyone has an explanatory model or system of health beliefs to explain or cope with symptoms. Kleinman's (Kleinman, Eisenberg, & Good, 1978) eight questions are as follows:

1. What do you call your problem? What name does it have?
2. What do you think has caused your problem?
3. Why do you think it started when it did?
4. What does your sickness do to you? How does it work?
5. How severe is it? Will it have a short or long course?
6. What do you fear most about your sickness?
7. What are the chief problems your sickness has caused for you?
8. What kind of treatment do you think you should receive? What are the most important results you hope to receive from the treatment? (p. 256)

Second Clinic Visit

During the second (or follow-up) clinic visit (see Table 18A-1), the practitioner reviews the patient's health status and laboratory test results and the recommended therapeutic interventions. The practitioner continues the Migration History and explores the act of migration itself. In the case of refugee patients, this may involve discussion of health status or events that occurred in the refugee camp, when symptoms might have emerged for the first time.

Third Clinic Visit

During the third visit (see Table 18A-1), the practitioner continues to evaluate the patient's symptoms and assess the efficacy of interventions. It is now appropriate to ask more probing questions about the migration, including the reason for leaving the homeland, the status of family and friends left behind, or specific details of the patient's flight. By now, a trusting relationship has likely been formed, and the patient may feel more comfortable disclosing painful portions of their migration history, such as imprisonment, torture, or other distressing memories. The medical evaluation is well under way, with symptoms evaluated by way of traditional medical, psychological, and cultural approaches.

PHYSICAL EXAMINATION

The physical examination is an opportunity for hands-on nursing care. Because nonverbal communication is the primary or only mode of communication between practitioner and patient when they do not speak the same language, the examination allows the nurse to provide touch and reassurance while gathering data. Even in follow-up clinic visits, when little new information might be gained from the physical examination, a maneuver that involves touch is helpful. Taking the pulse or blood pressure places the practitioner in direct contact with the patient and reinforces their nonverbal relationship. Otherwise, the pair is forced to rely only on verbal communication, which usually occurs through a third person: the interpreter (Sluzki, 1984).

Folk Treatments

The physical examination also allows the practitioner to examine the patient for the stigmata of folk treatments. In many Southeast Asian cultures, moxibustion, coin rubbing, or cupping are common treatments (Buchwald, Panwala, & Hooton, 1992). Moxibustion involves placing a burning herb stick over or onto an affected area of distress. A small superficial burn typically remains after the treatment, such as two symmetrical burns seen at either side of the umbilicus of young Cambodian children. The patients believe such treatment is useful for diarrhea, but practitioners may mistake the treatment as a sign of child abuse.

In coin rubbing, a coin is rubbed over the back in the linear configuration of the acupuncture meridians. A lubricant, such as tiger balm, facilitates the rubbing and leaves ecchymotic marks across the back. This treatment is common in adults and children, who believe it is useful for upper respiratory tract complaints. Unfortunately, practitioners unfamiliar with the practice have also mistaken it as evidence of child abuse.

Cupping is a treatment in which a small cup is warmed to create a vacuum and then placed over the area of complaint, usually the forehead, leaving a circular ecchymotic area that lasts for several days. This is a typical treatment for headache; it is not uncommon to see many patients in the waiting room with cupping marks on their foreheads.

Cultures vary in the types of treatments they consider useful. Some patients from East Africa, the Sudan, Ethiopia, or Eritrea use ritual scarification or folk surgery as treatments. Some patients from these cultures believe that vertical scars through the eyebrows are a useful treatment for trachoma. Patients consider uvulectomy as a treatment for dehydration. Perhaps the most controversial folk surgery is female circumcision or genital mutilation. Although this tribal custom has been outlawed, it persists, especially in rural areas. Women who have had sexual mutilation surgery may be ashamed and reluctant to be examined for fear of pain during the examination or of the practitioner's judgment. Painful sequelae and complications are associated with this practice, including increased frequency of infection, painful intercourse and childbirth, and decreased sexual sensitivity (El Dareer, 1983; Ntiri, 1993). Other tattoos and scars are visible on patients from many cultures, including our own.

Practitioners should ask patients if marks are for treatment, protection, or beauty. Practitioners must be aware of the marks some treatments leave. Because not all treatments leave marks, practitioners should inquire in a nonjudgmental way about the use of herbs, drugs, or other treatments as part of the assessment. It is important that practitioners present a nonjudgmental attitude about unfamiliar treatments and remember that Western medical treatments may be equally unusual to patients.

Dual Use of Healing Systems

Most patients are dual users of health systems, continuing to consult with folk or traditional healers while seeking help from Westerner practitioners. For example, they may believe Western medicines such as antibiotics are powerful and highly desirable treatments. One way of joining with the patient is to accept and promote the use of harmless traditional healing methods. This acceptance supports and validates the newcomer's health belief system and allows the practitioner to gradually introduce new concepts regarding health promotion, maintenance, or treatment from a Western perspective.

ASSESSMENT

At assessment, the practitioner can formulate a differential diagnosis and begin to join the Western paradigm with the patient's health belief system. The NP will have completed the history of the patient's illness, using several tools to determine the patient's immigration status and explanatory model or health belief system. The patient will have discussed the complaint and the practitioner will have noted what the patient calls the problem. The completed physical examination will include an assessment for signs of folk treatment. In discussing the assessment with the patient, the practitioner should use both the Western term for the problem and the patient's terminology; for example, "in this country, what you call heat in the belly we call cystitis or urinary tract infection. We believe it is caused by bacteria and is treated in the following manner." Or, "What you call 'wind in the back' we call bronchitis or an infection in the lungs." The assessment (and the problem list in the patient's medical record) includes the Western diagnostic language along with the patient's terminology for the problem.

CARE PLAN

For NPs, the patient care plan includes not only treatment for the patient's problem but also healthcare maintenance, health education, and preventive interventions. When working cross-culturally, the plan is expanded to include interventions that support the patient's health belief system and values. Such support enhances the practitioner–patient relationship and patient compliance and fosters an openness regarding dual healing philosophies. The practitioner should be explicit in discussing each facet of the patient care plan and not assume that the patient or family will understand expectations regarding medications, tests, diet, or consultation with other healthcare providers or folk healers.

Family

It is important to include the family in the care plan whenever possible because diagnoses affect the family as well as the patient. Furthermore, the family is the most important unit of care in most cultures; at times, it is the cohesiveness and integrity of the family unit that gives the patient the hope needed to survive serious illness or depression. The practitioner should ask the patient if particular family members (such as the head of the household) need to be present when the practitioner plans to make care recommendations. Including the family according to the patient's beliefs and wishes demonstrates the practitioner's respect for cultural values and enhances the prospects of compliance with the therapeutic regimen or plan.

Medications

Practitioners often incorrectly assume that patients from other cultures have ready access to remedies and over-the-counter medications. Consequently, practitioners may wait until arriving at a firm diagnosis, validated by quantifiable test results, before prescribing a therapeutic regimen. For newcomer patients, simple treatments such as acetaminophen or cough syrup may be unavailable because of the patient's income, inability to read labels written in English, or inability to speak the same language as the store clerk. For these reasons, it is helpful to provide the patient with simple over-the-counter remedies when possible. This demonstrates the practitioner's intention to care for the patient and to give help readily available to others.

Patients who do not speak or read English also have difficulty remembering medication instructions given verbally; practitioners can provide those patients with medication cards (Fig. 18A-1). Each medication card has an illustration representing morning, noon, early evening, and night. Medications are affixed to the cards with tape or glue under the appropriate time illustration, and the card is enclosed in a plastic envelope for protection. Patients are encouraged to bring the medication cards to each clinic session for review and revision with their practitioner. Use of medication cards illustrates a concrete way of educating patients about how and when to take their medications, even if they cannot read.

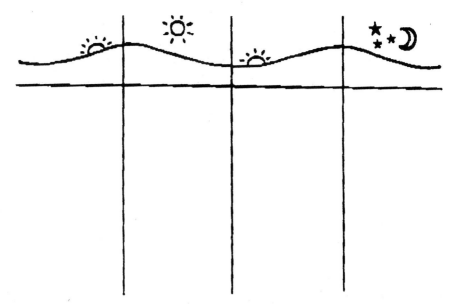

FIGURE 18A-1 Sample Medication Card for Patients Who Do Not Speak or Read English. Illustrations represent morning, noon, early evening, and night. Medications are affixed under the appropriate time illustration.

Blood Tests and Other Procedures

Blood tests present a particular problem in patient compliance. Because many patients may believe that blood embodies the life essence, they are fearful that they will become weak from blood loss or that their blood might be used for sinister purposes. It is helpful for the practitioner to explain that the body reproduces blood and to give the patient juice or water to help replenish fluids. The practitioner should reassure the patient that only clinic professionals will have access to the blood for testing.

Many highly technical medical tests used in the United States are unavailable in developing countries, so there may not be any equivalent terminology in the patient's language. To allay anxiety, the practitioner should take time to explain why the tests are being ordered and how the procedure will be done. The practitioner should also schedule a follow-up appointment soon after a test or any specialty referral to discuss further information, answer questions, and monitor compliance.

Diet

Diet interventions are common the world over, especially when other treatments are unavailable. Patients will often ask for dietary advice if the practitioner does not offer it. Cultures vary in their beliefs about what constitutes a healthy or therapeutic diet. Hot and cold theories abound but differ in which foods are assigned "hot" or "cold" status. Rather than memorize specific regimens for each culture, it is helpful for the practitioner to use sound nutrition information available in the United States, noting that some foods may be especially useful for a particular condition in the patient's culture. The practitioner should ask the patient about these foods and accommodate the patient's beliefs when making dietary recommendations that are sensible for the patient.

Folk Healers

Patients may also wish to continue to see folk healers or may choose to augment Western treatment with a religious ceremony or ritual (Shepherd & Faust, 1993). Continued use of folk healers and rituals can be especially helpful when patients suffer from unresolved grief or bereavement for the many losses they have endured (Eisenbruch, 1984). NPs encourage patients to participate in their care as much as possible, including using familiar, alternative therapies that are not harmful. The practitioner does not have to endorse an alternative therapy to acknowledge that the patient uses it. During each visit, the practitioner should discuss the patient's response to both the folk and Western treatments.

Communication Through Interpreters

Because most practitioners and newcomers do not share a common language, it is necessary to communicate through interpreters. Some clinics and hospitals maintain a staff of trained interpreters, whereas others use volunteer staff or rely on family and friends to provide this service. Medical interpretation, however, is different from word-for-word translation or from having a conversational familiarity with a language. The trained interpreter works not just as a translator of words but also conveys, across cultures, concepts for which there are no words. The interpreter also works as a "culture broker," bringing the patient's beliefs and cultural context to the provider (Faust & Drickey, 1986). Through the interpreter, the NP can explore personal and intimate concerns with patients who may be anxious and unfamiliar with English as well as the language and culture of healthcare.

In newcomer families, a school-age child often has the best grasp of English, and the family may proudly suggest that the child be the interpreter. Using a child as an interpreter, however, reverses the established parent–child roles and places unnecessary and often inappropriate responsibilities and burdens on the child. For this reason, it is recommended to use a trained interpreter when possible.

Cultural values make it difficult for patients to discuss issues of intimacy in the presence of interpreters, especially if the interpreters are of the opposite gender. To enhance reliability and respect, the best match apparently occurs when the interpreter is of the same gender and is older than the patient. The NP should reassure the patient during the first visit that the clinical encounters involving an interpreter are confidential, especially when the interpreter may also be a member of the patient's community.

It is often helpful for the practitioner to review the case with the interpreter before beginning the clinical encounter. They can exchange information about the patient's history and the goal of the visit. With pertinent information, the interpreter will be able to guide the visit, and a useful practitioner–interpreter alliance can be enhanced. It is helpful for the practitioner to face the patient and interpreter together. The practitioner will then be able to maintain eye contact and establish important nonverbal communication with the patient while checking easily with the interpreter. The practitioner can also ask the interpreter for a cultural explanation of the patient's beliefs or practices. For instance, it is common for an interpreter and patient to engage in lengthy conversations in which the provider cannot participate. If requested, the interpreter will explain to the practitioner the cultural context of the discussion that may have concerned a test or treatment unfamiliar to the patient or a healing practice commonly practiced by the patient's culture.

CASE VIGNETTES

The following clinical vignettes use the methods of cross-cultural care discussed in this exemplar. The Western medical tradition is not discussed in depth because it is assumed that the NP reader has considerable experience with this tradition.

Vignette 1

A 48-year-old Russian woman came to the clinic with a complaint of chest pain. A thorough history was taken to assess for a cardiac cause for her pain. After listening to the patient's explanation of the symptom, it became apparent that the complaint was not cardiac in nature but "heartbreak" over the losses she experienced as a result of migration. The aching pain over the heart began soon after arrival in the United States and now persists for hours or days. The pain did not radiate, and there was no diaphoresis, nausea, palpitation, or dizziness. She described the pain as being worse at night when she "thinks too much" and cannot sleep. She had been taking medicine for "nerves" from Russia, and valerian herbal tea to calm herself. She came to the United States as a refugee fleeing persecution for her Christian beliefs but wondered if this was the right thing to do. Life seemed so hard in this country. She was here with her husband and eight children, living on welfare and residing in public housing. Her husband had worked as a miner in Russia and she used to operate a machine in a Kiev factory. Neither spoke English. She requested medicine for her heart from the practitioner and perhaps a referral to a "heart specialist."

Her physical examination revealed borderline hypertension and obesity but otherwise was within normal limits. The assessment helped to shape the care plan as well as validated the patient's perception of her complaint. The NP's diagnosis included borderline hypertension, obesity, and possible angina. In addition, the problem list included "heartbreak" and anxiety caused by stresses of acculturation. The NP ordered appropriate laboratory tests, an electrocardiogram, and a exercise tolerance test. Furthermore, the practitioner discussed nutrition information and recommended a 24-hour diet recall or diary. Knowing that valerian tea is a harmless and common treatment for "heart pain" and nervousness, the NP encouraged the patient to continue its use because it gave some relief. The practitioner referred the patient to a social worker for vocational assessment and help locating an entry-level English class for her and her husband. Her follow-up appointment was set for 2 weeks later.

Vignette 2

A 62-year-old Vietnamese man, VN, came to the clinic with a complaint of generalized weakness and fatigue for the past year. A refugee who had resided in the United States for a little more than 1 year, VN had been an army officer imprisoned for 10 years in a "reeducation camp" in Vietnam before his arrival. He lost most of his family in the war but was here with his son and grandchildren, who were able to escape several years earlier. He believed that his weakness was caused by a problem with his brain and worried about "cancer."

He requested medicine to cure his problem because acupuncture treatments had given him no relief. He denied neurologic symptoms but, with further probing, complained of poor appetite, insomnia, nightmares, and intrusive thoughts about past events in prison. During times of intensified symptoms, he had palpitations, sweated profusely, and felt severe panic. Because of these episodes, he felt weak and fatigued and never seemed rested.

VN's physical examination revealed a thin older male who appeared worried and fatigued. His neurologic examination was completely normal, and he showed no signs of an endocrine disorder. Aside from being slightly underweight, his physical examination was otherwise within normal limits. Tests were ordered to rule out anemia and endocrine conditions. Benadryl and herbal tea were prescribed for sleep. He was advised to eliminate caffeinated beverages from his diet. A follow-up appointment was set for 2 weeks.

During the third visit, VN became tearful while recounting the history of his incarceration in the Vietnamese prison. He had considered taking his own life but felt he must remain strong for his grandchildren. At the time of the third visit, he had no active plan or means to commit suicide. VN's symptoms were consistent with a diagnosis of posttraumatic stress disorder (Hinton et al., 1993; Kroll et al., 1989). Because psychiatric terminology such as depression might be difficult for the patient to accept or comprehend, the practitioner discussed the "weakness" that the patient felt in terms of the suffering and worry he had endured, in addition to malnutrition. "Pain in the life can lead to pain in the body" was a phrase the practitioner found useful when discussing the patient's symptoms.

The assessment and problem list encompassed Western terminology—posttraumatic stress disorder—and also the patient's perception of the problem—weakness and fatigue. Symptomatic therapies were recommended at the third visit. The nurse also offered a contract and plan to minimize the risk of suicide. At future visits, the practitioner will discuss other interventions such as antidepressants or support group participation. In addition, the practitioner might advise the patient to see a counselor or psychiatrist, if available, if the patient agrees.

Vignette 3

A 13-year-old Iraqi girl, AP, came to clinic with the complaint of recent recurrence of bedwetting. She was accompanied by her mother, who stated that the girl had recently begun to wet the bed again, something she had not done since age 10. When this occurs, she gets up and changes the bed herself as her mother has instructed. Her older brother also wet the bed until early adolescence, as did her father when he was a boy. Currently, the patient denies urinary urgency, frequency, dysuria, or hematuria. She denies any endocrine symptoms such as polydipsia or uria and has no abdominal complaints. She states that she has never had sexual contact with anyone (she reiterates this when asked while alone with the practitioner). AP has recently reached menarche and has had two menstrual periods. Her last menstrual period (LMP) was 2 weeks ago.

AP came to the United States 8 months ago with her mother, father, and three brothers. They had escaped from Iraq into Saudi Arabia, where they waited for 6 months before they were granted asylum in the United States. AP's father was formerly a soldier in Iraq and suffered multiple gunshot wounds to the back and legs during the escape. He is also seen in this clinic for chronic pain and posttraumatic stress disorder. AP's mother often seeks counsel in the clinic because of her husband's rages and verbal violence against her and the children. He has not become physically abusive, and she has refused counseling or sanctuary at a women' shelter. She sees the same NP for her primary care as do her husband and other children.

Recently, conflict has escalated in this Muslim family since the onset of AP's menarche. The father believes that it is time to arrange a marriage for her to "keep her safe" now that she is a woman. Both AP and her mother are against this idea and feel helpless in the face of his decision. They feel that "traditions are different" in this country, even for Muslims, but also worry about his anger if they go against him.

On physical examination, AP appears well nourished, easily makes eye contact, and seems childlike in her demeanor. She is Tanner Stage 4, and the remainder of her examination (including external genitalia) is unremarkable. Her urinalysis is negative for blood, white blood cells, sugar, protein, or ketones. Her tuberculosis test (purified protein derivative) was negative 2 months ago.

On assessment, AP is described as having latency enuresis, common in her family but probably exacerbated by recent conflicts over acculturation and her coming maturity. The family's crisis of acculturation and the father's symptoms of posttraumatic stress disorder are centered on this conflict at present, so her symptoms were discussed in the context of the family.

The initial plan included behavioral techniques for addressing enuresis, such as fluid restriction in early evening, an alarm to awaken the patient to void, and instructions to maintain care for her clothes and bedclothes herself. A calendar was given with stickers for the "dry days." After several additional visits with minimal success, desmopressin acetate was given, with relief of her enuresis.

In addition, the NP met with the mother alone to discuss problems in the home. The father also came to the clinic and asked to discuss the difference in law in this country regarding the age of adulthood and marriage. He admitted to periods of rage, and expressed anxiety that he might lash out at his wife and family. He also requested help in dealing with his chronic pain and received some relief with acupuncture. The NP told him that she knew he was doing what he felt was best as the protector of his family but that cultural behaviors and laws were different here. He was also referred to an organization that provides therapy for victims of torture and war.

Summary

This exemplar discussed an approach to cross-cultural patient care based on the patient's explanatory model and the Migration History model. By understanding patterns in the patient's migration history and immigration status, the practitioner can become aware of psychological stressors that can affect the patient's health. Eliciting the patient's explanatory model of illness and examining for evidence of folk treatment enhance awareness of the patient's worldview and assist with supporting the relationship between NP and patient. Treatment options are expanded to include interventions from the patient's culture as well as Western medicine.

Perhaps the most important aspect of this approach is the acknowledgment of the patient as the cultural expert and as the practitioner's ally. It is critical to remember that behind each political event, wave of migration, or cultural worldview, resides an individual who has come for care. Patterns of culture and migration vary with each person, although some generalizations can be made about groups. Mindfulness of and respect for the individual as well as the cultural group of which he or she is a member can only deepen the NP's understanding and practice. The following prose poem illustrates the ability to look to the person for the biography of migration for the true story.

TOOLS OF THE TRADE

I turn my back as he unbuttons his shirt, the fifth article taken off (first a heavy coat brought from the old country, under that a new one—light flimsy—given at the point of entry, then a discarded suit jacket, a cardigan, now the flannel shirt).

His fingers, no longer supple, labor down the buttons. Sent to cobalt mines, he worked the Ukraine thirty years, hands curved around a pick and hammer. He tells this to the interpreter who in turn tells me. Something is lost. I imagine caves full of dark blue stone, blue glass that shatters with every hammer brought down.

They all come in with stories: Zina with her tired bones, Nadezda with her cough. Exposed to cobalt, to the regime, he places his body before me, offers it up. Given everything: how did this man survive? With the tools of my trade, a faith in the tangible, I search for clues (a strong constitution? a vigorous heart?), hold the stethoscope in my hands to warm it, to give his body one less shock. When I turn and lift the gown hospital—regulation, small blue stars against thin white cloth, a picture of the heavens—I find his body covered with faint blue lines, as if the gown were never raised. Looking closer, angels kneel on either side of his chest, face each other, hands clasped over the heart. As he breathes the wings on their backs expand, flutter. He tells the interpreter the angels were tattooed on long ago to protect him from Stalin. His life has been lifted on their wings. What lesser mystery could have guaranteed his passage to this examination room, my care, the soft rubber hammer at his knees?

(Mirosevich, 1994)

Key Points

Western health practitioners often do not understand the value new immigrant patients place on certain symptoms or treatment;

The Migration history model of migration is a helpful tool in the collection of historical information from the patient about his or her migration to the United States;

Most newcomer patients are dual users of health systems, continuing to consult with folk or traditional healers while seeking help from Western practitioners; and

By understanding patterns in the patient's migration history and immigration status, the practitioner can become aware of psychological stressors that affect the patient's health.

REFERENCES

Buchwald, D., Panwala, S., & Hooton, T. M. (1992). Use of traditional health practices by Southeast Asian refugees in a primary care clinic. *Western Journal of Medicine 156*(5), 507–511.

Chung, R. C., & Kagawa-Singer, M. (1993). Predictors of psychological distress among Southeast Asian refugees. *Social Science and Medicine 36*(5), 631–639.

DeLay, P., & Faust, S. (1987). Depression in Southeast Asian refugees. *American Family Physician 36*(4), 179–184.

Eisenbruch, M. (1984). Cross cultural aspects of bereavement: II. Ethnic and cultural variations in the development of bereavement practices. *Culture, Medicine and Psychiatry 8*(4), 315–347.

El Dareer, A. (1983). Complications of female circumcision in the Sudan. *Tropical Doctor 13*, 41–45.

Faust, S., & Drickey, R. (1986). Working with interpreters. *Journal of Family Practice 22*(2), 131, 134–138.

Hinton, W. L., Chen, Y. C., Du, N., et al. (1993). *DSM-III-R* disorders in Vietnamese refugees: Prevalence and correlates. *Journal of Nervous and Mental Disease 181*(2), 113–122.

Kleinman, A., Eisenberg, L., & Good, B. (1978). Culture, illness, and care: Clinical lessons from cross-cultural research. *Annals of Internal Medicine 88*(2), 251–258.

Kroll, J., Habenicht, M., Mackenzie, T., et al. (1989). Depression and post-traumatic stress disorder in Southeast Asian refugees. *American Journal of Psychiatry 146*(12), 1592–1597.

Maugham, W. S. (1944). *The razor's edge* (Introduction). New York: Farrar, Straus & Giroux.

Meucke, M. (1992). New paradigms for refugee health problems. *Social Science and Medicine 35*(4), 15–523.

Mirosevich, T. (1994). Tools of the trade. *Seattle Review 17*(1), 44.

Ntiri, D. W. (1993). Circumcision and health among rural women of Somalia as a part of a family life survey. *Health Care for Women International 14*, 215–226.

Nydegger, C. (1983). Multiple causality: Consequences for practice. *Western Journal of Medicine 138*(3), 430–436.

Patcher, L. (1994). Folk illness beliefs and behaviors and their implications for health care delivery. *Journal of the American Medical Association 271*(9), 690–694.

Shepherd, J., & Faust, S. (1993). Refugee health care and the problem of suffering. *Bioethics Forum 9*(2), 3–7.

Sluzki, C. (1979). Migration and family conflict. *Family Process 18*(4), 379–390.

Sluzki, C. (1984). The patient provider translator triad: A note for providers. *Family Systems Medicine 2*(4), 397–400.

Sluzki, C. (1992). Disruption and reconstruction of networks following migration/relocation. *Family Systems Medicine 10*(4), 359–363.

Westermeyer, J. (1990). Motivations for uprooting and migration. In W. H. Holtzmann & T. H. Bornemann (Eds.). *Mental health of immigrants and refugees* (pp. 78–89). Austin, TX: Hogg Foundation for Mental Health.

Westermeyer, J., Bouafuely, M., Neider, J., & Calleis, A. (1989). Somatization among refugees: An epidemiologic study. *Psychosomatics 30*(1), 34–43.

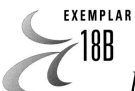

EXEMPLAR

18B

Beth Israel Deaconess Home Care:
A Model for Practice

Karen L. Dick
Susan Burns-Tisdale
Julie R. Knopp

The delivery of home health services continues to change and to respond to changes in the larger healthcare system. Services historically viewed as hospital-based continue to be routinely provided in the patient's home. Almost every treatment modality that can be made portable is a possible home care service (Council on Scientific Affairs, 1990). These modalities include caring for the ventilator-dependent patient, administering intravenous therapies, monitoring the patient with a high-risk pregnancy, and a variety of other care services. The expertise and equipment required to treat and sustain patients have been successfully implemented in the home, where patients, families, and diverse healthcare professionals work together in a less formal, structured environment (Mehlman and Younger, 1991). Care at home spans the continuum from prevention to rehabilitation to long-term maintenance. The most prevalent type of home health service is care of the older adult with a disabling chronic illness or illnesses.

Nurses have had a long history of providing care in the home. The basic assumptions underlying community health nursing practice described in the 1970s still hold great relevance in the practice of home care nursing in the 1990s. The emphasis on the environmental, social, and personal health factors affecting health status, as well as the care of the individual experiencing disease or disability, characterizes this practice. Nurses are most often the formal case managers for patients receiving home health services. The nurse completes an assessment, develops a plan of care, monitors the patient's care needs, and adjusts the plan accordingly. Much time and attention is given to teaching the patient and others in their life. They need information and support about how to care for the patient and effectively deal with issues related to patient care. The burden of care falls on the patient and family. Nurses and other health providers need to pay close attention to patients' and families' ability to manage the many components of care at home that are often overwhelming. This type of family-centered care, with interdependent relationships among the patient, the family, and the environment, is best coordinated by the professional nurse.

Older persons have long been the focus of home healthcare. The Medicare Home Health Benefit, introduced during the Johnson Administration in 1965, ensured access for older adults to home health services. The intent of the benefit was to cover patients' short-term needs, generally following a hospitalization. Thus, the home health benefit is grouped and administered under Medicare part A, which includes the hospital benefit. A few exceptions allow limited longer-term needs to be addressed. Patients must be homebound, have a skilled nursing or physical therapy need, and be under the care of a physician to qualify for services under this benefit. Other recipients of home health services include younger, homebound patients with disabling illnesses. These may include patients with illness related to human immunodeficiency virus (HIV), cancer, or multiple sclerosis. Patients requiring short-term intervention, following surgery or other invasive procedures, also require home health services. Most home health programs care for sick children and postpartum mothers and their infants.

In the late 1980s, most insurance plans began to offer home care as part of their healthcare benefits package, thus increasing access for a wider population. Both private and non-profit agencies that offer an array of specialized services and programs and compete for patients with complex medical and nursing needs have proliferated. The growth of managed care systems may limit the number of home care services that patients receive for a specific episode of illness. Managed care companies often hire internal case managers who, based on review of the patient's medical record, dictate the type and frequency of home care services offered. These companies also subcontract with specific home care companies to deliver home services, often at the most competitive prices. Many clients may be at risk of compromised care when assessment and delivery of care focuses on specific reimbursable services rather than on the establishment of a holistic plan of care (Benson and McDevitt, 1994). However, we have found that relationships and growing trust between the home care staff and the managed care case managers have facilitated the approval for necessary services. The instance that patients are well known by community case managers, home care length of stays can be shortened and patients can be transitioned more easily.

Expenditures for home healthcare have risen exponentially in recent years. In response to spiraling costs and focusing on the perception of widespread overutilization and wasteful spending in the Medicare system, the Balanced Budget Act of 1997 proposes to reduce payments to hospitals ($40 billion), managed care ($21.8 billion), skilled nursing services ($9.5 billion), and home healthcare ($16.2 billion) (Ettinger, 1998). Interim payment system puts a cap on home care reimbursement for 1998 and 1999 at 1993 rates. It establishes an interim payment system for home health services. Instead of payment for services provided at established per-visit rates, home health agencies are paid a capped per-beneficiary rate, regardless of the type and duration of services. According to the National Association of Home Care, these new per-beneficiary limits, although applied in the aggregate, may create perverse incentives. Agencies are faced with the financial disincentive to care for patients with intense needs. "The sickest and most fragile patients may have difficulty accessing and continuing services, experience reduction in services, or be shifted to less appropriate care settings" (National Association of Home Care, news release, March 16, 1998). The target of this reduction in payment is the "disproportionate users," who are the frailest, poorer, and older, and are of more limited mobility than the typical Medicare user. These are the patients who rely heavily on care provided by home care agencies and who otherwise would be institutionalized. The question that home health providers and other caregivers struggle with is "What is society's obligation to these patients who are living to ages unheard of, have multiple chronic illnesses which are limiting but manageable, and have limited financial resources and who want to remain in their homes?" (Home and Health Care Association of Massachusetts, 1998). Since Beth Israel Deaconess Home Care took on the mission many years ago of providing access and care to this same vulnerable population, we are struggling to provide essential care to a group of our current patients who require intensive oversight and services. We have had to reexamine our commitment to providing primary care to these patients with limited resources. In some cases, we have had to change payment sources, including transitioning patients to free care or Medicaid. We have had to force patients to self-sufficiency for tasks once the domain of the nurse. We have had to ask already burdened family members to take on greater caregiving responsibilities. It is clearly a difficult time for home health providers in maintaining a sense of satisfaction about practice, but we are committed to continuing to provide care to those most in need by exploring other options. These will be discussed at the end of this exemplar.

Beth Israel Deaconess Home Care

The Beth Israel Deaconess Home Care Department (Home Care) has been providing care for patients at home for more than 40 years. In the late 1970s, nurse practitioners (NPs) were integrated into the department with a physician practice, the Urban Medical Group. This group, an independent, nonprofit group practice of primary care physicians and mid-level providers, had been providing individualized care to the chronically ill, elderly, homebound, and nursing home residents of urban Boston. Their care was characterized by the elements of personalization and continuity. The group was committed to working with other providers, including NPs, to meet the complex needs of vulnerable populations (Master et al., 1980). NPs brought to the homes of generally frail, sick elders services that had previously required a trip to an ambulatory center. This was particularly important for this group of patients who had great difficulty leaving home. Although the program has grown in recent years to encompass a more diverse patient population, most of our patients continue to be older than 75 years, with several chronic illnesses. This population of patients continues to require ongoing monitoring and evaluation of the interplay of acute and chronic disease, social factors, function, and safety. We believe that our NP model provides for the delivery of care that best meets the needs of this vulnerable population. NPs are able to provide ongoing primary medical aspects of care, serve as case managers, provide linkages to the greater healthcare system, and provide direct hands-on nursing care (Burns-Tisdale and Goff, 1989). This type of care delivery model is in keeping with the need for the development of alternative programs and approaches to meet the needs of the underserved and at-risk populations. NPs have been providing this type of primary care service for many years now and have skill in triaging, coordinating, and managing healthy and unhealthy populations in primary care settings that equals and sometimes exceeds that of physicians in the same setting (OTA, 1986).

We believe that, given the current reimbursement crises in home health, the need for the advanced practice nurse (APN) in the home setting becomes even more essential to meet the needs of increasingly complex and challenging patient care situations, particularly in the absence of a consistent physician presence. These are the days when we no longer have the luxury of two or three visits to complete a thorough assessment and develop a comprehensive care plan: this has to be completed on the first visit. Like our colleagues on the acute care side, we now establish the discharge plan during that first visit. Instead of conceptualizing the duration of care on a monthly basis, we now think in terms of weeks. It is the APN who has the well-developed collaboration and communication skills necessary to ensure the delivery of safe, efficient, quality care to this population of patients. The critical question remains, though, who will pay for this service and for how long?

Beth Israel Deaconess Home Care is a certified home health agency that provides the customary skilled nursing and home health aide visits; physical, occupational, and speech therapies; social service; and physician visits. Although most of the nursing staff are NPs, baccalaureate-prepared nurses also provide care and work collaboratively with the NPs. All nursing visits, regardless of which nurse provider is providing them, are billed at the same rate: a separate charge is not incurred for NP visits. Primary nursing serves as the practice model for care delivery, with each nurse accountable for the coordination and provision of care to her primary patients. Both the clinical nurses and the NPs serve as both primary and associate nurses for the patients in the practice. The nurses, physicians, therapists, social workers, students, and other providers meet biweekly at team meetings to discuss problematic patient situations, explore alternative interventions, and pursue joint problem solving. It is clear that there is a high degree of trust and shared values in the group as the team comes together to plan for patient care, where all agree that promotion of function, safety, and quality of life is the principle that underlies and guides care decisions. In the past year, the imposed fiscal constraints forced us to be even more creative in our planning for patient care.

A hospital-wide online electronic mail system, as well as the use of fax technology, has greatly facilitated the communication between the Home Care staff and physicians and other providers. Our staff also has access to online patient information that includes information regarding past hospitalizations, medication histories, discharge summaries, and functional health pattern assessments. This type of information-sharing in a centralized database supports patient care continuity.

Most of our referrals come from the inpatient setting, with patients who are referred for posthospital services following the exacerbation and treatment of acute medical or surgical problems. The emergency department also refers patients who are not admitted to the hospital but who require follow-up for acute problems as well as for evaluation of the home environment. We also receive referrals from physicians, community agencies, and other providers. Our program has a reputation for providing a high level of coordinated care, focusing on promoting and maintaining patients' comfort, dignity, and function. We care for several terminally ill patients who choose to die at home and who often require nontraditional, innovative caring practices that are integrated and provided by both clinical nurses and NPs. We have seen a need to respond quickly to the earlier hospital discharge of patients who may require a higher level of intervention with more nursing visits, specific technologies such as intravenous therapy, complex medication regimens, and the need for intensive patient and family education that was not completed during the acute care stay. Because we are hospital-based, nursing staff can visit patients before discharge to help facilitate the transition to home, particularly when specific therapies, equipment, or wound care protocols may need to be followed. Often just the meeting of the home care provider while the patient is still hospitalized eases patients' fears and anxieties about their impending discharge. We also use and consult with various program-based APNs who may have been involved with patients in the inpatient setting and who work with us in planning for discharge. A spirit of partnership is evident as knowledge and resources are shared for optimizing patient care. We have also had situations in which we have had these inpatient APNs accompany us on home visits for help in problem identification and care planning for specific patient problems.

Our department also works collaboratively with NPs in the hospital-based ambulatory practice. We often receive referrals from them for patients who become terminally ill or homebound or are in need of additional supportive home services. We then may share patients with them, or entirely assume the care. Again, it is a colleagueship that is fostered and promoted through our professional practice model as well as a recognition of each practice's scope of responsibility and expertise.

CASE VIGNETTES

We are often asked to delineate how care provided by NPs differs from that provided by clinical nurses. There is a great deal of interest in the cost, efficiency, reimbursement mechanisms, and feasibility of this model, particularly in today's climate, which emphasizes controlling spiraling healthcare costs. Although we have no definitive data, we strongly believe that our patients have fewer hospitalizations, fewer emergency department visits, and fewer hospitalizations, with lower acuity rates, compared with patients managed by other nursing providers. We believe that the NP is effective in sorting out the physical, emotional, and social needs of patients and is skilled in assessing the multiple complicated illnesses and the interaction among the individual patient, illnesses, and therapies (Burns-Tisdale and Goff, 1989). Patient and family satisfaction is rated high as measured by our unit-based survey programs, as is physician satisfaction, as indicated by the increasing number of physician referrals. The key question is that of identifying up-front, at the time of intake, what are the patients' needs and who is the most appropriate provider? Patients with complicated medication regimens requiring frequent adjustment and titration of medications, patients with frequent emergency department visits, and patients with unpredictable presentation of illness are appropriate cases for the NP to manage. Although it is clear that we will need to continue to defend our practice model, from a fiscal perspective, the care examples from our practice give us a rich illustration of the kind of care that NPs provide. The following is one example of a critical incident, as told by a Home Care NP.

Vignette 1

I admitted WB, a 45-year-old HIV-positive woman, to Home Care in late fall. It was another busy Thursday, and I didn't get to her third floor loft apartment until late in the afternoon. She had returned home the previous afternoon after a 1-week Beth Israel Deaconess Hospital stay for evaluation of fatigue and severe jaundice. The diagnosis of viral hepatitis C was compounded by another dismal diagnosis—immunoblastic lymphoma—confirmed by a bone marrow biopsy. Diagnosed with HIV in 1987, it had become clear during this recent admission that her prognosis was poor. WB had been placed on high doses of prednisone, 100 mg every day, the day before hospital discharge, in an effort to address the lymphoma. She was not a candidate for chemotherapy.

When I climbed the stairs to her apartment, I found WB with a friend. Her friend had arrived only a couple of hours earlier to welcome her home. WB had been alone all night and morning. WB was not verbally communicative beyond an occasional "no." She mostly shook her head and sighed deeply. Her mouth and lips were extremely dry. I suggested that her friend make some soup, but WB seemed not to know what to do with a spoon or a glass of water. She had been discharged home with approximately four medications but indicated that she was confused about how to take them. They were all scheduled to be taken every day. I made her a new medication chart. She still didn't understand. Was this delirium or AIDS-related dementia? I didn't know at first. WB's referral made no indication of mental status changes. The pink intake sheet from Home Care noted that her insurance had approved her for only once-a-week skilled nursing visits. Her quiet friend was not much help either beyond stating that WB "didn't seem herself." I called the floor at Beth Israel Deaconess where she had been discharged. The primary nurse had left for the day, and no one who knew WB was on the floor. I called her physician who was unavailable by page. The registered nurse (RN) case manager at the community health center where WB received her care said that, if I had to send her back to the emergency department, I could, but she knew that WB did not want to go back to the hospital. And no, her behavior was not baseline per my description. Finally! Some information! My assessment was a steroid-induced psychosis. Unfortunately, I had no idea what the patient's real baseline was.

I was somewhat incredulous that WB had been discharged less than 24 hours earlier and that no one had seen this mental status change. I had never before been the first clinician on the scene to make the assessment of a new psychosis. I knew that WB could not be left alone. I also quickly assessed that her friend was overwhelmed and not able to manage the situation. I knew I wanted to avoid WB landing in the emergency department within 24 hours of discharge if possible. WB's friend had left the apartment within a half hour of my arrival, and I was awaiting the supposed visit of WB's sister, who was to arrive late in the afternoon. Fortunately, at 5:30, her sister HB, an RN, arrived and agreed to spend the night. HB was clearly torn between her role as an RN versus sister who was seeing her sibling slip away. I spent the next 30 minutes talking with HB about who her sister was, while she cried and hugged WB. I gently broached the role of RN with HB, trying to focus her and outline a plan of care, with a primary emphasis on safety issues. I felt that she was up to the task, despite her ambivalence, fear, and sadness. I asked HB not to administer any more prednisone until I spoke with the MD the next day, to presumably start a taper, which was, in fact, what happened. HB was adamant that she would "pinch hit" during this crisis, but that she had no intention of becoming the primary caretaker. She had to leave the following day. I had a crash course in case management issues with WB's managed care plan, as I worked hard to negotiate for 8 hours of home health aide time and skilled nursing visits every day. These were instituted on her second full day at home, and within a week her delusions cleared, her mental status returned to baseline, and I finally got to know my patient.

My initial feeling when I walked out of her loft after that second visit was that I had been lucky. On further reflection, I realize I had taken a lot of clinical information, cross referenced with a geriatric knowledge base of dementia versus delirium, and used my ability to communicate with families to pull together a plan that gave the patient her best shot at remaining home. Months after our initial meeting, WB would often laugh about how crazy she had been those first days at home. She had vivid recollections of her delusions. In an effort to acknowledge that it had been a shared experience, I told her I was a little scared not having sent her back to the hospital. She responded by telling me it wasn't fear or bravery, but that I was a professional who knew what I was doing. "Ah, fooled again," I told her, but I knew I had been paid a wonderful compliment.

This case is an illustration of the various functions that NPs practicing in the home are called on to carry out. Here the nurse used an advanced knowledge base to assess a medical condition, communicated with other providers, negotiated with third-party payers for increased services, formulated a workable plan with a family member, provided emotional support, and prevented a readmission to the acute care setting. This case illustrates the role of the NP as an autonomous provider who successfully intervened for a vulnerable patient.

Vignette 2

This second case describes a woman who, without a Home Care NP, would have had no care.

AF had a lifelong history of avoiding healthcare, especially physicians. She also had a long and active problem with alcoholism. Ten years before her Home Care admission, AF's daughter found her unconscious at home. She was admitted to the hospital, diagnosed with a left cerebrovascular accident that had occurred in the setting of an acute anemia caused by gastrointestinal tract bleeding caused by portal hypertension. She was treated and discharged but never returned for follow-up. Ten years of continued drinking ensued. AF began to have severe foot pain from gout and to self-medicate with aspirin. She also developed a large venous ulcer on her chronically edematous legs. Her daughter felt frantic and did not know where to turn for help because her agoraphobic mother refused to go out to see a doctor. At this point, her daughter approached me as I was visiting other patients in an elderly housing building. I agreed to meet the daughter at her mother's apartment with the goal of providing care.

On the appointed day, I arrived and was greeted by a frightened, elderly woman with severe ascites and mobility limitations who was shouting in an abusive manner that she would never under any circumstances come to the hospital. Using many different therapeutic approaches, I finally persuaded AF to allow care. It would be a long process to convince her to accept an MD, and ultimately she saw the MD only twice during a 2-year period marked by significant medical instability. Initially she was persuaded to allow venipuncture, which revealed a severe anemia and a probable active gastrointestinal tract bleed that needed to be assessed and treated in the hospital. She refused. I worked long and hard with AF to stop her drinking and aspirin use. I consulted with her MD and began treatment with an H2 blocker and iron for the gastrointestinal tract bleed and diuretics for the edema from the cirrhosis. Daily visits were made to treat the venous ulcer. Providing personal care required much therapeutic negotiation and limit setting, as AF was choosing to self-neglect out of her fear. The Home Care social worker was consulted and provided invaluable assistance and support with this difficult situation. Home health aides and the physical therapist provided maximal support as well. Ultimately, after another acute period of deterioration with a rebleed treated and managed at home, an unstable fluid status managed at home, and marked immobility supported by appropriate provider interventions, AF reached an level of optimum health and function for her. She had 2 good years before I found that she had a nonhealing mouth lesion that was eventually diagnosed as malignant. At this point, she was finally ready to see a physician and accept hospitalization, which she did. However, treatment options for her malignancy were limited, and she died peacefully on intravenous morphine therapy in a coma induced by liver failure.

This case is an example of a patient whose only access to healthcare occurred through her contact and relationship with her Home Care NP. AF is another example of the complex medically ill patient who can be managed primarily by an NP with appropriate consultation from a supportive MD.

Vignette 3

This last case example describes a complex patient who benefited from the ongoing relationship with the patient and his wife in detecting and managing his illnesses. AD is a 76-year-old man with chronic obstructive pulmonary disease (COPD), chronic heart failure, adult-onset diabetes mellitus, and peripheral vascular disease who was referred to Home Care after a January 1997 hospitalization for a COPD exacerbation and an infected leg wound. He had been followed by the visiting nurses but his wife was frustrated by the lack of communication between the RN and MD and his frequent hospitalizations. His MD suggested that Mr. D's care be transferred to us. Mrs. D's first request of me was that I be the only person to see her husband because she knew his lungs changed frequently and she wanted to have someone know him intimately. We agreed that I would keep the number of providers to a minimum but I also let her know that another nurse on my team would also follow him: we set up time for my colleague to meet Mr. D before I went on vacation. Because of his multiple, interconnected medical problems, frequent nursing visits were made to assess his cardiopulmonary status, evaluate and titrate medications for his diabetes, and ensure adequate skin care. Mrs. D finally agreed to a physical therapy evaluation and a home health aide to assist with bathing and the physical therapy exercises. She was an excellent caregiver: she was very involved in his care, and she felt that she was the cause of his long life in face of his severe chronic illnesses. They had three sons, one of whom was living at home. The sons were helpful and could be called on to help as needed. It took approximately 6 months for Mrs. D to trust me. It took a year for me to be able to make changes to his insulin doses without her insisting that I call the endocrinologist first.

During his admission to Home Care, Mr. D has been treated successfully for nine upper respiratory tract infections. His tenuous status required that I frequently adjust his insulin doses because of prednisone dosing, along with titration of diuretics and antihypertensives. Understanding the complexity and connectedness of his symptoms and subtle changes in status have led to early detection and treatment of these infections.

Since January 1997, Mr. D has been hospitalized twice, once for shingles and once for bronchitis. The hospitalization for shingles followed a visit to the pain clinic: he was admitted from the clinic. If he had been at home, I would have been able to treat him at home. I also sent him to the emergency department after a conversation with his MD once for back pain: I realize now it was my inexperience and lack of familiarity with his presentation of clinical symptoms that led to the emergency department visit. Mr. D now sees his primary care physician twice a year, his pulmonologist twice a year, and the endocrinologist twice a year. I visit him two to three times a month, with additional visits as needed. Before his admission to Home Care in 1997, Mr. D had had eight hospital admissions in 1996, and six in 1995. I feel strongly that our success in keeping him at home and out of the hospital works because of the prompt treatment for acute problems I am able to provide. I am also able to provide support to Mrs. D. She is often despondent about her lot in life, and my goal is to provide support for her because she is the primary caregiver in the family. Given her history of breast lumps, I provide frequent breast examinations and help her keep a record to follow her examinations over time. I also routinely check her blood pressure and provide flu shots for the family. I have found that this kind of support for the family benefits the patient in unseen ways, and as an NP providing home visits I have the means to provide this kind of care.

The Future

When we think about the future of the NP model in home care, it may become feasible to consider three alternative approaches. One is a care team model. These teams would include an NP, a clinical nurse, and a physician. When the NP is the primary nurse, the clinical nurse will be the associate nurse; and when the clinical nurse is the primary nurse, the

NP will be the associate. Our sense is that this will provide patients the best of what we have to offer in knowledge and skills. In addition, this model will facilitate coordination of complex patient care and intradisciplinary and interdisciplinary collaboration.

In another type of program, NPs can be paired with primary care physicians together in teams and collectively decide how to best follow a caseload of homebound patients. Unlike NPs in the Beth Israel Deaconess program, these NPs do not provide all the required nursing care. The practitioner may complete the assessment, develop the plan of care, and then refer the patient to a local Visiting Nurses' Association (VNA) for skilled nursing. These VNAs have a contractual agreement to this hospital-based program. The NP may then work closely with the VNA and depend on them to notify her of changes in the patient's condition (Mitiguy, 1994). This model has the advantages of accessing expert consultation and supervision at the individual case level, ensuring a mechanism for early referral of patient problems, and potentially decreasing the incidence of serious complications and hospital readmissions by this linkage to an APN (Soehren and Schumann, 1994).

With the ability to now bill under Medicare part B independently and without the "incident to" caveat, services furnished by NPs in the home can be reimbursed directly. These services would include services that would be reimbursable when provided by a physician. The development of a "house calls" type of program is under way. This would allow us to meet the needs of patients who may require episodic visits to assess and treat an acute problem. These patients may be those who become unable to come to the primary care ambulatory practice and instead come to the emergency department. Primary care physicians could refer high-risk patients to us for this purpose. We could also market to managed care programs to provide these types of visits to targeted at-risk groups. Finally, we would be able to transition patients off of the traditional home health benefit and on to this type of model. Although patients would not be eligible for the same services as provided under the home health benefit, we could meet our mission in continuing to provide primary care to the most vulnerable.

REFERENCES

Benson, E., & McDevitt, J. (1994). When third party payment determines service: The elderly at risk. *Holistic Nursing Practice 8*(2), 28–35.

Burns-Tisdale, S. & Goff, W. (1989). The geriatric nurse practitioner in home care. *Nursing Clinics of North America 24*(3), 809–817.

Council on Scientific Affairs. (1990). Home care in the 1990s. *Journal of the American Medical Association 263*(9), 1241–1244.

Ettinger, W. (1998). The Balanced Budget Act of 1997: Implications for the practice of geriatric medicine. *Journal of the American Geriatrics Society 46*, 530–533.

Home and Health Care Association of Massachusetts. (1998). *Position statement.*

Lerman, D., & Linne, E. (Eds.). (1993). *Hospital home care.* Chicago: American Hospital Publishing.

Master, R., Feltin, M., Jainchill, J., et al. (1980). A continuum of care for the inner city: Assessment of its benefits for Boston's elderly and high risk populations. *New England Journal of Medicine 302*(26), 1434–1440.

Mehlman, M., & Younger, S. (Eds.). (1991). *Delivering high technology health care.* New York: Springer Publishing Co.

Mitiguy, J. (1994). Caring for the elderly at home. *Boston Nurse 2*(9), 16.

Office of Technology Assessment, US Congress. (1986). *Nurse practitioner, physician assistants and certified nurse midwives: A policy analysis.* Washington, DC: US Government Printing Office.

Soehren, P., & Schumann, L. (1994). Enhanced role opportunities available to the CNS/nurse practitioner. *Clinical Nurse Specialist 8*(3), 123–127.

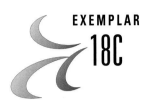

The Rural Nurse Practitioner

Leslie H. Rozier

The accident occurred at sunset. The call came in as I was closing the clinic after a long day that had started at 3 AM with an injured fisherman. They hit the dock piling as they brought the skiff onto shore. Blue and gasping for air he was pulled from the ice cold water of the bay. Faced with a fisherman with a ruptured diaphragm, broken ribs, collapsed lung, pelvic fractures, and significant alcohol intoxication, I faced one of the longest nights of my life. Darkness and sustained 50-mile-an-hour wind, with gusts to 90, prohibited the usual amphibious support to the neighboring island. Eighteen hours later, fighting fatigue and physiologic odds, we lifted off the island on a Coast Guard helicopter. As I looked down on the 30-foot waves in the Bering Sea, I wondered if we would make the first 100 miles of our 800-mile journey to the hospital. I began to wonder if my decision to practice in the Aleutian Islands was a sane one.

The Rural Community

Every rural community is unique. The nurse practitioner (NP) must carefully analyze the community characteristics that are expressed in the geographic location, the population demographics, local politics, religious groups, local board philosophies, and cultural hierarchies when considering a practice in a rural area. What are frequently overlooked during the anticipation phase of rural transition are the unrealistic expectations placed on the community by the practitioner.

CASE VIGNETTES

Vignette 1: The Rural Community
The village had no roads or cars. The clinic was situated near the center of the village next to the boardwalk that connected every building and home. I anticipated that the clinic's central location would be ideal for enhancing patient visits, but after 3 months, my expectations waned. I discovered that most

healthcare questions and referrals came during my walks from the clinic to the post office, the store, or a patient's home. Altering my expectations of a professional practice in a rural community, I locked the clinic and embraced what came to be known as "boardwalk rounds." My visibility in neutral territory augmented my success in the community. By 6 months, I had weekly home visits to the elders, weekly school visits, and bimonthly screening clinics in the post office lobby.

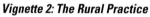 The Rural Practice

Rural practice is demanding and unforgiving. The responsibilities one accepts as the professional practitioner in the rural community are immense. Professional strengths must be diverse, as any weaknesses will be quickly exposed. It takes a unique personality to balance the professional and personal demands of the rural setting. Few individuals are willing to relinquish the resources of the urban environment to explore and experience their profession in a rural community. It is interesting that veteran practitioners often fondly describe the rural experience as the one that broadened the depth and dimension of their professional experience.

The rural practice provides the practitioner the occasion to study individuals, family units, health and disease processes, and health-related dynamics, not only in the clinic, but in the community and its stores, eating establishments, neighborhood library, school classrooms, churches, homes, parks, and roadways. One quickly learns that rural practice is a lifestyle, not a job.

Vignette 2: The Rural Practice

My professional dream was now a reality. I was going to be an NP providing healthcare in a remote, isolated practice. The professional package was perfect. The office hours were Monday through Friday, 8 to 5, with a full benefit package that included housing. What I failed to grasp before my arrival was the responsibility of being the only healthcare provider in 4000 square miles. Twenty-four–hour call took on a new dimension.

When I arrived, I was in awe of the clinic. There was a new portable x-ray machine, a state-of-the art x-ray processor, and a shrink-wrapped, covered computer sitting in its box. All of the basic equipment and supplies were there. I was ecstatic! What I didn't appreciate at the time was that they all required electricity. It took several weeks, but when the rain stopped, the water drained from the subtundra groundcover, and the hydroelectric plant ceased to run. On good days, the diesel generator would start up and the clinic lights would be reborn. If you were unlucky and the plane had delivered its precious cargo of alcohol, then flashlights and your professional savvy would suffice.

The Rural Nurse Practitioner

NPs have been providing primary care to isolated and underserved rural areas since the inception of the profession (Ford, 1994; Ford & Silver, 1967; Silver, Ford, & Day, 1968; Silver, Ford, & Stearly, 1967). The rural community has been the training ground for energetic and gifted nurses seeking the experiences of professional autonomy. It is the rare opportunity that many of us seek, but what the adventuresome NP rarely appreciates are the unspoken demands and expectations of "the nurse" by the rural community.

The rural NP engages in a specialized discipline that has its own dynamics, unique to the rural environment. The demands on the nurse require a resourceful and strong individual who must be highly skilled and competent in clinical practice while being sensitive to the unique cultural and social qualities of each community. It is a specialty that is concerned with the total well-being of the individual, the family, and the community.

Vignette 3: The Nurse Practitioner in the Isolated, Rural Community

As a family NP, I was hired to provide comprehensive healthcare to the residents of a remote, isolated island in the Aleutian Archipelago, a 1000-mile chain of islands off the coast of Alaska. NPs provide and coordinate most of the healthcare in bush Alaska, and professional isolation is the gold standard. I became the village nurse but in reality I was the mental health counselor, public health nurse, school nurse, social worker, pharmacist, dentist, optician, city sanitarian, clinic plumber, flight surgeon, and veterinarian; in retrospect, a nurse with many names.

I lived among the Russian Aleuts, whose families were taken from their homes by the U.S. government when the Japanese invaded the Aleutian Islands 6 months after the bombing of Pearl Harbor. During the Japanese occupation of Attu and Kiska, the villagers of the island were sent to internment camps and for 50 years have tried to rebuild their lives, as well as their children's lives. They have reclaimed their native lands and have rekindled their cultural ties despite their long-standing struggles with Russian fur traders, Scandinavian whalers, and American land dealers.

My primary professional task was to support their health and well-being, to encourage self-sufficiency, and to provide comprehensive medical care in their well-equipped clinic. My other task was to provide medical support to the fishing industry that gleans tons of ocean products daily: cod, crab, halibut, pollack, fingers, arms, lives. Alaska's fisherman works incredibly hard in a profession that holds the record for the highest death rate in America. Both tasks were challenging.

There are no days off in a rural practice. There is only 24-hour call. Professional relief is a concept known only to city dwellers. On the rare occasion that I left the island, all I saw from the plane window was worried faces; mothers who hoped their children would not fall or be injured while I was gone; elders who prayed that they would not die alone; fishermen expecting their luck would hold. Each time I returned I would pack my bags with courage and creature comforts, take a big breath, and welcome the challenges that I faced.

I grew. I thrived. I survived. They loved me. They hated me. I loved them. I hated them. Some grew. Some didn't. I loved it. I hated it. They changed. I changed. As the song goes, "Oz never did give nothin' to the tin man that he didn't, didn't already have" (America, 1975). In time, this tin man realized that NPs make a difference in the lives of Aleuts and fishermen. You live on the edge. You push the envelope. Your rewards have no words but are incredibly intense.

THE RURAL NURSE

"Rural nursing is defined as the practice of professional nursing within the physical and sociocultural context of sparsely populated communities. It involves the continual interaction of the rural environment, the nurse and his or her practice" (Bigbee, 1993, p. 132). Statisticians, the Census Bureau, scholars, and politicians debate what the delineators are that describe "rural," but the general sense is that rural represents few people, limited resources, and isolation, both culturally and geographically. The nurse in the rural environment has to creatively integrate the dimensions of the nursing profession into the rural context. Biegel (1983) described rural nursing as "the diagnosis and treatment of a diversified population of people of all ages and a variety of human responses to actual occupational hazards or potential health problems existent in maternity, pediatric, medical/surgical and emergency nursing in a given rural area" (p. 45). Lee (1991) described two characteristics unique to rural areas that challenge the nurse—low population density and diversity among rural areas—whereas Davis and Droes (1993) talked about the difficulties of practicing in geographically large and sparsely populated areas. What is represented is the variation of practice, professional autonomy, and diversity expected of the professional. Bigbee (1993) simplified the professional expansiveness recognized in rural practice as "a symbiotic relationship between the rural environment and professional practice" (p. 132).

Symbiotic relationships may be beneficial or detrimental, and it takes a creative and sensitive NP to make the relationship with a rural community work. Nightingale's reference to nursing as an art form fully realizes the creativeness that is required in this setting. "Nursing is an art; and if it is to be made an art, it requires as exclusive a devotion, as hard a preparation, as any painter's or sculptor's" (Florence Nightingale, cited in Donahue, 1985, p. 469).

The NP has evolved from this rich and diverse nursing history that is grounded in both art and science. Advanced practice nurses have aggressively sought the science aspect of their profession, but what is unique is their application of the science as nurses. They integrate personalized care, management of patient care services, and collaborative care with other professionals, without preference to their setting. They are nurses; they practice nursing.

There are moments when the rural NP is exposed, vulnerable, and alone, and has to devote incredible energy and diverse skills to the patient or circumstances surrounding a health crisis. What continually challenges the NP is the requirement of proficient skills that span the boundaries between nursing and medicine. It is the art form of nursing that Brush and Capezuti (1996) honor and describe: "Perhaps the reason why NPs consistently performed better than physicians in addressing the primary health care needs of their patients was because nurse practitioners were providing nursing rather than medical care" (p. 7).

The professional requirements are no different for the rural practitioner compared with the urban practitioner, but the degree of accountability and responsibility take on new dimensions in the rural environment. Material and human resources are scarce, and it takes a strong and creative individual to meet the demands of the rural practice. Ironically, some of Clement's (1914) qualities of the 1914 rural nurse are not dissimilar to those of the 20th and 21st century practitioner: courageous, firm, enthusiastic, cheerful, healthy, sympathetic, respectful of the open country with knowledge of country traditions, willing to forego the comforts of city living, possessing broad intelligence, patient, even-tempered, demonstrating a sense of humor, respectful of a discrete and silent tongue, and possessing a well-balanced and broad-minded character (p. 520).

THE EXPERT GENERALIST

Advanced practice in the rural setting has its own unique characteristics and dynamics. DeBella, Martin, and Siddall (1986) described the rural practitioner as an "expert generalist" whose area of practice is now considered a distinct specialty. "This specialty area is characterized by a unique style and approach to practice that requires an innovative, truly generalist approach characterized by as strong generalist role with multiple expectations" (Bigbee, 1993, p. 131). The practitioner whose generalist role provides first-contact care, primary or continuous care, family care, and comprehensive community care must integrate the clinical, biological, and behavioral sciences while engaging in a scope of practice that is not limited by sex, age, disease, or organ systems. It is the ultimate challenge, as the nurse must maintain professional proficiency and competency while being continually challenged professionally and personally.

Vignette 4: The Expert Generalist

I had just finished starting an intravenous infusion on a 6-month-old with dehydration when the schoolchildren came into the clinic. The fourth grader's bicycle tire had missed the ramp to the top of their homemade jump, and he crashed in the salmonberry bushes. Radiographs confirmed a fracture dislocation. The surgeon would take care of him, but the major challenge would be getting him to the surgeon. He had no health insurance. His parents were unemployed. The round-trip plane ticket from the island to the mainland was $890, a significant amount that doubled if his mother accompanied him. They could stay with friends once in town, and if the weather cooperated they could leave the island tomorrow. As his parents talked about their resources, I slipped into the next room and rechecked the infant's intravenous infusion before making phone calls to secure emergency funding.

When I heard the front door of the clinic open, I expected to see another family member. When I

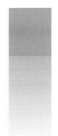

looked up she was standing in front of me, tears rolling down her face, holding her limp cat in her arms. Her cat had encountered a four-wheeler on the boardwalk. After radiographs confirmed a fractured pelvis, the cat was gently placed in the cardboard box that was strapped to the back of my bicycle, fondly known by the villagers as "The Ambulance." I was not optimistic, but I gave her my recommendations for good nursing care as I watched her roll the bicycle and her cat down the boardwalk to her home.

As I slipped back into the clinic to wash off the remnants of the cat, I glanced at the fluid in the infant's intravenous bag and headed back to my office when another call came in. There was a fisherman who had been caught in "the chopper" and had amputated four fingers. The vessel was due north in the Bering Sea—estimated time of arrival was 2 hours. It was going to be a long day.

A NURSE BY NO OTHER NAME

The NP will have an intimate relationship with each patient and will eventually appreciate that most relationships are intertwined with the community. Patients and their community are inseparable. The close, personal, long-term relationship with family and friends reduces professional anonymity and blurs professional, social, and personal roles. The in-depth personal knowledge one gains from working in rural practice can be extremely beneficial in balancing one's professional and personal life. Dolphin (1984) and Benson, Sweeney, and Nicolls (1982) suggested that personal and professional challenges were considered by some nurses as advantages of rural practice, whereas others considered them disadvantages.

> Although lack of anonymity and in-depth interpersonal knowledge are similar and interrelated themes, they each have a different focus. Lack of anonymity is perceived as the sense of knowing who and what everyone is by their name and their community role. In-depth interpersonal knowledge is knowing someone on a person-to-person basis, what their family structure is, their health problems and how to intervene (or the difficulty of intervening) on a professional basis. Lack of anonymity is a public concept, and in-depth interpersonal knowledge is a private one. (Davis & Droes, 1993, p. 168)

How the rural practitioner handles the loss of anonymity in the rural community and the wealth of in-depth interpersonal knowledge gained in rural practice will predict the success of the experience.

THE PASSIVE OBSERVER

The care that the NP provides in the rural community must be mindful. If there is lack of attention to details, the problem will present itself again and again. Innovative creativity is required. The NP must market healthcare services after careful consideration of the needs of the community and the appropriateness of the services to be rendered. The NP must be sensitive to professional, personal, and community relationships. Observing patients in the clinical environment is as important as observing them in the world in which they live. The keys are simple: (1) passively observe your patients, (2) listen carefully to their complaints, (3) gently explore their feelings and perceptions of what they think is wrong, (4) avoid passing judgment, and (5) integrate the information into your evaluation and treatment plan.

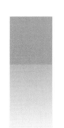

Vignette 5: Passive Observation
I could not understand why he was not getting better. I spent several hours a week working with him. He was compliant with his stretching exercises. He came to the clinic three times a week for my rendition of a physical therapy program. He seemed to thrive on the attention, but his symptoms persisted. It happened one afternoon as I was sitting at my desk looking out the window onto the boardwalk. He was hunched over and tentative in his ataxic gait as he made his way to the store from his home. With each step, he was leaning down onto a very short wooden cane . . . a cane that he had shorted 3 inches without telling anyone.

THE RESOURCEFUL PROVIDER

It is easy to prescribe a balanced lifestyle but more difficult to live one. Veteran practitioners describe various survival techniques, but the astute practitioner will find the combination that works best if care is taken to be objective. "There is no burden so heavy, no night so long that it cannot be eased by music. The members of the Army Nurse Corps should be encouraged to sing, for in song there is a contentment that means happier times, good fellowship, better care for their patients and a more optimistic outlook for the entire Corps" (Aynes, 1973, p. 243).

Vignette 6: Resourcefulness

I was standing in the front of the elementary class timing the 60 seconds of their fluoride rinse. They were fidgeting, making faces, trying to laugh, some choking, and, finding nothing to focus their attention, I began to sing. The change was magical. My voice was a gift that I had been given, a gift that had been silent for years but one that had to be shared. Perhaps it was for my own survival. Health class turned into music class and mental health was entered into the curriculum, theirs and mine.

Rural Wisdom/Rural Rewards

Intellectual curiosity is the mainstay of survival in rural practice. When you stop studying, inquiring, learning, or exploring you become mentally old. Your most valuable resource is your clinical practice, your patients your greatest teachers. Your interactions will bring you your greatest rewards. "The way to prevent fixation of mind is to keep intellectual curiosity alive. Men have sought in vain the fountain of perpetual youth: what they needed to seek instead was the fountain of perennial adventure" (Miller, 1955, p. ii). The perennial adventurer, however, must be mindful and sensitive to personal health and well-being. Honor your health. Honor what you believe. Live what you teach.

Vignette 7: Rural Wisdom/Rural Rewards

I grabbed the radio, called the dog, and stomped out of the clinic. I was angry, frustrated, and discouraged that another weekend was coming to a close and I had not had the opportunity to play, to do something that I wanted to do. We had made plans to climb the peak overlooking the harbor, but the clinic calls prevented my escape. It was a dreary, gray day, and the spring flowers were attempting to open their faces to a warmer sky. I started to climb the hill behind the clinic and knew that within 50 yards my tennis shoes would be wet, and by the time I hit the 1000-ft mark, the Aleutian wind would be howling. Good way to vent my frustrations—poor me.

   As I climbed out of the village watershed, the sun grew brighter, the clouds disappeared, and the sky was a magnificent blue. The dog was chasing eagles and ptarmigan, and the ravens were chasing him. Wildflowers were everywhere. The cinder cone of the volcano was steaming and the entire rim was glistening with wet snow. It was a glorious day. As I turned to look down the mountain, the village was completely buried under dense, gray clouds. It was a kind and symbolic reminder of how important it was to take care of myself.

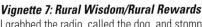

The Rural Adventure

Ruralness is a matter of perspective. It is as complex and diverse as the NPs who find themselves living in its midst. The rural environment is not for the meek and mild but the brave and courageous. The demands are great yet the rural journey will challenge the creativeness and resourcefulness of the individual seeking rewards in unusual places. Accept the ultimate professional challenge. Dare to be a rural adventurer.

Acknowledgment: A special thank you to the Qigiigun Aleuts who honored my innocence and shared their wisdom.

৬ *Essential Points to Remember*

- Each rural community is unique.
- Rural practice is a lifestyle, not a job.
- Rural practice requires commitment to professional proficiency.
- The rural practitioner's specialty is characterized by a strong generalist role.
- The rural NP role requires a hardy, independent individual.
- Rural NPs must be realistic in their expectations.
- Rural NPs work hard, take risks, and listen.

REFERENCES

America. (1975). Tin man. On *America History/America's Greatest Hits* (Warner Bros. Records Inc., Cassette Recording No. WB-M5–3110). Burbank, CA: Warner Communications Co.

Aynes, E. A. (1973). *From Nightingale to eagle.* Englewood Cliffs, NJ: Prentice-Hall, Inc.

Benson, A., Sweeney, M. & Nicolls, R. (1982). A faculty learns about rural nursing. *Nursing Health Care 3*(2), 78–82.

Biegel, A. (1983). Toward a definition of rural nursing. *Home Healthcare Nurse 1*(1), 45–46.

Bigbee, J. L. (1993). The uniqueness of rural nursing. *Nursing Clinics of North America 28*(1), 131–143.

Brush, B.L., & Capezuti, E.A. (1996). Revisiting "A nurse for all settings": The nurse practitioner movement, 1965–1995. *American Academy of Nurse Practitioners 8*(1), 5–11.

Clement, F. E. (1914). American Red Cross town and country nursing service. *American Journal of Nursing 14*, 520.

Davis, D. J., & Droes, N. S. (1993). Community health nursing in rural and frontier counties. *Nursing Clinics of North America 28*(1), 159–169.

DeBella, S., Martin, L., & Siddall, S. (1986). Rural health: Special area of need for nurses in health services and rural development. In *Nurse's role in health care planning.* Norwalk, CT: Appleton-Century-Crofts.

Dolphin, N. (1984). Rural health. In B. B. Logan & C. E. Dawkins (Eds.). *Family-centered nursing in the community* (p. 515). Menlo Park, CA: Addison-Wesley.

Donahue, M. P. (1985). *Nursing: The finest art.* St. Louis, MO: C. V. Mosby.

Ford, L. C. (1994). Myths and misconceptions regarding the nurse practitioner. In D. H. Stapleton & C. A. Welch (Eds.). *Critical issues in American nursing in the 20th century: Perspectives and case studies* (pp. 109–115). North Tarrytown, NY: Rockefeller Archive Center.

Ford, L. C., & Silver, H. K. (1967). Expanded role of the nurse in child care. *Nursing Outlook 15*, 43–45.

Lee, H. (1991). Definitions of rural: A review of the literature. In A. Bushy (Ed.). *Rural nursing* (p. 7). Newbury Park, CA: Sage Publications.

Miller, R. C. (1955). Foreword. In *C. G. Wilson's Alice Eastwood's wonderland: The adventures of a botanist.* San Francisco: California Academy of Sciences.

Silver, H. K., Ford, L. C., & Day, L. R. (1968). The pediatric nurse-practitioner program. *Journal of the American Medical Association 204*, 298–303.

Silver, H. K., Ford, L. C., & Stearly, S. G. (1967). A program to increase health care for children: The pediatric nurse practitioner program. *Pediatrics 39*, 756–760.

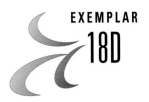

Healthcare for Persons
with HIV/AIDS

Anthony J. Adinolfi

Historical Perspective

In the early 1980s, patients were being seen in hospitals, offices, and clinics with an array of infections and cancers that were not seen in previously healthy people. Men who had sex with men, people who used intravenous drugs, people who received blood and blood products, and hemophiliacs were being treated for medical conditions that usually affected patients with compromised immune systems (e.g., transplant recipients and patients undergoing chemotherapy). *Pneumocystis carinii* pneumonia, a rare form of pneumonia, had never been seen in the general population. Along with Kaposi's sarcoma, a rare cancer of the lining of the blood vessels, affecting young, healthy men, demonstrated that a new disease, or actually a syndrome, was killing young people in the prime of their lives.

The Centers for Disease Control and Prevention in Atlanta, GA, in 1981, notified the country in the weekly *Morbidity and Mortality Weekly Review* that there might possibly be a new disease to be reckoned with. The earliest cases of the as-yet-unknown disease were primarily seen in California and New York and were connected to the sharing of blood and bodily fluids. The disease was called Gay-Related Immune Deficiency because a number of men who became sick had a history of having sex with other men. A couple of years later, the name of the syndrome was changed to acquired immunodeficiency syndrome (AIDS), and this name is used to identify the myriad infections, cancers, and immune system destruction that occurs with the disease. Scientists, physicians, and researchers began their quest for the identification of the causative agent of this syndrome, and in 1985 identified the human T-cell lymphotropic virus, or HTLV III, a virus. A blood test was created to identify antibodies to HTLV III, and all blood that was used throughout the United States was tested for the presence of these antibodies and the blood supply became safer. The virus was then renamed the human immunodeficiency virus (HIV).

At the same time this was occurring, the relationship between sex and the transmission of the virus was strongly identified, and the concept of "safer sex" was created and adopted by many gay men. Campaigns to include condom use with all sexual activity became the norm, and the incidence of HIV among men who have sex with men declined. The population that was to become the new group to be infected was people who injected drugs and their sexual partners. This population of HIV-infected people today includes those people for whom healthcare is a luxury, not a right. African-Americans and women are overrepresented in the numbers of people infected. The U.S. population is composed of approximately 12% African-Americans, although 57% of the new cases of AIDS are in African-Americans. The common denominator of new cases of AIDS in the United States is poverty. Also, AIDS may be the last thing that people worry about after food, housing, substance abuse, and poverty. There is still a stigma around AIDS, and many people are reluctant to be tested and are afraid to be seen attending an "AIDS clinic" for fear of disclosure. Many new cases of HIV infection are discovered when a woman attends a prenatal clinic and has routine testing for her pregnancy.

The U.S. healthcare system is one of the best in the world, although the AIDS crisis is demonstrating the inadequacies of the system. Nurse practitioners (NPs) trained in HIV/AIDS care may be able to reach some patients that slip through the cracks, in HIV/AIDS clinics, or in primary care clinics.

The Nursing Response

Nurses have been leaders in HIV and AIDS care. In San Francisco, Bobbi Campbell, a nurse, the sixteenth person diagnosed with AIDS, was the first person to publicly announce that he had AIDS. He had Kaposi's sarcoma and helped start the first support group for people living with AIDS. At San Francisco General, Cliff Morrison, a clinical nurse specialist, was the first manager of the country's first inpatient unit for people with AIDS. Morrison brought nursing ideas to the management of the unit by allowing the patient to participate in decision making regarding their care and allowing family and friends to visit during "nontraditional times." There is controversy about having patients in a dedicated AIDS ward, although the San Francisco experience proved to be a valuable and viable one.

In 1982, also in San Francisco, it was nurses who organized the Shanti Project. The first AIDS clinic, counseling program, and support services were started by Helen Schietinger, also a nurse. The Visiting Nurses Association of San Francisco, under the leadership of Jeannee Parker Martin, also a nurse, developed and implemented a comprehensive and coordinated approach to caring for persons with AIDS at home.

In New York City, in the early 1980s, it was nurses who initiated educational programs to assist the public in their understanding of AIDS. Also, nurses provided information for professional and lay caregivers to provide sensitive and comprehensive care to persons with AIDS.

In the late 1980s, a group of nurses who were caring for patients with HIV infection met and proposed that a special nursing group be started to represent nurses in HIV care. The Association of Nurses in AIDS Care therefore was started, and in 1999 it celebrates 12 years in existence and offers a certification examination for nurses to become AIDS certified registered nurses (ACRNs). More than 1000 nurses have passed the examination, are nationally credentialed, and use the initials "ACRN" after their names.

My Story

In 1983 I lived in Columbia, SC, and I worked in the Department of Corrections and part-time in a critical care setting. I was taking graduate courses in the school of public health and was examining health issues that were important to gay men. At the time, hepatitis posed a major problem because it was sexually transmitted and it caused major morbidity. I had just begun to hear of a new syndrome affecting previously healthy gay men in San

Francisco, Los Angles, and New York. I moved back to Durham, NC, and joined the North Carolina Lesbian and Gay Health Project, a grassroots organization designed to improve the healthcare of gay men and lesbians. I was working in a large North Carolina hospital as a staff nurse in the coronary care unit. In November 1983, a young man was admitted to the general medical unit of the hospital with *Pneumocystis carinii* pneumonia. He was living in San Francisco and moved back to North Carolina to be closer to his family, who lived in the mountains. Because I was known as the "nurse interested in gay issues," I was asked by the nursing staff to visit Walter (his name has been changed). On my first visit to his room I observed gowns, gloves, masks, and booties outside his door and his room in disarray. As I introduced myself, I realized that this patient needed someone to talk with because the staff quickly performed their tasks and did not spend any extra time with him. He had been diagnosed in San Francisco and had lived in the Shanti Project, a facility that cared for persons with terminal illnesses with no other place to live. He had also participated in death and dying workshops with Dr. Elizabeth Kubler-Ross, and he was home to die. He mentioned to me that in San Francisco there were groups formed to provide "buddies," that is, people who would do things for you like your family would do when you are sick. He asked me if such a group existed in Durham. I said no, but if you help me we can start one here.

A Buddy Support Group grew from a small group of gay men and lesbians who met in my living room on a Sunday in 1983. We had collected information from New York on what buddies were all about and how best to use community resources. We arranged for a Buddy to visit Walter regularly at the hospital, bring him food and toiletries, and, when he was ready to be discharged, find him a place to live. We were able to find him a very pleasant apartment not far from the hospital where he could spend the time that he had left. We also arranged to pick his family up at the bus station when they came to town to visit him and to transport him to and from the hospital for his appointments. This initial buddy project became the first buddy program for people living with AIDS in North Carolina.

The next patient that I met with AIDS was a young man from a small farming community in eastern North Carolina. He was the youngest of eight children, who left home to experience "life in the big city of Atlanta." During early 1984, he came down with a series of infections and suffered severe weight loss. He came home thin and tired and his parents drove him to the local hospital for care. I cared for Chad (his name has been changed) in the coronary care unit because there were no beds in the medical intensive care unit. Chad ended up on a ventilator with acute pneumocystis pneumonia. During his care, the treatment of choice was a medication, pentamidine, and it had to be shipped from the Centers for Disease Control and Prevention in Atlanta. I was assigned to Chad every shift that I worked. I got to know his mom, dad, brothers, sisters, and their families. I provided updates to them and held their hands while they visited Chad and quietly held them when they left the room to cry in the hallways. We all knew that things would not get better. Although Chad remained alert, he experienced episodes of confusion (now looking back he may have had AIDS dementia) that led to him extubating himself and suffering anoxia. He lived a couple of weeks, clinically brain dead, and died on Mother's Day in 1984. The same week, Walter died from complications of Kaposi's sarcoma. It was a rough week.

I continued to volunteer as the coordinator of the buddy program. In late 1985, some of my friends who were HIV-positive asked me if there was a venue where they could talk about their experiences and meet other people with AIDS. I called a friend who was a nurse at another hospital working with AIDS patients, a physician friend, and a psychologist friend to ask them if they would be willing to start a support group for people with AIDS. The first meeting in early 1986 brought together four healthcare providers and two persons with AIDS. This was the start of the first support group in North Carolina for people with AIDS.

Part of my role as buddy coordinator was to meet with physicians in Durham who cared for AIDS patients. The chief of infectious diseases at another major hospital asked me to come and talk with him about the possibility of working with him. I became the first nurse hired by infectious diseases and coordinated clinical drug trials, including the phase II trial of zidovudine (AZT). I was a nurse clinician, that is, trained by my supervising physicians to assist them in providing care. Later, we became members of the National Institutes of Health's AIDS Clinical Trials Group, conducting clinical trials on new and promising AIDS drugs. We also opened a full-time clinic to meet the growing needs of patients with HIV infection, and I was the clinic manager. We went from a staff of 3 to more than 20 and provided interdisciplinary care, which included physicians, physician assistants, NPs, social workers, treatment nurses, research nurses, and ancillary staff.

The early 1980s were heartbreaking. We had few drugs, and those we did have were toxic and expensive. Our patients died in large numbers, and we found that the best thing that we could offer them was kindness, compassion, and fair treatment. We watched as up to 20 patients a month died. We became the extended family of many patients as they were abandoned and rejected by their families and friends.

The late 1980s were better. We were able to prevent opportunistic infections and provide better treatment for HIV. Patients still died, although we had more options for care and better understanding of the infections that occurred.

In 1990, I realized that I could provide better nursing care to my patients if I had an advanced degree. The Duke School of Nursing offered a master's degree with a specialty as a clinical nurse specialist in oncology. I thought that this was the closest I would get to studying HIV, so I enrolled part-time in the graduate school while working full-time in the infectious diseases clinic. The faculty of the clinical nurse specialist program allowed me to pursue study in HIV as it paralleled cancer as the needs that the patients had and the concept of some cancers as a terminal illness. I began to meet and talk with caregivers of persons with AIDS and listened as they talked about how hard it was to care for their loved ones. I proposed to do my master's thesis on the burden of caregiving experienced by caregivers of persons with AIDS. Interestingly, the burden of caring for a person with AIDS paralleled the burden of care that caregivers of cancer patients experience. The number one burden identified by both groups is difficulty in providing transportation for the person they are caring for.

After completing the master's program, I took a job with a clinical research organization, which provided drug companies with the resources to conduct clinical trials. I wrote protocols, reviewed and completed documents for regulatory agencies, and initiated the clinical sites and met with the study coordinators and personnel so they could conduct the trials. During my tenure with the a clinical research organization, I discovered that the Duke School of Nursing offered a new NP option to become an oncology/HIV/AIDS NP. I entered the adult oncology/HIV/AIDS NP program as a part-time, post–master's certificate student in the spring of 1994 and completed the program in 1995. During the program, I worked part-time in the sexually transmitted diseases clinic of the local health department and in the county jail. I was fortunate to be able to do my residency with an oncologist in West Palm Beach, FL. I spent 6 weeks learning more about the medical management of patients with hematologic disorders and cancer.

During my stay in Florida, I attended an AIDS update in Fort Lauderdale and met a physician who was fascinated by the idea that there was an NP who specialized in oncology and HIV. He hired me and I started in private practice with him in December 1995. I saw patients daily in the office, rounded on the inpatients in a designated HIV unit, and coordinated the outpatient treatment room in our practice. The physician was a member of a company that managed HIV practices throughout South Florida, and another physician in the group needed help. I was assigned to work in the office of a physician in Miami when he was not there. At this practice, I cared for patients with HIV infection and AIDS. This practice was unique in that most of the patients were people of color, mostly woman, and almost all without insurance. Many of the patients were Spanish or Creole speaking, and, I have to admit, I spoke neither. Fortunately, the practice had a nursing assistant who spoke Creole and a secretary who spoke Spanish. I really enjoyed this assignment—2 days a week I saw mostly gay men with insurance in Fort Lauderdale and the other 3 days, the Miami patients.

During my stay in South Florida, a colleague who I worked with in 1986 at Duke contacted me. She was working with a large drug company in the Care Management Division where her group was developing a program for people living with AIDS and their caregivers and she wanted me to assist them in identifying caregiver issues based on my thesis work. I became a consultant to a project that was designed to empower patients and their caregivers through information and access to resources. This innovative program was called T.H.E. Course, or Tools for Health and Empowerment. My role was to review all the content for accuracy and applicability. I also became a trainer to train clinicians to take T.H.E. Course back to their communities and teach it. During this time, I missed the interactions that I had with both patients and their families and realized that I was a good NP and should practice as one.

I approached the dean of the school of nursing with the proposition that I teach in the NP program, and I also approached the director of AIDS Treatment and Research at Duke University Medical Center to see patients. The dean and the director of the AIDS programs designed a position where I was funded by the medical center with 3 days in the nursing school teaching in the NP programs and 2 days in the medical center seeing adult patients with HIV infection. I also mentor students in that program and am a preceptor for graduate students while in my clinical practice.

In my practice, 1 day per week is spent in a rural outreach clinic for persons with HIV infection. The outreach arrangement was facilitated through the joint efforts of Duke University Medical Center and the local HIV/AIDS coordinating agency, the Piedmont Consortium. The Piedmont Consortium coordinates the distribution of resources that the Ryan White Care Fund distributes to the state of North Carolina in a specific geographic area. Financial support for this project was obtained through a grant from the AIDS Control Program of North Carolina. The grant provides the salaries for the physicians, the NPs, a case manager, and a chaplain. The chaplain is well known to the community because she conducts a family support group and coordinates a program for area clergy that provides education and support for clergy through workshops and seminars. She provides a vital link to the community because of her credibility and compassion. The host hospital provides physical space, including a private entrance to preserve confidentiality for the HIV/AIDS patients. Support staff includes a medicating licensed practical nurse, secretary, laboratory facilities, and x-ray availability. The clinic is in close proximity to the emergency department, with 24-hour physician coverage. This outreach clinic is approximately 45 minutes from Duke, which affords patients the opportunity to be followed for their HIV infection within their own community. Patients have reported that they are pleased with this arrangement because they spend less time traveling (especially when they are not feeling well), are able to take less time off work, and have the benefit of an expert in assisting with their care. Some patients have a primary care provider in the community, and we work with their primary care provider to coordinate continuity of care. The clinic is staffed by three adult NPs, all of which are graduates of the Duke University School of Nursing Oncology/HIV/AIDS NP program. We see patients in all stages of HIV infection, and patients who attend the clinic usually are from the surrounding rural counties. At the completion of each clinic day, an infectious diseases attending physician attends the clinic to review the patients seen and cosign charts. A physician is always available by telephone should we need consultation.

The rural outreach clinic, called the Northern Outreach Clinic, provides the opportunity for the NPs to be autonomous, and we are guided by standing protocols that have been developed at other major HIV/AIDS centers. Patients are also allowed to participate in clinical trials that Duke is conducting, thus improving their access to new and promising HIV/AIDS treatments.

As an advanced practice nurse in HIV/AIDS I speak at local, regional, and national workshops and conferences on the care of persons with HIV infection. I helped start the North Carolina Triangle Chapter of the Association of Nurses in AIDS Care and am currently the chapter president. With support of the Dean, I am actively involved in writing articles and chapters in books and am a consultant to pharmaceutical companies in both clinical and educational endeavors.

Role of the Nurse Practitioner

In her *New York Times* piece, Anna Quindlen (1994) writes, "It is clearly the future of health care in a system that must be reconfigured around needs, not job titles." She writes about healthcare reform and how NPs are able to provide services traditionally reserved for physicians. Martha Orr (1994), executive director of the New York State Nurses Association, states that NPs can provide all kinds of care in a more humane and cost-effective way.

The oncology/HIV/AIDS NP is a fairly new specialized advanced practice role. As mentioned previously, the practice of caring for persons with HIV infection and AIDS did not come about until the early 1980s. The HIV/AIDS NP role was created when schools of nursing began examining the possibilities of advanced practice specialization in fields such as oncology, acute care, and neonatal care. The oncology/HIV NP was also created to meet the demands of changing healthcare needs of the population.

At Hunter-Bellevue School of Nursing in New York City, a subspecialty option in HIV/AIDS began in the fall of 1990. The subspecialty option is offered to graduate nursing students in all of the advanced practice programs, with the terminal objective of the program being to prepare the graduate students to become leaders in HIV/AIDS care.

It is well supported in the literature that when physicians have experience in caring for HIV/AIDS patients, the patients have a better chance of survival. A group of primary care physicians trained in internal medicine were found to be slower to adopt new therapies for AIDS, and physicians with more experience had patients living longer, probably because of their familiarity with HIV and AIDS care (Kitahata et al., 1996). There are reasons to suggest that NPs trained in HIV/AIDS can provide care to patients that may increase their chances of survival. This is because the training that the oncology/HIV NP receives, including an intensive residency program that allows the NP to devote time and attention to keeping up to date with the latest in treatment options for HIV/AIDS.

At the Owen Clinic in San Diego, the NP is involved in fundamental delivery of care and is the primary care provider in the multidisciplinary program. Patients at the Owen Clinic have chronic and multisystem disorders, for which the NP is prepared to provide comprehensive care. According to Nuffer (1991), the NPs and the physician assistant provide primary care, conduct follow-up visits, and, following up on laboratory tests and procedure results, coordinate home care and respond to telephone calls from patients and their caregivers. The NPs also make hospital rounds, provide home care for end-stage patients, and assist in the delivery of continuing education programs to all the staff. The NPs are guided by protocols, and these protocols are updated on a regular basis.

Primary care is important because it allows for continuity, coordination, and comprehensive follow-through for a vulnerable population group. The primary care NP has a broad knowledge base and experience in managing complex chronic problems. The authors go on to describe the multifaceted components of the NP's responsibilities, which include appraising risk, staging of infection, conducting an HIV-focused history, conducting an HIV-focused review of systems, performing HIV-focused physical examinations, ordering and interpreting diagnostic and laboratory evaluations, and providing health maintenance interventions, including medical management (Aiken, Lake, & Semaan, 1993).

Nursing students benefit from having a faculty role model to develop positive attitudes toward AIDS care. An NP who is providing care to patients with HIV infection and also teaching has the unique opportunity to demonstrate state-of-the-art care and to share knowledge, skills, and attitudes that are important in assisting the student in role development and future perspectives in the care of persons with HIV infection.

CASE VIGNETTE

At the beginning of 1998, the rural outreach clinic described previously was ready to open. I looked at this as an opportunity to use my training and education to the fullest. The first couple of weeks that we met, we had few patients. At the third week, we each had a patient to see, and by the fourth week, patients were being asked to wait for an appointment. We observed this slow start as the time that the community was taking to make sure that they could trust us. The support groups were meeting regularly, and the chaplain, who had credibility within the community, spoke highly of us. It was not until a patient who was an "informal leader" in the community was seen and her positive experience was shared with other members of the support group that it was "OK" for patients to attend the clinic. Each of the NPs developed a caseload, seeing patients who were previously being followed at Duke and also seeing new patients who were referred to us.

In January 1998, about 4 weeks after the clinic opened, a young man presented to the clinic after being referred by a local gastroenterologist. The referral letter stated that the patient had been evaluated in the emergency department in December 1997 and was found to have oral candidiasis and weight loss. Based on his presentation, the local doctor requested that the patient be tested for HIV, which turned out to be positive. The patient, Michael, was a 25-year-old, married, white male. He presented to us with profound weight loss, fatigue, pallor, and oral candidiasis. Red flags were raised because he looked like he had advanced HIV disease. I obtained a thorough history and conducted a physical examination. On taking the history, I discovered that the patient had injected drugs intravenously about 10 years before his visit; other than that, he had no risk factors for HIV. He was in a marriage that was monogamous and had not had sex with any other person in the last 5 years. On physical examination, he had hepatomegaly, enlarged cervical and axillary lymph nodes, and thrush. From my experience and training, my differential diagnosis included disseminated mycobacterium avium complex (MAC), lymphoma, hepatitis, and advanced HIV infection. My clinical intuition told me that he was sick. I ordered a STAT complete blood cell count, which revealed a hemoglobin of 7 g and a white blood cell count of 2000. I also ordered a chemistry panel, syphilis serology, hepatitis panel, blood cultures (to include acid-fast bacillus), a CD4 cell count, HIV-RNA viral load, and a tuberculosis skin test. An important component of my role as an NP is to work with all disciplines of the care team. I contacted the referring physician and asked him if he could arrange for the patient to receive a transfusion, and it was arranged. The patient received blood in the hospital the next day. During this outpatient visit for transfusion, one of the nurses in the treatment area spoke with the patient about his HIV infection. At church the following Sunday, this nurse spoke to Michael and told him that there was another member of the church who had "the same disease that you have." She proceeded to point out the other person. Michael paged me to tell me that he believed that his confidentiality had been breached. Because of this incident, we had many meetings with hospital administration, and the nurse who breached Michael's confidentiality was reprimanded.

The next visit that the patient made to the clinic was spent discussing his HIV disease. Laboratory tests that were obtained on the last visit revealed a CD4 cell count of 1 and an HIV-RNA viral load of 2 million. A lot of time was spent educating him about HIV because he had a low level of understanding of HIV disease. He said that he was totally shocked about his diagnosis but now that he knew, it was time to do something about it. I knew that he would benefit from antiretroviral medication at this time. In choosing appropriate medications for him, I discussed his work and home schedule and the feasibility of taking many drugs throughout the day. A potent antiretroviral regimen was prescribed for him, a triple combination of drugs called highly active antiretroviral therapy or HAART. He was placed on two reverse transcriptase inhibitors and one protease inhibitor. He was also given a prescription for topical treatment for thrush. Also at this time, his liver functions were reviewed and were found to be elevated (SGOT and SGPT). After discussing this with my attending physician, we decided that the patient would benefit from HAART and that we would keep a close eye on his liver function. The blood cultures were still pending at this time.

On the next visit, empiric therapy was started for MAC and prophylaxis for *P. carinii* pneumonia. After 1 week, Michael's liver function test results were even more markedly elevated, he was more leukopenic, and he was experiencing anemia again, requiring another transfusion. The MAC treatment was changed to a less hepatotoxic regimen, and he was taken off trimethoprim sulfa and switched to aerosolized pentamidine (we do not use pentamidine as often because it doesn't provide systemic prophylaxis against pneumocystis). His local doctor was contacted, and it was arranged for Michael to receive another transfusion. At the same time I was changing medications, his insurance carrier notified the patient that he had "maxed out" his drug reimbursement benefits. The case manager was consulted and appropriate paperwork was completed to enter Michael into drug procurement programs through the drug companies. Although he and his wife both work, together they made just enough money to pay their mortgage and bills and to feed and clothe their children. In the state of North Carolina, the program that usually helps people obtain their HIV medications is no longer enrolling new patients and even is threatening to close.

On the fourth visit, Michael appeared very sad. He said that he was feeling a little better and that his appetite had increased. I ordered another complete blood cell count and he again was anemic and also, for the first time, thrombocytopenic. I contacted a colleague at Duke, an oncologist, and we arranged for Michael to go to Duke the next day for a bone marrow aspiration. After listening to him, I realized that there was something he was not sharing with me. I confronted him and he started crying, stating that he was worried that he might have infected his wife and what could be done. I provided him with options, including having his wife tested. Because his wife was in the waiting room, I asked Michael if I could spend some time with her after we were through, and he agreed. Joanne appeared calm and concerned, and I obtained the appropriate consent, drew her blood, and told her to come with Michael on the next visit.

During the bone marrow aspiration, I assisted the physician, mainly by providing moral support for Michael. This was his first time away from the outreach clinic in an area that was unfamiliar to him. Fortunately, the bone marrow went well and the results showed that Michael did not have cancer, although it looked like MAC. My hunch to treat him paid off. Michael understood that the empiric treatment he was on was appropriate and was relieved with the results of the bone marrow.

On the next visit, I gave Joanne the results of her HIV test—positive. She took the news quite well and wanted to know what she should do. I suggested we assess her immune status and the status of the virus through laboratory testing. I obtained a CD4 cell count and HIV-RNA viral load and would share the results of those tests in 2 weeks. For Michael, his liver function test results returned to baseline, his white blood cell count was within normal limits, and he was no longer anemic. I attributed this to the antiretroviral therapy strengthening his body.

After 6 weeks, the blood cultures returned, confirming what the bone marrow had shown—definite acid fast bacillus. Now Michael was on a regimen that seemed to be working—treatment for MAC, HAART, topical therapy for thrush, and *P. carinii* pneumonia prophylaxis. His laboratory tests were within normal limits and he was gaining weight. Unfortunately, because he was unable to work and the family was used to two incomes, they lost their home and moved into an apartment. The case manager again was called in to assist him in obtaining money for rent. His wife Joanne was placed on three drugs also and I decided to place them both on the same regimen to make compliance and adherence easier.

About 8 weeks after I first saw Michael, he was doing much better. The myriad of medical problems were sorted out and he was on appropriate therapies. His social situation was being assisted with help from the case manager.

It has now been 1 year, 4 months since I first met Michael. I try not to become personally involved with patients, but he and his wife have touched my heart. Michael tries his hand at art, and he presented me with a framed sketch of Spiderman with the inscription "to a real-life superhero." I think that is one of the nicest compliments I have ever received. He has gained 20 lb, and his immune system is stronger based on his CD4 cell count of over 100 and a viral load that is nondetectable. I would like to see his CD4 cell count higher and his viral load remain nondetectable. I feel that we have made some headway making him stronger and healthier.

This scenario represents only one couple with HIV infection. The rural outreach clinic afforded both Michael and Joanne the opportunity to be followed for their HIV infections in the community where they live, with Duke available for more complicated tests and procedures. The multidisciplinary team approach to care has paid off with input from the chaplain and the case manager. At the beginning I was paged at least weekly, but I now get called infrequently to help sort things out, and Michael returns to the outreach clinic monthly for routine laboratory tests, reassurance, and a hug.

REFERENCES

Aiken, L., Lake, E., & Semaan, S. (1993). Nurse practitioner–managed care for persons with HIV infection. *Image 25*(3), 172–177.

Association of Nurses in AIDS Care, 11250 Roger Bacon Dr., Suite 8, Reston, VA 20190, 1-800-260-6780.

Kitahata, M., Koepsell, T., Deyo, R., et al. (1996). Physicians' experience with the Acquired Immunodeficiency Syndrome as a factor in patient's survival. *New England Journal of Medicine 334*(11), 701–706.

Nuffer, K. (1991). Creating a care system for the HIV-infected. *Nurse Practitioner Forum 2*(2), 104–107.

Orr, M. (1994). In Nursing hospitals toward the future. The New York Times, June 2, 1994.

Quindlen, A. (1994). "Nursing hospitals toward the future." *The New York Times,* June 2, 1994.

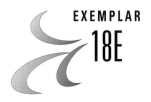

Women's Health

Janine J. Sherman

History of Women's Healthcare

Since the early 1900s, nurses have played an important role in women's healthcare, helping to deliver prenatal care (Thompson, Walsh, & Merkatz, 1900). Many physicians and hospitals initiated home visits by nurses to provide prenatal care and education, hoping to decrease the infant and maternal mortality rate. In 1920, Ann Stevens, the director of the Maternity Center Association in New York, helped provide prenatal care to as many women as possible by canvassing neighborhoods and coordinating nurses to make home visits. The nurse performed urinalysis; auscultated fetal heart tones; assessed for danger signals; and provided education on diet, hygiene, exercise, and infant care. With mandatory pasteurization of milk and the development of prenatal care provided by nurses, the maternal mortality rate dropped by 21.5%.

One of the most effective nurse-oriented prenatal care programs has been the Frontier Nursing Service, begun in 1925 and continuing to the present. Started by a wealthy woman named Mary Breckinridge, who ultimately became a nurse–midwife, the service promoted complete family health in rural Kentucky, which included prenatal care and family planning. Over time, physicians were incorporated as consultants, but most healthcare was provided by nurse practitioners (NPs) and certified nurse–midwives.

Women's healthcare programs came into their own as formal NP training programs in the 1960s, educating healthcare providers for rural and other underserved areas. Many of these early training programs for women's healthcare NPs were certificate programs sponsored by Planned Parenthood or the armed services. By the 1970s, family planning and well-women gynecologic care became part of the responsibilities of the women's healthcare NP (Nagle, 1988).

Today, the role of the women's healthcare NP continues to expand, necessitating the evolution of master's degree training programs for providers. Women's healthcare NPs now provide an array of services for women, which include prevention and treatment of women throughout various stages of life.

Preparation of Women's Healthcare Nurse Practitioners

To practice as a women's healthcare NP, a registered nurse must complete a training program leading to either an advanced NP certificate or a graduate nursing degree, qualifying the candidate to sit for the National Certification Corporation examination for the obstetric, gynecologic, and neonatal specialties. These programs usually require a 1- to 2-year course of study with both didactic and clinical experiences, including a holistic approach to both gynecology and obstetric care at all developmental stages. Preventive healthcare is emphasized in preparing women's healthcare providers.

Role of the Women's Healthcare Nurse Practitioner

The role of the women's healthcare NP should include a holistic approach to prevention and treatment of disease, addressing psychological and educational needs. Much of the responsibility of the NP is to deliver primary healthcare throughout a woman's life. Nagle (1988) points out that a woman's contact with a healthcare professional is often related to a normal life process or event, rather than illness. An example of this form of interaction is a woman who is consulting an NP about hormone replacement therapy for menopause, a naturally occurring process in a woman's life. Appropriate referral to other members of the healthcare team is also an important part of the NP's practice.

Presently, women's healthcare NPs continue to provide healthcare to underserved and rural areas. Further practice developments have included expansion into the managed care setting, a movement and creation of private practices in collaboration with physicians.

Careers in Women's Healthcare

After graduating from a master's degree NP program, I have found endless employment opportunities as a women's healthcare NP. I have had the opportunity to work in four different settings simultaneously, each with its own unique aspects. The four positions that I have held are in a private, primarily Medicaid-based practice; a not-for-profit, hospital-supported prenatal program for indigent patients; an upper-middle-class suburban practice; and a master's-level women's health NPs program. In the first three settings, I worked with physicians in a collaborative practice. The theoretical framework for working in three such diverse settings was Madeline Leininger's (1991) cultural care theory. This construct is particularly applicable to women's healthcare as women approach many of their life cycle events, such as childbirth or menopause, with varied cultural ideas and customs that need to be considered when delivering care. An example of the application of this theory was my care for an African-American patient who was trying to make the decision whether to breastfeed her newborn child. Her cultural feelings instead of mine needed to be considered in this decision, especially because we had different cultural beliefs. Other situations in which I have used this theory included discussions about contraception, pregnancy, and sexuality, to name a few. I certainly believe that adequate holistic care cannot be provided without taking into consideration the patient's cultural background and beliefs.

MEDICAID PRACTICE

The physician with whom I worked in the Medicaid-based practice had previous experience working with NPs during his duty in the public health service; he has allowed me to practice independently. His desire to employ an NP in a part-time collaborative practice was partially based on his workload of more than 30 deliveries monthly. Thus, he sought an NP to work in the office so that he would be more readily available to attend childbirths. For me, I learned a considerable amount about the delivery of women's healthcare, and I quickly was capable of making independent decisions even when faced with difficult situations in the physician's absence. The physician has been highly supportive of my decisions about patient care. The practice population is approximately 75% obstetric and 25% gynecologic, and I often see as many as 25 patients a day, including five or six new patients. My clinical practice has incorporated primary prevention through Pap smear screening and breast examinations, high-risk antenatal care, and routine as well as complicated gynecologic care. The socioeconomic issues inherent in caring for a Medicaid population require a holistic approach. The prenatal patients that I care for in this practice are often adolescent, with no financial or emotional support from the baby's father, and are often unable to achieve their own personal development goals because of lack of family support. The patients frequently have had numerous children fathered by several different boys or men. This patient population often has many concurrent medical issues, such as a high rate of sexually transmitted diseases. Many patients have received minimal antenatal care, often beginning prenatal care late in pregnancy, and frequently they have had little previous education regarding health and pregnancy. To provide adequate physical as well as psychological care for these patients, complete medical and social assessments are required. In fact, many patients who have had little access to care before their pregnancy generally require what may be their first complete physical examination. Initially we see patients free of charge for the first visit and provide them with the means to apply for and obtain Medicaid with the assistance of an on-site caseworker. During this first visit, we perform a prenatal risk assessment, begin to educate the patient about pregnancy, and supply prenatal vitamins. Unless acutely indicated, laboratory studies may be deferred at this initial visit until Medicaid coverage has been activated. If a patient has significant risk factors and requires more urgent care, we send them to a hospital-based clinic. The on-site caseworker works with the providers to assess personal educational needs, such as schooling to obtain a Graduate Equivalence Degree, and often performs home visits to assess living conditions. The collaboration with the caseworker (who also trained as a registered nurse) has significantly improved patient outcomes because it helped complete the delivery of holistic healthcare.

The office has a well-equipped laboratory in which I can perform wet mounts, urine dipstick analyses, and pregnancy tests. The office also has a fetal monitor and an ultrasound machine. The ability to do nonstress tests in the office allows us to prevent unnecessary admissions to the hospital and to monitor more closely high-risk patients. An ultrasound technician comes to the office weekly to perform routine prenatal ultrasounds. Both the physician and the ultrasound technician taught me basic ultrasound skills that I use to check for fetal viability and for pregnancy dating. In this practice, we use a large network of physicians for referral purposes. This has been particularly important for the many patients who require the services of other physicians and specialists. For example, we have had numerous patients with asthma who required concurrent care by pulmonary physicians during their pregnancies.

*C*ASE VIGNETTE

Vignette 1
A 16-year-old G1P0 with an LMP 6/10 and an EDC 3/17 presents to the clinic for her first prenatal visit at 26 2/7 weeks by dates. The patient has not received previous prenatal care and denies problems with this pregnancy until this point. She is single and lives at home with her mother and two siblings. She states that the father of the baby is no longer involved in her life but that her mother is helping her out.

She states that she has been sexually active since age 14 years, has never used birth control, and is not worried about sexually transmitted diseases. She states that she has had only two sexual partners. She denies alcohol, tobacco, or drug abuse, and she denies a significant past medical history. She states that she has a brother with sickle cell anemia but that she is unsure of sickle cell history in the family of the baby's father. She is a sophomore in high school and would like to remain in school if possible. She has not applied for Medicaid and Women, Infants, and Children (WIC) services but should be eligible for both. On physical examination, she is 5' 5" tall and weighs 152 lb. Her pelvic examination revealed a large amount of mucopurulent discharge from a friable cervix, and the wet mount revealed leukocytes too numerous to count. Her cervix was 2 to 3 cm dilated and 80% effaced. The fundal height was 24 cm.

This case is fairly typical in this practice. The patient was sent to the hospital to be monitored for contractions and to rule out intrauterine growth retardation. She was treated for a chlamydial infection and for preterm labor. After hospital discharge, she was followed up in the office and the caseworker helped get the paperwork for Medicaid and WIC completed and submitted. The caseworker and I also assisted her in finding ways to complete her schoolwork. We followed her closely for preterm labor and intrauterine growth retardation, with frequent nonstress tests and education. Hemoglobin electrophoresis revealed that she was a carrier of the sickle cell trait. We tracked down the father of the baby, and sickle cell test results for him were negative. Eventually, a healthy 37-week baby girl was born and the patient was placed on Depo Provera injections for birth control.

HOSPITAL-BASED CLINIC

The hospital-supported clinic in which I work is based in a freestanding family planning clinic. This program provides care to indigent patients who are often illegal immigrants. The philosophy that underlies the hospital's support of this clinic states that provision of adequate prenatal care lowers overall healthcare costs by increasing the likelihood of delivering full-term healthy babies instead of premature babies. These patients are usually eligible only for emergency Medicaid coverage at the time of delivery or in the case of a needed hospitalization. The clinic has multilingual counselors, health educators, medical assistants, Medicaid insurance specialists, phlebotomists, and ultrasound technicians. The counselors perform the initial assessment to determine the patient's risk factors and to begin discussion of postpartum contraceptive options. The health educators spend time in the waiting room addressing various prenatal topics such as normal body changes in pregnancy, breast self-examination, and infant care. The medical assistants take vital signs and a screening history regarding problems the patient may be experiencing. The Medicaid specialist assists the patients with the paperwork required to apply for emergency coverage, key to the financial survival of the hospital's support for the clinic. An ultrasound technician attends each afternoon session, and a formal interpretation is provided by a consulting radiologist. With all of these support personnel, I can see 60 to 70 patients in a day, often seeing up to 15 new patients. The pregnancies of these patients frequently can be characterized as extremely high risk, yet I often see most of these patients without direct input from a physician. The physician with whom I work is often at the hospital performing deliveries but remains accessible by phone and beeper. This physician had not previously worked with NPs but is supportive of the role.

Vignette 2

A 45-year-old G6P4014 pregnant woman (7 5/7 weeks by dates) came into the clinic for prenatal care. She had recently emigrated illegally from South America and therefore was not eligible for Medicaid or WIC. She had moved here with two of her children, ages 12 and 14 years, and she lived with one of her sisters. The father of the baby remained in South America. Her past pregnancies were uncomplicated except that the last baby was apparently much bigger than her previous children. She did not speak English and was unemployed. She denied past medical problems or relevant family history. This patient's pregnancy was high risk based on her age, and she was offered genetic counseling. Through the clinic's in-

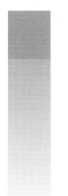

terpreter, we explained her risk status because of her older age, and she decided to have genetic counseling arranged at a nearby hospital. The clinic's Medicaid specialist helped her prepare the application for emergency coverage that would be submitted when her child was born, ensuring reimbursement for both the hospital and physicians involved in her delivery. She had genetic counseling and was found to be carrying a normal male child. She had an uneventful pregnancy until the 3-hour glucose tolerance test performed in her 29th week revealed that she had gestational diabetes. She was referred to the hospital's diabetes center, where plans were made to manage her blood glucose with diet modification. She was followed closely in the clinic to ensure that the recommended dietary changes were consistent with her cultural attitudes toward food and pregnancy and to minimize the age-related risks that accompanied the pregnancy. We also introduced her to other members in the community from her country to help her adjust to her new environment. Her sister was in attendance for the delivery, which was uneventful. She was followed up in the postpartum family planning clinic and attended infant care classes. Born as an American citizen, the baby received Medicaid for 1 year and was followed up by a local pediatrician.

PRIVATE PRACTICE

The suburban private practice in which I work has a single obstetrician–gynecologist as my collaborative physician. The initial contact with the practice occurred during my graduate school training. A friend who obtained her care from this physician mentioned to him my need for a preceptor. This led to a meeting in which we agreed that he would serve as my clinical preceptor during the last stage of graduate school. The typically middle-class patients in this practice usually have private insurance and often have had a long-term professional relationship with this physician. Initially, we were concerned about how the patients in this practice would respond to a mid-level provider. The physician instructed the office staff to ask patients who were scheduling appointments if they would see the NP student under his supervision; at least 75% of the patients were receptive to seeing me. During this preceptorship, I was given my own examination room and my own daily appointment schedule. About 25% of the patients in the practice were receiving obstetric care, and the remaining patients were being seen for routine or problem-oriented gynecologic examinations. I would present each patient to the physician and we would jointly develop a course of action. When the clinical plan that I presented differed from his, I was often allowed to pursue my approach, provided I could support my decision with an appropriate rationale. I would often observe particularly interesting deliveries or procedures when time was available.

The preceptorship was so successful and rewarding that I joined the practice after graduating with my master's degree. Once a week, I see 15 to 20 patients in the office on the day that the physician is scheduled to perform surgery. As I began to see patients independently, women would call the office specifically requesting appointments with me. In this practice, patient education is a priority, despite the high level of information that the patients already have about health issues. The women would often bring with them the latest information about new drugs and treatments or health prevention. In addition to the considerable amount of preventive care that I deliver, many patients are seen for problems such as breast lumps detected by breast self-examinations or concern about the risk of developing breast cancer after hormone replacement therapy. Some common psychosocial problems that are addressed include body image issues and depression developing in the perimenopausal period. A medical assistant takes vital signs and assists with necessary specimen collection. The two receptionists and medical insurance specialists make sure appropriate steps are followed regarding insurance coverage, all of which supports the NP role. Interacting with many different insurers can be problematic, given the widely differing rules for coverage of charges for tests and procedures. For example, to perform an endometrial biopsy, approval may be needed from a referring primary care physician, or the health care plan may require referral to another specialist.

I attribute my success in this practice to the attitude of the physician and the staff's support of my role as an NP. Although he had never worked with a NP before working with me, the physician has developed into being my mentor, a role that will likely continue for many years to come. Our relationship is collaborative, based on mutual respect for each other's roles. When he is in surgery and I am seeing patients, he remains available and helpful. On days that I am not in the office, he will often page me to discuss a case or get my opinion on an issue. In addition, the medical community and hospital to which the physician refers patients have been helpful and accepting of my role.

Vignette 3

A 43-year-old G3P2012 presented to the office for a routine annual examination. She had been a long-term patient in this practice. She described heavy vaginal bleeding and abdominal cramping occurring as often as every 2 weeks for the previous 3 to 4 months; she stated that she was not having hot flashes or vaginal dryness but that she noted moodiness and decreased libido that she attributed to the bleeding. She is married, reporting a good relationship with her spouse, and has two teenaged children who live at home with her. She stated that she was satisfied with her life except for the stress and anxiety associated with trying to meet the needs of everyone in her family. Her obstetrical history was uneventful except for an early first-trimester missed abortion for which a dilation and curettage was performed. She had been seen annually for her examination, without detection of any abnormality, and her past medical and family histories were otherwise noncontributory. On examination, she had a slightly irregular uterus with some enlargement estimated at 6 weeks in size. After taking the patient's history and completing her examination, we decided that she needed an endometrial biopsy and a transvaginal ultrasound. When the insurance company was notified of these recommendations, we were informed that the procedures could not be done that day because her visit was only approved for the annual examination. I discussed with the patient how to reduce stress in her life through exercise and relaxation techniques. It took approximately 3 weeks to get insurance approval for the tests that we recommended to determine the cause of her bleeding. After diagnosing uterine fibroid tumors, therapy was started for anemia (hemoglobin 9.8%) as well as fibroids. During follow-up, we also discussed the effectiveness of the stress-reduction techniques we had previously recommended.

EDUCATOR

I began my role as a nurse educator about 6 months after completing graduate school, by having baccalaureate-candidate nursing students attend the hospital-based clinic with me as part of their obstetrics training. I would have one student during a clinic session working with me throughout the day. After several more months, I began serving as a preceptor for women's healthcare and perinatal master's-level students who were generally in the early stages of their graduate school careers. These students worked with me in both the Medicaid and clinic-based practices. I was also asked to help teach the didactic and clinical portions of the women's healthcare and perinatal programs at the school of nursing. My responsibilities include clinical placements and evaluation of students' performance in their clinical settings.

This role has rounded out my career because it allows me to serve as a mentor in a career that has personally rewarded and satisfied me. I believe that part of our mission is to increase the awareness and success of the women's healthcare and perinatal NP roles. I am able to achieve this goal through interaction with students and their successful placement with new preceptors. I have also been encouraged to develop a research program, and I have undertaken to evaluate the understanding and acceptance by local physicians of NPs. Furthermore, being in an academic role makes it imperative that I remain up-to-date in my specialty.

Aside from the activities at the university, I have served as a consultant to help set up an osteoporosis teaching program for a large, private obstetrician–gynecologist practice. I established a comprehensive teaching program for patients who were undergoing bone density screening. The teaching program included risk assessment, counseling about nutrition and physical activity, safety assessments, and education on prevention and treatment of osteoporosis. I used resources provided by pharmaceutical companies and designed information brochures for patients. This teaching program was well received by the group of physicians, and now their patients receive appropriate assessment and education.

Future Trends in Women's Healthcare

As Sinclair (1997) points out, redefining nursing roles is an ongoing phenomenon related to all of the changes in the healthcare delivery system. Today in women's healthcare, many opportunities are available to serve in capacities ranging from hospital-based settings to various forms of private practice. Spatz (1996) points out that improved access to advanced practice nurses will also help to break down the many barriers that currently prevent patients from seeing NPs. As healthcare continues to change, the women's healthcare NP role will continue to grow. Furthermore, increasing acceptance of the NP's role in medical communities will expand the availability of collaborative practices to help meet patients' needs and to improve the delivery of cost-efficient care. However, despite the increasing medical practice of the NP, it is critically important to maintain the fundamental orientation and education in nursing. It is important for NPs not to be viewed as an extension of a physician but as unique complements to the medical world. By maintaining the emphasis on our nursing roots, we will also allow ourselves to remain open to alternatives to traditional therapies such as relaxation techniques, and to maintain the nursing approach to providing culturally appropriate care.

REFERENCES

Leininger, M. M. (1991). *Cultural care diversity and universiality: A theory of nursing.* New York: National League for Nursing Press.

Nagle, M. (1988). Nurse practitioners: Primary health care nursing for women. *Imprint 35*(4), 115–117.

Sinclair , B. P. (1997). Advanced practice nurses in integrated health care systems. *Journal of Obstetrics, Gynecology and Neonatal Nursing 26*(2), 217–223.

Spatz, D. L.(1996). Women's health: The role of advanced practice nurses in the 21st century. *Nursing Clinics of North America 31*(2), 269–277.

Thompson, J. E., Walsh, L. V., & Merkatz, I. R. (1990). The history of prenatal care: Cultural, social, and medical contexts. In I. R. Merkatz & J. E. Thompson (Eds.). *New prospects on prenatal care* (pp. 9–30). New York: Elsevier Science Publishing Co.

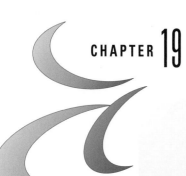

CHAPTER 19

Pushing the Boundaries of Advanced Practice Nursing

Exemplars

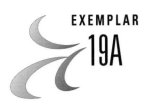

The Nurse Anesthetist: A Pioneer in Advanced Practice Nursing

Joseph T. Kanusky

Nurse anesthetists are advanced practice nurses who have been providing quality anesthesia for more than 100 years. They administer approximately 65% of the 28 million anesthetics given annually in the United States and more than 70% of anesthesia services in rural areas (Foster, 1998). Nurse anesthetists must be certified as certified registered nurse anesthetists (CRNAs) within 2 years of graduation to be eligible for Medicare reimbursement. After the 2-year grace period, those not certified are excluded from Medicare reimbursement. In the average practice, at least 30% of cases are paid for by Medicare. Therefore, employing persons who are not CRNAs is not financially practical. In this exemplar, CRNA will be used to represent all nurse anesthetists.

CRNAs provide all types of regional and general anesthesia to patient populations from pediatric to geriatric age groups and for all patient classifications listed by the American Society of Anesthesiologists (ASA). Nurse anesthetists practice in a variety of settings where surgery is performed, such as hospitals, ambulatory surgery centers, diagnostic centers, and physicians' offices. CRNAs are the primary anesthesia providers for the military services. Some CRNAs choose to practice independently, whereas most choose to work with an anesthesiologist or an anesthesiology group in a "team concept" model of practice.

History of Anesthesia and Nurse Anesthetists

Crawford Long, a Georgia physician, first used diethyl ether in 1842 for removal of a tumor from a patient's neck, but he did not publish his work until 1849. The first public demonstration of diethyl ether for surgical anesthesia is attributed to William T. G. Morton, a dentist and medical student. This event occurred at Massachusetts General Hospital in Boston on October 16, 1846 (Atkinson, Rushman, & Davies, 1993).

Anesthesia was recognized as an important aspect of surgery, but administering anesthesia lacked prestige and financial incentive for the anesthesia provider to be a physician (Gunn, 1997). The surgeon was in charge and was the provider who collected the fee (Bankert,

1989). Medical students, junior house officers, nurses, and nonprofessionals, under the guidance of the surgeon, would drop ether or chloroform. Not surprisingly, anesthesia-related morbidity and mortality was high. Surgeons encouraged nurses to become "professional anesthetists" to prove themselves as reliable and competent assistants.

The first nurse anesthetist was Sister Mary Bernard, who assumed anesthetist duties at St. Vincent's Hospital in Erie, PA, in 1877 (Bankert, 1989). Alice Magaw, a nurse anesthetist who worked with the Mayo brothers, was later named the "Mother of Anesthesia" by Dr. Charles Mayo, one of the brothers who founded the Mayo Clinic in the 1890s (Bauer, 1998). Magaw published on the topic of open-drop inhalation with ether and chloroform. She also published a paper in the *St. Paul Medical Journal* describing patient outcomes between 1899 and 1906, during which time she administered more than 14,000 anesthetics without a single death directly attributed to the anesthesia (Bankert, 1989).

Nurses most likely learned how to administer anesthesia as part of their basic nursing training. Bankert (1989) identifies this practice in Isabel Adams Hampton Robb's textbook entitled *Nursing: Its Principles and Practices for Hospital and Private Use* (1893), in which a chapter was devoted to "The Administration of Anesthetics." In 1909, St. Vincent's Hospital in Portland, OR, began the first formal anesthesia program for nurses. From an international perspective, Dr. George Crile and Agatha Hodgins, his nurse anesthetist, went to France in 1914 and taught English and French physicians and nurses how to administer anesthesia. Since World War I, nurse anesthetists have been primary anesthesia providers for the U.S. military (Gunn, 1997).

Nurse anesthetists have faced legal challenges regarding their practice. In 1916, the Louisville Society of Anesthetists passed a resolution stating that only physicians should administer anesthesia, an opinion supported by the state attorney general. In the same year, the Kentucky State Medical Association passed a resolution stating that it was unethical for a physician to employ a nonphysician anesthetist or to refer patients to hospitals that permitted nurses to give anesthetics. This resolution led Dr. Louis Frank, a Louisville surgeon, and his nurse anesthetist, Margaret Hatfield, to ask the State Board of Health to join them in a suit against the State Medical Association. The original ruling was against Frank and Hatfield, but on appeal, the decision was reversed when the judge confirmed the right of nurses to administer anesthesia and confirmed that Hatfield was not engaged in the practice of medicine (Bankert, 1989). The definitive test case of whether nurse anesthetists are practicing medicine or nursing when they engage in the delivery of anesthesia services occurred in California in 1933 and involved Dagmar Nelson, a nurse anesthetist charged with practicing medicine without a license. The case was decided in favor of the defendant, and the California Supreme Court ruled that she was not diagnosing and treating within the meaning of the medical practice act and, therefore, was practicing nursing and not medicine (Gunn, 1997).

Nurse Anesthesia Programs and Certification

In 1931, the American Association of Nurse Anesthetists (AANA) was founded by Agatha Hodgins. A certification program was developed in 1945, and the first qualifying examination for AANA members was administered later that year. In 1952, an accreditation program for nurse anesthesia schools was established. Accreditation of nurse anesthesia educational programs by the AANA has been recognized by the Department of Health, Education, and Human Services since 1955. Mandatory recertification was established in 1978 (Jordan, 1994).

Today, 85 nurse anesthesia educational programs are offered in the United States, ranging from 24 to 36 months. Curricula are governed by the accreditation standards of the Council on Accreditation of Nurse Anesthesia Educational Programs. These programs reside in a variety of schools and disciplines, including nursing, health science, biology, biomedical science, education, management, and nurse anesthesia. Each program leads to a master's degree in the respective discipline. Admission criteria include graduation from an approved nursing program, a baccalaureate degree in nursing or another appropriate discipline, current licensure as a registered professional nurse, and a minimum of 1 year of professional nursing experience in an acute care setting (Council on Accreditation of Nurse Anesthesia Educational Programs, 1990). Requirements for course content are specific and include advanced anatomy, physiology, and pathophysiology; biochemistry and physics related to anesthesia; advanced pharmacology; and principles of anesthesia practice. University-required core courses, specific to the discipline awarding the degree, are also taken. In addition to the didactics, a rigorous clinical component ensures that the graduate meets the requirements for entry-level practice.

Graduates of a nurse anesthesia program must meet all the requirements prescribed by the Council on Certification of Nurse Anesthetists to write the certification examination. Eligibility requirements for CRNA candidates include the following:

1. Maintain current and unrestricted licensure as a registered professional nurse and, where applicable, authorization to practice nurse anesthesia in all states in which the candidate currently practices; and
2. Have completed a nurse anesthesia educational program accredited by the Council on Certification of Nurse Anesthesia Educational Programs (Council on Certification of Nurse Anesthetists, 1997).

A transcript that includes actual class hours and documentation of clinical experience is required (Council on Accreditation of Nurse Anesthetists, 1993). For example, the minimum acceptable hours for course work in professional aspects of anesthesia is 45 hours, whereas a minimum of 135 hours is required in anatomy and physiology and pathophysiology. The minimum clinical experience hours is also outlined in detail. For example, total minimum number of cases must be 450, and the total hours of anesthesia time must be 800 hours. Requirements are also set by age (geriatric patients, 30; pediatric patients 2–12 years, 15), anatomic area (intra-abdominal, 50; extracranial, 15), type of anesthetic agent (nitrous oxide, 150; inhalation agents, 100; intravenous induction agents, 200), type of anesthesia (inhalation anesthesia, 300; endotracheal anesthesia, 175), and regional techniques (administration or maintenance, 30).

In 1969, a bylaws change was adopted by the members of the AANA making continuing education an optional program for CRNAs; this became a mandatory program in 1978. The Council on Recertification of Nurse Anesthetists recertifies qualified CRNAs on a biennial basis. Recertification criteria include (1) initial certification; (2) current licensure as a registered nurse with no restrictions; (3) completion of 40 hours of continuing education in the preceding 2 years; (4) substantial engagement in a practice of anesthesia; (5) no mental or physical conditions that may cause or interfere with practice; (6) no convictions for a felony and not under indictment; and (7) not subject to any documented allegations of misconduct, incompetent practice, or unethical behavior (Council on Recertification of Nurse Anesthetists, 1998).

Scope of Practice

CRNAs are involved in the care of patients preoperatively, intraoperatively, and postoperatively. Some CRNAs participate in pain management services. CRNAs serve as consultants in airway management, respiratory care, resuscitative care, and fluid and electrolyte problems. Scope of practice, similar to other advanced practice roles, includes serving on institutional committees, participating in staff development, quality improvement, and risk management programs. Some CRNAs serve as administrative officers for departments of anesthesia and assume administrative and budgetary responsibilities (AANA, 1996).

Preoperative Anesthesia Care

Preoperative evaluation of the patient is essential to the nursing process of assessing, planning, implementing, and evaluating the plan of care. The conduct of the preanesthesia visit is important in establishing rapport with the patient and to allay fear and anxiety. The CRNA collects a health history, with special emphasis on the patient's pathophysiologic features and health habits, including medications as they relate to the anesthetic experience. A physical examination appropriate to anesthetic practice is conducted. An airway examination is always performed whether a regional or general anesthetic is planned. The range of motion of the patient's head and neck is examined because it is essential to determine whether hyperextension is possible for intubation. Identifying potentially difficult intubation situations is facilitated using a few techniques. First, determine the distance between the tip of the patient's mandible and the thyroid notch when the neck is fully extended. Normally this is 6.5 cm, or 4 fingerbreadths, or more, in the adult. If the measurement is less than 6 cm, it will be impossible to visualize the larynx (Mallampati, 1997). A second strategy is called the Mallampati classification. This approach compares the ratio of the tongue to pharyngeal size, and it has been moderately successful in identifying potentially difficult-to-intubate patients (Fleisher, 1997). With the patient in a sitting position and the tongue protruding, the CRNA looks at the size of the tongue in relation to the size of the oral cavity and grades it based on how much of the pharynx is obscured by the tongue according to the following classification:

> Class I denotes visualization of the soft palate, hard palate, fauces, uvula, tonsillar pillars, and tongue;
>
> Class II denotes visualization of the soft palate, hard palate, fauces, uvula, and tongue;
>
> Class III denotes visualization of the soft palate, hard palate, base of the uvula, and tongue; and
>
> Class IV denotes visualization of the hard palate and tongue (Morgan & Mikhail, 1996).

The higher the class, the more difficulty expected in visualizing the glottis for laryngoscopy. Next, the CRNA evaluates the patient for signs of airway obstruction, for example, chest retractions or stridor and hypoxia. Finally, determination is made about the last time food or drink was consumed. The patient is not given anything by mouth to decrease the chance of aspiration pneumonitis.

The anesthesia history is obtained in relationship to past anesthesia experience and problems with anesthesia. It is important to obtain a family history of anesthesia problems. This may alert the CRNA to the possibilities of atypical pseudocholinesterase and malignant hyperthermia. Diagnostic results such as complete blood cell count, blood gases, liver enzymes, urinalysis, chest radiographs, drug levels (aminophylline or digitalis), and pulmonary function tests are reviewed. The nurse anesthetist not only interprets the results but may also request additional diagnostic tests depending on findings of the health history or physical examination. The CRNA evaluates the patient's anesthetic risk and makes decisions regarding the fitness for anesthesia at the proposed time. Risk is defined in terms of ASA status and ranges from Class 1 to Class 5. For example, Class 1 designates no organic pathology, or patients in whom the pathologic process is localized and does not cause any systemic disturbance or abnormality (i.e., a patient presenting for open reduction of a tibial fracture). By comparison, Class 5 designates a moribund patient not expected to survive 24 hours with or without surgery. Emergency surgery also presents a risk. An emergency operation is defined as a surgical procedure that, in the surgeon's opinion, should be performed without delay. In this case, one precedes the classification number with an "E" for "emergency surgery" (Fleisher, 1997).

In the planning phase, an anesthesia nursing care plan based on the patient's physical condition and proposed surgical or diagnostic intervention is developed. The CRNA must obtain informed consent for anesthesia, advise the patient of possible risks and complications, and answer all questions concerning anesthesia care. Next, the CRNA selects premedications and evening sedation, if appropriate. Decisions to withhold or continue administration of prescribed medications are also made.

From the point of good-quality anesthesia care and continuity, the CRNA who is scheduled to provide anesthesia to the patient should make the preoperative visit the day before the scheduled procedure (Kachnij, 1997). In today's practice setting this is not always possible. Most cases are performed either as outpatient procedures or as same-day admissions, necessitating another member of the team to conduct the preoperative visit. In some practice settings, preoperative visits are assigned to an individual for that day, or the visit is made by whomever is not administering anesthesia. This departmental decision is usually made in an attempt to prevent unnecessary patient waiting or delay.

Intraoperative Anesthesia Care

The intraoperative care and services afforded the patient by the CRNA creates an optimal environment for the surgical intervention (AANA, 1996). These services include rendering the patient insensitive to pain, with or without the loss of consciousness. It also means maintaining the patient's physiologic functions within acceptable ranges. The CRNA implements the anesthesia nursing care plan using a variety of regional or general anesthetic techniques. It is here in the operating room that most individuals think the practice of anesthesia is performed. They do not realize the comprehensive scope of practice that CRNAs provide before and after surgery.

Before the patient's arrival in the operating room, certain basic equipment, such as monitors and an anesthesia machine, must be made ready. The mnemonic "MS MAID" guides preparation. The "M" is for machine. The anesthesia machine must be thoroughly checked every day using the appropriate checklist (Willenkin & Polk, 1994). The breathing circuit must be checked to ensure that a means of delivering positive-pressure ventilation exists. Most CRNAs breath through this circuit to ensure that the gases flow freely. The "S" represents suction. The suction equipment must be attached to the central line and functioning and placed within easy reach of the nurse anesthetist. The "M" is for monitor and includes a precordial stethoscope, automatic blood pressure apparatus, electrocardiogram, pulse oximeter, capnogram, anesthetic gas analyzer, temperature, and peripheral nerve stimulator. The "A" is for airway. This includes the mask, oropharyngeal airways, tongue blade, and endotracheal tube. The "I" is for intravenous access and includes intravenous catheters, solution, tubing, tourniquet, alcohol wipes, antibiotic ointment, and tape. The "D" represents drugs, including sedatives, intravenous induction agents, opioids, neuromuscular blocking agents, antimuscarinics, reversal agents for the neuromuscular blocking drugs, and emergency medications.

After the preparation is complete, the CRNA is now ready to focus on the patient and to attend to aspects of care related to administration of the anesthetic. He or she greets the patient and reintroduces himself or herself as the CRNA who will provide the anesthesia care. The patient's identity is verified by asking his or her name and the surgical procedure for which he or she is scheduled and by checking the identification bracelet and the chart for a match. The chart is reviewed to reaffirm that the procedure permit has been signed, dated, and witnessed. The patient is continuously reassured in a calm, professional manner. Every attempt is made to allay fear and apprehension. A check for the presence of dentures, prostheses, and jewelry is conducted. The nothing-by-mouth status is verified. An intravenous infusion is then started using an adequately sized catheter—the smallest acceptable is an 18 gauge—and it is secured with tape. The patient is then moved into the operating room. After locking both the operating room table and the gurney, and securing adequate help on both sides of the patient, the patient positions himself or herself supine on the operating room table. Once a safe transfer is completed, the CRNA ensures that all safety straps are properly attached. All monitoring equipment is applied and includes the blood pressure cuff, pulse oximeter, electrocardiographic pads, precordial stethoscope, and peripheral nerve stimulator. The patient is now ready for preoxygenation. The CRNA records the baseline vital signs on the anesthesia record. Once everything is in order, the induction of anesthesia is begun.

The patient is preoxygenated for 5 minutes with 100% oxygen. Some CRNAs give incremental doses of a sedative-hypnotic such as midazolam and also an opioid such as fentanyl. A test dose of sodium pentothal (25–50 mg) is administered, and after two to three circulation times, the vital signs are checked. If vital signs are stable, a sleep dose of sodium pentothal (1–4 mg/kg) is administered. Once the lid reflex is obtunded, the mask is secured and ventilation is assessed. An oral pharyngeal airway is inserted, if indicated. The gas flows of nitrous oxide and oxygen are adjusted to deliver a fraction of inspired oxygen of 0.33 or higher. The volatile anesthetic agent—halothane, enflurane, isoflurane, desflurane, or sevoflurane—is titrated at a rate of 0.5% every three to five breaths as tolerated, using blood pressure, heart rate, and respiratory rate as signs of increasing depth of anesthesia. The CRNA must continually assess the airway, using the principles of airway management to maintain patency. Concentrations of drugs that exceed 2% halothane, 4% enflurane, 3% isoflurane, 10% desflurane, and 4% sevoflurane are given with extreme caution. It takes about 6 to 8 minutes with this technique to adequately induce the patient.

If the patient requires intubation, the CRNA administers a defasciculating dose of a nondepolarizing neuromuscular blocking drug such as d-tubocurare during this 6- to 8-minute induction sequence and 3 to 5 minutes before the patient is intubated. The fraction of inspired oxygen is increased to 1.0 for a minimum of 1 minute before intubation. Succinylcholine, 1.5 mg/kg, is then administered. The patient is intubated when appropriate. The endotracheal tube is connected to the breathing circuit, the presence of carbon dioxide on the capnogram is ascertained, and the breath sounds are checked to ensure equality bilaterally. The endotracheal tube is taped in place. The anesthetic concentration is adjusted according to the vital signs of the patient. The patient's eyes are lubricated and taped closed. A nasal or oral gastric tube is passed, if appropriate. An esophageal temperature probe with an esophageal stethoscope is also placed at this time.

The surgical preparation now takes place. After a return of motor function following stimulation by the peripheral nerve stimulator, a paralyzing dose of a nondepolarizing neuromuscular blocking drug, such as vecuronium, is administered. The initial and subsequent doses of a neuromuscular blocking agent are kept to the minimum necessary to produce the desired relaxation. The volatile inhalational anesthetic agent concentration is increased 1 to 2 minutes before skin incision in anticipation of the greater stimulation. During the surgical procedure, the depth of the anesthetic agent is adjusted in response to surgical needs. Opioids and neuromuscular blocking drugs are administered incrementally as appropriate.

The CRNA anticipates the end of the surgical procedure by decreasing the anesthetic agent concentration as tolerated and then discontinuing the agent completely as appropriate. Each anesthetic agent has different elimination characteristics, such as blood/gas solubility coefficients, that the CRNA must consider in timing the elimination of the anesthetic agent. Emergence tends to be shortest with desflurane and sevoflurane, short with isoflurane, intermediate with enflurane, and longest with halothane. The nondepolarizing neuromuscular blocking agent must be reversed, allowing for full reversal before the patient awakens. An example of medications used for reversal of the neuromuscular blocking agents is the use of neostigmine, 0.07 mg/kg, and glycopyrrolate, 0.014 mg/kg, with an onset time of 3 to 10 minutes. As the last skin clip or suture is applied, the fraction of inspired oxygen is increased to 1.0, and this is maintained until the patient demonstrates the return of reflexes, reactivity, and consciousness. The CRNA uses the following criteria to determine adequate reversal: an adequate, spontaneously breathing tidal volume of 5 to 7 mL/kg; a vital capacity of 15 to 20 mL/kg; and either a sustained head lift of at least 5 seconds' duration or a sustained handgrip.

Timing of extubation is one of the most crucial judgments facing a CRNA in the anesthetic experience. The decision is made taking into account the evidence of adequate reversal of the neuromuscular blockade, spontaneous breathing, the patient's responsiveness to commands, and the presence of protective reflexes. These protective reflexes include the gag reflex, the cough reflex, and the swallowing reflex. Extubation coincides with end-inspiration to ensure adequate oxygenation. After extubation, the patient is encouraged to breathe deeply while the nurse anesthetist gently holds a mask over his or her face with 100% oxygen. Ventilation is continually assessed by observing chest movement, vital signs, and pulse oximeter readings. A nasal oxygen cannula is then inserted, and the patient is made ready for transfer to the recovery bed. Before transfer, the intravenous bag is moved to the bed pole, all invasive monitor lines are connected to a portable monitor, all drains are free, restraining straps are removed, and the operating room table and stretcher are locked. The CRNA controls transfer to the recovery room bed. Adequate help to make the transfer must be available; at least four people are necessary. The transfer should be a smooth and coordinated effort, with the CRNA managing the head and shoulders.

Postanesthesia Care

All patients are transported to the postanesthesia care unit (PACU) with oxygen and a pulse oximeter. Awake patients are transported in the semi-Fowler's position with the anticipated goal of increasing the functional residual capacity above the closing volume. During transfer, the CRNA is constantly assessing the patient.

After arrival in the PACU, the monitors are replaced and oxygen is connected to the wall outlet by the recovery room staff. The electrocardiogram, blood pressure, respiratory rate, and pulse oximeter are continually monitored. The CRNA gives a report about the patient's history and course of anesthesia to the PACU nurse. The history includes the patient's name and age, surgical procedure, and any pertinent medical history. The anesthesia report includes the agents used and the reversals used, blood loss and replacement of fluids, currently infusing drugs, complications, and areas of concern. The CRNA remains with the patient until he or she is stable, and then the patient's care is turned over to the PACU staff.

Practice of Anesthesia

Most CRNAs are employed by either a hospital that bills for their services or a physician anesthesia group contracted to the particular hospital in which the nurse anesthetist practices. The average salary for a CRNA in all practice settings is approximately $85,000 per year plus benefits. This figure includes base salary plus overtime and call differential. Some CRNAs practice as independent contractors and bill for their professional services.

Historically, anesthesia charges were based on direct time involvement in anesthesia patient care (Simonson & Garde, 1994). By charging for time spent caring for the patient, the final cost was determined by the number of minutes the anesthesia provider was involved in the anesthesia care multiplied by a dollar amount, called a *conversion factor*. This billing procedure did not take into account the complexity of the anesthesia procedure in terms of the skill, preparation, or risk involved. The Relative Value Scale was developed in

1966 by the California Society of Anesthesiologists to arrive at a charge based on a combination of time and the complexity of the anesthesia (Simonson & Garde, 1994). Several Relative Value Guides are available for determination of anesthesia fees. An example of a Relative Value Guide for anesthesia services is published by the ASA.

What is charged by the provider and what is paid by the third-party payers are different. Many insurers, including Medicare, base payments on their own fee schedule, which may be determined by what the average charge is for the service. In non-Medicare cases, CRNAs may directly bill the patient for the balance of charges to make up the difference between what was billed and what was paid by the third- party insurer.

It is a matter of simple mathematics to calculate the fee to be charged for a particular anesthetic. Base units are determined by referring to the particular surgical procedure in the Relative Value Guide. Time units are determined by dividing the anesthesia time by 15-minute intervals. Base units are then added to time units to determine the total number of units for the procedure. The number of units is multiplied by the CRNA's own conversion factor to arrive at the cost of the anesthetic. The conversion factor is based on the cost of living, cost of education, cost of practice, availability to secure a patient base, and quality of life (Simonson & Garde, 1994).

Example 1: A 40-Minute Cataract Procedure

Anesthesia for lens surgery	4 units
Time: 40 minutes (@ 15 minutes/unit)	3 units
Total units	7 units
Conversion factor	$28/unit
Charge for the anesthetic	$196

Example 2: A $2^3/_4$-Hour Coronary Artery Bypass Graft

Anesthesia for procedure on heart, pericardium, and great vessels of chest, with pump oxygenator	25 units
Time: 165 minutes (@ 15 minutes/unit)	11 units
Total units	36 units
Conversion factor	$28/unit
Charge for anesthetic	$1008

Direct reimbursement for CRNA services from Medicare became effective January 1, 1989. All CRNA services are subject to Medicare assignment, which means no balance billing (Simonson & Garde, 1994). *Balance billing* refers to the practice of billing the patient for the remainder of the fee greater than the insurer's allowable charges. The following is an example of balance billing for a 40-minute cataract procedure. Medicare payment is based on the 1998 Medicare-participating CRNA/physician anesthesia conversion factors for Houston, TX.

The charge for anesthesia provided by a CRNA	
7 units @ $28/unit	$196.00
Medicare allows @ $17.63/unit	$123.41
Medicare pays 80%	$98.73
Patient is responsible for	$24.68
Balance (difference between what CRNA charges and Medicare allows	$72.59

It is important for the CRNA to know how to determine the exact worth of his or her professional services. The average number of anesthetics administered by a CRNA per year is 600, or an average of 2.5 per day. The average units per case, time and base, is 10 units. Therefore, the nurse anesthetists can bill for 6000 units per year. By comparing three different practice settings, consider anesthesia charges for those 6000 units.

Example 1: CRNA only provides anesthesia care for Medicare patients
100% Medicare	6000 units @ $17.63/unit	$105,780

Example 2: CRNA is an independent contractor for anesthesia services
30% Medicare	1800 units @ $17.63/unit	$31,734
10% Noncollectible	600 units @ $0/unit	$0
60% Fee for service	3600 units @ $28/unit	$100,800
Total fees collected	$132,534	

Example 3: CRNA is employed in a physician group in a large Texas city
30% Medicare	1800 units @ $17.63/unit	$31,734
10% Noncollectible	600 units @ $0/unit	$0
60% Collectable charges	3600 units @ $55/unit	$198,000
Total fees collected	$229,734	
CRNA salary ($85,000) and benefits	($21,250)	$106,250
CRNA earned for the group	$123,484	

These examples demonstrate the net worth of the CRNA in three different practice settings. The first setting only provides anesthesia services for Medicare patients, which is one of the lowest payers in healthcare. The second example represents a realistic mix of payers for a self-employed CRNA. The last example represents a higher unit charge because it is billed at the anesthesiologist's rate. From these examples, one can see the cost-effectiveness of using CRNAs to provide anesthesia care.

CRNAs have been providing quality anesthesia care in the United States for more than 100 years. Studies comparing anesthesia care outcomes between physician anesthesiologist and CRNAs have demonstrated that no significant difference exists between the two providers (Abenstein & Warner, 1996). The most common anesthesia accidents concern the respiratory system, such as lack of oxygen supply to the patient, intubation of the esophagus instead of the trachea, and disconnection of the oxygen supply to the patient. All of these accidents result from lack of attention to monitoring, not from lack of education (AANA, 1996).

The Future of Nurse Anesthetists

The outlook for the future of nurse anesthesia practice is bright. One only has to look at the increase in the Positions Available section of the *AANA News Bulletin* to be encouraged. In the next 14 years, 53% of practicing CRNAs will reach retirement age (Garde, 1997). Based on current AANA membership, this means that at least 14,500 nurse anesthesia positions will be available in 2012, not counting those who leave the work force for other reasons besides retirement. Currently, approximately 1,200 individuals are certified as CRNAs each year. In 1990, the U.S. Department of Health and Human Services estimated the need for more than 35,000 CRNAs by the year 2010 (Maree, 1990). Based on current figures of new graduates, projected retirements, and estimated need, a shortfall of about 4,000 CRNAs will exist by the year 2010. In light of the rewards of independent practice, earning potential, and job opportunities, this exciting advanced practice nursing option holds great promise for the future.

Key Points

- Nurse anesthetists are advanced practice nurses who have been providing quality anesthesia care for more than 100 years;
- Nurse anesthetists must be certified as CRNAs within 2 years of graduation to be eligible for Medicare reimbursement;

- CRNAs are involved in the care of patients preoperatively, intraoperatively, and postoperatively;
- CRNAs serve as consultants in airway management, respiratory care, resuscitative care, and fluid management; and
- CRNAs provide all types of regional and general anesthesia to patient populations from pediatric to geriatric age groups.

REFERENCES

Abenstein, J. P., & Warner, M. A. (1996). Anesthesia providers, patient outcomes, and cost. *Anesthesia and Analgesia 82*(6), 1273–1283.

American Association of Nurse Anesthetists. (1996). *Professional practice manual for the certified registered nurse anesthetist.* Park Ridge, IL: Author.

Atkinson, R. S., Rushman, G. B., & Davies, N. J. H. (1993). *Lee's synopsis of anaesthesia* (11th ed.). Oxford: Butterworth-Heinemann.

Bankert, M. (1989). *Watchful care: A history of America's nurse anesthetists.* New York: The Continuum Publishing Co.

Bauer, J. C. (1998). *Not what the doctor ordered* (2nd ed.). New York: McGraw-Hill.

Council on Accreditation of Nurse Anesthesia Educational Programs (1990). *Standards and guidelines for accreditation of nurse anesthesia educational programs.* Park Ridge, IL: Author.

Council on Certification of Nurse Anesthetists. (1993). *Member administrative manual.* Park Ridge, IL: Author.

Council on Certification of Nurse Anesthetists. (1997). *1998 Candidate handbook.* Park Ridge, IL: Author.

Council on Recertification of Nurse Anesthetists (1998). *Criteria for recertification.* Park Ridge, IL: Author.

Fleisher, L. A. (1997). Preoperative evaluation. In P. G. Barash, B. F. Cullen, & R. K. Stoelting (Eds.). *Clinical anesthesia* (3rd ed.). Philadelphia: Lippincott-Raven Publishers.

Foster, S. (1998). An open letter to congress. *AANA News Bulletin 52*(5), 5.

Garde, J. F. (1997). Report of the executive director: Our ongoing journey into the knowledge age. *AANA News Bulletin 51*(10), 13–15.

Gunn, I. P. (1997). Nurse anesthesia: A history of challenge. In J. J. Nagelhout & K. L. Zaglaniczny (Eds.). *Nurse anesthesia.* Philadelphia: W. B. Saunders Co.

Jordan, L. M. (1994). Qualifications and capabilities of the certified registered nurse anesthetist. In S. D. Foster & L. M. Jordan (Eds.). *Professional aspects of nurse anesthesia practice.* Philadelphia: F. A. Davis Co.

Kachnij, J. M. (1997). Preoperative evaluation and preparation of the patient. In J. J. Nagelhout & K. L. Zaglaniczny (Eds.). *Nurse anesthesia.* Philadelphia: W. B. Saunders Co.

Mallampati, S. R. (1997). Airway management. In P. G. Barash, B. F. Cullen, & R. K. Stoelting (Eds.). *Clinical anesthesia* (3rd ed.). Philadelphia: Lippincott-Raven Publishers.

Maree, S. M. (1990). *National commission on nurse anesthesia education.* Chicago: American Association of Nurse Anesthetists.

Morgan, G. E., & Mikhail, M. S. (1996). *Clinical anesthesiology* (2nd ed.). Stamford, CT: Appleton & Lange.

Simonson, D. C., & Garde, J. F. (1994). Reimbursement for clinical services. In S. D. Foster & L. M. Jordan (Eds.). *Professional aspects of nurse anesthesia practice.* Philadelphia: F. A. Davis Co.

Willenkin, R. L., & Polk, S. L. (1994). Management of general anesthesia. In R. D. Miller (Ed.). *Anesthesia* (4th ed.). New York: Churchill Livingstone.

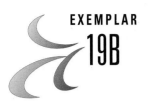

The Evolution of the Nurse–Midwife Role

Margaret A. Edmundson

Midwives have been a valued and respected part of society since the beginning of time. The term *midwife* is an Anglo-Saxon word meaning "with woman." Women have assisted other women during their pregnancies and births since the beginning of time in all cultures and societies. Certainly, midwives have been an important part of American history since the settlement of the colonies. However, as physicians became a more integral part of the healthcare system in our society, particularly after 1900, midwives became a less-valued and important part of our society.

The evolution of the practice of midwifery care in the United States is fascinating. Midwives were an important part of the settlement of the American colonies, having immigrated with the other settlers to this country. As the adventurous Americans moved westward, the midwives moved with them as part of the community and provided healthcare to women and children. These women were highly respected members of the new communities.

In the early 1900s, however, it was recognized that maternal and infant care was inadequate in the United States. The maternal mortality rates at the beginning of the 20th century were as high as they are in developing countries today. Between 1900 and 1930, the maternal mortality rate reached a high level of 600 to 700 maternal deaths per 100,000 births. These rates dropped sharply with the advent of blood transfusions, antibiotics, and medications for pregnancy-induced hypertension (Rooks, 1997, p. 30).

Midwives were considered contributors to the high maternal and child mortality rates because of their lack of education, medical support, and facilities available to physicians providing maternity care. Women in the 1930s, therefore, started having their babies delivered in hospitals by physicians, and the need for "untrained" midwives and home births decreased.

Today, several different kinds of midwives practice in this country—lay midwives, direct-entry midwives, foreign-trained midwives, and certified nurse–midwives (CNMs). Lay midwives have generally apprenticed with other, more experienced midwives and without a formalized educational program. Direct-entry midwives, on the other hand, usually complete a professional midwifery program and have clinical experience. They are not necessarily registered nurses before becoming midwives (Rooks, 1997, p. 6).

I became a nurse–midwife because I had always enjoyed obstetrical nursing. I wanted to broaden the scope of my nursing skills and get to know families before the births of their babies. I wanted to provide labor support as well as assist with the birth process (deliver the baby) for a woman and her family. I wanted to help the family adjust to a new family member. I wanted to continue the healthcare of a woman with family planning and annual gynecologic examinations. I wanted to be part of this circle of healthcare. I have found this circle of care to be very rewarding. Midwifery is more than a job to me. It is with a sense of awe that I assist these births, a wonderful joy of helping babies enter the world, and experiencing the amazement and excitement of the new parents.

Nurse–midwives were probably the first group of advanced practice nurses in the United States. There were several schools of midwifery operating in the early 1900s in New York City, including Bellevue Hospital and the Lobenstine Midwifery School. However, these schools did not cater to registered nurses—they were for women who chose to be midwives.

The Frontier Nursing Service of Hyden, KY, was founded in 1928. Mary Breckinridge, one of the founders, was from a wealthy and prominent Southern family. Widowed at the young age of 25 years and losing two young children through early deaths, she decided to study nursing in New York City. She saw the impoverished conditions in the city where poor women gave birth. The prenatal care provided to these women was also minimal. Mrs. Breckenridge also spent some time visiting her family living in the mountains of Kentucky and viewed the conditions where most women gave birth and healthcare was provided for their children. She was appalled at the lack of adequate healthcare in the land of wealth and plenty. After studying the healthcare system of England, she went there and enrolled in a midwifery program to learn this specialized healthcare. Along with several nurses from England, she started the Frontier Nursing Service of Hyden, KY, providing much-needed healthcare to poor families in that area. Mrs. Breckinridge and the other nurses rode on horseback to visit families and to deliver babies. This service found that by keeping detailed records of their clients' outcomes, they could show that adequate prenatal care by well-educated nurse–midwives, normal births of babies in prepared homes, and postpartum and well-child care in strategically placed clinics in the mountains markedly decreased the maternal–infant mortality rate.

The philosophy of nurse–midwives is different from that of most physicians. Physicians are more likely to view pregnancy as a pathologic event that must be "managed" by a healthcare provider (i.e., physician), whereas nurse–midwives see pregnancy as a normal life event in which the pregnant woman is the primary decision maker unless complications occur. Nurse–midwives see their role as educators of women, giving them the information and power to make informed decisions regarding healthcare.

CNMs work in a variety of settings in this country. Some work in independent private practices with generally middle-class families. Others work for large hospitals in clinics or "private" practices within the organization; many CNMs work for the Indian Health Service on reservations scattered throughout the country; several CNMs work as employees of private physicians in their practices. CNMs also teach in many different programs in universities to educate the new nurse–midwives in the United States.

As of 1998, approximately 4500 CNMs were practicing in this country. This is a great increase since 1963, when only 11% of CNMs practiced the full scope of midwifery services (i.e., antepartum, intrapartum, postpartum, and well-woman gynecology). In 1967, the percentage had increased to 23%. In 1995, 77% of nurse–midwife respondents reported practicing full-scope midwifery care (Roberts, 1998).

Many people ask me why a woman would seek maternity care from a CNM as opposed to seeing an obstetrician in the same building. One of the main issues is control. As mentioned, nurse–midwives consider pregnancy to be a normal process of life, whereas physicians often consider pregnancy to be a pathologic condition needing to be "managed" by a healthcare provider (i.e., physician) to realize a good outcome. Many women recognize the normalcy of pregnancy and have a desire to maintain control over their own bodies as much as possible. Women who want control over their birth experiences want to ambulate during labor, eat and drink liquids as desired, not have intravenous tubes routinely, have intermittent fetal monitoring (external), and only use internal fetal and intrauterine monitoring when necessary. They want to have family members and friends present, prepared siblings at the birth, and use of a birth plan when desired. They have availed themselves of the lay and professional literature regarding pregnancy and have attended various childbirth classes with different points of view. Some women desire a birth at home with family and friends present, others prefer a birth center setting, and still others want the security of a hospital and the flexibility of a nurse–midwife. Many families are concerned about the legality of a home birth; I remind them that babies can be legally born anywhere (even a car); it is really a matter of where the parents feel most comfortable. Another issue is time spent with a care provider. Often physicians are scheduled very tightly and have little opportunity to sit and listen to concerned clients. CNMs try to spend as much time with clients as necessary. In some settings this is difficult because of other time constraints; however, this is a goal of most CNMs. It is important to listen to women's concerns and fears as well as their preparations for the new family. Education of families is a primary task of all nurse–midwives; the needs of one couple are often completely different from those of the next.

I have been a CNM for more than 20 years and have been privileged to be involved in more than 1300 births. It truly has been a fascinating career! It amazes me that some of "my babies" are older than 20 years and may even have children of their own. It has been demanding at times, helping families have the kind of birth experience they desire (some labors and births are not always the way they should be). If the birth does not go as planned, my partners and I still work hard to provide a satisfying and fulfilling experience for families.

The annual statistics in our practice have been outstanding compared with the national obstetric statistics. The cesarean section rate is about 5% to 7%, the preterm birth rate is approximately 3%, and the use of forceps and vacuum extractions is 2% to 3% (Colorado Nurse Midwives, personal communication, 1997). We are extremely pleased that these numbers are better than the national statistics. Our consulting physicians of Denver-Evergreen Ob-Gyn, P.C., are conservative and bide their time before acting quickly and thus performing unnecessary procedures. The above-mentioned numbers include women who have low-risk pregnancies but develop complications as the pregnancy progresses.

CNMs in our practice have a close working relationship with our consulting physicians. Often the consultation is an informal "hallway chat" whereby the CNM asks the physician a quick question regarding a treatment plan; at other times the consultation is more formal in which the CNM will have the physician see the client and he or she will develop a medical plan of care. Sometimes a woman will develop a serious health problem—gynecologic, prenatally, or postpartum—and the physician needs to take over the care of that client. The CNM will remain involved in the care to provide emotional support and education to the client and family.

Our practice is unusual in that it has been involved in nurse–midwifery in some way for 20 years. Two of us were instrumental in starting a nurse–midwifery practice in the Denver metropolitan area in the late 1970s. As the practice evolved, different forms of the practice developed. For many years, this practice was part of the University of Colorado Health Sciences Center in Denver and was funded by the University of Colorado and federal funds in the form of grants. This practice was also the beginning of the nurse–midwifery educational program at the University of Colorado Health Sciences Center and provided a clinical educational site for student nurse–midwives. Another aspect of this practice is the job-sharing of the work. All of us are wives and mothers; therefore, we want to spend time with our families. We are allotted two full-time equivalent positions that are then divided into various percentages of time as desired by the practice members. Presently, we are employed by the Columbia Presbyterian/St.Luke's Hospital in Denver, which pays for our malpractice insurance, health insurance, and other benefits usually offered by a major company. This is helpful to practice members. When one CNM is ill, the other CNMs provide coverage for her to provide care for the clients.

As stated previously, nurse–midwives work in a myriad of different settings and receive payments from several different sources. Private insurers, such as Blue Cross/Blue Shield, pay for a number of clients as they provide payment for physicians. Sometimes CNMs are included in the lists of approved providers; or their consulting physicians may be on the approved provider list, which allows payment for mid-level care providers.

Health maintenance organizations (HMOs) are prevalent in many areas of the country. CNMs can be employed by these companies in several different positions or the HMOs may pay CNMs as they pay physicians. Managed care organizations are another form of payers that often provide jobs for CNMs. It seems that new forms of payments are developed every day; and new rules and regulations are promulgated for each organization. Therefore, healthcare providers must continue to be aware of changes that occur almost daily within the healthcare system.

As with all ACNPs, several barriers must be constantly dealt with to start or continue a practice. These include education of the public, education of insurance companies, privileges at various healthcare facilities, and developing strong relationships with consulting physicians. With these major categories of barriers are smaller barriers that are daily battles that must be coped with.

Nurse–midwifery is certainly a challenging and exciting profession. I never get over the cry of a newborn baby. Or those wiggly arms and legs. Or the excitement of new parents and grandparents. Or the look of the newborn seeing bright light for the first time. I think of the baby smiling for the first time for his mom and dad. Taking those first few steps. The look of joy of the mother successfully breastfeeding and watching the baby grow on her own milk. The father watching this baby turn over on the rug and seeing the baby smile for the first time. What delights! What excitement! Nurse–midwifery is truly an exciting profession.

CASE VIGNETTE

Vignette 1

Brenda and Chris, a couple expecting a baby

This is Brenda's first pregnancy. She and Chris have been married 4 years and felt it was time for them to start a family. She decided to see the CNMs in our practice because she had heard positive comments from one of her friends who had recently had a baby delivered by us. Brenda liked the idea of a healthcare provider spending time with Chris and her to answer their questions, provide classes for pregnancy, and spend more time with her in labor. She also liked the idea of having more control over the management of her care. The pregnancy progressed well without any complications, the birth of her baby was relatively easy (she said *after* the birth), and they were anxious to go home and begin their new roles as parents. Brenda stated that she felt such support throughout her pregnancy, labor, and birth. She felt that she received ample information regarding breastfeeding and infant care that she was confident in her new role as a mother. She also felt like she could call us at any time with questions and concerns.

Vignette 2

Marianne, a sexually-active adolescent

Marianne, 16 years old, was brought in by her mother, who suspected that Marianne had a sexually transmitted disease. Marianne slouched in the chair, kept her eyes from mine, and answered my questions with one word. I ascertained that she had some vaginal discharge, itching, and a foul odor in the vagina. She did say, after some careful questioning, that in fact she was sexually active. I completed a wet mount slide and found clue cells indicating bacterial vaginosis. After giving her the diagnosis and the treatment (Cleocin cream intravaginally for 7 days), I talked with her at length about contraception, potential sexually transmitted diseases, and the possible sequelae as well as her feelings about herself and her expectations for the future. She left the office with several sample packs of oral contraceptives, a prescription for Cleocin cream, and a follow-up appointment in 2 months.

Vignette 3
Rita, a woman entering the menopausal years

Rita, a 53-year-old woman, is experiencing several signs and symptoms of menopause. These include hot flashes, irritability, fatigue, and skipped menses. She states that her husband of 25 years has been more than sympathetic but is concerned about her health. Generally, they have a good relationship and a satisfying sex life, but she experiences occasional dyspareunia and decreased libido. She wants to know what she can do to make this transition in her life easier. Following a complete history and physical examination, the results of which were normal, I sat down and talked with her regarding various management plans. We discussed the use of vitamin and mineral supplements, particularly calcium. Exercise is an important part of daily life and helps one cope with the bodily changes that occur in menopause. Hormone replacement therapy risks and benefits were carefully discussed. I gave her suggestions about reading material that might help her decide whether hormone replacement therapy was right for her. She left the office after making another appointment for a month later. No prescriptions were given.

Key Points

- Midwives have assisted women during pregnancies and births since the beginning of time in all cultures and societies;
- CNMs view pregnancy as a normal life event in which the pregnant woman is the primary decision maker unless complications occur;
- In 1998, 4500 CNMs were practicing in America; and
- Positive outcomes of CNM practice include low caesarian section rates, low preterm birth rates, and low rates of use of forceps and vacuum extractions.

Definitions

Midwife (international definition): "A midwife is a person who, having been regularly admitted to a midwifery educational program, duly recognized in the country in which it is located, has successfully completed the prescribed course of studies in midwifery and has acquired the requisite qualifications to be a registered or legally licensed to practice midwifery" (Varney, 1997).

Certified nurse–midwife: A registered nurse who has completed accredited nurse–midwifery education programs, passed a national certification examination, and met other criteria for certification by the American College of Nurse–Midwives (ACNM) or the ACNM Certification Council (Rooks, 1997).

Lay midwives: Women who have apprenticed with more experienced midwives but generally have not completed a formalized midwifery educational program. These midwives deliver babies in homes (Rooks, 1997).

Direct-entry midwives: Persons who enter midwifery without being a nurse first. Most have completed a midwifery educational program and some have taken and passed a midwifery examination and call themselves certified professional midwives, which is controlled by the North American Registry of Midwives (Rooks, 1997).

Licensed midwives: Used in some states to designate a direct-entry midwife who is licensed by the state in which she practices. Standards vary a great deal in various states (Rooks, 1997).

Birth attendants and doulas: Women who attend births to provide support for the laboring woman and assist the primary birth attendant (either physician or midwife) (Rooks, 1997).

Practice sites:
Hospitals
Birth centers
Domiciliary settings (home births)
Universities—as faculty
Indian reservations
Clinics

Professional organizations:
American College of Nurse–Midwives (ACNM)
Midwives Association of North America (MANA)
International Confederation of Midwives (ICM)

REFERENCES

Roberts, J. President's pen. *Quickening May–June,* 1998.

Rooks, J. P. (1997). *Midwifery and childbirth in America.* Philadelphia: Temple University Press.

Varney, H. (1997). *Varney's midwifery.* Boston: Jones and Bartlett Publishers.

Reemphasizing the "Clinical" in the Clinical Nurse Specialist Role

Anne W. Wojner

The clinical nurse specialist (CNS) role was designed as an expert clinical nursing role with a focus on developing the expertise and skill set of clinical nurses working in high-acuity settings. The role was originally conceived as one that included four subroles that were integrated by the CNS to meet the needs of staff and clients (Fig. 19C-1). The CNS was described as fluently moving between each subrole to achieve optimal clinical care delivery (Hamric & Spross).

Despite the original *clinical* intent supporting the design of the CNS role, research on role execution has revealed that many CNSs spend much of their time in subroles other than clinical practice. Education, consultation, and special project development have been commonly identified by CNSs and their administrators as primary consumers of their time. Rarely has the research subrole been identified as commonly used by CNSs (Fenton, 1985; Hart, Lekander, Bartels, & Tebbitt, 1987; Taristano, Brophy, & Snyder, 1986; Wyers, Grove, & Pastorino, 1985).

Informally then, CNSs have reported a hierarchy of subrole execution dominated by education and consultation, with the clinical and research subroles serving in less important capacities. This form of subrole execution resulted in movement of the CNS away from the clinical setting that the role had initially been developed to serve.

Clinical inaccessibility, coupled with the lack of a program of research to guide role execution, placed the CNS role in a vulnerable position in the early 1990s. Without data to support the impact of the CNS role on achievement of key patient outcomes, the position was eliminated in many institutions across the United States as administrators attempted to reduce fixed operating costs in a climate of managed health care (Wojner & Kite-Powell, 1997).

Since that time, many programs that eliminated the CNS role have come to recognize the need for an expert nurse *clinician* and *researcher* to guide interdisciplinary care delivery for a variety of complex patient populations. Retooled from its original design, the CNS role that was once near death has now emerged as one of the most powerful roles in acute care, when guided by a *clinically based* framework that supports the measurement and on-going management of patient outcomes (Wojner, 1999).

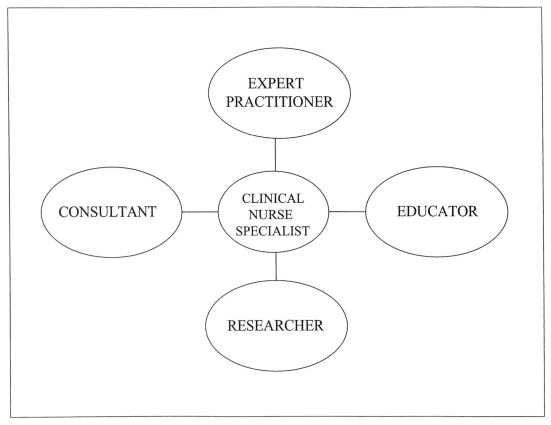

FIGURE 19C-1 The Traditional Clinical Nurse Specialist Role.

Aligning the Clinical Nurse Specialist Role With Outcomes Management

Outcomes management (OM) is the "enhancement of physiologic and psychosocial patient outcomes through development and implementation of exemplary health practices and services, as driven by outcomes assessment" (Wojner, 1997a, p. 5). Paul Ellwood (1988) first theorized the process of OM, suggesting that quality measures should be anchored to outcome analyses. Ellwood defined OM as a "technology of patient experience designed to help patients, payers and providers make rational medical care–related choices based on better insight into the effect of these choices on the patient's life" (p. 1549). Ellwood cited four key components for inclusion in an OM initiative:

1. Emphasis on standards that physicians can use to select appropriate interventions;
2. Measurement of patient functioning and well-being along with disease-specific clinical outcomes;
3. Pooling of clinical and outcome data on a massive scale; and
4. Analysis and dissemination of the database to appropriate decision makers (Ellwood, 1988).

OM programs must be supported by a strong research arm. Outcomes research facil-

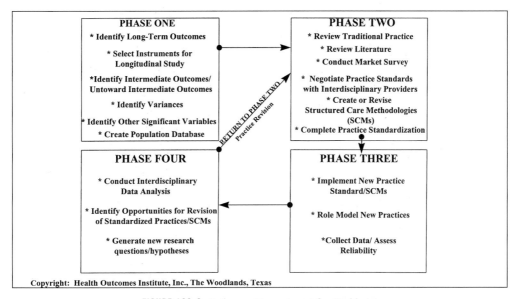

FIGURE 19C-2 Outcomes Management Quality Model.

itates the study of interdisciplinary interventions (care processes) aimed at achievement of specified goals (physiologic and psychosocial outcomes). A favorable outcome is defined as one that results in achievement of a specified goal (Davies et al., 1994). Because the definition of an "acceptable" or "desirable" outcome varies by patient, payer, and provider, interdisciplinary providers engaging in OM must agree on the health outcomes to be measured and how each variable will be defined at the start of the initiative (Wojner, 1999).

Figure 19C-2 illustrates a model that provides a framework for describing the OM process. Diagnostic groups within a practice setting are identified for OM based on patient volume, the existence of untoward outcomes, and clinical interest. In *phase one,* goals are defined and a database, or outcomes data repository, is constructed. The process then progresses to *phase two,* in which practices are standardized through use of a variety of structured care methods (Table 19C-1). In *phase three,* interdisciplinary providers work to achieve mastery of the standardized practices, and data are collected. *Phase four* involves analysis of the outcomes data and determination of the next steps in the improvement of clinical care. The process then returns to *phase two,* in which new interventions are designed and standardized (Wojner, 1997b).

A FRAMEWORK FOR CLINICAL NURSE SPECIALIST PRACTICE

As inpatient days continue to drop, and inpatient acuity continues to rise, the need for clinical expertise driven by clinical outcomes research will gain in significance. The CNS position has been identified as one capable of meeting current and future high-acuity clinical needs through use of a clinically based framework that promotes excellence in interdisciplinary healthcare and patient outcomes (Wojner & Kite-Powell, 1997).

Figure 19C-3 presents a hierarchy of CNS subroles that supports the clinical needs of patients, families, and interdisciplinary staff, as well as optimizing institutional financial outcomes. The following assumptions support the framework:

1. The growing complexity of acute care patients requires expert attending nurse oversight to ensure optimal, interdisciplinary healthcare delivery;
2. The complexity of current and evolving healthcare technology and medicinal therapies, coupled with increased nurse–patient care requirements, challenges the ability of the bedside nurse to provide expert nursing care, patient and familial advocacy, and clinical oversight;
3. Inpatient acuity will continue to rise, whereas inpatient length of stay will continue to drop in traditional acute care settings;
4. Research serves as the foundation for identification and utilization of best practices in healthcare;

TABLE 19C-1 *Characteristics of Structured Care Methods*

Structured Care Method	Characteristics
Critical pathway	Represents a sequential, interdisciplinary, minimal practice standard for a specific patient population
	Provider flexibility to alter care to meet individualized patient needs
	Abbreviated format, broad perspective
	Phase- or episode-driven
	Lack of control prohibits ability to measure the cause-and-effect relationship between pathway and patient outcomes; changes in patient outcome are directly attributable to the efforts of the collaborative practice team
Algorithm	Binary decision trees that guide stepwise assessment and intervention
	Intense specificity; no provider flexibility
	Useful in the management of high-risk subgroups within the cohort
	May be "layered" on top of a pathway to highly control care practices used to manage a specific problem
	May use analytical research methods to measure cause and effect
Protocol	Prescribes specific therapeutic interventions for a clinical problem unique to a subgroup of patients within the cohort
	Multifaceted; may be used to drive practice for more than one discipline
	Broader specificity than an algorithm; allows for minimal provider flexibility by way of treatment options
	May be "layered" on top of a pathway to control care practices used to manage a specific problem
	May use analytic research methods to measure cause and effect
Order set	Preprinted provider orders used to expedite the order process once a practice standard has been validated through analytic research
	Complements and increases compliance with existing practice standards
	Can be used to represent the algorithm or protocol in order format
Guideline	Broad, research-based practice recommendations
	May or may not have been tested in clinical practice
	Practice resources helpful in the construction of structured care methods
	No mechanism for ensuring practice implementation

Reprinted with permission from the Health Outcomes Institute, Inc., The Woodlands, TX.

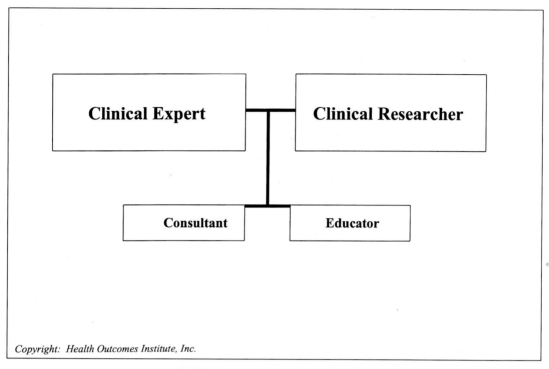

FIGURE 19C-3 A Hierarchy of CNS Subroles.

5. Complications are the primary drivers of increased healthcare costs in acute care settings;
6. Clinical expertise and relevance is a necessary prerequisite to conducting clinical outcomes research;
7. Hands-on clinical expertise and a highly visible clinical presence promote increased CNS effectiveness; and
8. CNSs use their expertise in clinical practice and research to act as change agents, promoting interdisciplinary practice improvement.

CLINICAL NURSE SPECIALIST AS EXPERT CLINICAL PRACTITIONER

CNSs must assume the role of attending nurse within their acute care setting, overseeing delivery of complex interdisciplinary patient care for a specific population. As a *specialist,* the CNS brings an expert body of knowledge—coupled with hands-on clinical expertise—to the care setting, enhancing delivery of highly complex, technical care. CNSs collaborate and consult with interdisciplinary providers, role-modeling expert nursing practice; trouble-shooting complex patient care issues; providing impromptu education for patients, family members, and interdisciplinary staff; and continuously assessing the results of interventions through the eyes of a clinical researcher (Fig. 19C-4) (Wojner & Kite-Powell, 1991). Table 19C-2 lists performance criteria specific to the clinical realm of the CNS.

The CNS role requires true hands-on clinical expertise and is an unsuitable role for a clinical impostor. Approximately 60% to 70% of the CNS's time should be dedicated to clinical practice, working toward development of relationships with bedside providers that will later facilitate their ability to manipulate the practice environment (Wojner, 1999). Role-modeling expert clinical practice ensures not only credibility but respect for the CNS and makes a strong statement in support of advanced practice nursing roles.

High-quality clinical care improves patient outcomes, which in turn reduces cost and length of stay. CNSs should be held accountable for both the patient population and financial outcomes that result from the quality of clinical practice within their care settings (Wojner, in press). Outcomes accountability represents one of the most powerful aspects of the CNS role and fosters acknowledgment of a cause-and-effect relationship between use of a CNS and program results.

Traditional staff development responsibilities should not be part of the CNS role. Instead, the education provided by CNSs should reflect their clinical assessment and research findings within their assigned care settings. When findings suggest a need for a new practice standard and additional staff education, CNSs should take responsibility for constructing the standard in concert with other provider disciplines and actively be involved in disseminating staff education. As attending nurses, CNSs may also need to spend a considerable amount of time imparting education to patients and families given the current staffing demands that limit the bedside nurse's ability to teach and counsel (Wojner & Kite-Powell, 1997).

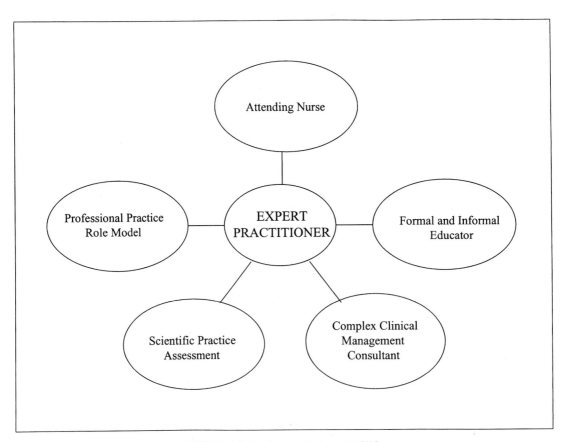

FIGURE 19C-4 The Clinical Realm of the CNS.

TABLE 19C-2 *Performance Criteria for Clinical Nurse Specialists Related to Outcomes Management*

Effective	Exceeds Effective	Highly Effective
Expert Clinical Practice—Analyses practice and designs interdisciplinary interventions for implementation and testing toward achievement of best practice for an assigned patient population		
1. Demonstrates and communicates clinical expertise in an assigned patient population, role-modeling application of clinical practice standards 2. Responds to interdisciplinary requests for evaluation and management of complex patients as they move across the continuum 3. Analyzes contributors to variable cost, making recommendations for change in clinical practice to facilitate cost-effective, quality care 4. Provides informal education to interdisciplinary providers and consumers as indicated by patient outcomes	1. Supports development of business and marketing plans for assigned patient population 2. Provides formal educational programs to interdisciplinary providers and consumers 3. Practices beyond the boundaries of his or her assigned patient population as requested, to enhance quality and financial outcomes 4. Mentors graduate nursing students in the provision of expert, research-based, clinical care 5. Supports the ongoing professional growth of his or her peer group within the OM department.	1. Demonstrates increased efficiency and quality in clinical practice 2. Impacts community wellness through development and implementation of continuum-based services 3. Achieves a balance between clinical quality and financial outcomes that positively impacts the institution's bottom line 4. Develops service or divisional policy and procedures as driven by OM
Clinical Researcher—Facilitates enrichment of the body of science and research-based care, leading to the identification of best practice for the assigned patient population		
1. Facilitates development, implementation and ongoing revision of structured care methods based on scientific evidence 2. Establishes outcomes measures and methods for data collection 3. Builds an OM database to describe quality and efficiency of care 4. Participates in the development of descriptive research 5. Engages members of the interdisciplinary team in the generation of research questions or hypotheses for study within the population of interest 6. Shares findings from OM database with interdisciplinary grassroots providers	1. Participates as a co-investigator in the development of research proposals suitable for submission to the institutional review board 2. Implements well-conducted observational studies related to assigned population 3. Implements a research-based change in practice that results in improved quality and financial outcomes 4. Provides formal education regarding the research process to interdisciplinary providers	1. Serves as a principal investigator in the development of research proposals 2. Implements well-conducted randomized controlled trials or cohort studies 3. Serves as an administrator for a funded research project 4. Submits grant proposal(s) for funding of proposed research study 5. Publishes original research in peer-reviewed journals 6. Mentors interdisciplinary providers in the process of research proposal development 7. Coordinates a service-based journal club charged with research utilization for assigned patient populations

Reprinted with permission from the Health Outcomes Institute, Inc., The Woodlands, TX.

CLINICAL NURSE SPECIALIST AS CLINICAL RESEARCHER

The use of a CNS fosters an ability to conduct ongoing outcomes research for defined patient populations, enabling changes in clinical practice that are guided by science. CNSs spearheading an OM initiative facilitate interdisciplinary movement toward the discovery and implementation of best practices (Wojner, 1999). Table 19C-2 identifies performance criteria for CNSs as clinical outcomes researchers.

CNSs must remain current with practice literature, assessing the quality of published research findings, identifying conceptual difficulties in research, and recognizing implications for interdisciplinary practice and opportunities for research utilization. The significant concentration of time spent in clinical practice by CNSs promotes their ability to generate clinically significant, interdisciplinary research questions and hypotheses and identifies opportunities for intervention development and testing (Wojner, 1999).

CNSs with entry-level master's preparation should enlist the support of a doctorally prepared research mentor to assist them with building a program of research. Mentors may represent a variety of disciplines, functioning as nurses, physicians, epidemiologists, or other health science professionals. The CNS's need for research mentorship is likely to vary and may lessen over time as research ability develops. Doctorally educated CNSs should function as independent outcomes researchers in collaboration with the other practice disciplines in their care setting.

The consultant and educator subroles are used by the CNS clinical researcher to share study results and invite interdisciplinary staff ownership of study findings. By focusing on scientifically guided clinical improvement, CNSs are able to steer bedside interdisciplinary providers toward delivery of care strategically aimed at enhancing outcomes, thereby achieving institutional goals for cost reduction through prevention of untoward patient outcomes (Wojner, 1999).

COREQUISITES FOR SUCCESSFUL CLINICAL NURSE SPECIALIST ROLE ACTUALIZATION

Several corequisite professional and personal characteristics are necessary to support success in the CNS role. The CNS candidate must possess hands-on clinical expertise, the ability to act as a leader and change agent, sound teaching and consultation skills, experience with research methods, a collaborative practice philosophy, tenacity, political astuteness, and a willingness to take risks. A commitment to continuous self-reflection, evaluation, and role improvement is necessary to foster effective interdisciplinary team relationships and improved clinical outcomes (Wojner, in press; Wojner & Kite-Powell, 1997).

Summary

The process of OM optimizes outcomes through provision of care guided by research. CNS education positions these advanced practice nurses to spearhead an outcomes initiative by supporting development of specialized clinical expertise, research skills, and mastery of change process. The flexibility of the CNS role accommodates ongoing staff development through education and consultation that support a program of expert clinical practice and research. Returning the CNS role to the clinical domain ensures a powerful impact on patient and institutional outcomes.

Key Points

- The CNS role has emerged as one of the most powerful roles in acute care when guided by a clinically based framework that supports the measurement and ongoing management of patient outcomes;

- OM must be supported by a strong research arm;
- Interdisciplinary providers engaging in OM must agree on the health outcomes to be measured;
- CNSs should be held accountable for both the patient population and financial outcomes that result from the quality of clinical practice within their care settings; and
- CNSs facilitate interdisciplinary movement toward the discovery and implementation of best practice.

REFERENCES

Davies, A. R., Doyle, M. A., Lansky, D., et al. (1994). Outcomes assessment in clinical settings: A consensus statement on principles and best practices in project management. *Journal on Quality Improvement* 20(1), 6–16.

Ellwood, P.M. (1988). Outcomes management: A technology of patient experience. *New England Journal of Medicine 318*(23), 1549–1556.

Fenton, M. V. (1985). Identifying competencies of clinical nurse specialists. *Journal of Nursing Administration 15,* 31–37.

Hart, C., Lekander, B., Bartels, D., & Tebbitt, B. (1987). Clinical nurse specialists: An institutional process for determining priorities. *Journal of Nursing Administration 17,* 31–35.

Taristano, B. J., Brophy, E. B., & Snyder, D. J. (1986). A demystification of the clinical nurse specialist role: Perceptions of clinical nurse specialists and nurse administrators. *Journal of Nursing Education 25,* 4–9.

Wojner, A. W. (1997a). Outcomes management: From theory to practice. *Critical Care Nursing Quarterly 19*(4), 1–15.

Wojner, A. W. (1997b). Widening the scope: From case management to outcomes management. *The Case Manager 8*(2), 77–82.

Wojner, A. W. (1999). *Outcomes management: Application for clinical practice.* St. Louis, MO: Mosby-Yearbook.

Wojner, A. W., & Kite-Powell, D. (1997). Outcomes manager: A role for the advanced practice nurse. *Critical Care Nursing Quarterly 19*(4), 16–24.

Wyers, M. E. A., Grove, S. K., & Pastorino, C. (1985). Clinical nurse specialist: In search of the right role. *Nursing and Health Care April,* 203–207.

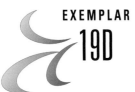

EXEMPLAR
19D

A Nurse Practitioner–managed Cardiovascular Intensive Care Unit

Michael H. Ackerman
Jean Clark
Teresa Reed
Lauren Van Horn
Maria Francati

The acute care nurse practitioner (ACNP) role is relatively new compared with other advanced practice roles. To date, few practice models exist to guide new ACNPs in developing their practices. The purpose of this exemplar is to describe a group practice in the cardiovascular intensive care unit (CVICU). The foundation of the practice is based on the Strong Model of Advanced Practice (Ackerman et al., 1996). The Strong model identifies five domains of practice: direct care, education, system support, research, and professional publications and leadership. Common threads that influence each domain of the model include, scholarship, collaboration, and empowerment. It is expected that within each domain practitioners will possess different strengths as well as areas for improvement. Each domain has as its foundation a novice-to-expert framework to recognize the uniqueness of each practitioner. The model is illustrated in Figure 19D-1. This article uses the Strong model as a guide to exemplify a ACNP–managed ICU.

Direct Care

ACNPs in the ICU provide direct care using a holistic approach. ACNPs are responsible for complete management of patient care issues. In addition, ACNPs act as an important communication link for the family, attending surgeons, and surgical residents. Daily rounds are made with the physicians to review the patient's progress and to formulate a plan. The ACNPs know each patient in detail and collaborate fully in the formulation of the plan for each patient. Laboratory values, radiographs, and physical examinations are performed and evaluated daily. Treatments, consults, procedures, and plans are made based on these assessments. Each patient and family is treated as an individual with special needs. Daily meetings are held with each family to discuss concerns and progress. Problems and complications are communicated to the residents, consultants, and attending physicians.

Direct patient care is the primary aspect of the ACNP in the CVICU. Advanced skills

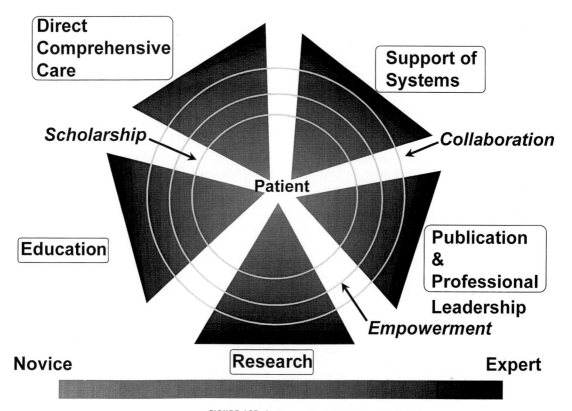

FIGURE 19D-1 Strong Model of Advanced Practice.

are needed for interpreting laboratory and radiologic test results, performing surgical and diagnostic procedures, and ordering treatments and medications. Physicians rely on the ongoing assessments and planning of ACNPs to provide the care needed for these patients. Families need daily information and emotional support. The ACNP has the unique ability to coordinate and case-manage patients in the ICU and to play a major role in patient outcomes. This includes ordering tests and interpreting their results, prescribing medications, and collaborating with physicians and consultants to develop an individualized plan for patient care.

The performance of invasive procedures is a function of the role that has traditionally been done by physicians. Specialty-specific procedures include placement of arterial lines, pulmonary arterial catheters, and central venous catheters; thoracentesis; and tube thoracostomy. The credentialing process for ACNPs is similar to the process for credentialing physicians.

In the CVICU, the two categories of patients are those who "fast-track" and those who do not. For those patients who fast-track, the care is directed by preestablished protocols developed by the cardiothoracic team. It is the responsibility of the ACNP to make sure the protocols are implemented and carried out. However, a certain number of patients do not fast-track, and it for these patients that the ACNP must use more complex knowledge and skills. A more complex patient is the ultimate challenge for the practitioner. Intervention for complications of surgery may be as simple as fluid replacement for hypovolemia or as complex as patients who hemorrhage or who have hemodynamic instability, low cardiac output, arrhythmias, infection, or ultimately multisystem failure. Once the patient has "fallen off track," it then becomes the ACNP's responsibility to case-manage that patient.

C ASE VIGNETTE

To demonstrate a typical scenario facing the ACNP, a case vignette will be used. This case vignette exemplifies the scope, standards, and direct care role of the ACNP.

The call comes from the operating room that the cardiac surgery patient is about to arrive in the CVICU. The patient arrives and is admitted. The patient is assessed by the ACNP immediately on arrival to the unit. The initial assessment includes hemodynamics, volume issues (blood loss), surgical sites, and current intravenous medications. A brief operative report is given to the practitioner by the anesthesiologist. This report can provide vital information regarding the operative course that will guide the postoperative management. The patient's medical record can now be reviewed, and the physical examination is completed. The plan of care is developed holistically to include the physical, psychological, and social needs of the patient. The medical interventions are based on the Cardiovascular Intensive Care Unit Guidelines for Adult Cardiac Surgery Patients (see Table 19D-1 and 19D-2 on page 479 for sample guidelines). These guidelines are a suggested approach for treating patients in the immediate postoperative period and were established based on the issues that are most common and life-threatening in the immediate postoperative period. Current guidelines include management of bleeding, hypotension, hypertension, and hypothermia; epicardial pacing and removal of wires; short-term mechanical ventilation wean protocol; transfer criteria; and stress ulcer and deep venous thrombosis prophylaxis.

The patient is a 73-year-old man with a past medical history of renal insufficiency, is admitted to the emergency department with chest pain. An electrocardiogram revealed acute ST changes, and the patient was ruled in for an anterior wall myocardial infarction. Three days later the patient developed acute shortness of breath. A cardiac catheterization revealed severe three-vessel disease. An echocardiogarm revealed a ruptured papillary muscle with severe mitral regurgitation. His estimated ejection fraction was 40%. The patient was taken urgently to the operating room, where an intra-aortic balloon pump was placed and had coronary artery bypass grafts of four vessels with a mitral valve replacement.

Postoperative Day 1

On arrival to the CVICU, the patient was neurologically awake and following commands off sedation. The decision was made to extubate the patient. The patient's cardiac index off epinephrine was 2 L/min per square meter, and dobutamine therapy was started. The patient's blood pressure was persistently low, in the 90 systolic range. The patient's urine output was approximately 30 mL/h. Five hundred milliliters of colloid replacement was ordered, and a dopamine drip was started. Following these interventions, the cardiac index increased to 2.4 L/min per square meter.

The patient's hemodynamic status continued to stabilize. A furosemide drip was initiated in an attempt to mobilize the third space fluid. Throughout the night the patient continued to diurese. His blood pressure remained stable. The patient's right foot became more mottled with increased neurovascular changes. The ACNP initiated a vascular surgery consult for this problem. The IABP was weaned and removed by the ACNP.

Postoperative Day 2

The patient's hemodynamic status remained stable overnight. The patient started to complain of shortness of breath with activity, with a respiratory rate of 28 and an oxygen saturation of 92%. A chest radiograph revealed small bilateral pleural effusions. The rest of postoperative day 2 was unremarkable. However, it was clear that this patient was not a fast-track candidate.

Postoperative Day 3

Vital signs remained stable on dobutamine and renal dose dopamine. Blood urea nitrogen and creatinine levels remained high but stable. Urine output was good. After collaboration with the surgical attending, a renal consultation was called to help manage the patient's worsening renal function. The ACNP is responsible for making the referral and for communication between the services.

The patient developed atrial fibrillation and was started on diltiazem therapy, which stabilized his heart rate. The ACNPs, cardiologist, and surgeons have designed a formal protocol for atrial fibrillation. The pulmonary artery catheter was removed and physical therapy was started to increase mobility. Full movement and sensation returned to the right foot. He had generalized weakness in that extremity. Clear liquids were advanced to a low-sodium diet after extubation.

Bilateral pleural effusions were enlarged on a chest radiograph. By radiograph, the right effusion was large and the left effusion was moderate. A thoracentesis drained the left effusion, but a chest tube was inserted on the right to drain the large effusion. Procedures were carefully explained to the patient. Emotional support and pain control were provided. These decisions and procedures are common in patients after cardiac surgery and are done independently by ACNPs certified to perform them.

The patient was awake and alert but continued to have episodes of extreme anxiety and restlessness. Medications to control these periods were helping, but these episodes were interfering with his oxygenation and pulmonary status. The patient developed wheezes and became dyspneic at these times. The arterial line was pulled out during one of these episodes. The line was reinserted by the ACNP. A family conference was arranged and held by the ACNP; we found that he liked to listen to classical music and watch television to relax. The patient was taught relaxation techniques, and the television and music were played for him. These diversion techniques to control his anxiety and medications helped him control his anxiety. This also helped the family and provided them with a means to get involved with the patient's care. Daily meetings were held with the family to answer questions and keep them informed of the progress.

Postoperative Day 4

The patient was doing much better. He remained calm with minimal sedation. Patient and family education was started on heart disease, diet, and anticoagulation therapy. Cardiac rehabilitation was started. Vital signs remained stable; he converted to normal sinus rhythm. The epicardial wires were removed by the ACNP. A plan was made to convert intravenous medications to the oral route. The diltiazem was weaned off and started orally. Light diuresis was started and dopamine therapy was continued per the nephrology service. The patient developed a fever and an elevated white blood cell count. The ACNP then made the decision to remove the old central line and place a new one. These types of decisions are typical of those made independently by the ACNP.

The patient's chest radiograph began to show significant improvement with no infiltrates and the triple lumen catheter in superior vena cava. The chest tube drained a total of 1800 cc of pleural fluid in 24 hours. Because of the large amount of pleural drainage, the chest tube remained in place. After discussion with the attending physician, a decision was made to continue ICU care 1 day longer. Cardiac rehabilitation was progressing. A social work evaluation was done for discharge planning. The patient was progressing well with physical therapy, pulmonary toilet, and diet.

Postoperative Day 5

The patient was ready for transfer to the floor. The CVICU ACNP is responsible for conferring with the step-down unit ACNPs to ensure that the care for this patient remains seamless. All relevant information was shared with the receiving ACNPs. The patient was transferred to the step-down unit and was subsequently discharged from the hospital.

Conclusion

This case vignette provided an overview of the many responsibilities involved in the management of a patient after cardiac surgery. The coordination of these activities is the major responsibility of the ACNP as part of the direct care domain. As can be seen from this case vignette, many activities of the ACNP ensure continuity of care. This case management and constant surveillance of the patient's status are key components in ensuring quality outcomes for patients.

Systems Support

ACNPs in the CVICU are engaged in many activities that can be identified as systems support or "indirect" patient care activities. These activities, from the unit level to the hospital level, share the goal of improving patient care. This section explores the systems support domain and provides several examples of tasks specific to the CVICU.

CONSULTATION

Consultation with others regarding conduct of projects or presentations is one task within the domain. A prime example of consultation and interdisciplinary collaboration was the creation of the CVICU. The ACNPs were an integral part of the design team for the new ICU. The team members consisted of nursing administrators, staff nurses, physicians, engineers, and ACNPs, to name a few of the participants. The ACNPs dealt with everything from product selection to design layout to decorating, ensuring that everything necessary for patient care was at hand.

STRATEGIC PLANNING

Strategic planning for the unit and the department is another important task of the ACNP. ACNPs attend monthly meetings with cardiothoracic surgeons to plan goals for the service and evaluate progress on previously set goals. Examples of service goals include decreasing length of stay and reducing intubation times. Any problems in the process of care—including preoperative, intraoperative, or postoperative issues—are discussed and solutions are brainstormed by the team. Quarterly meetings are also held with the ACNPs responsible for the care of the patients once they leave the ICU. The goals of these meetings are to improve continuity of care and to facilitate the "flow" of patients to the step-down unit.

QUALITY IMPROVEMENT

Many of the quality improvement projects that ACNPs are involved with are at the unit level. This involvement extends from identification of problem issues to development of programs to implementation and evaluation. Infection control and reduction of nosocomial infections is a continuing project in the CVICU. The reevaluation of our central line dressing procedure is a recent example of an attempt to decrease line sepsis. Frequently changing invasive catheters such as central lines and arterial lines is another way we reduced infection rates.

ACNPs also participated in a hospitalwide quality assurance project called the PICOS project. This project was a quality improvement program, in collaboration with General Motors, that looked at improving quality in prehospital care for cardiac surgery patients. A few of the outcomes of that project were providing valet parking for patients the day of admission to reduce the stress of the parking garage and improving the flow of paperwork throughout the hospital system.

STANDARDS OF PRACTICE

Developing standards of practice is another task that ACNPs share with nurse leaders on the unit. ACNPs recently helped redesigned the care maps to direct the patient's care throughout hospitalization. The ACNP group, in collaboration with the surgeons, developed protocols to guide patient management. These protocols include management of hypertension, hypotension, and postoperative bleeding, as well as many other problems common to the postoperative cardiac surgery patient.

PRECEPTORSHIP

ACNPs in the CVICU act as preceptors for critical care ACNP students, ICU nurses, and surgical interns involved in their first critical care rotations. The university has both a critical care concentration for the ACNP students and a unit, the CVICU, where the ACNP functions as the primary care provider. This provides the students with a unique opportunity for clinical experience.

ADVOCATE FOR THE ACUTE CARE ACNP ROLE

Because the ACNP role is relatively new, and few models exist of ACNP practice in which patients in the ICU are managed primarily by ACNPs, it is important for the ACNP to advocate for the role. This advocacy is done at many levels. Advocacy can occur at the individual level, where ACNPs interact with a variety of healthcare professionals. It is important to let others know what the scope and responsibilities are for ACNPs. Advocacy can also occur at the patient level, where ACNPs discuss their role in patient care with patients and their families. The ACNP is also responsible for advocating for the role to the lay and professional public. This can be accomplished by attending and presenting at professional meetings, attending legislative functions, or writing for lay and professional journals.

Education

Another domain of the ACNP role—education—involves a multitude of activities, including program evaluator, formal classroom educator, clinical preceptor to graduate students and residents, and informal educator, while providing direction for direct patient and family teaching.

EVALUATE EDUCATION PROGRAMS

Some ACNPs are responsible for providing clinical expertise as the liaison to the education programs in schools of nursing. They are able to articulate the changing needs in the clinical area to the educators who are teaching the didactic portion of the program. Ideally, the educators/professors will have a dual appointment as both clinician and educator. Several authors have supported this concept for the past 5 years or more (Kraus et al., 1997). This advisory role is key to the success of the program in meeting the needs of the medical community and ultimately the patient.

FORMAL EDUCATOR

Formal classroom teaching occurs when the ACNP provides education to student ACNPs in the school of nursing or as part of the new critical care nurse orientation program. It is important for ACNPs to have a strong relationship with a school of nursing. The ACNP lectures on specific topics as the "expert" on that clinical topic. For example, the ACNP in cardiac surgery would provide the lecture on cardiac diseases and surgery, whereas the pulmonary ACNP would lecture on care of the ventilated patient. This is a vital link to the credibility of the program when clinicians who are active in the role provide the education.

Precepting graduate students in the work place can be a rewarding experience. The challenge for schools of nursing is in finding clinical areas with qualified preceptors to teach students in the acute care program. Few ICUs are using ACNPs in this capacity. Currently, our institution employs five ACNPs in the CVICU. In addition, three ACNPs provide preoperative evaluation, postoperative management on the step-down unit, clinic visits, and field phone consultations from visiting nurses and patients. This complement of ACNPs provides a rich resource for graduate students.

EDUCATIONAL RESOURCE

The ACNP also "assumes a leadership role in establishing and monitoring standards of practice to improve client care" (American Nurses Association [ANA], 1997). This occurs on two levels. One level is continually staying abreast of advances in research to ensure optimal treatment modalities for the patient population. An example of this is the ever-changing recommendations for stress ulcer prophylaxis in postoperative patients. Historically, histamine antagonists have been used. Based on a study by Erstad, Camama, and Miller (1997), a practice change was made to use sucralfate. This change has also resulted in a 67% cost savings.

The second level involves working with the nursing staff who gather data on quality of care. One issue has been achieving earlier extubation times by implementing a ventilator weaning protocol for postoperative cardiac surgical patients. Data are recorded by the critical care staff nurses, who also collate and report the results. The ACNP serves as a resource for ensuring that guidelines have been created using research-based practices. In the above example, the ACNP acted as the communication link between the surgeons, the respiratory care department, and the staff.

INFORMAL EDUCATOR

The ACNP has a wonderful opportunity to be an informal educator to staff while providing direct care services. The constant presence at the bedside ensures that practices are consistent among critical care nurses. An example of this role is when a new nurse was performing cardiac indices and obtained a systemic vascular resistance of -20 and wondered how that was possible. This becomes the time to reinforce the components required to calculate systemic vascular resistance (mean arterial pressure minus right arterial pressure divided by cardiac output times 80). This opportunity brings the classroom to the bedside, where values involving formulas begin to make sense.

Another example of the ACNP as informal educator is preparing simple one-page information sheets when new procedures begin to occur, such as the Ross or Bentall procedures. These can be quick 10-minute in-services that inform the staff and ultimately help the patient and family as this information is passed on.

PATIENT AND FAMILY EDUCATOR

Providing appropriate patient and family education is sometimes seen as a challenge. However, when ACNPs are visible 7 days a week, they become a daily resource to the patient and family. As questions and concerns arise, they can be clearly answered by the ACNP. Families view the ACNP as the "spokesperson" for their surgeon. They no longer have to wait and hope to "catch" the surgeon to have their questions addressed. The ACNP becomes "the perfect link and complement between surgeons, residents, patients and their families, and nursing staff" (Hicks, 1998).

Patient and family education can also take the form of printed material. This includes instruction sheets for procedures, booklets for various types of surgery, care maps for families, and discharge instructions. Continually updating these resources can be a challenging job. It is helpful if an annual review of written materials is maintained.

Publication and Professional Leadership

DISSEMINATE NURSING KNOWLEDGE

The role of the ACNP has only been around since the late 1960s (Ford & Silver, 1967), and the ACNP role is still in its infancy. Therefore, it is imperative that information about the role is disseminated at the national and international level. Although the location of the ACNP as a caregiver is different from that of the ACNP as a primary care provider, many of the role expectations are the same. The ANA defines the ACNP role as "a skilled health care provider who utilizes critical judgment in the performance of comprehensive health assessments, differential diagnosis, and the prescribing of pharmacologic and nonpharmacologic treatments in the direct management of acute and chronic illness and disease" (ANA, 1997). It is important that the ACNP model is communicated to institutions that could benefit from the constancy of care, communication, and quality that ACNPs can provide (Hicks, 1998).

PROFESSIONAL ORGANIZATIONS

Membership in professional organizations serves as a means of sharing information, comparing treatment strategies, and learning new ideas. For ACNPs working in critical care units, it is important to be held to the same standards as the staff nurses; therefore, participation in the American Association of Critical Care Nurses is advisable. Critical care registered nurse certification should also be an expectation, as well as national certification as an ACNP.

Local American Association of Critical Care Nurses chapter involvement is a prime place for disseminating information with nurses from surrounding institutions. At the regional, national, and international level, sharing techniques and procedures assists everyone in seeing situations through different eyes. The involvement beyond our own institutions provides stimulation of new ideas or confirmation that existing treatments are effective elsewhere.

The Society of Critical Care Medicine provides a wealth of information contained in journals, which is helpful in remaining current on the latest research for critical care. The Society of Critical Care Medicine Annual Symposium provides the ACNP with an opportunity to meet with critical care physicians to discuss treatment modalities across the country.

One of the interesting forums for disseminating information is to the lay public. Gatherings such as ambulance groups, Mended Hearts, or church groups are rewarding to the ACNP as well as informative. Public groups are usually eager to hear of new techniques such as total arterial revascularization or minimally invasive procedures. It is a means of educating the public both formally, through lecture, and informally, through elicitation of personal questions.

PUBLIC POLICY

Not every ACNP is skilled at articulating issues involved with public policy, just as not all ACNPs can insert a pulmonary artery catheter with ease. ACNPs who are skilled at understanding legislative concerns and shaping public policy should be provided the administrative support to take the lead with healthcare issues. It is not only good for the institution, it is also good for patients in the long run when issues are brought to the forefront by a healthcare professional active at the bedside. Issues such as third-party reimbursement, economic inequity, hospital privileges, and allocation of health education and resources provided by the government will continue to be controversial (Anonymous, 1997; Koch, Pazaki, & Campbell, 1992; Davis, 1994). These are all areas in which the ACNP can help influence legislation and public policy.

PUBLICATION

Many subjects unique to the ACNP role are in need of publishing. Implementing the role in the various environments is a subject in need of description. Each medical or surgical discipline has treatment options in need of research. For instance, postoperative cardiac surgery patients historically were not extubated for 24 hours. In recent years that time frame has decreased by ICUs using fast-track weaning protocols. Currently, 2 to 6 hours is the norm, but the medical literature has reported patients being extubated in the operating room (Acuff, Landreneau, Griffith, & Mack, 1996). Obviously, this is an area that requires a collaborative approach among the surgeon, anesthesia, nursing, and the ACNP. ACNPs need to take an active role in adding to the nursing and medical literature.

As an expert in a particular field, the ACNP becomes recognized as a prime resource to the institution in which they work. As specific experts, ACNPs may be asked to provide expert witness for legal cases. Publishing articles increases their recognition on a national level, and they may be sought out to lecture to an ever- broadening audience. Journal editors seek knowledgeable clinicians as reviewers for journal articles. Clearly, many demands may be placed on ACNPs as their visibility increases. The need to *balance* the multitude of requests placed on the ACNP's time becomes imperative. Direct delivery of care takes priority. With a cooperative ACNP team, many of these other demands can be met.

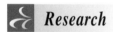 *Research*

RESEARCH UTILIZATION

The final domain of the model is the research domain. This domain is divided into two different, but related, types of activities. The first type of activities are those that have to do with research utilization. It is imperative that the practice of the ACNP is evidence-based. Therefore, it is essential that the ACNP stay abreast of the current literature in their specialty and practice accordingly. The ACNP must move away from practicing according to tradition and commit to practicing according to evidence. It is also important to role-model this behavior for the staff nurses that the ACNPs interface with. The ACNP in the ICU must be one of the strong proponents of change in the nursing practice. The ACNP must assist the staff to search for the evidence, analyze the results, and finally implement the changes, based on the findings.

Journal clubs are a good way to accomplish research utilization projects and disseminate research information. In addition, the ACNP has the advanced skills to do literature searches and also provide the staff with a constant update of information.

PERFORMING RESEARCH

The research utilization activities of the ACNP are activities that should be expected from all ACNPs. However, the actual performance of research is something that may or may not be possible, depending on the practitioner's skills as well as the practice setting. The performance of research can be at a variety of levels. ACNPs may be involved in data collection for a clinical trial their team is involved with or may be principal investigators on a study they design. The level of activity will depend on the level of skill and the ability of the ACNP. The ACNP is in an ideal situation to do research with the patients they are car-

TABLE 19D-1 *Cardiovascular Intensive Care Unit Guidelines for Adult Cardiac Surgery Patients*

Guidelines for Bleeding Following Cardiac Surgery

The following is a **suggested** approach for the patient who is bleeding following cardiac surgery:
Bleeding will be defined as: mediastinal or chest tube drainage greater than 100cc in 30 minutes.

1. Obtain coagulation studies.
2. The following therapies may be initiated if the patient meets the defined bleeding criteria:
   a. Amicar is to be used for bleeding exceeding 200cc/hr. **No Amicar is to be used if the patient has received Aprotinin.**
   b. Fresh frozen plasma is to be used for an elevated aPTT in the presence of bleeding.
   c. Packed red blood cells are to be used for patients who are bleeding, over 70 years old, with a hematocrit less than 25.
      For patients less than 70 years old, with a hematocrit less than 25, check with the surgeon.
   d. Platelets are to be used for patients with a platelet count less than 100,000 who are actively bleeding.
   e. Cryoprecipitate is to be used for a fibrinogen less than 200 in patients who are bleeding.
   f. Protamine sulfate is to be used for patients with an elevated aPTT who are bleeding. Dosage: 50 mg IV over 10 min.
   g. PEEP may be used up to 10 cm if the Cardiac Index is over 2.0 liters/min.
3. Notify the Cardiac Fellow and/or Cardiac Surgeon for bleeding in excess of 200cc/hr.

 TABLE 19D-2 *Cardiovascular Intensive Care Unit Guidelines for Adult Cardiac Surgery Patients*

Guidelines for Hypertension Following Cardiac Surgery

The following is a **suggested** approach for the patient who is hypertensive following cardiac surgery, within the first 12 hours:

Hypertension will be defined as: systolic blood pressure over 150 and/or SVR over 1500.

1. Administer morphine sulfate at 0.05 mg/kg.
2. If no response within 10 minutes, repeat dose of morphine.
3. If still no response within 10 minutes, initiate a Cardene infusion. Start at 2.5 mg/hr and titrate upward as needed to a maximum of 15 mg/hr.
4. If shunting occures, as evidenced by a SaO2 less than 90%, discontinue Cardene.
5. Consult surgeon for choice of antihypertensive, such as Nipride, Nitroglycerin, or Labetolol.

ing for. They are also in an ideal situation to get involved with industry-sponsored clinical trials. Although the direct care component of the practice has the potential to be time-consuming, with some creativity and thought, a clinical research study could be nicely integrated into a practice setting.

Conclusion

This chapter described an ICU practice in which ACNPs are the primary providers of care. Practice is based on the Strong Model of Advanced Practice. Described have been the domains of practice within the model and exemplars of how the model is operationalized. It is imperative for a successful practice to have strong collaboration among team members. The success of the model described in this chapter is grounded in a strong collaborative model of practice.

REFERENCES

Ackerman, M. H., Norsen L., Martin B., et al. (1996). Development of a model of advanced practice. *American Journal of Critical Care 5*(1), 68–73.

Acuff, T. E., Landreneau, R. J., Griffith, B. P., & Mack, M. J. (1996). Minimally invasive coronary artery bypass grafting. *Annals of Thoracic Surgery 61,* 135–137.

American Nurses Association. (1997). *Scope and standards of advanced practice registered nursing.* Washington, DC: Author.

Anonymous. (1997). Pulse: The evolving health care team: Nonphysician clinicians and the medical student. *Journal of the American Medical Association 277*(13), 1089–1095.

Davis, A. R. (1994). ACNPs today and tomorrow. *ACNP 19*(1), 74–76.

Erstad, B. L., Camama, J. M., Miller, M. J., et al. (1997). Impacting cost and appropriateness of stress ulcer prophylaxis at the university medical center. *Critical Care Medicine 25,* 1678–1684.

Ford, L. C., & Silver, H. K. (1967). The expanded role of the nurse in child care. *Nursing Outlook 15*(8), 43–45.

Hicks, G. L. (1998). Cardiac surgery and the acute care ACNP—"the perfect link." *Heart & Lung 27*(5), 283–284.

Koch, L. W., Pazaki, S. H., & Campbell, J. D. (1992). The first 20 years of ACNP literature: An evolution of joint practice issues. *ACNP 17*(2), 62; 64–66; 68 passim.

Kraus, V. L., Felten, S., Burton, S., et al. (1997). The use of ACNPs in the acute care setting. *Journal of Nursing Administration 27*(2), 20–27.

Index

Page numbers in *italics* denote figures; those followed by a "t" denote tables.

Denise Johnson

Den